Contents

Contents

Citation Index

Contributors

Robert H Anderson
Cardiac Unit, Institute of Child Health, University College London, London, UK

S G Ball
Institute for Cardiovascular Research, Leeds General Infirmary, Leeds, UK

Mark A de Belder
South Cleveland Hosptial, Middlesbrough, UK

K E Berkin
St James's Hospital, Leeds, UK

Stephen J Brecker
Department of Cardiology, St George's Hospital Medical School, London, UK

Morris J Brown
Clinical Pharmacology Unit, Addenbroke's Hospital, Cambridge, UK

Norman Chan
Centre for Clinical Pharmacology, University College London, London, UK

Hugh Collins
Johns Hopkins Hospital, Baltimore, Maryland, USA

Jack M Colman
University of Toronto Congenital Cardiac Centre for Adults, University Health Network and Mount Sinai Hospital, Toronto, Ontario, Canada

Derek T Connolly
The Cardiothoracic Centre - Liverpool NHS Trust, Liverpool, UK

Raimund Erbel
Department of Cardiology, Division of Internal Medicine, University Essen, Germany

S J Eykyn
Department of Microbiology St Thomas' Hospital, London, UK

Andrew J S Coats
National Heart and Lung Institute, Imperial College of Science, Technology and Medicine, Royal Brompton Hospital, London, UK

Nazzareno Galiè
Institute of Cardiology, University of Bologna, Italy

Anthony H Gershlick
Glenfield Hospital, Leicester, UK

Michael R Gold
University of Maryland School of Medicine, Baltimore, Maryland, USA

Roger J C Hall
Imperial College School of Medicine, Hammersmith Hospital, London, UK

E William Hancock
Stanford University School of Medicine, Stanford, California, USA

Peter Hanrath
Medical Clinic I, University Hospital RWTH Aachen, Germany

Siew Yen Ho
National Heart & Lung Institute, Imperial College School of Medicine, London, UK

D Horstkotte
Department of Cardiology, Department of Thoracic and Cardiovascular Surgery, Heart Center, North Rhine-Westphalia, Ruhr University, Bad Oeynhausen, Germany

Alan G Jardine
University Department of Medicine & Therapeutics, Western Infirmary, Glasgow, UK

R Korfer
Department of Cardiology, Department of Thoracic and Cardiovascular Surgery, Heart Center, North Rhine-Westphalia, Ruhr University, Bad Oeynhausen, Germany

Kevin McLaughlin
University of Calgary, Calgary, Alberta, Canada

Karen A McLeod
Department of Cardiology, Royal Hospital for Sick Children, Glasgow, UK

John J V McMurray
Clinical Research Initiative in Heart Failure, Wolfson Building, University of Glasgow, Glasgow, UK

Aldo Pietro Maggioni
Research Center of the Italian Assocation of Hospital Cardiologists (ANMCO), Firenze, Italy

Celia M Oakley
Imperial College School of Medicine, Hammersmith Hospital, London, UK

Contributors

Dudley Pennell
Cardiovascular Magnetic Resonance Unit, Royal Brompton Hospital, National Heart and Lung Institute, Imperial College, London, UK

Gaietà Permanyer-Miralda
Servei de Cardiologia, Hospital Universitari Vall d'Hebron, Barcelona, Spain

C Piper
Department of Cardiology, Department of Thoracic and Cardiovascular Surgery, Heart Center, North Rhine-Westphalia, Ruhr University, Bad Oeynhausen, Germany

Shahbudin H Rahimtoola
Division of Cardiology, Department of Medicine, University of Southern California and LAC+USC Medical Center, Los Angeles, California, USA

Martin Riedel
German Heart Center, Munich, Germany

Jaume Sagristà-Sauleda
Servei de Cardiologia, Hospital Universitari Vall d'Hebron, Barcelona, Spain

Leonard M Shapiro
Department of Cardiology, Papworth Hospital, Cambridge, UK

Samuel C Siu
University of Toronto Congenital Cardiac Centre for Adults, University Health Network and Mount Sinai Hospital, Toronto, Ontario, Canada

Adam D Timmis
Department of Cardiology, Barts London NHS Trust, London, UK

Adam Torbicki
Department of Chest Medicine, Institute of Tuberculosis and Lung Diseases, Warsaw, Poland

Alec Vahanian
Bichat Hospital, Paris, France

Patrick Vallance
Centre for Clinical Pharmacology, University College London, London, UK

Hein JJ Wellens
Interuniversity Cardiology Institute of the Netherlands (ICIN), Utrecht, The Netherlands

James L Wilkinson
Royal Children's Hospital, Parkville, Victoria, Australia

Felix Zijlstra
Department of Cardiology, Hospital De Weezenlanden, Zwolle, The Netherlands

Introduction

In this book we have collected together all the articles from the second year of "Education in *Heart*". We have been encouraged by the feedback from readers of all levels of seniority. The relevance to day-to-day practice, general interest, and attractive presentation has helped to make postgraduate education enjoyable.

In the second year we have continued the policy of covering the spectrum of subjects in cardiology. We have also sought authors of international repute to provide the highest possible standard of education writing.

My thanks are due to the authors whose articles are a testament to their thoughtful work. I am also most grateful to the Section Editors who have given a great deal of their time to matching the broad range of subjects with appropriate authors.

I hope you will find this collection of articles valuable, as the commissioning team continues to work on the third year of "Education in *Heart*".

PETER MILLS
SERIES EDITOR

Section editors: Michael J Davies (cardiomyopathy), Christopher Davidson (general cardiology), John L Gibbs (congenital heart disease), Roger Hall (valve disease), David Lefroy (heart failure, imaging techniques, electrophysiology), Janet M McComb (electrophysiology), R Gordon Murray (coronary disease)

SECTION I: CORONARY DISEASE

1 Acute myocardial infarction: failed thrombolysis

Mark A de Belder

Reperfusion strategies in the early phase of treatment of acute myocardial infarction aim to rapidly normalise and maintain tissue perfusion. Primary angioplasty is probably the best current treatment but it can only be applied to a minority of patients and has its own problems. Thrombolysis remains the most commonly used treatment. It has well demonstrated benefits, saving lives and reducing left ventricular damage, but is far from perfect.[1] The mega-trials have sent a clear message that the greatest benefits are seen with patients who are treated early. Clinical efforts have therefore been concentrated on educating the population to heed the early symptoms, encouraging rapid admission to hospital (sometimes with thrombolytic treatment being administered in the ambulance) and minimising "door to needle" times. Continuous and widespread use of audit increases the number of patients treated and the speed with which treatment is administered.

Having been treated with thrombolytic therapy and aspirin (and heparin if tissue plasminogen activator (t-PA) is used), patients fall into two groups—those who do benefit, and those who do not benefit. The former can be further categorised into those who respond rapidly and those who appear to reperfuse relatively late. The management of lytic failures and slow reperfusers is perhaps the most vexing current problem facing doctors working in coronary care units and interventional catheter laboratories.

The use of terminology should be precise in this context.[2] *Reperfusion* implies perfusion at tissue level. This can only be assessed accurately by modern imaging techniques (not conventional coronary angiography) or by near complete normalisation of the 12 lead ECG. Vessel *patency* implies that there is flow down the vessel, however ineffective. *Recanalisation* implies that a previously occluded vessel has re-opened. Recanalisation and patency are best assessed by angiography. Tissue perfusion does not necessarily imply patency, as sometimes tissue is supplied by collateral vessels. Conversely, patency does not necessarily imply perfusion—for example, as with the "no-reflow" phenomenon.

Mechanisms of failed thrombolysis

Certain clinical features predisposing to failure of thrombolysis have been identified, but the precise mechanisms are not well established.

Some possible mechanisms of failure of thrombolytic treatment

- As yet unspecified genetic differences
- Varying levels of circulating factors
    - fibrinogen
    - lipoproteins
    - thrombin/antithrombin III complexes, etc
- Mechanical factors
    - arterial pressure proximal to occluding thrombus
    - myocardial wall tension
    - thrombus burden
    - lesion complexity when reperfusion starts
    - residual stenosis after initial reperfusion
    - subintimal haemorrhage

Patients with failure of thrombolysis are generally older, non-smokers, more likely to have had a previous infarct, and have a greater delay to lytic treatment.[3 4] A number of mechanisms of lytic resistance have been postulated, separable into two groups:

(a) *Resistance to thrombolysis*. Proposed factors implicated in resistance to thrombolysis are shown in the box above. Genetic differences between patients may exist but have not been studied in depth. Varying levels of circulatory factors and thrombin release in response to thrombolysis are likely to be important.[5] Mechanical factors are also implicated.

(b) *Resistance to tissue perfusion*. It is well recognised that tissue flow can be impaired even with normal epicardial flow, and that no- or slow-flow appearances can be found in the absence of a significant epicardial coronary obstruction. A number of reasons are thought to be responsible. The most plausible relates to embolisation of platelet aggregates, cholesterol crystals, and other atheromatous debris after plaque rupture. Endothelial swelling and distal vessel vasoconstriction may also play a role.

Incidence of failed thrombolysis

It is difficult to define the incidence of failed thrombolysis precisely as it is dependent on multiple factors, not least the timing and method of evaluation of efficacy and the definition of success and failure. Others include the thrombolytic agent used, the dosing regimen, the clinical characteristics of the patients being treated, and the time from symptom onset to start of treatment.

Studies using angiography and contrast echocardiography have been performed on selected groups of patients. For those patients eligible for thrombolytic trials, overall patency is achieved with current agents in 60–85% of patients, but only 50–60% achieve TIMI 3 flow and significantly fewer achieve this in the first 90 minutes

4

(between 25–50%). Of the most commonly used drugs, alteplase and reteplase achieve earlier patency and TIMI 3 flow than streptokinase, but there is a catch up phenomenon with the latter over the next few hours. Overall, only 25–40% achieve normal perfusion; many patients shown to have normal angiographic flow can be shown to have incomplete tissue perfusion. In addition, over 10% will reocclude while still an in-patient (overtly or silently) and 30% by three months.[1][2][5–7]

On this basis, currently used thrombolytic agents fail to achieve patency in at least 15–40% of patients (the average is about 30%); they fail to achieve normal TIMI 3 flow in approximately 40–50% (50–75% at 90 minutes), and fail to achieve normal tissue perfusion in 60–75%. Figures for all comers (including those not eligible for trials) are likely to be significantly worse.

Significance of failed thrombolysis

However defined, failed thrombolysis is associated with a much higher chance of early death and greater left ventricular dysfunction.[3]

Following the GUSTO angiographic trial, other studies have evaluated the relation between angiographically defined TIMI flow and outcome. In a meta-analysis, TIMI 3 flow was associated with a 4–6 week mortality of 3.7%, compared to 7% for TIMI 2 and 8.8% for TIMI 0 and 1 combined.[8] Although TIMI 2 is associated with a numeric value of mortality between that of TIMI 3 and TIMI 0/1 flow, it is far nearer the result of no patency than full flow. Thus, when angiography is performed, TIMI 3 flow is the desired end point. Angiographic studies, however, have been performed on a selected group of patients treated relatively early after symptom onset. One study investigating a consecutive series of unselected patients suggests that the early mortality of failed reperfusion defined electrocardiographically is associated with a mortality of 16–20%.[9]

Diagnosis of failed thrombolysis

Patients whose ECGs return to normal early do well with low mortality and preserved left ventricular function. Unfortunately this situation is not common. Relief of chest pain together with normalisation of ST segments and the identification of reperfusion arrhythmias only occur together in 15% of patients. Also, chest pain is diminished or abolished with opiates in many, including those with a persistently occluded vessel. Conversely, a persistent ache often occurs in those with an open vessel (possibly because of lack of tissue perfusion). As age, diabetes, pain threshold, and the development of pericarditis also influence pain, then the presence or absence of pain is limited as a diagnostic test. However, consideration of rescue techniques for those with continuing ischaemic pain may be one method of targeting those most likely to benefit. The situation is

further clouded by the fact that reperfusion is sometimes characterised by an increase in pain and further temporary elevation of ST segments; patients with these features usually have large infarcts.

There is an obvious need to define failed thrombolysis clinically, as then efforts can be made to treat patients with an alternative strategy. As time is essential, a successful diagnostic technique must be simple, easy to use, and the results must be made available rapidly. It may not matter which test is applied within a single coronary care unit as long as the diagnostic limitations of the chosen test are understood. A sensitive test will detect all those with failed reperfusion but may have low specificity—that is, it may lead to further investigation or treatment of many patients who have reperfused. A specific test (that is, if positive, failed reperfusion is almost certainly the correct diagnosis) may have low sensitivity, so a compromise is needed.

TISSUE PERFUSION
The ideal method of diagnosing failure of thrombolytic treatment would be some test of myocardial perfusion. Possibilities include positron emission tomography and contrast echocardiography. Although they have been used to demonstrate the inadequacies of thrombolysis as well as its angiographic analysis, they have not been used prospectively in studies of diagnostic power. In addition, they require equipment or training that is not commonly available.

ANGIOGRAPHIC FLOW
Although angiography has been considered by many to be the gold standard for diagnosis, it has major limitations. The act of angiography itself can influence the efficacy of thrombolytic agents, opening up some occluded vessels.[10] Although the TIMI flow rate is the established method of analysis, this does not actually measure tissue perfusion. However, until techniques for measuring the latter are perfected, this will probably remain the methodology used for analysing new reperfusion strategies.

ELECTROCARDIOGRAPHIC TECHNIQUES
Many ECG criteria have been examined. These include the ratio of the height of maximum ST elevation before and after treatment (usually measured 80 ms after the J point), the ratio of sums of ST segment elevation and/or depression, and the height of the T wave. There are few prospective studies where the ECG has been analysed at predetermined times following thrombolytic treatment with respect to the results of angiography. The criterion that appears to be most established is failure of the elevated ST segment (measured 80 ms after the J point in the lead of the 12 lead ECG with maximal ST elevation at baseline) to fall by 50% or more (figs 1.1 and 1.2). If measured two hours after the start of thrombolysis the diagnostic accuracy is about 80–85% for failure to achieve TIMI 3 flow.[10] This means that 15% of patients will, however, be wrongly classified. Some patients will have a

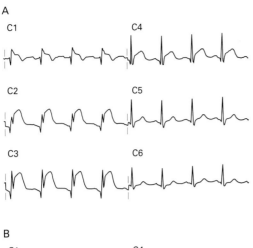

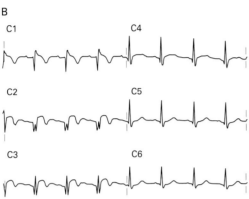

Figure 1.1 ECG diagnosis of successful thrombolysis. The baseline ECG before thrombolytic treatment shows significant ST elevation in the anterior leads, with maximal ST elevation of 7 mm in lead V3 80 ms after the J point (A). Two hours after the start of thrombolysis with streptokinase, the ST segments have reduced (B). Although the ST elevation in C3 is 2–3 mm, the fall in ST elevation from baseline is greater than 50% of the initial elevation. The patient was shown at angiography to have TIMI 3 flow in the left anterior descending artery (the infarct related vessel).

fall in ST elevation but the vessel remains occluded (false negative for failed thrombolysis). It has been demonstrated, however, that those who have early ST falls are in a good prognostic group, and so it is possible that those who fail to achieve patency are protected in some way (possibly by collaterals). If the 12 lead ECG is used, an ECG recorded at 60 minutes after onset of thrombolysis identifies a high risk group with as much accuracy as one recorded at 90 and 180 minutes.[9]

Continuous ST monitoring using a varying number of ECG leads has been studied by several groups. This technique has revealed the very dynamic nature of the reperfusion process. ST segment monitoring is attractive in concept as this provides a means of assessing peak ST elevation, rather than its baseline level just before treatment starts. This could improve accuracy, but additional equipment is necessary and results must be available on-line for meaningful clinical use. ST segment and QRS vector analysis are other methods under evaluation but are not in routine clinical use.

Reperfusion arrhythmias are well recognised but are very insensitive for prediction of reperfusion. The early and frequent appearance of automatic idioventricular rhythm is perhaps the most useful marker of reperfusion and the absence of this rhythm can be incorporated as one of several criteria to help make the diagnosis of failed reperfusion.[10]

BIOCHEMICAL MARKERS

Measurement of cardiac enzyme release has become an integral part of the retrospective diagnosis of myocardial infarction, and the peak concentrations are useful in the process of risk stratification. In general, though, they have not proved very useful for immediate decision making in the management of acute myocardial infarction. Although enzyme concentrations can now be measured rapidly, a single measurement is not useful and even sequential

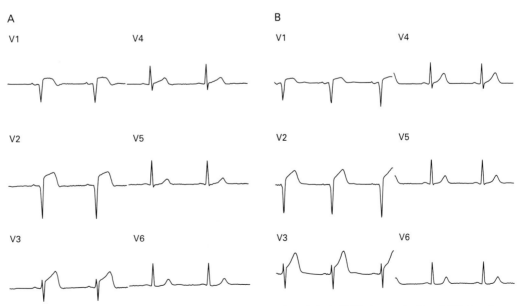

Figure 1.2. ECG diagnosis of failed thrombolysis. The pre-thrombolysis ECG shows significant ST elevation, maximal at just over 4 mm in lead V3 (A). Two hours after the start of thrombolysis, there is no change in the ST elevation in this lead (B). The patient was shown to have an occluded left anterior descending artery at angiography just after the ECG was taken.

measurements are difficult to interpret as the shape of the release curve relates to the time from onset of infarction (which is very variable) and, of course, to the thrombolytic agent used.

Early peaking of creatine kinase or its isoforms is seen with reperfusion (the "washout" phenomenon), but the time course is such that its identification occurs too late to add a second treatment, and there is considerable overlap with non-reperfused patients. Moreover, its assessment needs multiple blood tests and rapid delivery of laboratory results. More productive research has aimed at investigating the concentrations of enzymes and the rate of change of plasma enzyme concentrations in the first two hours or so, making use of the fact that those patients who reperfuse have a much earlier and a higher peak than those who do not. Early studies investigated creatinine kinase isoforms but predictive accuracy was disappointing. More recently, attention has turned to the use of myoglobin or troponin (T or I) concentrations.[4] These proteins can be identified earlier and the hope has been that their measurement would lead to greater accuracy in assessing the efficacy of thrombolysis. This has not yet proved to be the case and they are unlikely to be used on a widespread basis until studies comparing their predictive accuracy with ECG markers are performed.

Timing of diagnosis

Lytic trials have shown that the greatest impact of treatment is seen in those individuals treated within three hours of onset of symptoms, with a smaller impact for those presenting within 3–6 hours. Thereafter, although benefit can be identified out to 24 hours, the magnitude of benefit is considerably less—the number needed to treat increases exponentially with time. With relatively inexpensive therapy such as thrombolytic treatment, cost effectiveness issues are not so important, especially as relatively few patients nowadays present late. However, with more expensive strategies such as angioplasty, the cost effectiveness arguments become a real issue. With this in mind, and given our current lack of knowledge, it is probably inappropriate to offer rescue angioplasty to patients who are more than 12 hours into infarction, and some might argue that there may be little to gain for those considered after eight hours.

Although the concept of "time is muscle" might argue in favour of a rescue strategy being offered early after thrombolytic treatment, a number of issues should be considered.

First, reperfusion rates after thrombolysis increase with time, and providing a second treatment too early may result in it being offered to patients who were going to do well anyway. If offered too late, then many patients are denied any potential benefit, and there is less myocardium to salvage.

Secondly, success rates and risks of rescue treatment, and the way these may change with time after thrombolytic treatment, are poorly

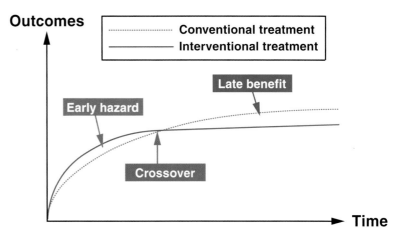

Figure 1.3. Theoretical considerations in evaluation of interventional treatment in acute myocardial infarction. The treatment will only be justified if the late benefit greatly exceeds early hazard. Currently, the areas between the curves and the time to crossover in relation to rescue angioplasty are unknown.

characterised. Repeat thrombolysis carries an obvious potential for increasing the risk of clinically important bleeding. Potential problems related to rescue angioplasty include those associated with angiographic contrast load, late reperfusion injury, and embolisation. Previous studies of angioplasty used as a routine after thrombolysis demonstrate a potential for doing harm—the need for targeting those who will benefit is clear. If the risks of rescue angioplasty are not time dependent, then offering it relatively late aims to benefit a truly high risk subset of patients (but success rates might be low for this subset). If the risks increase with time, then offering it late may worsen the outcome of this already high risk group. The balance between early risks and late benefits is crucial to the overall efficacy of treatment (fig 1.3).

A third factor that must be considered is the time delay between a decision to offer a second treatment and the ability to provide it. Repeat thrombolysis can be delivered immediately (although it will take time to be effective), but rescue angioplasty will often require the calling out of an out-of-hours cardiac catheterisation laboratory team and/or the transfer of the patient from one hospital to another. This time delay would argue for a decision being made earlier than might be the case for repeat thrombolysis.

Fourthly, most of the studies looking at the non-invasive diagnosis of failed thrombolysis have looked at the results of tests obtained 60–180 minutes after the onset of treatment. The diagnostic accuracy of tests performed later is not known.

Previous studies have not helped provide the answer for the optimal time for a second treatment (whether angioplasty or repeat thrombolysis), and current studies are not designed to look at this point. Although there is an intrinsic desire to open vessels as fast as possible, rushing in to do so may be inappropriate, particularly if angioplasty is then offered routinely to all patients, including those whose vessels have already recanalised with normal flow (see below). Either a delay might be appropriate or angioplasty should only be offered to those with occluded vessels, as both might swing the risk:benefit ratio in favour of the treatment.

Arguments for immediate rescue treatment can thus be countered to some extent by an argument for delay. Our current understanding suggests that the timing of intervention should be as follows: (a) should repeat thrombolysis be considered, then fibrinogen concentrations should be measured at 60 minutes and a 12 lead ECG recorded at 90 minutes and treatment targeted at those who appear not to have reached a lytic state (see below); (b) should rescue angioplasty be offered, two diagnostic strategies can be considered. In one, a non-invasive diagnostic test performed at 60–120 minutes allows the treatment to be delivered to selected patients at a reasonable time after thrombolysis. The other offers immediate angiography as soon as possible after thrombolysis, with rescue angioplasty being offered only to those with persistently occluded vessels.

Management options

In the majority of coronary care units, failure of thrombolysis is either not looked for or a second treatment is not considered. Even if the early response to thrombolysis is poor, many hope that, given more time, the thrombolytic agent will be effective. Although these patients are clearly at a disadvantage for the reasons outlined above, the lack of activity cannot be unduly criticised as current research does not clearly identify a "correct" strategy. The other options are considered below.

Repeat thrombolysis
Although further thrombolysis can be offered successfully to those who reinfarct after initial reperfusion, there has been only one study of a strategy of repeat thrombolysis for failure of initial treatment.[11] The Newcastle protocol was to record a 12 lead ECG 90 minutes after streptokinase. Failure of the baseline ST elevation to fall by 25% or more in the lead showing the greatest elevation was used to define failed reperfusion. These patients were randomised to receive either standard dose alteplase or placebo. Improved left ventricular function was seen in the treatment group, but only in those with failed fibrinogenolysis, defined as a 60 minute fibrinogen level > 1 g/l. This small study (37 patients) was not powered to look at survival benefits, nor for an adequate analysis of bleeding risks (it should be remembered that the combined thrombolytic arm of GUSTO-I doubled the risk of haemorrhagic cerebral events). At this stage, this study cannot be used to support a widespread use of this strategy.

Rescue angioplasty
The literature on rescue angioplasty is dominated by observational series and the few randomised studies have been on relatively small groups of patients.[12-15] Current knowledge of rescue angioplasty can be summarised as follows:

(1) transferring patients from community hospitals to revascularisation centres in the setting of acute myocardial infarction is associated with an acceptably low risk;

(2) unless delivered very early after thrombolysis, rescue angioplasty is less likely to achieve patency compared to primary angioplasty (80–90% v 90–95%) and less likely to achieve TIMI-3 flow; moreover, reocclusion rates with standard balloon angioplasty are higher in this setting (15–30%) than after primary angioplasty (5–15%);

(3) rescue angioplasty is applied later than primary angioplasty (because of the time taken for thrombolytic treatment to be administered and the additional delay until the diagnosis of failed thrombolysis is made);

(4) by definition, rescue angioplasty is associated with the downside of the thrombolytic agent initially administered (allergy, hypotension, and haemorrhage);

(5) although patients with successful rescue angioplasty do relatively well (in-hospital mortality between 5–10%), failed rescue is associated with a high mortality (25–40%)—overall, the mortality of the entire cohort undergoing rescue angioplasty is higher than the mortality associated with primary angioplasty (probably because the treatments are offered to patients with different risk profiles, but an early hazard associated with rescue angioplasty cannot be excluded).

The latter possibility is suggested particularly from data obtained in the GUSTO-1 angiographic substudy, in which rescue angioplasty was a prespecified end point. Operators performing angiography at 90 or 180 minutes were permitted but not required to perform rescue angioplasty if the vessel was occluded. The overall mortality for the whole rescue group was actually 11.1% (8.6% for successful rescue, 30% for failed rescue), which was higher than the 7.9% for the lytic failure, no rescue group. Although this may simply have represented a higher risk group, it is suggestive that rescue angioplasty may be associated with early harm in some patients.[16]

The most favourable data come from the TAMI phase 5 and the RESCUE studies. In both, angioplasty was targeted at those with failed thrombolysis, although randomisation to rescue angioplasty or conservative treatment was performed only in the RESCUE study (fig 1.4). Other smaller studies have not shown consistent results with some suggesting a worse outcome for patients treated with a strategy of early invasive assessment with a view to rescue angioplasty.

Considerable gaps in our knowledge concerning rescue angioplasty can be summarised as follows.

● The risk:benefit ratio of rescue strategies for allcomers is still unknown. The overall benefits of this strategy are currently being evaluated in the UK in the REACT and the MERLIN trial. The REACT trial has three arms: (1) thrombolysis with rescue angioplasty being offered to those with ECG

8

evidence of failed thrombolysis; (2) thrombolysis with continuing standard conservative care; and (3) thrombolysis with repeat thrombolysis with reteplase offered to those in whom the first lytic agent fails. The MERLIN study compares a rescue angioplasty arm with a conservative care arm.

- As discussed above, the optimal timing for a diagnosis of "failed reperfusion" after initial thrombolysis is unknown. Current trials may not answer this question.

- The risks and benefits of various adjuncts to rescue angioplasty (stenting, intra-aortic balloon counterpulsation, glycoprotein IIb/IIIa receptor blockers, and embolisation protection devices) are unclear.

- The management of patients with TIMI 3 flow at angiography post-thrombolysis is not clear. We have shown that those with a very tight residual stenosis (> 85%) are highly likely to require urgent re-intervention during the recovery period, suggesting that these patients should be offered early intervention, but that those with residual stenoses < 85% (and certainly those with < 75%) do not need immediate intervention.[17]

- Patients with TIMI 2 flow at angiography post-thrombolysis present a particularly difficult problem. Some might have reduced flow because of a tight residual stenosis, but many have no significant residual obstructive lesion. The slow-flow phenomenon is probably associated with problems in the distal vasculature. Some of these may subsequently improve to TIMI 3 flow but others may subsequently reocclude. Whether the various factors that contribute to distal problems can be overcome is unknown. Although local vasodilator agents might help, mechanical devices are unlikely to reverse embolisation that has already occurred, and may even lead to further embolisation.

- The duration of follow up needed to demonstrate benefit is unclear. Early risks may be acceptable if the benefits later are evident and sustained. Longer term follow up may be necessary to demonstrate the efficacy of treatment (fig 3). It is possible that any benefit of rescue angioplasty will remain hidden if follow up to only 4–6 weeks or even six months is considered.

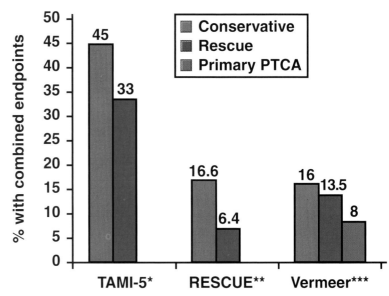

Figure 1.4. Results from three studies of rescue angioplasty: *TAMI-5[12]; **RESCUE[13]; ***Vermeer et al.[14] Combined end points: TAMI-5—death, stroke, reinfarction, reocclusion, heart failure or recurrent ischaemia during hospitalisation (rescue v conservative, p = 0.004); RESCUE—death or congestive failure at 30 days (rescue v conservative, p = 0.05); Vermeer et al—death or recurrent infarction within 42 days (comparison between groups, p = NS).

The timing of crossover from potential harm to potential benefit is unknown.

Coronary artery bypass grafting

There are no randomised trials of surgery in this context, nor are there likely to be. Angioplasty is less risky and easier to deliver. The concept of major surgery in the face of active thrombolysis or combined thrombolytic/antiplatelet treatment is clearly undesirable. Surgery, if indicated, should be delayed as much as possible. Given the lack of knowledge in this setting, the only comments to be made are based on common sense and experience.

In the face of left main stem disease or multivessel disease unsuited to total revascularisation by angioplasty, the culprit artery should be treated where possible, allowing stabilisation and delayed surgery when the risks are much lower. For multivessel disease suited to angioplasty, most operators stabilise the patient by treating the culprit vessel acutely and then deal with other lesions electively at a later date. Where anatomy precludes any attempt at angioplasty, then augmentation of the thrombolytic agent with intra-aortic balloon pumping and possibly with glycoprotein IIb/IIIa agents should be considered and surgery contemplated when bleeding risks have minimised.

Future directions

Improve vessel patency with new lytic regimens

A number of approaches are under evaluation. New thrombolytics (reteplase, saruplase, TNK-tissue plasminogen activator, and lanoteplase) have either been introduced into the clinical arena or are under investigation. Results to date, however, do not show a clear advantage over the most commonly used agents. Combinations of different thrombolytics, or combinations of lytics with antithrombotic treatments, have also been studied, but the most promising results have been seen with low dose thrombolytics and glycoprotein IIb/IIIa inhibitors.[18] Further trials are underway. The efficacy of thrombolytics can also be enhanced by intra-aortic balloon pumping, but it is not clear whether this could be easily utilised as a routine in all coronary care units.[19]

Early thrombolysis and angiography for all, with selected rescue angioplasty

In the past, immediate balloon angioplasty for all patients treated with thrombolytics was not shown to be beneficial and there was a suggestion of early harm. However, these studies can be criticised in a number of ways. First, angioplasty was sometimes delivered relatively late after the onset of chest pain. Some patients did not receive antiplatelet treatment in the early stages. Stenting and glycoprotein IIb/IIIa inhibitors were not available, and there was minimal use of intra-aortic balloon pumping. Angioplasty was also performed on patients with patent vessels and good flow, a group who, in retrospect, almost certainly did not benefit from the strategy. However, this approach is currently undergoing reappraisal with earlier (pre-hospital) thrombolysis, early angiography, and rescue angioplasty only where necessary but not as a routine.[20 21] Early results of this approach are encouraging and suggest that a combination of thrombolysis and appropriate rescue angioplasty may achieve a reduction in mortality after myocardial infarction close to that achievable with primary angioplasty, and clearly offers the potential of increasing the number of patients who might achieve successful reperfusion without having to increase dramatically the facilities for angioplasty. Randomised trials of this strategy versus primary angioplasty are warranted.

Conclusions

In patients with acute myocardial infarction, the direct effect on tissue perfusion depends on mechanical, rheological, metabolic, and haematological factors. Mechanical factors include the occlusion of the vessel, the complexity of the residual stenosis once flow restarts as well as the extent of embolisation of platelet aggregates, thrombus, and atheromatous debris. Metabolic factors include reperfusion injury, the deleterious effect of activated neutrophils and tissue effects of inadequate oxygenation, enzymatic processes, and the presence of toxic metabolites. Haematological factors include the extent and type of thrombus (which themselves may be influenced by the interplay of thrombogenic and intrinsic thrombolytic factors), the haemodynamic status of the patient, and mechanical and other factors which influence rheology. Some factors may be irreversible, but an optimal management strategy for patients with infarction probably requires combinations of measures to overcome some or all of these. Coronary flow should be restored with the least possible embolisation, minimising reperfusion injury and ensuring that maximal blood flow is maintained during the healing process. It is likely that the best approach will require a combination of coronary interventional and pharmacological approaches, together with the ability to support the haemodynamic status of the patient where necessary in the early period.

Currently, however, most patients are treated with either thrombolytic agents *or* primary angioplasty. Thrombolytic agents on their own do well but not well enough. The reestablishment of coronary flow helps many patients, but for others these agents either do not restore flow, or do it too slowly. Patients

---

Key points

- Failure of thrombolytic treatment at 1–2 hours is associated with a 30 day mortality > 15%

- The diagnosis of failed thrombolytic treatment is currently best achieved with repeat 12 lead ECGs

- The absence of chest pain 1–2 hours after the onset of thrombolytic treatment does not imply reperfusion

- Conversely, the presence of chest pain does not imply failure to achieve TIMI-3 flow at coronary angiography

- Angiographic coronary patency at 60–90 minutes is achieved more frequently after t-PA or r-PA compared with streptokinase, but there is no significant difference in vessel patency at 6–12 hours between these agents

- Angiographic TIMI-3 flow is achieved in only 25–50% of patients with modern thrombolytic agents at 90 minutes after onset of treatment

- Normal tissue perfusion is achieved in < 40% of patients treated with current thrombolytic agents

- Repeat thrombolysis has not been shown to reduce mortality associated with failure of initial treatment

- Rescue angioplasty has been shown to confer some clinical benefits in patients with first time anterior infarction as long as it is delivered within 6–8 hours of onset of chest pain

- The optimal timing of rescue angioplasty after the onset of thrombolysis is unknown

- Rescue angioplasty has not yet been shown to reduce the mortality associated with failure of thrombolysis

- Ongoing clinical trials hope to establish the role of repeat thrombolytic treatment and rescue angioplasty

with the diagnosis of "failed thrombolysis" fare badly, even if it is diagnosed early (one hour after onset of treatment). A number of methods are available to identify these patients, and although they are imprecise, a convenient and easy-to-use method is to examine the ST segments on the standard 12 lead ECG.

Having made the diagnosis, rescue angioplasty probably offers the best hope of restoring flow and improving the survival of these patients. Overall results are encouraging but the outcomes of larger ongoing trials and an analysis of cost effectiveness are needed before this strategy will be widely accepted.

Current management

A number of guidelines are suggested to aid the management of patients in whom thrombolytic treatment is deemed unsuccessful.

(1) Make the diagnosis only if it will alter management. You cannot be criticised for considering no action with the current state of knowledge, but there probably is some benefit for rescue angioplasty if offered early enough, especially for first time anterior infarction.

(2) Have a policy concerning the timing of the diagnosis. This may need to change as new information becomes available. Treatment considered and offered on an ad hoc basis is not likely to offer patients a good deal.

(3) If rescue angioplasty is chosen, ensure that the management protocol is shared by both those administering the thrombolytic agents as well as those providing angioplasty.

(4) If repeat thrombolysis is considered, monitor the results. More information is needed about the efficacy of this strategy and its associated bleeding risks. It is probably NOT appropriate to use repeat thrombolysis and *then* to ask for rescue angioplasty when that fails. As further time will have passed and with less myocardium to salvage, rescue angioplasty will probably not carry much benefit. Choose repeat thrombolysis or rescue angioplasty—but not both.

(5) If rescue angioplasty is considered, accept its limitations and the uncertainties outlined above. If used, measures should be taken to minimise time of transfer and "door-to-balloon" times—measurement of both should be monitored in an audit process. Transfer for rescue angioplasty from one hospital to another is associated with an acceptably low risk.

(6) Patients who are more than 8–12 hours into an infarct are unlikely to gain much benefit from a rescue strategy. It is likely (but not proved) that efficacy and cost efficacy of a rescue angioplasty service will be greatest if the rescue angioplasty is offered early.

(7) Enroll patients into trials whenever possible as further information on this common but difficult question is urgently needed.

(8) Widening the scope for intervention in acute myocardial infarction will certainly increase the number of patients achieving TIMI 3 flow. It is likely, but not yet proved, that this will reduce mortality.

1. **Topol EJ.** Acute myocardial infarction: thrombolysis. *Heart* 2000;**83**:122–6.
• *A current overview of the benefits and limitations of thrombolytic strategies and the move towards combining thrombolytic agents with glycoprotein IIb/IIIa receptor blockers.*

2. **Lincoff AM, Topol EJ.** Illusion of reperfusion. Does anyone achieve optimal reperfusion during acute myocardial infarction? *Circulation* 1993;**88**:1361–74.
• *An overview of the limitations not only of thrombolytic agents but also the angiographic assessment of their efficacy.*

3. **Califf RM, Topol EJ, George BS,** *et al* **and the TAMI Study Group.** Characteristics and outcome of patients in whom reperfusion with intravenous tissue-type plasminogen activator fails: results of the thrombolysis and angioplasty in myocardial infarction (TAMI) I trial. *Circulation* 1988;**77**:1090–9.
• *Analysis of the characteristics of patients with failed thrombolytic treatment.*

4. **Stewart JT, French JK, Theroux P,** *et al.* Early noninvasive identification of failed reperfusion after intravenous thrombolytic therapy in acute myocardial infarction. *J Am Coll Cardiol* 1998;**31**:1499–505.
• *A study of the diagnosis of failed thrombolysis with biochemical markers and the characteristics of patients with this diagnosis.*

5. **Davies CH, Ormerod OJM.** Failed coronary thrombolysis. *Lancet* 1998;**351**:1191–6.
• *An excellent review of the subject up to 1998.*

6. **The GUSTO Angiographic Investigators.** The effect of tissue plasminogen activator, streptokinase, or both on coronary artery patency, ventricular function, and survival after acute myocardial infarction [erratum *N Engl J Med* 1994;**330**:516]. *N Engl J Med* 1993;**329**:1615–22.
• *The GUSTO angiographic substudy confirming the importance of achieving TIMI-3 flow early after thrombolytic treatment.*

7. **Cannon CP.** Overcoming thrombolytic resistance. Rationale and initial clinical experience combining thrombolytic therapy and glycoprotein IIb/IIIa receptor inhibition for acute myocardial infarction. *J Am Coll Cardiol* 1999;**34**:1395–402.
• *A review of studies leading to the rationale for combining thrombolytic treatment with new antiplatelet strategies.*

8. **Anderson JL, Karagounis LA, Califf RM.** Metaanalysis of five reported studies on the relation of early coronary patency grades with mortality and outcomes after acute myocardial infarction. *Am J Cardiol* 1996;**78**:1–8.
• *A meta-analysis of the GUSTO angiographic substudy and subsequent studies investigating the relation of TIMI angiographic flow with early outcome.*

9. **Purcell IF, Newall N, Farrer M.** Change in ST segment elevation 60 minutes after thrombolytic initiation predicts clinical outcome as accurately as later electrocardiographic changes. *Heart* 1997;**78**:465–71.
• *A study investigating the outcome of unselected patients treated with thrombolytic therapy on a coronary care unit in a district hospital and investigating the role of ECG markers of reperfusion.*

10. **Sutton AGC, Campbell PG, Price DJA,** *et al.* Failure of thrombolysis by streptokinase: detection with a simple electrocardiographic method. *Heart* 2000;**84**:149–56.
• *A prospective study of ECG markers of reperfusion with angiography and diagnostic ECGs performed two hours after onset of thrombolytic treatment.*

11. **Mounsey JP, Skinner JS, Hawkins T,** *et al.* Rescue thrombolysis: alteplase as adjuvant treatment after streptokinase in acute myocardial infarction. *Br Heart J* 1995;**74**:348–53.
• *The only (but small) study of the use of repeat thrombolysis after failure of the first thrombolytic agent suggesting that fibrinogen concentrations help determine which patients might benefit from this strategy.*

12. **Califf RM, Topol EJ, Stack RS,** *et al,* **for the TAMI Study Group.** Evaluation of combination thrombolytic therapy and timing of cardiac catheterization in acute myocardial infarction. Results of thrombolysis and angioplasty in myocardial infarction—phase 5 randomized trial. TAMI study group. *Circulation* 1991;**83**:1543–56.
• *Trial of 575 patients randomised to t-PA, urokinase, or both as well as immediate or delayed catheterisation with angioplasty for failed thrombolysis.*

13. **Ellis SG, da Silva ER, Heyndrickx GR,** *et al,* **for the RESCUE Investigators.** Randomized comparison of rescue angioplasty with conservative management of patients with early failure of thrombolysis for acute anterior myocardial infarction. *Circulation* 1994;**90**:2280–84.
• *Trial of 151 patients with first anterior myocardial infarction randomised to conservative treatment or intervention as long as cardiac catheterisation could be offered within 6–8 hours after the onset of chest pain.*

14. **Vermeer F, Oude Ophuis AJM, vd Berg EJ,** *et al.* Prospective randomised comparison between thrombolysis, rescue PTCA, and primary PTCA in patients with extensive myocardial infarction admitted to a hospital without PTCA facilities: a safety and feasibility study. *Heart* 1999;**82**:426–31.

- *Randomised trial of the above three strategies (approximately 75 patients per group) in patients with large infarcts, but underpowered.*

15. Ellis SG, Ribeiro da Silva E, Spaulding CM, *et al.* Review of immediate angioplasty after fibrinolytic therapy for acute myocardial infarction: insights from the RESCUE I, RESCUE II, and other contemporary clinical experiences. *Am Heart J* 2000;**139**:1046–53.
- *Review of data from nine randomised trials of rescue angioplasty versus conservative treatment after thrombolytic therapy for acute myocardial infarction and a number of registries suggesting that rescue and immediate angioplasty may have an important role in reducing mortality.*

16. Ross AM, Lundergan CF, Rohrbeck SC, *et al* **for the GUSTO-1 Angiographic Investigators.** Rescue angioplasty after failed thrombolysis: technical and clinical outcomes in a large thrombolysis trial. *J Am Coll Cardiol* 1998;**31**:1511–7.
- *Lessons from the GUSTO-1 angiographic substudy suggesting a low mortality of successful rescue angioplasty, but the overall mortality of the rescue group (including the high mortality of the failed rescue group) was higher than the mortality for patients with failed thrombolysis without rescue angioplasty—suggesting the possibility of harm with rescue angioplasty, at least in some patients.*

17. Grech ED, Sutton AGC, Campbell PG, *et al.* Reappraising the role of immediate intervention following thrombolytic recanalization in acute myocardial infarction. *Am J Cardiol* 2000;**86**:400–5.
- *A study looking at the clinical reocclusion rate and requirement for urgent revascularisation in patients with angiographically demonstrated successful reperfusion two hours after thrombolysis but with a tight residual stenosis.*

18. Antman EM, Giugliano RP, Gibson CM, *et al.* Abciximab facilitates the rate and extent of thrombolysis: results of TIMI-14 trial. *Circulation* 1999;**99**:2720-32.
- *Study showing the potential benefits of reduced dose t-PA and bolus/infusion treatment with abciximab.*

19. Ohman EM, George BS, White CJ, *et al* **and the Randomized IABP Study Group.** Use of aortic counterpulsation to improve sustained coronary artery patency during acute myocardial infarction: results of a randomized trial. *Circulation* 1994;**90**:792–9.
- *Study demonstrating the potential to enhance the efficacy of thrombolysis with intra-aortic balloon counterpulsation.*

20. Ross AM, Coyne KS, Reiner JS, *et al* **for the PACT Investigators.** A randomized trial comparing primary angioplasty with a strategy of short-acting thrombolysis and immediate planned rescue angioplasty in acute myocardial infarction: the PACT trial. *J Am Coll Cardiol* 1999;**34**:1954–62.
- *A study suggesting that immediate angiography after thrombolysis and rescue angioplasty for only those with failed thrombolysis could achieve patency rates close to those achievable with primary angioplasty.*

21. Juliard J-M, Himbert D, Cristofini P, *et al.* A matched comparison of the combination of prehospital thrombolysis and standby rescue angioplasty with primary angioplasty. *Am J Cardiol* 1999;**83**:305–10.
- *Another study suggesting that immediate angiography after thrombolysis and rescue angioplasty for only those with failed thrombolysis could achieve patency rates close to those achievable with primary angioplasty.*

11

2 Acute myocardial infarction: primary angioplasty

Felix Zijlstra

The treatment of myocardial infarction has evolved considerably over the past decades. Reported mortality rates have fallen as a result of a variety of factors, including earlier diagnosis and treatment of the acute event, improved management of complications such as recurrent ischaemia and heart failure, and general availability of pharmacological treatments such as aspirin, β blockers, and angiotensin converting enzyme inhibitors.[1] Most attention, however, has been focused on treatments that may restore antegrade coronary blood flow in the culprit artery of the patient with evolving acute myocardial infarction. The two methods to achieve this goal are thrombolytic treatment and immediate coronary angiography followed by primary angioplasty if appropriate.[1]

History of angioplasty for acute myocardial infarction

Angioplasty for acute myocardial infarction was first described as a rescue treatment in the case of failed intracoronary thrombolysis, and was studied extensively as adjunctive therapy, performed immediately (within hours), early (within 1–2 days), late (after two days), or elective for inducible ischaemia and/or postinfarction angina, after intravenous thrombolytic treatment. Primary angioplasty, without the use of thrombolytic treatment, was described in 1983.[2] It can be applied as an alternative reperfusion therapy in candidates for thrombolytic treatment, and is the only reperfusion option in many patients with acute myocardial infarction ineligible for thrombolytic treatment.

Pathophysiological considerations and concomitant pharmacological treatment

Studies based on necropsy, angiography, and angioscopy have shown that formation of a coronary thrombus on an atherosclerotic plaque, leading to total or subtotal occlusion of the coronary artery, is the key event that causes acute ischaemic syndromes. The initial event in coronary thrombus formation usually is disruption or fissuring of the plaque. Typically this is a lipid laden plaque with a thin cap, and most of these plaques are not haemodynamically significant before rupture. At the site of rupture, platelets adhere to the arterial wall and release vasoconstricting and aggregating substances. A platelet thrombus is formed, the coagulation system is activated, and the end product is a coronary thrombus consisting of aggregated platelets stabilised by fibrin. The result of a mechanical approach to reperfusion is therefore critically dependent on the concomitant use of adjunctive pharmacotherapy to counterbalance the many factors that predispose to further thrombus formation, distal embolisation, and reocclusion of the coronary artery. A brief overview is given in table 2.1. Meticulous attention to the clinical and haemodynamic condition of the patient and strict adherence to guidelines for the adjuvant treatments will have a profound beneficial effect, irrespective of the mode of reperfusion therapy.

Advantages of acute coronary angiography

The safety and diagnostic potential of coronary angiography during the early hours of acute myocardial infarction have been reported more than 20 years ago.[3] In addition to being a prelude to angioplasty, acute coronary angiography offers several advantages. Patient management after the acute event is facilitated by the knowledge of the coronary anatomy, and allows identification of a large subgroup of patients that can be discharged very early (2–3 days) after the acute event,[4] as well as the 5–10% of patients who have an indication for elective coronary artery bypass grafting on anatomical grounds, such as left main disease and/or triple vessel disease with involvement of the proximal left anterior descending coronary artery.[5] Some patients presenting with symptoms and signs of acute myocardial infarction should not undergo reperfusion therapy and this can only be ascertained by angiography—for example, patients with spontaneous reperfusion of the infarct related coronary artery, or patients with a cardiac event without thrombotic occlusion of a coronary artery or non-cardiac condition, that may mimic acute myocardial infarction.

Finally, patients with aortic dissections extending into the aortic root or with a coronary anatomy unsuitable for angioplasty can be considered for acute surgical intervention.

Table 2.1 *Adjunctive pharmacotherapy during and after primary angioplasty*

Drug	Target	Acute	Chronic
Aspirin	Platelets	+	+
Glycoprotein IIa/IIIb antagonists	Platelets	+	–
Clopidogrel (after stenting)	Platelets	+	4 weeks
Nitrates ic and/or iv	Vasospasm	+	–
Heparin	Thrombin	+	–
β Adrenergic blockers	Sympathetic receptor	+	+
ACE inhibitor	Heart failure prevention	?	+

Do not forget adequate sedation and pain relief!
ic, intracoronary; iv, intravenous; ACE, angiotensin converting enzyme.

Primary angioplasty in patients eligible for thrombolytic treatment

An overview of short term results of 10 comparisons[6] of the two approaches has shown that, compared to thrombolysis, primary angioplasty results in a lower mortality (4.4% v 6.5%; relative risk 0.66, 95% confidence interval (CI) 0.46 to 0.94), translating into an absolute benefit of two lives saved per 100 patients treated with angioplasty compared with thrombolysis. The reduction in the combination of death or non-fatal reinfarction after angioplasty compared with thrombolysis is even more striking (11.9% v 7.2%; relative risk 0.58, 95% CI 0.44 to 0.76). With respect to safety, stroke was reduced from 2.0% with thrombolysis to 0.7% with angioplasty (relative risk 0.35, 95% CI 0.14 to 0.77).

Recently, long term follow up data were published of 395 patients randomly assigned to treatment with angioplasty or intravenous streptokinase.[7] Clinical information was collected for a mean (SD) of 5 (2) years, and medical charges were compared. A total of 194 patients were assigned to undergo angioplasty and 201 to receive streptokinase. Mortality was 13% in the angioplasty group, as compared with 24% in the streptokinase group (relative risk 0.54, 95% CI 0.36 to 0.87). Non-fatal reinfarction occurred in 6% and 22% of the two groups, respectively (relative risk 0.27, 95% CI 0.15 to 0.52). The combined incidence of death and non-fatal reinfarction was lower for early events (within the first 30 days), with a relative risk of 0.13 (95% CI 0.05 to 0.37), as well as for late events (after 30 days), with a relative risk of 0.62 (95% CI 0.43 to 0.91). The rates of readmission for heart failure and ischaemia were lower in patients from the angioplasty group than in the streptokinase treated patients. Total medical charges per patient were similar in the angioplasty group ($16 090) and the streptokinase group ($16 813).

That costs are not higher, and in fact may even be lower for primary angioplasty than for thrombolysis, has been shown in several settings.[8] Given the superior safety and efficacy of primary angioplasty, this treatment is now preferred when logistics allow this approach. The results of primary angioplasty are in part dependent on the setting in which it is performed, and therefore the results from various hospitals may differ considerably. This a consequence of the fundamental difference between a procedure and pharmacotherapy,[9] and has also been shown for angioplasty for stable and unstable angina. Quality control, outcome monitoring, and adherence to guidelines and recommendations of task forces of the European Society of Cardiology[1] and the American College of Cardiology/American Heart Association are therefore of crucial importance.

Table 2.2   Additional data* from the overview of 10 comparisons between angioplasty and thrombolysis[6]: outcome of patients with early (< 2 hours), intermediate (2–4 hours), and late (> 4 hours) presentation

	Early	Intermediate	Late
30 days mortality (%)			
Angioplasty	3.9	4.1	4.7
Thrombolysis	5.0	6.3	12.1
Death and reinfarction (%)			
Angioplasty	6.0	8.2	7.7
Thrombolysis	12.5	13.4	20.0
Death, reinfarction and stroke (%)			
Angioplasty	6.5	9.0	8.8
Thrombolysis	13.9	15.7	22.5

*Presented at the American College of Cardiology annual meeting, Anaheim 1999.

Stents

In the early years of coronary stenting the presence of an intraluminal thrombus was considered a relative contraindication for stenting. The anticoagulation regimens that were used resulted in a high risk of bleeding and vascular complications. Stenting was therefore restricted to bail-out situations, such as flow limiting dissections or severe residual stenosis despite balloon dilatations. Despite these two problems, the initial results of stenting were quite favourable. In particular, after the development of safe and effective antiplatelet agents, stenting has had a profound effect on the performance and results of primary angioplasty both in the acute phase and during follow up (table 2.1). Randomised trials have shown a lower adverse event rate after stenting compared to balloon angioplasty.[10] The impact of stenting is also pertinent to the costs; by reducing the rate of restenosis, stent eligible patients have a reduced need for repeat hospitalisation and procedures.

Nevertheless, there are important caveats in our current knowledge of the role of stenting for acute myocardial infarction. Firstly, the benefit of stenting to reduce the rate of restenosis and the need for repeat revascularisation procedures is clear, but the effect of stenting on mortality seems to be absent.

Secondly, (almost) all stent trials have enrolled patients after diagnostic angiography, and excluded many patients after diagnostic angiography, deemed "not suitable" for stenting. Results of trials that enroll all patients with acute ST elevation myocardial infarction, and with randomisation before vascular access is obtained, are urgently needed. At the present time, stenting can be advocated for bail-out situations, and to reduce restenosis in selected suitable candidates. Further improvements will come from new stent designs and possibly from stents covered with drugs or materials that prevent thrombosis or restenosis, or both.

Which patients benefit most?

Only a minority of patients with acute myocardial infarction are presented to a hospital with the facilities to provide primary angioplasty to

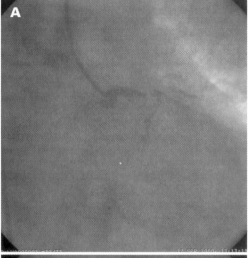

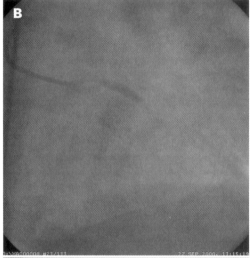

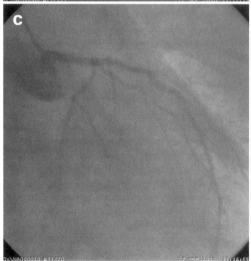

Figure 2.1. A 46 year old male patient presented in profound cardiogenic shock. His ECG showed a sinus rhythm, right bundle branch block with left axis deviation, and ST elevation in all anterior and lateral leads. Following referral and transportation to our hospital, coronary angiography showed a normal right coronary artery (not shown), and a total occlusion of the left main coronary artery (A). After balloon angioplasty and stenting (B), patency was restored (C). The patient was supported for three days with an intra-aortic balloon pump. He made a full recovery and currently, more than a year after the acute event, he is asymptomatic and has resumed his former activities, except smoking.

Priority list for referral for primary angioplasty

(1) Patients with signs of a large myocardial infarction ($\geq$ 15 mm cumulative ST segment elevation and/or $\geq$ 7 leads of the 12 lead ECG with $\geq$ 1 mm ST segment deviation), and contraindications for thrombolytic treatment

(2) Patients eligible or not eligible for thrombolytic treatment, and two or more high risk characteristics:
- age > 70 years
- anterior wall myocardial infarction
- heart rate > 100 beats/min
- systolic blood pressure < 100 mm Hg
- previous myocardial infarction
- previous coronary artery bypass grafting
- diabetes

(3) Patients eligible or not eligible for thrombolytic treatment, with one or fewer high risk characteristics, but with signs of a large (see 1) myocardial infarction.

Whether all patients with acute ST elevation myocardial infarction should be referred is currently being investigated in the DANAMI-2 study (a large multicentre, almost nationwide trial in Denmark comparing thrombolysis in the nearest facility (including transportation) with primary angioplasty, which is expected to be completed in 2001), and also in the PRAGUE-2 study (a similar nationwide trial in the Czech Republic).

---

all patients with acute myocardial infarction. Most patients are presented in settings—at home, in an ambulance, an emergency room or another hospital facility—that permit the immediate use of thrombolytic treatment, but need additional referral and transportation to allow primary angioplasty. This can be organised safely, but the additional time delay will offset some of the benefit, even though time to therapy is less important for clinical outcome after primary angioplasty compared to thrombolytic treatment (table 2.2).

One of the first attempts to provide and study primary angioplasty from a community perspective has recently been published, and several larger trials are underway.[11] Furthermore, reports have consistently shown that the risk of transportation for primary angioplasty is lower than the risk of stroke associated with the use of thrombolytic treatment. In general, it can be stated that the higher the risk of the patient, the greater the potential benefit of primary angioplasty.[12] This is illustrated in fig 2.1, and a clinical priority list is given in the box above.

Patency of the artery and reperfusion of the myocardium

In experiments with temporary occlusion of a coronary artery in animals, it has been shown that restoration of antegrade flow in the epicar-

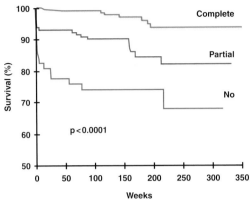

Figure 2.2. The importance of myocardial reperfusion. Kaplan-Meier survival curves of 398 patients who underwent successful primary angioplasty. ST-T segment elevation resolution on the 12 lead ECG one hour after angioplasty. Complete, complete normalisation of the ST segments; Partial, partial normalisation of the ST segments; No, continuing ST segment elevation. Adapted with permission from AWJ van 't Hof, thesis.

15

Key points

- Restoration of antegrade coronary blood flow in the culprit artery of the patient with evolving acute myocardial infarction is of paramount importance

- Primary angioplasty can be applied as an alternative reperfusion therapy in candidates for thrombolytic treatment and is the only reperfusion option in all other patients

- Primary angioplasty results in two lives saved per 100 patients treated compared with thrombolysis

- Primary angioplasty results in a lower risk of stroke and reinfarction compared with thrombolysis

- The higher the risk of the patient, the greater the potential of primary angioplasty compared with thrombolysis

dial coronary artery does not always result in effective reperfusion of the affected myocardium, because of damage to the distal microvasculature. This has been called the "no-reflow" phenomenon. Studies of the ST segment changes on the ECG, the appearance of radiographic contrast during angiography in the myocardium, intracoronary Doppler flow measurements, contrast echocardiography, and magnetic resonance imaging have shown that in a considerable number of patients, flow into the distal myocardium is not normal or even absent despite a patent epicardial coronary artery.[13] Clinical data show that patients with evidence of adequate myocardial perfusion have an excellent clinical outcome, whereas almost all major adverse clinical events after reperfusion therapy occur in patients with signs of the "no-reflow" phenomenon.[13] The prognostic importance of signs of myocardial reperfusion is illustrated in fig 2.2. In day-to-day clinical practice 12 lead electrocardiography, in particular resolution of the ST segment elevations after reperfusion therapy, is an excellent and simple method[14 15] that can be applied after all forms of reperfusion therapy. Several approaches are under investigation to improve myocardial perfusion and to maintain or restore microvascular integrity in infarct patients—for example, with adjuvant antiplatelet agents, metabolic support or mechanical devices that may prevent distal embolisation.

Future developments

Developments in both mechanical and pharmacological treatments for acute myocardial infarction will continue. If we define our goal for the future as effective myocardial reperfusion within two hours after symptom onset in all patients with acute infarction, it is clear that we still have a long way to go. Earlier diagnosis by 12 lead electrocardiography at home or in the ambulance, rapid transportation, and institution of the best available option should be the first priorities. Prehospital diagnosis allows

preparations before the arrival of the patient and results in an important improvement in the delivery of reperfusion therapy. In patients treated with primary angioplasty it results in a reduction in time to first balloon inflation by 30–40 minutes,[16] and where angioplasty is not available it allows the prehospital and more rapid administration of thrombolytic treatment. Prehospital diagnosis offers as an additional advantage the possibility to consider pharmacological pretreatment on the way to the catheterisation laboratory. Trials with very high doses of heparin[17] and with thrombolytics[18] have been reported, but did not show clear clinical benefits in spite of a somewhat higher initial patency of the infarct related artery, at the expense of higher bleeding rates. Glycoprotein IIb/IIIa antagonists are an attractive option[19] and should be studied for this specific purpose,[20] as well as various forms of metabolic support, such as glucose–insulin–potassium.

Although more research is required into many facets of primary angioplasty, it is clear that this treatment is here to stay. Planning for infarct angioplasty needs to be coordinated and clinical protocols agreed by all involved in the care of patients with acute myocardial infarction. The additional benefits and limitations of new drugs, devices, and combinations of both will be investigated and may lead to improved patient outcome, but in the years to come, most benefit for our patients will come from dedicated application of the therapeutic possibilities that are available today.

1. **The Task Force on the Management of Acute Myocardial Infarction of the European Society of Cardiology.** Acute myocardial infarction: pre-hospital and in-hospital management. *Eur Heart J* 1996;**17**:43–63.

2. **Hartzler GO, Rutherford BD, McConahay DR,** *et al.* Percutaneous transluminal coronary angioplasty with and without thrombolytic therapy for treatment of acute myocardial infarction. *Am Heart J* 1983;**106**:965–73.
- *The first description in a large series of patients of primary angioplasty without the concomitant use of thrombolytic drugs. It established the safety and efficacy of angioplasty in order to obtain a patent infarct related artery.*

16

3. **DeWood MA, Spores J, Notske R,** *et al.* Prevalence of total coronary occlusion during the early hours of transmural myocardial infarction. *N Engl J Med* 1980;**303**:897–902.
- *The first large study that documented the safety and diagnostic potential of coronary angiography during acute myocardial infarction. It showed that most patients presenting with acute ST segment elevation myocardial infarction have a total occlusion of a major epicardial coronary artery and that thrombosis is involved in many patients.*

4. **Grines CL, Marselese DL, Brodie B,** *et al* **for the PAMI-II Investigators.** Safety and cost-effectiveness of early discharge after primary angioplasty in low risk patients with acute myocardial infarction. *J Am Coll Cardiol* 1998;**31**:967–72.

5. **Every NR, Maynard C, Cochran RP,** *et al* **for the Myocardial Infarction Triage and Intervention Investigators.** Characteristics, management, and outcome of patients with acute myocardial infarction treated with bypass surgery. *Circulation* 1996;**94** (suppl II):81–6.
- *A report from the MITI investigators, describing 1299 patients who underwent bypass surgery early in the course of acute myocardial infarction. In selected patients with acute myocardial infarction, bypass surgery is associated with a low repeat procedure use and excellent long term survival.*

6. **Weaver WD, Simes RJ, Betriu A,** *et al* **for the Primary Coronary Angioplasty vs. Thrombolysis Collaboration Group.** Comparison of primary coronary angioplasty and intravenous thrombolytic therapy for acute myocardial infarction: a quantitative overview. *JAMA* 1997;**278**:2093–8.
- *An overview of 10 randomised comparisons of thrombolytic treatment and primary angioplasty.*

7. **Zijlstra F, Hoorntje JCA, de Boer MJ,** *et al.* Long-term benefit of primary angioplasty as compared with thrombolytic therapy for acute myocardial infarction. *N Engl J Med* 1999;**341**:1413–9.

8. **Lieu TA, Gurley RJ, Lundstrom RJ,** *et al.* Projected cost-effectiveness of primary angioplasty for acute myocardial infarction. *J Am Coll Cardiol* 1997;**30**:1741–50.

9. **Canto JG, Every NR, Magid DJ,** *et al.* The volume of primary angioplasty procedures and survival after myocardial infarction. *N Engl J Med* 2000;**342**:1573–80.
- *A nice illustration of the fact that angioplasty is a procedure, and that therefore the results are dependent on both the operator and the general setting in which the procedure is performed. Hospitals with the greatest number of interventions had a lower mortality (2.0 fewer deaths per 100 patients treated). There was no relation between the number of thrombolytic interventions and mortality among patients who received thrombolytic treatment.*

10. **Grines CL, Cox DA, Stone GW,** *et al* **for the Stent Primary Angioplasty in Myocardial Infarction Study Group.** Coronary angioplasty with or without stent implantation for acute myocardial infarction. *N Engl J Med* 1999;**341**:1949–56.
- *Important stent trial that shows unequivocally that stents result in a reduced rate of recurrent ischaemic events. However, TIMI flow after the procedure and mortality were at least as good after "plain old balloon angioplasty" with some bail-out stenting compared to primary stenting.*

11. **Widimsky P, Groch L, Zelizko M,** *et al* **on behalf of the PRAGUE Study Group Investigators.** Multicentre randomized trial comparing transport to primary angioplasty vs immediate thrombolysis vs combined strategy for patients with acute myocardial infarction presenting to a community hospital without a catheterization laboratory: the PRAGUE study. *Eur Heart J* 2000;**21**:823–31.
- *One of the first attempts to deliver and study primary angioplasty on a "nationwide" scale. The results of the ongoing DANAMI-2 and PRAGUE-2 studies may have a profound impact on the care of the many patients with acute myocardial infarction presenting to a community hospital without a catheterisation laboratory.*

12. **O'Neill WW, de Boer MJ, Gibbons RJ,** *et al.* Lessons from the pooled outcome of the Pami, Zwolle and Mayo Clinic randomized trials of primary angioplasty versus thrombolytic therapy of acute myocardial infarction. *J Invasive Cardiol* 1998;**10**:4A–10A.
- *Observations based on pooled data from three randomised trials performed a decade ago. Two of the conclusions are that the results of angioplasty are less time dependent in comparison with the results of thrombolytic treatment, and that the benefits of angioplasty compared to thrombolysis are most pronounced in patients with high risk characteristics.*

13. **Iliceto S, Marangelli V, Marchese A,** *et al.* Myocardial contrast echocardiography in acute myocardial infarction: pathophysiological background and clinical applications. *Eur Heart J* 1996;**17**:344–53.
- *A nice example of one of the many ways by which we can study myocardial reperfusion after the restoration of patency of the epicardial infarct related coronary artery.*

14. **Schröder R, Dissmann R, Bruggemann T,** *et al.* Extent of early ST segment elevation resolution: a simple but strong predictor of outcome in patients with acute myocardial infarction. *J Am Coll Cardiol* 1994;**24**:384–91.
- *One of the first reports that showed the prognostic importance of ST segment elevation resolution after thrombolytic treatment. It was subsequently established that this simple electrocardiographic parameter is of similar value after successful primary angioplasty.*

15. **van 't Hof AWJ, Liem AL, de Boer MJ,** *et al* **on behalf of the Zwolle Myocardial Infarction Study Group.** Clinical value of 12-lead electrocardiogram after successful reperfusion therapy for acute myocardial infarction. *Lancet* 1997;**350**:615–9.

16. **Zijlstra F.** Long-term benefit of primary angioplasty compared to thrombolytic therapy for acute myocardial infarction. *Eur Heart J* 2000;**21**:1487–9.

17. **Liem AL, Zijlstra F, Ottervanger JP,** *et al.* High dose heparin as pretreatment for primary angioplasty in acute myocardial infarction: the heparin in early patency (HEAP) randomized trial. *J Am Coll Cardiol* 2000;**35**:600–4.

18. **Ross AM, Coyne CS, Reiner JS,** *et al* **for the PACT Investigators.** A randomized trial comparing primary angioplasty with a strategy of short-acting thrombolysis and immediate planned rescue angioplasty in acute myocardial infarction; the PACT trial. *J Am Coll Cardiol* 1999;**33**:1528–33.

19. **Brener SJ, Ban, LA, Burchenal JEB,** *et al* **on behalf of the RAPPORT Investigators.** Randomised, placebo-controlled trial of platelet glycoprotein IIb/IIIa blockade with primary angioplasty for acute myocardial infarction. *Circulation* 1998;**98**:734–41.

20. **van den Merkhof LFM, Zijlstra F, Olsson H,** *et al.* Abciximab in the treatment of acute myocardial infarction eligible for primary percutaneous transluminal coronary angioplasty. Results of the glycoprotein receptor antagonist patency evaluation (Grape) pilot study. *J Am Coll Cardiol* 1999;**33**:1528–33.

3 Role of stenting in coronary revascularisation

Anthony H Gershlick

Percutaneous treatment for atheromatous coronary disease has developed rapidly in the last 5–10 years. Some technologies, such as laser therapy, have fallen by the wayside as clinical trials and clinical experience demonstrates lack of efficacy or excess complications. Others devices such as intravascular ultrasound are no longer used routinely. Stent use has grown exponentially, however, initially because operators perceived that angioplasty with adjunctive stenting was safer. Developments allowed the procedure to be increasingly undertaken quickly and safely with short inpatient stay. However, treating patients needs to be evidence based. This article highlights the evidence that underpins the clinical impression that stent deployment is now central to percutaneous treatment of coronary artery disease.

Background

Atheromatous coronary artery disease (CAD) has a major impact on health and on medical economics. There are 150 000 admissions for acute myocardial infarction in the UK annually, and the prevalence of angina has been estimated to be between 1–3% (up to 1.8 million for a population of 60 million). The incidence of new angina varies from 3.6–7.9%. Gandhi[w1] has published an annual incidence of 0.44/1000/year in the younger age group (26 000/year) and 2.32/1000/year in patients aged 61–70 years (139 000/year or 2320/million/year). Much of the presentation of CAD is the result of progression, or dynamic change, in the coronary atheromatous plaque. Important treatment aims should be stabilisation of the plaque, restoration of flow, and the alleviation of any flow limitation. Mechanical means to negate the effects of atheromatous obstruction (be they coronary surgery or percutaneous intervention) play an important part in improving the outcome in those patients with CAD.

Percutaneous coronary intervention (PCI) has become an increasingly used and successful treatment option over the last 20 years. It has undergone various evolutionary changes and "came of age" in 2000 with the endorsement of routine stent use by the National Institute for Clinical Excellence.

Why stents?

The development of stenting and its current position in PCI came about to some degree by accident. Until the mid 1990s balloon angioplasty alone was the main method of undertaking PCI. A number of studies had demonstrated its superiority over medical treatment alone, but results varied when it was compared to coronary artery bypass surgery (CABG). The ACME trial compared angioplasty with medical treatment for patients with single vessel disease and exercise induced myocardial ischaemia. At six months 64% of the medically treated group still had angina compared to 46% (p < 0.01) of the angioplasty group who were largely not taking anti-anginal medication.[w2] The value of intervention in improving symptoms was further supported by the RITA-2 trial,[w3] with a significant improvement in exercise tolerance in those treated with angioplasty. The longer term results versus surgery were, however, less convincing.

The RITA-1 trial data compared outcome in patients with single or multivessel disease considered suitable for angioplasty or coronary surgery who were then randomised to one or other treatment. The results[w4] showed that early mortality was similar, but at six months those patients randomised to coronary angioplasty (PTCA) had a higher incidence of angina (32% v 11%), a greater need for repeat coronary angiography (31% v 7% for surgery), and a higher need for revascularisation (38% v 11%) compared to those patients who underwent surgery. This supported previous published observational data on the early natural history of angioplasty, which reported restenosis following PTCA in up to 40% of patients.[w5] This recurrence rate did not fall despite multiple drug trials designed to test whether the response of the vessel wall to balloon damage could be attenuated.[w6] It had been established that restenosis, if it was going to happen, would occur within the first 4–6 months. The two year follow up data from the RITA trial supported this, when the angina rate for PTCA had not changed (31% v 32% at six months), but it had risen in the surgical group from 11% to 22%.

Despite the possible equalisation of outcome with time, PTCA alone remained an unsatisfactory treatment. Published meta-analyses[1 2] of other comparative trials indicate that while there is no notable difference in mortality between PTCA and surgery at one and three years, further intervention is required more frequently in the angioplasty patients; in the first year 33.7% of patients initially treated with angioplasty required a further procedure compared to 3.3% of those treated with surgery (p = 0.006) (fig 3.1). While angina rates were higher early after angioplasty, by three years the incidence of angina was the same. It has been proposed that longer term results may favour non-surgical intervention since there is a 2.5% vein graft attrition rate per year with only 50% of grafts patent at 10 years. Up to 15% of angioplasty procedures are undertaken in patients who have had previous coronary artery bypass grafts. The results of balloon angioplasty alone were still unacceptable, however.

- **Consensus**—Balloon angioplasty alone improves symptoms compared to medical treatment, but because of early failure the procedure is worse than surgery in the short and medium term follow up.

The problems of balloon angioplasty

ACUTE

Balloon intervention suffers two major problems. Firstly, high pressure inflation induces "controlled" disruption of the atheromatous plaque, which sometimes becomes less controlled. At these times acute coronary closure may result. Published data suggest that outcome after surgery in such circumstances is worse than the outcome following stenting and worse than that after routine "cold" operations. Some authors[3] have reported mortality rates of between 5–10% in such circumstances, depending on the patient's clinical condition at the time of urgent surgical referral. Kioka and colleagues[4] reported an astonishing 15.8% mortality.

By the mid 1990s stent use was being advocated to improve outcome following acute coronary closure, the concept being that scaffolding of the loose and potentially obstructive intima would restore flow and reduce the need for emergency coronary surgery. While there are few large observation studies or any randomised trials, outcome following stent placement for bailout appeared good, with mortality rates of less than 5%.[5] Roubin has published data on bailout stenting indicating an optimal angiographic result can be obtained in 93% of patients and a mortality rate of 1.7%.[6] Clinical evidence suggests that the earlier the stent is deployed after a poor angiographic result, the better the outcome. Indeed, one reason for the increase in stent use was the desire not to wait until the artery closed, at which time stenting is more difficult and potentially unsuccessful. Two year survival following stenting for acute bailout has been reported to be 95%, but event-free survival was only 70.7%.[7] Recent changes in stent design, deployment techniques, and treatments to prevent thrombotic occlusion and restenosis in higher risk patients will, it is hoped, improve this longer term outcome, but it highlights the issue of restenosis.

- **Consensus**—Acute closure after balloon angioplasty carries a high complication rate.

CHRONIC PROBLEMS: RESTENOSIS FOLLOWING ANGIOPLASTY

Initial concepts on recurrence or restenosis after balloon angioplasty centred on the neointimal (smooth muscle cell) response. However, clinical drug trials to limit the impact of smooth muscle cell hyperplasia were generally unsuccessful. Concepts evolved to include the importance of the acute luminal diameter gain, recoil, and the impact of negative remodelling[8] (whereby the restenosing artery gets smaller rather than bigger to accommodate the intraluminal tissue) (fig 3.2). It was generally

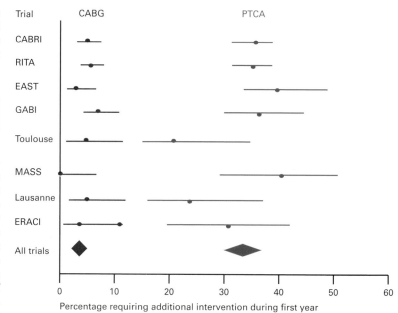

Figure 3.1. Trials of percutaneous transluminal coronary angioplasty (PTCA) versus coronary artery bypass graft (CABG) surgery. When angioplasty alone is used, the need for intervention during the first year is much greater than for surgical patients.

felt that such mechanical issues were more important than the impact of tissue in-growth. This meant that stent deployment could have an impact on recurrence since it would deal with three of the four factors thought to be important.

The larger the lumen that can be achieved and maintained after PCI, the less impact any restenotic tissue might have.[9] Additionally 60% or so of the loss of lumen is caused by elastic recoil and negative remodelling. Quantitative angiographic data from a number of trials clearly showed that stents produced a significantly greater acute luminal gain,[10] and prevented recoil. Although tissue response to stenting is exacerbated it has less impact since the arterial lumen is larger. Trial data[10] indicate that the difference in final acute minimal luminal diameter can be increased from about 1.7 mm with angioplasty to about 2.7 mm (158%) with stents.

- **Consensus**—Evolving concepts on restenosis suggest a mechanical solution is likely to reduce recurrence rates.

Is the use of stents justified?: clinical trials

STENTING VERSUS ANGIOPLASTY ALONE

Two major trials were designed to assess the medium term angiographic and clinical outcome following de novo (primary) stenting. Angioplasty in these trials was the preliminary procedure to stent delivery but could be used to optimise the post-stent lumen. The two trials (BENESTENT I and STRESS) have clearly shown that stenting in native vessels reduces the incidence of recurrence. In terms of reduction in restenosis rates, the results were remarkably similar in both trials.[10] In the BENESTENT study, the primary clinical end points of myocardial infarction, need for

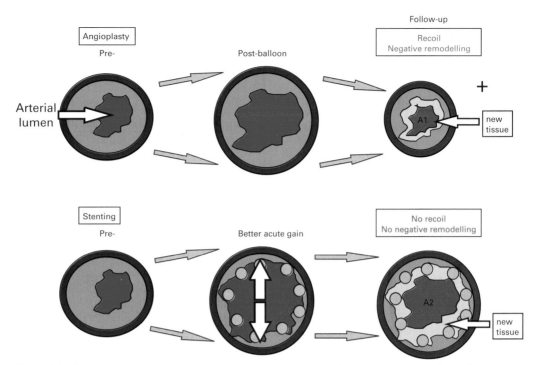

Figure 3.2. Stents improve outcome by improving the acute gain and by reducing recoil and negative remodelling, although tissue growth is not affected and may even be greater with stents than balloon angioplasty. Even so, the eventual lumen diameter is still larger after stenting (A2 > A1).

CABG or re-PTCA, and stroke had a relative risk of 0.68 (95% confidence interval 0.5 to 0.92) in those patients randomised to stenting compared to those undergoing PTCA alone (p = 0.02). The angiographic restenosis rate, measured quantitatively on follow up angiogram, was 22% for stenting and 32% for PTCA. For the STRESS trial[11] the restenosis rate was 29.1% for stenting versus 42% in the PTCA arm (p = 0.011).

A number of equivalence studies have now been published comparing newer stents with the stents used in these trials. Any stent which produces a good acute result leads to recurrence rates of between 15–20% compared to historical results of 35% for PTCA.[12] The WEST,[w7] MUSIC,[w8] and FINESS[w9] trials have confirmed even lower restenosis rates. Use of intravascular ultrasound to optimise the best possible result leads to restenosis rates of < 10%, but this cannot be justified in terms of time and costs.

Effect of stent use on clinical practice

While appropriately conducted clinical trials have shown a clear benefit of stenting compared to angioplasty, such trials are sometimes criticised for not being "real life" in that there is always some degree of patient selection. The case for stents in reducing the need for subsequent reintervention is supported further by indirect evidence from the British Cardiovascular Intervention Society (BCIS) audit data. From 1992 to 1998 there was an increase in angioplasties from 11 575 to 24 661 (113%) with an increase in case complexity. During the same period there was a reduction in reintervention rates for restenosis (from 11.6% to 5.2%) mirrored by an increase in stent use from 2.7% of all cases to 69%. This suggests that an increase in stenting reduces the clinical need for reintervention (table 3.1).

Is there too much stenting?

It has been suggested that stenting is used uncritically and unnecessarily.[13] A study designed to assess the potential added value of stenting once a good angioplasty result had been obtained has been published.[w10] In this trial (involving only 116 patients) if residual stenosis was less than 0.3 mm, patients were randomised to either stent or no stent; 13.5% of patients developed recoil at 30 minutes and crossed over to the stent group. The results showed that there was no difference in restenosis rate, event-free survival, and target lesion revascularisation between the two groups at follow up. There are a number of important issues related to this study. Firstly, interventionists do not generally stent when they achieve a stent-like result. There are certain other messages, however. Of 953 angioplasties considered for this trial only 116 (12%) met the criteria for the study, suggesting that achieving a "stent-like" result in everyday practice is difficult. It is unclear from the cost benefit analysis whether the excess number of balloons that are frequently required to achieve a stent-like result have been included. Finally, one of the stents that was used predominantly

Table 3.1 Coronary stenting: impact on requirement for emergency CABG and the need for reintervention in the UK 1992–98

Year	Number of PCIs	Stent rate (%)	Emergency CABG rate (%)	PCI for restenosis (%)
1992	11575	2.7	2.0	11.6
1993	12937	5.6	2.0	12.3
1994	14624	13.5	1.8	11.4
1995	17344	27.6	1.9	9.6
1996	20511	45.9	1.5	9.4
1997	22902	60.0	1.1	7.4
1998	24661	69.0	0.6	5.2

CABG, coronary artery bypass graft; PCI, percutaneous coronary intervention.

was the GR II stent, which is a coil stent and as such has been associated with a higher restenosis rates. Certainly for the lesions included, stent restenosis rates would be expected to be lower than that cited in this study.

It is clear that if a "stent-like" result can be achieved with one or two balloons then stenting (which with contemporary units requires only one predilatation balloon) need not be necessary. Such immediate success with angioplasty alone is, however, uncommon and attempts to obtain the + 5% to −5% residual stenosis routinely seen after stenting is not without attendant risks of dissection and acute vessel closure, since larger balloons and higher pressure may be needed.

● **Consensus**—Stenting improves outcome compared to balloon angioplasty alone. Achieving a stent-like result with angioplasty alone is difficult.

Stents versus surgery in 2001

Previous trials of angioplasty versus surgery quoted were in the pre-stent era. Stents should have made an impact, reducing or negating the difference between PCI and coronary surgery. There are a number of randomised studies comparing stenting with surgery for multi-vessel disease.

The one year results of the ARTS trial (n = 1200), which compared stenting (mean (SD) 2.7 (0.2) stents per patient) to surgery (2.8 (1.1) anastomoses per patient) in multi-vessel disease have been published.[14] Ninety three per cent of patients received an arterial graft, and the percentage incidence of patients with unstable angina was similar in each group (37% and 36%, respectively). The average duration of the procedures was 1.5 hours for stenting and 4 hours for surgery. The in-hospital stays were 3.4 days and 11.3 days, respectively.

Treatment according to randomisation was successful in 97% of patients treated with stents and 96% of those treated with surgery. Only 0.5% of stented patients needed urgent bypass grafting and a further 1.7% needed elective surgery. At one year the rates of death, acute myocardial infarction or stroke were low and did not differ between the groups (9.5% for stented patients and 8.8% for surgical patients).

However, the event-free survival was higher in the surgical patients (87.3% *v* 73.3%) entirely because of the need for reintervention in the stented patients (fig 3.3). While eliminating in-stent restenosis is the current research aim for many groups worldwide, even when as in this study it results in a 14% difference in need for reintervention, stenting remains cost effective compared to surgery. In the ARTS study stenting saved 4278 Euro in initial procedure costs compared to surgery, and although part of these savings were lost because of a higher need for revascularisation, the net savings at one year were 2965 Euro.[w11]

The UK based SOS trial is shortly to be published in full.

Comparisons between angioplasty plus stenting and minimally invasive surgery to the left anterior descending artery are underway. Others such as the AMIST study have now had substantial funding approval and are recruiting.

● **Consensus**—In-stent restenosis caused by intimal hyperplasia remains a problem.

Problems with stenting

One problem with stenting is the residual incidence of restenosis. While this may be < 10% for intravascular ultrasound (IVUS) direct selected cases and 15% for trial BENESTENT lesions, even if these were real life the impact on the need for repeat procedures would be high. For the 1.2 million angioplasties carried out worldwide each year at a stent rate of 85%, repeat procedures would be required in 153 000 patients. The situation, however, is worse than this. Certain patient subsets have a higher incidence of in-stent restenosis. Data suggest that the rates are higher for both small vessels stented (up to 45%)[15] and for multiple stents (32%).[16] Diabetics are a particular at risk group, and pre-stenting surgery was advocated based on the BARI trial data. In-stent restenosis rates of up to 55% have been quoted.[17]

Dealing with in-stent restenosis

In-stent restenosis remains one of the challenges for investigators. There is no doubt that treatment in the form of vascular brachytherapy is available. In-stent restenosis rates are reduced by about 60% and the clinical (target revascularisation) rates by about 50% irrespective of whether this is delivered as a β emitter or a γ emitter.[w12-15] Two recently published trials (START[18] and INHIBIT[19]) specifically demonstrated that compared to placebo the use of ^{90}Sr/Y and ^{32}P radionucleotide post reballooning to deliver 18 Gy at 2 mm from the source

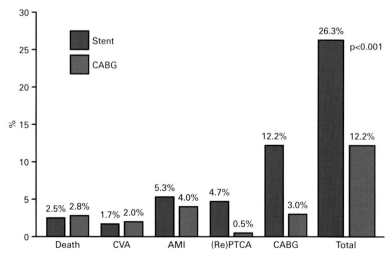

Figure 3.3. Residual problems with stenting relate to in-stent restenosis requiring repeat angioplasty (RePTCA) or bypass surgery (CABG). CVA, cerebrovascular accident; AMI, acute myocardial infarction.

wall reduced the in-stent recurrence from 42.2% to 14.2% (p < 0.001) and from 48% to 16% (p < 0.0001), respectively. The incidence of tissue re-growth is greater at the edges of the stent (28.8% and 26%, respectively) which, although less than for placebo (45.2% and 52%, respectively), highlights one of the problems with the use of vascular brachytherapy. Others include the worry about long term outcome and in-stent thrombosis. The main problem, however, is that vascular brachytherapy is secondary treatment, and patients have to have developed in-stent restenosis first. A better approach would be primary prevention.

There is no doubt that it is the aim of all clinical investigators to eliminate or significantly reduce the incidence of in-stent restenosis, if only to reduce further the gap between PCI and surgery (currently around 14% (ARTS)[14]). Local delivery of an anti-restenotic drug with the stent has the major advantage of being local and potentially cost effective. Two agents are currently in clinical trial.

Paclitaxel, an extract of the yew tree, has clinical use in ovarian cancer. It has specific properties with regard to microtubules, promoting polymerisation of tubulin. It inhibits the disassembly of microtubules, which thus become very stable and dysfunctional, so inhibiting cell division.[w16] We have now been able to coat stents with paclitaxel. In the work undertaken at John Hopkins using the pig coronary stent model, the inhibitory effects on smooth muscle activity appear to be dose related with an inhibitory, but not necessary linear, response at a dose of between 10 µg and 187 µg per stent. This, together with the dose related inhibitory effects on post-traumatic endothelial cell regeneration, have led at this stage to the initiation of a European pilot safety study (ELUTES). The trial completed recruitment in April 2001.

A large European based trial of sirolimus is also almost completed. Sirolimus is a naturally occurring macrocyclic lactone. It has been used as an immunosupressive agent in renal and islet grafting and for bone marrow transplantation. It binds to a specific cytosolic protein (immunophilin) found in target cells. This complex then binds to a specific regulatory kinase called the "mammalian target of rapamycin" (mTOR), inhibiting its activation, which in turn through inhibition of cell cycle progression suppresses cytokine stimulated T cell proliferation. However, it has other effects, including inhibition of translation of cdk4/cyclin D and cdk2/cyclin E complexes, that are perhaps of greater potential for inhibiting in-stent restenosis. The RAVEL study will be reporting mid 2001. Early results are exciting.

Paclitaxel is being studied in the QUANUM study, being delivered on a specially designed stent (as opposed to the other studies involving a routine stent).

- **Consensus:** Vascular brachytherapy is the treatment of choice for diffuse in-stent restenosis. Trials on the use of drug eluting stents are currently underway.

Stenting in certain patient subgroups

Stenting following previous CABG

Long waiting lists for first time surgery, the success of the procedure, and the lower mortality and morbidity associated with angioplasty compared to re-do operation makes non-surgical intervention an attractive method of treating post-CABG patients (about 15% of all PCI). Restenosis rates after angioplasty to vein grafts are known to be higher than in native vessels, however, although the reasons are unclear. Rates of up to 60% have been reported.[w17] In some small observational studies the rate of restenosis following stenting has been shown to be less (range 14–34%).[w18] A further observational study by the Palmaz-Schatz study group[w19] suggests that the clinical outcome and restenosis rates for stented grafts are comparable to those for angioplasty undertaken on native vessels. In other words, the excess rates associated with angioplasty to vein grafts may be "normalised" by stenting. A recently published study (saphenous vein de novo trial) confirmed a better clinical outcome in that the end points of freedom from death, myocardial infarction, repeated bypass surgery or revascularisation were reached less frequently in stented patients (73% v 58%, p = 0.03).[w20] One further challenge for the treatment of old grafts with stents is the incidence of no reflow, where atherosclerotic debris occludes the distal vessel. A recent trial (SAFER[w21]) suggests that the outcome (in terms of enzyme defined myocardial infarction) is better if a distal protection device is used.

Stents for treating occluded vessels

There is good evidence that using stents in the setting of balloon angioplasty for chronic total occlusions improves the outcome. This was shown in the SICCO trial[20] which reported that 57% of 119 stented patients were angina-free compared to 24% treated with angioplasty alone (p < 0.001). Angiographic restenosis occurred in 32% of stented patients compared to 74% of the PTCA group (p < 0.001) and reocclusion occurred in 12% and 26%, respectively (p = 0.058). Target lesion revascularisation within 300 days was also less frequent in the stented patients (22% v 42%, p = 0.025). The TOSCA study[w22] confirmed the value of stenting in chronic total occlusions. Stenting produced a 45% reduction in clinically driven target lesion revascularisation at six months (15.4% v 8.4%, p = 0.03).

Stents in unstable angina.

Despite some evidence that lesions in patients with unstable angina are more thrombogenic and are therefore potentially at higher risk, intervention for acute coronary syndromes accounts for 40% of the angioplasty workload. Support for the use of stents in the setting of unstable angina is available in the literature. Marzocchi and colleagues have recently published their experience of stenting in the setting of unstable angina.[w23] Of 266 consecutive patients stented either electively (24%), for bailout (11%) or for suboptimal angioplasty result (65%), the overall 30 day mortality was 0.3% (one patient with cardiogenic shock), and the incidence of non-fatal myocardial infarction was 2.2% (six patients). At longer term follow up (mean (SD) 17.7 (9.4) months) the cardiac mortality was 0.4%, the myocardial infarction rate was 1.5%, and the target lesion revascularisation rate was 9.3%. Again certain subgroups, such as patients with diabetes or those who had longer stents implanted, adversely influenced the outcome.

STENTS AND ACUTE MYOCARDIAL INFARCTION

Thrombolysis remains the mainstay of treatment for acute infarction. Intervention in the form of primary angioplasty has been shown to be better than angioplasty in terms of patency and longer term follow up.[w24][w25] However, primary angioplasty has a major drawback. Most patients with acute infarcts present to district general hospitals with no interventional facilities. However, in those that do undergo PCI a number of studies have shown that the use of stents appears to confer significant advantage despite the potentially thrombogenic combination of the stent and disrupted thrombogenic atheromatous plaque. The GRAMI trial[w26] randomised 104 patients to either balloon angioplasty alone or to balloon angioplasty followed by stent deployment. While procedural success was equally high in both groups (94.2% v 98%, respectively), in-hospital adverse events were significantly less in the stented group (3.8% v 19.2%, p < 0.03), and at late follow up event-free survival was 83% for the stented group versus 65% for the angioplasty group (p < 0.002). Other small observational studies appear to show that restenosis rates in patients stented during acute infarction are no higher than for routine stented patients.[w27][w28]

The use of angioplasty with stenting, if considered necessary, as compared to repeat thrombolytic or conservative treatment in patients with failed thrombolysis is being tested in the UK based REACT trial being funded by the British Heart Foundation. A similar trial (MERLIN) is comparing repeat thrombolysis and intervention.

Adjunctive pharmacological treatment

The use of adjunctive drug treatment was addressed in a previous article in this series.[21] In summary, the FANTASTIC, STARS, ISAR, and most importantly the CLASSICS study showed that antiplatelet treatment following stenting should include ADP receptor blocking agents (clopidogrel loading dose 300 mg and then 75 mg per day for a month) as well as aspirin.

The use of the glycoprotein IIb/IIIa inhibitors is more controversial. The various trials have assessed the monoclonal antibody abciximab (c-7 E3 Fab, ReoPro) (EPIC, EPILOG, CAPTURE, EPISTENT trials[w29–32]) and the synthetic small molecules tirofiban (Aggrastat) (PRISM–PLUS, RESTORE[w33][w34]), and eptifibatide (Integrilin) (IMPACT, PURSUIT[w35][w36]). There is no doubt that these agents have an impact on trial end points, in particular that of enzyme defined myocardial infarction, in those patients with acute coronary syndromes who are troponin T/I positive (CAPTURE[w31]), and are especially valuable in this regard in those going on to PCI (CAPTURE,[w31] PRISM-PLUS,[w33] PURSUIT[w36]). Patients at high risk undergoing intervention undoubtedly benefit irrespective of the agent used (EPIC,[w29] EPILOG (few stents used),[w30] PRISM-PLUS,[w33] PURSUIT[w36]). Debate is ongoing concerning the true benefit of these agents in *routine* PCI, despite it being advocated by the National Institute for Clinical Evidence, and also whether one agent is "better" than any of the others. The EPISTENT study suggested benefit in stable patients, but it is less clear if the placebo group included patients who would have received this agent normally. However, if there is the belief that the glycoprotein IIb/IIIa inhibitors are to be used in "all PCIs" then two recent trials would support the use of abciximab. The recently presented ESPRIT study (eptifibatide)[w37] indicated benefit only in patients with acute coronary syndrome of < 2 days' duration (5.75% v 11.1%, p = 0.013), with no benefit in stable patients (5.4% v 7.2%, NS), and the TARGET study (abciximab v tirofiban) demonstrated superiority of abciximab over tirofiban in all patient groups (6.01% v 7.55%, p = 0.037).[w38]

There is still the belief, however, that these agents may not be necessary in the routine treatment of patients and the trial to demonstrate this is still needed. While their benefit in those with acute coronary syndrome going onto PCI has been shown, the situation is complicated by the fact that the recent GUSTO IV ACS trial[w38] failed to show a benefit with abciximab in acute coronary syndromes, whereas trials of tirofiban and eptifibatide have.

How a patient presenting with acute coronary syndrome should be treated is unresolved. The evidence suggests that they should be given either tirofiban or eptifibatide (there are unlikely to be any head to head comparisons) but not abciximab, but that if they go on to PCI then abciximab is the preferred agent. There are concerns about both cost and receptor occupancy (and bleeding) if a policy of transferring over from the small synthetic molecules to the antibody is proposed. Most will attempt to triage patients, and transfer and intervene with PCI during the infusion of the small molecule agent (first 72 hours). The debate continues.

Stenting and areas of contention

Small vessel disease

Previous trials have suggested high restenosis rates (> 45%) in those patients with small vessel disease. Four recent studies have produced

Summary of trials utilising glycoprotein IIb/IIIa inhibitors in patients requiring percutaneous coronary intervention (PCI)

Abciximab

EPIC Most benefit in subgroup considered higher risk (acute coronary syndrome) (predominantly balloon angioplasty)

EPILOG Lower dose heparin during the procedure leads to less bleeding with these agents

CAPTURE The benefits, albeit to a lesser degree, occur before PCI in patients with acute coronary syndrome

EPISTENT The use of these agents improves stenting outcome predominantly through a reduction in enzyme defined acute infarction, but additionally there is some mortality benefit especially in diabetics

GUSTO IV ACS Abciximab has no benefits in patients with acute coronary syndrome

Eptifibatide

PURSUIT Predominantly a study of acute coronary syndrome showing a small absolute benefit (14.2% v 15.7%)

IMPACT I and II Predominantly dosing studies

ESPRIT Patients receiving eptifibatide who have acute coronary syndrome do better when undergoing PCI compared to placebo. No benefit was seen in those with stable angina

Tirofiban

PRISM-PLUS Tirofiban of benefit in those presenting with acute coronary syndrome (probability of death/acute myocardial infarction 0.9% v 2.6%), and especially beneficial in those patients going onto PCI (about a quarter in this study)

RESTORE 98% of patients with acute coronary syndrome went on to PCI in this study and an early benefit was seen but this was lost by six months, although retained if re-analysed according to the EPOIC data

TARGET Incidence end point reached significantly less with abciximab compared with tirofiban

The resolved and unresolved problems of stenting

- Stents have been shown to be beneficial in:
  - acute post-angioplasty vessel closure
  - BENESTENT type lesions (short, simple lesions)
  - PCI in coronary vein grafts
  - chronic total occlusions
  - acute coronary syndromes (unstable angina and acute myocardial infarction)

- Stent use remains problematic in:
  - vessels with reference diameter < 3 mm (restenosis rates >25% compared with approximately 15% BENESTENT lesions)
  - diabetics
  - bifurcation disease

- Stent use is as yet unproven in:
  - left main stem disease
  - preventing restenosis with drug elution

revascularisation rate of 13% versus 25%, respectively (p = 0.016). ISAR-SMART showed no benefit from stenting (35.7% v 37.4%, vessel size 2.0–2.8 mm) whereas RAP (Garcia) (vessel size 2.2–2.7 mm) demonstrated a restenosis rate 27% in the stent group versus 37% in the balloon group. The average restenosis rates for these studies in stents deployed in vessels of between 2.2–2.9 mm is 27.5%, double that of BENESTENT lesions. It is clear that physicians will wish not to exclude patients from the potential benefit of stenting based on vessel size. It is likely therefore that it is in this group that drug eluting stents may have most impact since intimal hyperplasia will always have greater impact on the smaller lumen.

Left main stem stenting

It has always been regarded as taboo to undertake PCI on unprotected left main stem disease. However, a number of groups world wide are, through the use of registries, identifying the risk and the patients in whom such intervention could be deemed acceptable. In general early studies such as that by Park suggested excellent results in those at low risk (100% success rate, 17% clinical recurrence at six months and only one death),[w41] although Barragan reported three deaths out of 15 high risk patients.[w42] Ellis has reported on the ULTIMA registry and the outcome appeared dependent on patient characteristics, ranging from those with stable angina to those deemed inoperable, as well as left ventricular function status. Two hundred and seventy nine consecutive patients who had left main stem PCI at one of 25 sites between 1993 and 1998 were studied. Forty six per cent of these patients were deemed inoperable or at high surgical risk. Thirty eight patients (13.7%) died in hospital, and the rest were followed for a mean of 19 months. The one year incidence was 24.2% for all cause mortality, 20.2% for cardiac mortality, 9.8% for myocardial infarction, and 9.4% for CABG. Independent corre-

conflicting results. A number of studies have recently been published. The SISA trial[w39] (n = 325) showed a trend only towards less adverse outcome with stent (Bestent) versus balloon in vessels < 2.9 mm. This was because the acute gain with stenting (1.37 mm v 0.91 mm, p = 0.0001) was offset by the greater late loss in the stent group (28.5% v 18.4%, p = 0.0002). In the setting of small vessels such loss cannot be accommodated so easily. The BESMART study[w40] (n = 381) on the other hand (also Bestent) showed a restenosis rate of 22.7% in the stent group versus 48.8% in balloon group (p < 0.0001) and a target lesion

24

lates of all cause mortality were: left ventricular ejection fraction (LVEF) ≤ 30%, mitral regurgitation grade 3 or 4, presentation with myocardial infarction and shock, creatinine ≥ 2.0 mg/dl, and severe lesion calcification. For the 32% of patients aged < 65 years, with LVEF > 30% and without shock, the prevalence of these adverse risk factors was low. No periprocedural deaths were observed in this low risk subset, and the one year mortality was only 3.4 %. It is likely that PCI for unprotected left main stem disease will be kept for those at high risk from surgery.

Bifurcation lesions

The best treatment for bifurcation disease is unresolved. Some would question whether PCI is the treatment of choice, because of technical issues and a high incidence of acute and chronic subsequent events. Stent deployment in both arms of the bifurcation, or the stenting of one and ballooning of the other depending on the presence of disease or the result of intervention, are current topics for debate. While some authors have reported very high restenosis rates, Lefevre[w43] reported major adverse cardiac event rates of 17.1–29.2% depending on the learning curve. The use of so-called "kissing" balloons appeared to have a beneficial influence on the outcome. Others have shown that stenting of the side branch may not be essential but choosing which to stent and which to leave is the subject of several proposed studies.

Direct stenting

Direct stenting may have significant advantages over routine procedure where there is predilatation with a balloon first. There appears little doubt that tissue response to the vessel wall is the result of the damage induced by the balloon inflation (and stent deployment). If this damage could be reduced, less tissue response should occur. Additionally the procedure would be cheaper requiring a balloon-stent unit only. There have been a number of reports outlining the feasibility of such a strategy. Hamon recently published the outcome of 122 "carefully selected" patients. Factors such as calcification and tortuosity need to be taken into account when direct stenting is considered. Procedural success was 96%.[w44] In five cases it was not possible to deliver the stent through the undilated lesion and the stent was retrieved, but in two cases the stent was lost in the peripheral circulation. The authors rightly reported the need for a controlled trial and one UK study (the SLIDE trial) is underway.

Future directions

There are three areas of future direction for stents. Firstly, radiation is likely to be incorporated into clinical practice to deal with in-stent restenosis.

The second area of development is the use of stents that carry drugs to inhibit the tissue responses. The use of such stents is likely to be

Trial acronyms

ACME Angioplasty Compared with Medicine
AMIST Angioplasty versus Minimally Invasive Surgery Trial
ARTS Arterial Revascularization Therapy Study
BARI Bypass Angioplasty Revascularization Investigation
BENESTENT Belgium-Netherlands Stent Study
BESMART Bestent in Small Arteries
CABRI Coronary Angioplasty versus Bypass Revascularisation Investigation
CAPTURE Chimeric 7E3 Anti-Platelet in Unstable Angina Refractory to Standard Treatment
CLASSICS Clopidogrel plus Aspirin Stent International Cooperative Study
EAST Emory Angioplasty versus Surgery Trial
ELUTES Evaluation of Taxol Eluting Stent
EPIC Evaluation of IIb/IIIa platelet receptor antagonist 7E3 in Preventing Ischemic Complications
EPILOG Evaluation of PTCA to Improve Long-term Outcome by c7E3 GP IIb/IIIa receptor blockade trial
EPISTENT Evaluation of Platelet GP IIb/IIIa Inhibitor for Stenting
EPIC Evaluation of 7E3 for the Prevention of Ischemic Complications
ERACI Argentine Randomized Trial Coronary Angioplasty versus Coronary Artery Bypass Surgery in Multivessel Disease
ESPRIT European Study of Prevention of Reocclusion after Initial Thrombolysis
FANTASTIC Full Anticoagulation versus Ticlopidine plus Aspirin After Stent Implantation
FINESS First International New Intravascular Rigid-flex Endovascular Stent Study
GABI German Angioplasty Bypass Surgery Investigation
GRAMI GRII stent in Acute Myocardial Infarction
GUSTO Global Use of Strategies To Open Occluded Coronary Arteries
IMPACT Integrilin to Manage Platelet Aggregation to Combat Thrombosis Trial
INHIBIT Inhibit Restenosis Intervention with β-Radiation Trial
ISAR Intracoronary Stenting and Antithrombotic Regimen
ISAR-SMART Intracoronary Stenting or Angioplasty for Restenosis Reduction in Small Arteries.
MASS The Medicine, Angioplasty or Surgery Study
MUSIC Multicenter Ultrasound Stenting in Coronaries
PRISM–PLUS Platelet Receptor Inhibition in Ischemic Syndrome Management in Patients Limited by Unstable Signs and Symptoms
PURSUIT Platelet IIb/IIIa Underpinning the Receptor for Suppression of Unstable Ischemia Trial
RAVEL Randomized study with sirolimus coated BX Velocity balloon Expandable stent in the treat of patients with de novo native coronary Lesions
REACT Rescue Angioplasty versus Conservative treatment or repeat Thrombolysis
RESTORE Randomized Efficacy Study of Tirofiban for Outcomes and Restenosis
RITA Randomized Intervention Treatment of Angina
SAFER Saphenous vein graft Angioplasty Free of Emboli Randomized trial
SICCO Stenting In Chronic Coronary Occlusion
SISA Stents In Small Arteries
SLIDE Selected Lesion Indication for Direct Stenting
SOS Stent Or Surgery
START Stents and Radiation Therapy Trial
STARS Stent Anticoagulation Regimen Study
STRESS Stent Restenosis Study
TARGET Do Tirofiban And Reopro Give similar Efficacy outcomes Trial
TOSCA Total Occlusion Study of Canada
ULTIMA Unprotected Left main Trunk Intervention Multi-center Assessment.
WEST West European Stent Trial
WIDEST Wiktor Stent in de Novo Stenosis

cost beneficial because of the small amount of drug required in comparison to systemic treatments, provided the "overall" cost of the stent is not too high and the technology can be applied to longer stents. If shown to be effective in upcoming clinical trials then stents will deal with all four aspects of restenosis; good acute result, recoil, negative remodelling, and in-stent tissue growth.

Finally, there is likely to be an increase in the combined approach to treating multivessel disease, with the interventionist dealing with lesions in the right coronary and circumflex arteries while the surgeon performs a minimally invasive operation on the left anterior descending artery. The rationale for the combined approach is based on the increased difficulty the surgeon has in using arterial conduits to graft the right and circumflex arteries compared to the left anterior descending artery, which may be best treated with a minimally invasive procedure. If this can be done then angioplasty and stenting of the other diseased vessels rather than using the vein as a conduit may be a good option. Clinical trials of such a combined approach are required.

1. **Pocock SJ, Henderson RA, Rickards AF,** *et al.* Meta-analysis of randomised trials comparing coronary angioplasty with bypass surgery. *Lancet* 1995;**346**:1184–9
   • *Important meta-analysis demonstrating the medium term disadvantages of balloon angioplasty versus surgery in terms of need for revascularisation.*

2. **Rickards AF, Davies SW.** Coronary angioplasty versus coronary surgery in the management of angina. *Curr Opin Cardiol* 1995;**10**:399–403.
   • *An overview of balloon angioplasty versus surgery using registry data as well as trial data.*

3. **Zapolanski A, Rosenblum J, Myler RK,** *et al.* Emergency coronary artery bypass surgery following failed balloon angioplasty: role of the internal mammary artery graft. *J Cardiac Surg* 1991;**6**;439–48.
   • *This study highlighted the risk of acute coronary closure following angioplasty and the failure to use best surgical treatment.*

4. **Kioka Y, Dallan L, Oliveira S,** *et al.* Clinical experience of emergency coronary artery bypass grafting following failed percutaneous transluminal coronary angioplasty. *Jpn J Surg* 1991;**21**:643–9.
   • *Showed just how high risk failed balloon angioplasty could be.*

5. **Scott NA, Weintraub WS, Carlin SF,** *et al.* Recent changes in the management and outcome of acute closure after percutaneous transluminal coronary angioplasty. *Am J Cardiol* 1993;**71**:1159–63.
   • *Indicated that there was a problem with balloon angioplasty and set the scene for stenting.*

6. **Roubin GS, Cannon AD, Aggarwal SK,** *et al.* Intracoronary stenting for acute and threatened closure complicating percutaneous transluminal coronary angioplasty. *Circulation* 1992;**85**:916–27.
   • *Indicated that stenting may be the answer to acute balloon failure.*

7. **Schomig A, Kastrati A, Mudra H,** *et al.* Four-year experience with Palmaz-Schatz stenting in coronary angioplasty complicated by dissection with threatened or present vessel closure. *Circulation* 1994;**90**:2716–24.
   • *Important in the development of stenting, suggesting that the treatment of choice for acute problems was the deployment of stents.*

8. **Mintz GS, Mehran R, Waksman R,** *et al.* Treatment of in-stent restenosis. *Seminars in Interventional Cardiology* 1998;**3**:117–21.
   • *Highlighted the importance of negative remodelling in the development on in-stent restenosis.*

9. **Kuntz RE, Baim DS.** Defining coronary restenosis. Newer clinical and angiographic paradigms. *Circulation* 1993;**88**:1310–23.

   • *A seminal paper indicating that the better the acute gain the more room there was for the development of any in-stent restenosis, irrespective of device used. Stenting was shown to produce and retain the best acute result.*

10. **Serruys PW, de Jaegere P, Kiemeneij F,** *et al.* A comparison of balloon-expandable-stent implantation with balloon angioplasty in patients with coronary artery disease. Benestent study group. *N Engl J Med* 1994;**331**:489–95.
   • *Demonstrated that stenting produced less recurrence than balloon alone, but also that this was caused by the acute benefit. This study also showed that tissue in-growth was greater with stenting.*

11. **Fischman DL, Leon MB, Baim DS,** *et al.* A randomised comparison of coronary stent placement and balloon angioplasty in the treatment of coronary artery disease. Stent restenosis investigators. *N Engl J Med* 1994;**331**:496–501.
   • *This study also showed the benefits of stenting versus angioplasty, but interestingly the restenosis rates were 10% higher than in the Benestent trial because of differences in case selection.*

12. **Dirschinger J, Schuhlen H, Boekstegers P,** *et al.* Equivalence or difference? One year follow up of a randomised trial of five different slotted-tube stents [abstract]. *Circulation* 1998;**98**:I-661.
   • *Suggested that for whatever reason a stent might be chosen, in general most stents are the same in terms of outcome, providing they are of the same design—that is, slotted tube rather than coil tube design.*

13. **Karsch KR, Newby A.** Stent magic! The genie has escaped from the bottle. *Heart* 2000;**84**:469–70.
   • *An important recent commentary expressing the belief, based on the WIDEST study, that there is too much stenting.*

14. **Serruys PW, Unger F, van Hout BA,** *et al.* The ARTS study (arterial revascularisation therapies study). *Seminars in Interventional Cardiology* 1999;**4**:209–19.
   • *Trial of multivessel stenting versus angioplasty. Previous comparisons had been between balloon angioplasty alone and surgery.*

15. **Nunes G, Pintto I, Mattos L,** *et al.* Coronary stenting in vessels smaller than 3 mm is associated with higher restenosis rates [abstract] *Eur Heart J* 1996;**17**:173.
   • *Highlighted the problems when there is insufficient room, as with small reference vessels, for the intimal hyperplasia to be accomodated.*

16. **Ponde CK, Watson PS, Aroney CN,** *et al.* Multiple stent implantation in single coronary arteries: acute results and six month angiographic follow up. *Cathet Cardiovasc Diag* 1997;**42**:158–65.
   • *Found higher risk of restenosis in patients receiving multiple stents, but reason unknown.*

17. **Lau KW, Ding ZP, Johan A,** *et al.* Midterm angiographic outcome of single-vessel intracoronary stent placement in diabetic versus non-diabetic patients: a matched comparative study. *Am Heart J* 1998;**136**:150–5.
   • *Diabetics remain at high risk of in-stent restenosis, especially in small vessel reference diameter.*

18. **Popma J, Heuser R, Suntharalingam M,** *et al* **for the START Investigators.** Late clinical and angiographic outcomes after use of $^{90}Sr/^{90}Y$ beta radiation for the treatment of in-stent restenosis. Results from the stents and radiation therapy (START) trial [abstract]. *J Am Coll Cardiol* 2000;**35**.
   • *Definitive study demonstrating the benefit of β emitter radiation for treatment of in-stent restenosis.*

19. **Waksman R, Raizner A, Lansky A,** *et al.* Beta radiation to inhibit recurrence of in-stent restenosis: study design, device and dosimetry details of the multicenter randomised double blind study [abstract]. *Circulation* 2000;**102**(suppl):II-667.
   • *A second trial showing benefit of a β emitter (32 P) in in-stent restenosis compared to balloon angioplasty alone.*

20. **Sirnes PA, Golf S, Myreng Y,** *et al.* Stenting in chronic coronary occlusion (SICCO): a randomised controlled trial of adding a stent implantation after successful angioplasty. *J Am Coll Cardiol* 1996;**28**:1444–51.
   • *An important study which suggested that in the short term at least those patients with chronic occlusion were better off receiving a stent than just being treated with balloon angioplasty alone.*

21. **Windecker S, Meier B.** Intervention in coronary artery disease. *Heart* 2000;**83**:481–90.
   • *Previous article in the Education in Heart series addressing adjunctive pharmacological treatment in PCI.*

SECTION II: HEART FAILURE

4 Treatment strategies for heart failure: β blockers and antiarrhythmics

Aldo Pietro Maggioni

The role of β blockers and antiarrhythmic drugs in the management of patients with heart failure is reviewed.

β Blockers

Although several investigators since the 1970s proposed β adrenergic blocking agents as a possible treatment for patients with heart failure,[1] the simple observation that they can reduce myocardial contractility confined them to being absolutely contraindicated for the treatment of this condition. However, the medical approach to heart failure has changed dramatically over the past 10 years, progressing from a haemodynamic to a neurohormonal pathophysiological paradigm.[2] Since activation of the sympathetic system is recognised as one of the cardinal pathophysiologic abnormalities in patients with chronic heart failure,[3] the effects of β adrenergic receptor blockers have been specifically tested in randomised clinical trials. Consequently, over a relatively brief period of time, a treatment that was once contraindicated is now an established, evidence based recommended treatment for heart failure.

Rationale for use

The concentrations of circulating catecholamines are increased in patients with chronic heart failure.[3] The adrenergic activation observed in these patients can be useful initially to maintain an acceptable cardiac performance by increasing contractility and heart rate, but ultimately the increase in the adrenergic drive can damage the failing human heart.[4] In the human cardiac myocyte, there are three adrenergic receptors—β1, β2, and α1—whose activation can lead to cardiac myocyte growth (β1, β2, α1), positive inotropic response (β1, β2), positive chronotropic response (β1, β2), myocyte toxicity (β1, β2), and myocyte apoptosis (β1).[5] Therefore, the continuously increased activation of the adrenergic system leads to several adverse biological signals to the cardiac myocytes through the adrenergic receptors. The rationale for the use of β adrenergic blocking agents in patients with heart failure is based mainly upon these observations.

Effects on physiologic end points

Left ventricular function and remodelling processes
All available trials testing β blockers versus placebo showed that, apart from short term negative inotropic effect, β blocker treatment given for at least three months is always associated with an improvement in left ventricular systolic function.[6 7] Further, after longer treatment periods, normalisation of ventricular shape and regression in myocardial hypertrophy can occur.[7] These modifications are generally called "reverse remodelling". This phenomenon has been observed with different β blockers, and, together with the improvement in ventricular function, is unique among all the other "evidence based" recommended treatments for heart failure patients.

Effects on exercise capacity

The long term effect of β blockers on exercise tolerance remains controversial.[8] Several trials have shown a significant improvement in maximal exercise tolerance, while others report no change[9] or even a detrimental effect.[8] A more consistent improvement was seen with metoprolol than with carvedilol or bucindolol.

Effects on neurohormones

There are sparse data on the long term effects of β blockers on neurohormonal activation, the majority of studies suggesting a reduction in the circulating noradrenaline (norepinephrine) concentrations.[10] Recently, the RESOLVD study specifically addressed the issue of neurohormonal modifications induced by long term (23 weeks) metoprolol treatment.[9] Metoprolol did not modify plasma catecholamine, aldosterone, and endothelin concentrations but decreased significantly renin and angiotensin II concentrations, which is in agreement with other reports. Interestingly, circulating concentrations of atrial natriuretic peptide (ANP) and brain natriuretic peptide (BNP) increased significantly in patients allocated to metoprolol treatment. The reasons for this modification are not readily apparent, though an increase in left ventricular filling pressure determined by metoprolol is a possible explanation.

Effects on hospital admissions and quality of life

Hospital admissions are now generally considered in clinical trials as one of the most relevant end points, both for their relation to patient quality of life and for cost implications. In this context, large scale clinical trials testing carvedilol,[11] bisoprolol[12] or metoprolol[13] consistently showed that the hospitalisation rate for heart failure among patients allocated to β blockers was significantly reduced in comparison to that observed in placebo allocated patients. This benefit was not counterbalanced by a significant increase in other causes of hospital admission, resulting in a significant reduction of all cause hospitalisations.

When quality of life was evaluated with specific questionnaires, results obtained with β blocker treatment were conflicting.[9] While the MDC trial showed an improvement of quality of life, the RESOLVD trial[10] and the US carvedilol studies[11] did not show any difference. The Australian–New Zealand study showed a trend toward worsening quality of life scores.

Table 4.1   Characteristics of randomised trials testing β blockers in patients with heart failure

Trial	Drug	Number of patients	NYHA class	Mean age (years)	Ejection fraction (%)	Annual mortality placebo group (%)	Primary end point	Mean follow up (months)	Run-in phase
US Carvedilol Program[11]	Carvedilol	1094	II–IV	58	≤ 35	12	Total mortality	6.5*	Yes
CIBIS-II[12]	Bisoprolol	2,647	III-IV	61	≤ 35	11.2	Total mortality	16	No
MERIT-HF[13]	Metoprolol	3,991	II-IV	64	≤ 40	9.4	Total mortality or hospitalisations	12	No

*Median.

Effects on survival

Over the last five years clear evidence has accumulated to show that β blockers improve the morbidity and mortality of patients with symptomatic heart failure and decreased ejection fraction. As a result, editorials, reviews, and official guidelines now consistently suggest that these drugs should be added to conventional treatment with angiotensin converting enzyme (ACE) inhibitors and diuretics. A meta-analysis of placebo controlled, randomised trials on 3023 patients, recruited in 18 published small scale studies, showed that β blockade reduced the combined risk of death and hospitalisation for heart failure by 37%.[14] These encouraging observations were confirmed by the US Carvedilol Program which showed that in 1094 patients with heart failure carvedilol reduced the risk of total mortality by 65%.[11] This very impressive finding led the data and safety monitoring board of the study to recommend the early termination of the trial because of a clear evidence of benefit. On the basis of this study, carvedilol was approved for the clinical use in patients with chronic heart failure in several countries. Carvedilol has pharmacological properties in addition to β adrenergic blockade. It has been claimed that its favourable effects could be due to the peculiar characteristic of the drug and that this favourable evidence could not allow the conclusion that similar effects can be obtained with all the other β blockers.

More recently, two adequately powered, well conducted, large scale clinical trials, testing bisoprolol[12] and metoprolol,[13] confirmed that β blockade does reduce total and sudden deaths of patients with symptomatic heart failure and impaired ventricular function. Table 4.1 shows the characteristics of the above trials, and fig 4.1 summarises the results on total mortality and sudden death. While the US Carvedilol Program[11] pools data from four different studies to provide statistically reliable information on total mortality, CIBIS-2[12] and MERIT-HF[13] are the only two randomised clinical trials specifically powered to test the effects of β blockers on survival.

CIBIS-2, a multicentred, double blind, placebo controlled trial conducted in eastern and western Europe, enrolled 2647 patients with severely symptomatic (New York Heart Association (NYHA) functional class III and IV) heart failure with an ejection fraction of 35% or less receiving standard treatment with ACE inhibitors and diuretics.[12] Patients allocated to treatment with bisoprolol, a β1 selective adrenoreceptor blocker, showed a total mortality reduction of nearly 34%. Sudden death—one of the most common types of death in patients with chronic heart failure—was reduced by more than 40%. Hence, β blockers can be considered as complementary to ACE inhibitor treatment, whose effects on sudden death are not established. The trial was stopped after a planned interim analysis which showed a significant difference in all cause mortality between the two treatment groups.

MERIT-HF was a randomised, double blind controlled trial which tested metoprolol (a β1 adrenoreceptor blocker) versus placebo in 3991 patients enrolled in 14 countries in North America and Europe. Patients must have been symptomatic (NYHA class II–IV) with a left ventricular ejection fraction of 40% or less. The incidence of the most relevant predefined end point was significantly lower in the metoprolol group. Specifically the combined end point of total mortality or heart transplantation was reduced by 32%, and sudden death by nearly 50%. Similarly to the US Carvedilol Program and the CIBIS-2 trial, the MERIT-HF trial was

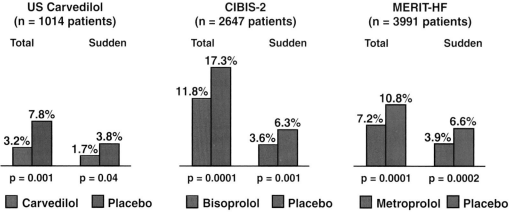

Figure 4.1. β Blockers in patients with heart failure: effects on total mortality and sudden death.

Trial acronyms

AVID: Antiarrhythmic Versus Implantable Defibrillator trial

BEST: β Blocker Evaluation Survival Trial

CIBIS-2: Cardiac Insufficiency Bisoprolol Study

COMET: Carvedilol or Metoprolol European Trial

COPERNICUS: Carvedilol Prospective Randomised Cumulative Survival Trial

DIAMOND: Danish Investigators of Arrhythmia and Mortality On Dofetilide

GESICA: Grupo de Estudio de la Sobrevida en la Insuficiencia Cardiaca en Argentina

MADIT: Multicenter Automatic Defibrillation Implantation Trial

MDC: Metoprolol in Dilated Cardiomyopathy

MERIT-HF: Metoprolol CR/XL Randomized Intervention Trial in congestive Heart Failure

RESOLVD: Randomized Evaluation of Strategies for Left Ventricular Dysfunction Pilot Study

SCD-HeFT: Sudden Cardiac Death in Heart Failure Trial

STAT-CHF: Survival Trial of Antiarrhythmic Therapy in Congestive Heart Failure

Table 4.2 Summary of the recommendations for β blocker use in patients with heart failure

Indications
Which patients with congestive heart failure are suitable for β blocker treatment?
- Patients with symptomatic heart failure of any cause, with depressed left ventricular function (ejection fraction ≤ 40%), in NYHA class II/III, clinically stable, already on treatment with ACE inhibitor, diuretic, and digitalis

Which patients are more likely to benefit?
- History of hypertension
- Heart rate > 90 beats/min

Which patients are less likely to benefit?
- Severe biventricular dysfunction
- Systolic blood pressure < 100 mm Hg
- Heart rate < 60 beats/min

Uncertain indications
For which patients do uncertainties still exist (scarce data from trials)?
- Elderly patients (> 75 years)
- NYHA class IV
- Asymptomatic left ventricular dysfunction
- Heart failure caused by valvar disease or diastolic dysfunction
- Comorbidities (diabetes, mild to moderate obstructive pulmonary disease, renal failure, peripheral vasculopathy)

Contraindications
What are the contraindications?
- Severe chronic obstructive pulmonary disease
- First degree AV block (PQ > 0.28 seconds) and second degree AV block (Mobitz 2 or advanced)
- Heart rate < 50 beats/min
- Systolic blood pressure < 90 mm Hg

AV, atrioventricular.

prematurely terminated because of a clear evidence of benefit.

Clinical recommendations

Which patients should be treated with β blockers?
On the basis of the evidence available, all patients with chronic, stable, mild to moderate symptomatic heart failure with depressed left ventricular function should be treated with β blockers. Benefits from β blockers appear to be similar in patients with heart failure caused by ischaemia or dilated cardiomyopathy. β Blocker treatment should be prescribed in addition to the other recommended treatments, such as ACE inhibitors and diuretics.

There is scant information on the effects of β blockers in patients with more severe (NYHA functional class IV) heart failure and in those with preserved left ventricular function. Furthermore, although in existing trials there were generally no age limits, elderly patients are poorly represented. Table 4.2 summarises the recommendations for β blocker use in patients with heart failure.

Which β blocker agent should be used?
Similar results in terms of morbidity and mortality reduction have been obtained with second or third generation β adrenergic blockers. Therefore, carvedilol, metoprolol or bisoprolol are the suggested agents to be used in patients with heart failure. In the absence of studies which directly compare the different compounds, there are no definite reasons to prefer any particular one of these three agents. The COMET trial, which is still ongoing, is comparing the effects of carvedilol versus metoprolol.

Table 4.3 summarises the pharmacological characteristics and the proposed dosages of the β blocker compounds most frequently studied in patients with heart failure. While for carvedilol, bisoprolol, and metoprolol there is clear evidence of a favourable effect in terms of mortality reduction, up to now bucindolol and nebivolol cannot be considered as evidence based recommended treatments for heart failure patients.

Table 4.3 Characteristics and proposed dosages of β blocker agents tested in patients with heart failure

Drug	Generation	β1 selectivity	Vasodilator	Starting dose	Maximal maintenance dose
Metoprolol	Second	+ +	No	5 mg twice daily 25 mg once daily**	75 mg twice daily 200 mg once daily**
Bisoprolol	Second	+++	No	1.25 mg once daily	10 mg once daily
Carvedilol	Third	±	Yes	6.25 mg twice daily	50 mg twice daily
Bucindolol	Third	0	yes	12.5 mg once daily	200 mg once daily
Nebivolol	Third	+++	yes	1.25 mg once daily	10 mg once daily

** CR/XL formulation.

32

> ## Evidence from β blocker trials
>
> - Long term treatment with different types of β blockers results in normalisation of left ventricular shape, regression in myocardial hypertrophy, and an improvement in ventricular function ("reverse modelling")
>
> - Effects of β blockers on exercise tolerance remain controversial, with some trials showing a significant improvement in maximal exercise tolerance and others showing no change or even a detrimental effect
>
> - Clinical trials consistently show that the hospitalisation rate for heart failure is significantly reduced by β blocker treatment
>
> - When quality of life for heart failure patients is evaluated using specific questionnaires, results of the effects of β blockers are conflicting
>
> - Adequately powered clinical trials testing different types of β blockers (carvedilol, bisoprolol, metoprolol) clearly demonstrate that total and cardiovascular mortality are significantly improved by each of these agents

Initiation of treatment

Since the adrenergic system is activated to support the reduced contractility of the failing heart, the administration of a β blocker in a patient with heart failure can induce myocardial depression that can be associated with different degrees of symptom manifestations. This possible initial deterioration of the clinical conditions could occur with any β blocking agent, although with non-selective first generation agents, such as propranolol, this phenomenon can be more evident. Second generation, β1 selective agents, such as metoprolol or bisoprolol—which leave β2 receptors unblocked and thus capable of supporting myocardial function—are generally better tolerated. Metoprolol or bisoprolol, started at very low dosages (table 4.3), are associated with a tolerability rate of more than 80%. The third generation compounds (carvedilol, bucindolol, nebivolol) have an acceptable initial tolerability rate, reducing the afterload and thus counteracting the negative inotropic properties of adrenergic blockade. While these vasodilating properties can play a favourable role at the initiation of treatment, it is less likely that vasodilation can give a substantial contribution to the long term effects of third generation compounds. Once treatment is started and the maintenance dosage is reached, the treatment should be continued indefinitely at the maximal tolerated dosage.

Open issues

Subgroups of patients not yet adequately studied

Uncertainties still exist on the effects of β blockers in patients with *advanced heart failure*—that is, those in NYHA functional class IV. The COPERNICUS trial, which specifically addressed this question, has been prematurely stopped because of an evidence of benefit, but the results have not yet been published. The only study that was terminated early because there was no likelihood of demonstrating a beneficial effect of treatment on mortality is the BEST trial, which tested bucindolol, a potent non-selective β blocker with sympathomimetic activity. This trial included 2708 patients with advanced heart failure. The less favourable effect observed in this trial could be explained by the fact that bucindolol may be less effective than metoprolol, carvedilol or bisoprolol. However, the most likely reason for the differing results is that the BEST trial randomised more patients with advanced heart failure than the other β blocker trials.

Furthermore, the BEST trial enrolled a large number of black patients. Black patients are already known to be poorly responsive to β blockade for the treatment of hypertension. The trend toward a detrimental effect of bucindolol observed in the BEST trial underscores the paucity of information in this population of patients.

There is not yet clear evidence of benefit from β blockers in the treatment of two other very important categories of patients: (a) the patients with overt heart failure but with *preserved left ventricular function*; and (b) *elderly patients*, who are today the largest majority of patients with heart failure as revealed by epidemiological surveys conducted in community settings. For all these categories of patients, further adequately powered studies are necessary.

Transferability of results to clinical practice

Finally, despite the impressive results in terms of morbidity and mortality reduction, and the increasing availability of β blockers in appropriate formulations, the transfer of these results into clinical practice is certainly difficult, mainly because of a distorted perception which clinicians have about the efficacy and tolerability of β blockers in congestive heart failure. International data show that only a minority of patients are treated with β blockers in clinical practice in the "real world". It is commonly perceived that β blockers are difficult to initiate and uptitrate, and that they have multiple contraindications so that very few patients can be considered eligible and only highly selected patients can tolerate them. The explanation for this discrepancy lies in part in the large differences which exist between the populations of patients with heart failure enrolled in clinical trials and those patients commonly encountered in clinical practice with respect mainly to age, sex distribution, and presence of comorbidities. Methods of implementing the results of trials in clinical practice should be developed to overcome these barriers and to start β blocker treatment in the huge number of patients with heart failure who could benefit from this treatment.[15]

β Blockers: summary

- At one time contraindicated in the treatment of heart failure, β blockers have become an established, evidence based, recommended treatment for patients with this condition

- The increased activation of the adrenergic system induced by heart failure—which leads to transmission of several adverse biological signals to the cardiac myocytes through the adrenergic receptors—provides the rationale for the use of β blockers in heart failure

- While the effects of β blockers on exercise capacity, quality of life, and the neurohormonal profile are still controversial, clinical trials clearly show that left ventricular shape and function, and the need for hospitalisation are improved by β blocker treatment

- Three adequately powered trials—US Carvedilol Program, CIBIS-2, and MERIT-HF—testing carvedilol, bisoprolol, and metoprolol, respectively, showed that these β blockers significantly reduce total and sudden mortality in heart failure patients

- On the basis of all available evidence, all patients with chronic, stable, mild to moderate, symptomatic heart failure (NYHA functional class II/III) and with depressed left ventricular function should be treated with β blockers

- Uncertainties still exist about the use of β blockers in heart failure patients in NYHA functional class I or IV, in those patients of advanced age, and/or in those patients with preserved left ventricular function

- β Blocker treatment should be started in stable patients with a very low initial dosage and then uptitrated to the maximal tolerated dosage

- Once treatment is started and the maintenance dosage is reached, treatment should be continued indefinitely and at the maximal dosage tolerated

- Despite the impressive results in terms of morbidity and mortality reduction, and the increasing availability of β blockers in appropriate formulations, the transfer of these benefits to the clinical practice setting in the "real world" is difficult, with international data showing only a minority of patients being treated

Antiarrhythmic drugs

Despite the clear evidence of benefit in terms of mortality reduction obtained with ACE inhibitors and β blockers, the prognosis of heart failure has remained a major issue. The five year mortality rate has been estimated to be at least 50%, and, besides progressive pump dysfunction, sudden death is the most common reason, being considered responsible for 25–70% of all deaths. The relative rate of sudden death is generally higher in patients with less severe functional status.[13] The majority of sudden deaths are generally caused by ventricular arrhythmias. In this context, the potential role of antiarrhythmic strategies has been considered of primary relevance for a long period of time. Over the last two decades, antiarrhythmic drugs have been tested by specific clinical trials to evaluate their role in improving survival of patients with congestive heart failure. It must be noted that almost all trials testing antiarrhythmic agents have been conducted when ACE inhibitor treatment was not yet largely adopted in clinical practice and β blockers were still a contraindicated treatment.

The use of antiarrhythmic agents in patients with heart failure has two potential serious adverse consequences: depression of left ventricular function and, in some cases, exacerbation of ventricular arrhythmias. Consistent with these unfavourable effects, several class I antiarrhythmic agents—such as encainide, flecainide, moricizine, and propafenone—have been demonstrated to increase mortality.[10] Apart from β blockers, only amiodarone among all antiarrhythmic drugs seems to have a potentially beneficial effect in terms of total mortality reduction.[16]

Amiodarone

In the presence of left ventricular dysfunction, amiodarone appears to be haemodynamically well tolerated even in the cases of more advanced heart failure. For this reason, several trials investigated the role of amiodarone in patients with congestive heart failure. Two of these trials were specifically powered to evaluate the effect of amiodarone on total mortality—the GESICA[17] and the STAT-CHF[18] trials.

The Argentinian GESICA study was an open, randomised trial testing amiodarone (600 mg/day for two weeks followed by a maintenance dose for 300 mg/day) versus placebo in 516 patients with severe heart failure: mean ejection fraction was 20%, and nearly 80% of the total population was in NYHA functional class III or IV. The mean period of follow up was 24 months. Amiodarone treatment was associated with a significant reduction of total and sudden mortality of 28% and 27%, respectively. The benefit appeared after only three months following initiation of treatment, and was consistent across subgroups defined by symptomatic severity.

Less favourable results have been shown by the STAT-CHF trial.[18] This randomised, double blind trial included 674 patients with symptomatic heart failure, with an ejection fraction of 40% or less, cardiac enlargement, and at least 10 premature ventricular beats per hour. During the median follow up period of 45 months, there was no significant difference in terms of either total or sudden deaths. While

5 Angiotensin receptor blockers for chronic heart failure and acute myocardial infarction

John J V McMurray

Two landmark clinical trials, CONSENSUS I and SOLVD-T, have shown, unequivocally, that angiotensin converting enzyme (ACE) inhibitors reduce all cause mortality in patients with chronic heart failure (CHF) and underlying left ventricular systolic dysfunction.[1][2] These and other trials have also confirmed that ACE inhibitors reduce morbidity, as manifest by hospital admission, in patients with CHF.[3]

A number of other key randomised, controlled, trials have also shown that ACE inhibitors reduce the risk of all cause mortality and major clinical events (sudden death, reinfarction, heart failure) after myocardial infarction.[w1-3] These benefits are most clearly seen in patients with left ventricular systolic dysfunction or clinical evidence of heart failure.[w4]

The ATLAS study has shown that higher doses of ACE inhibitor give greater morbidity/mortality benefits.[w5]

Recently, another drug known to block a component of the renin-angiotensin-aldosterone system (RAAS), spironolactone (an aldosterone antagonist), has also been shown to reduce mortality and morbidity in CHF, even when added to an ACE inhibitor (this was demonstrated in RALES).[w6]

The question arises, therefore, as to what the role of the newest agents available for RAAS inhibition, the angiotensin II receptor antagonists or blockers (ARBs), might be in CHF and acute myocardial infarction?

ARB–ACE inhibitor comparison studies

Though, logically, the first question to ask of ARBs might be whether these new drugs are better than placebo, the first comparison actually made in a large scale trial was with an ACE inhibitor. The first of these—the ELITE-1 trial—addressed tolerability, whereas the hypothesis of the larger ELITE-2 trial was that losartan would be more efficacious than captopril. The approach of the ELITE trials was based on the belief that: (1) ARBs are more effective inhibitors of the RAAS than ACE inhibitors; and (2) bradykinin, the breakdown of which is blocked by ACE inhibitors, is directly or indirectly responsible for cough and possibly other adverse effects of these agents.[4] There is some scientific basis for the view that ARBs might be more efficacious than ACE inhibitors at blocking the RAAS. If it is accepted that ACE inhibitors bring about benefit through reducing the actions of angiotensin II, then the recent demonstration that angiotensin II generating pathways that bypass ACE exist in human myocardium and arteries is of some significance (fig 1).[w7-9] Clearly, these observations suggest that ARBs offer a potentially more effective means of inhibiting the actions of angiotensin II. Arguably, the ATLAS and RALES trials also support the view that more intense inhibition of the RAAS might be better.[w5 w6] This hypothesis, however, needed to be tested in one or more definitive morbidity/mortality trials—for example, ELITE-2 (see below). Selective blockade of the angiotensin (AT) II receptor subtype, with hyperstimulation of the unblocked AT_2 receptor by displaced angiotensin II, is also more attractive, theoretically, than reduced stimulation of both receptor subtypes with an ACE inhibitor (fig 5.1). This is because the AT_2R may mediate biological actions which are the opposite of those that follow AT_1R activation (and, hence, potentially favourable in CHF). How have these hypotheses stood the test of clinical trials?

Tolerability: SPICE and ELITE-1
If ARBs are no more efficacious than ACE inhibitors, but are better tolerated, then there may be potentially substantial public health benefit to be gained. Though we do not yet know if ARBs are as efficacious as ACE inhibitors (see below), we do know ARBs are better tolerated. ARBs do not cause cough and do not seem to cause more of any other adverse effect

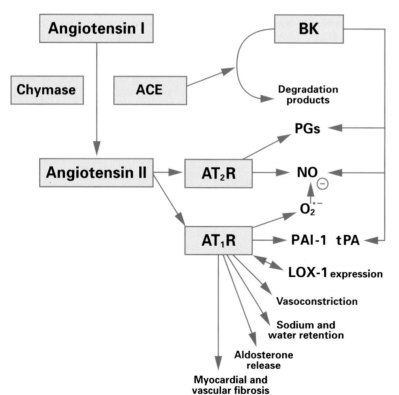

Figure 5.1. Known and postulated actions of angiotensin converting enzyme (ACE) and angiotensin II, and pathways for angiotensin II generation. tPA, tissue plasminogen activator; PAI-1, plasminogen activator inhibitor 1; BK, bradykinin; $O_2^{\cdot-}$, superoxide anion radical; NO, nitric oxide; LOX-1, lectin-like oxidised low density lipoprotein (LDL) receptor-1, $\ominus$, $O_2^{\cdot-}$ neutralises nitric oxide;◄─►, oxidised LDL induces AT_1R expression/angiotensin II induces LOX-1 through AT_1R.

Table 5.1 Angiotensin receptor blocker (ARB) trials in chronic heart failure (CHF): number of patients and main inclusion criteria

	ELITE-2	Val-HeFT	CHARM
Number of patients	3152	5010	7601
Entry criteria	• ≥ 60 years (85% ≥ 65) • NYHA class II–IV • > 70% IHD • LVEF ≤0.40 • No ACE-I/ARB within 3 months • ≤ 25% β blocker	• NYHA class II–IV • LVEF < 0.40 and LVIDD > 2.9 cm/m² • Usual background therapy (most ACE-I)	• NYHA class II–IV (1) LVEF ≤ 0.40 ACE-I intolerance arm (n=2028) (2) LVEF ≤ 0.40 ACE-I/ARB combination arm (n=2548) (3) LVEF > 0.40 arm (n=3025)
Treatment groups	Captopril v losartan	Placebo v valsartan (background ACE-I)	Placebo v candesartan—no ACE-I (1) placebo v candesartan-background ACE-I (2 + 3)

LVEF, left ventricular ejection fraction; NYHA, New York Heart Association; ACE-I, angiotensin converting enzyme; IHD, ischaemic heart disease; LVIDD, left ventricular internal dimension.

Table 5.2 Angiotensin receptor blocker (ARB) trials in chronic heart failure (CHF): hypotheses tested

	Non-inferiority	Superiority		
	ARB ≤ ACE-I	ARB > placebo	ARB > ACE-I	ARB + ACE-II > ACE-I
ELITE-2	No	No	Yes (25%, P 90%)†	No
Val-HeFT	No	No	No	Yes (20%, P 90%)††
CHARM	No	Yes (LVEF ≤ 0.40* 18%, P 94% LVEF > 0.40** 18%, P 86%)	No	Yes (18%, P 90%)†††

P, power—that is, power of study to detect that risk reduction (for example, Val HeFT has a 90% power to detect a 20% relative risk reduction in mortality with valsartan compared to placebo). *Assuming an annual placebo group event rate of 24%; **assuming an annual placebo group event rate of 13%; ≤ not significantly inferior to; †assuming a captopril group annual mortality rate of 9.4%; ††assuming placebo group annual mortality rate of 12%; †††assuming an annual placebo group event rate of 18%.
See table 1 for key to abbreviations.

than ACE inhibitors. Certainly, the SPICE trial found that candesartan was well tolerated by patients deemed to be ACE inhibitor intolerant by their physician.[5] In the ELITE-1 study 20.8% of captopril treated patients discontinued treatment because of an adverse event (excluding death) compared to 12.2% of losartan treated patients (p ≤ 0.002).[4 6] The more recent ELITE-2 study supports this finding, reporting that 14.5% of patients withdrew from captopril because of adverse effects, compared to 9.4% from losartan (p < 0.001).[7 8]

Efficacy: ELITE-1, RESOLVD, and ELITE-2
The ELITE-1 study reported the surprising finding that patients with CHF treated with losartan had a lower mortality than patients treated with captopril.[4 6] This trial was not designed to test this hypothesis and was too small to prove, with confidence, that ARBs have superior efficacy to ACE inhibitors. The RESOLVD study, comparing candesartan cilexetil (candesartan) to enalapril did not support the findings of ELITE-1.[9 10]

Recently, a large, prospective, properly powered, study has compared an ACE inhibitor (captopril) to an ARB (losartan).[7 8] ELITE-2 was designed to test the hypothesis that losartan was more efficacious than captopril (tables 5.1, 5.2, and 5.3).[7 8] This hypothesis was not proven— that is, losartan was not superior to captopril (table 5.4). ELITE-2 cannot, strictly speaking, answer any more questions than the one asked. It cannot tell us whether losartan is "as good as" (equivalent to) captopril or, at least, no worse than (not inferior) to captopril. These terms have strict statistical and regulatory definitions that the design and results of ELITE-2 do not fulfil.[w10] [w11] Indeed, ELITE-2 cannot even tell us if losartan is superior to placebo.[w12]

ARB–ACE inhibitor combination studies

The second question, addressed by a major clinical trial, was whether ARB–ACE inhibitor combination therapy is better than ACE inhibitor monotherapy. The hypothesis underlying this approach is very different from that underlying the ELITE studies. While the belief that ARBs are better inhibitors of the RAAS is shared by both hypotheses, the combination therapy approach takes the view that bradykinin is "good" rather than "bad".[11] This is because bradykinin may enhance the production of nitric oxide and possibly other vasoactive mediators, such as vasodilator prostanoids in vascular and other tissues.[w13-15] Bradykinin may also stimulate tissue plasminogen activator release from the endothelium and favourably influence coagulation/fibrinolysis balance.[w16] Consequently, combination ARB–ACE inhibitor therapy may give optimum RAAS inhibition *and* the putative benefits of bradykinin accumulation, through inhibition of its breakdown.

A number of relevant "mechanistic" and "pilot" clinical studies preceded what was

Table 5.3 Clinical characteristics of the patients enrolled in ELITE-2 and Val-HeFT

	ELITE-2	Val-HeFT
Number of patients	3152	5010
Mean age (years)	71	63
Males (%)	70	80
NYHA class (%)		
II	52	62
III	43	36
IV	5	2
LVEF (%)	31	27
Concomitant diagnoses (%)		
Coronary aetiology*	79	57
Hypertension	49	–
Atrial fibrillation	30	12
Diabetes mellitus	24	24
Drug treatment (%)		
Diuretic	78	86
ACE inhibitor	–†	93
Cardiac glycoside	50	67
β Blocker	22	34

*"History of ischaemia" in ELITE-2.
†Patients randomised to either losartan or captopril (23% of patients had received prior ACE inhibitor)

Trial acronyms

AIRE Acute Infarction Ramipril Efficacy
ATLAS Assessment of Treatment with Lisinopril And Survival
CHARM Candesartan in Heart failure: Assessment of Reduction in Mortality and Morbidity
CONSENSUS-1 Co-operative North Scandanavian Enalapril Survival Study
ELITE Evaluation of Losartan In The Elderly
HOPE Heart Outcomes Prevention Evaluation
OPTIMAAL Optimal Therapy in Myocardial infarction with the Angiotensin II Antagonist Losartan
PEP-CHF Perindopril for Elderly People with Chronic Heart Failure
RALES Randomised Aldactone Evaluation Study
REPLACE Replacement of angiotensin converting enzyme inhibition
RESOLVD Randomized Evaluation of Strategies for Left Ventricular Dysfunction
SAVE Survival and Ventricular Enlargement
SOLVD-T Treatment arm of the Studies Of Left Ventricular Dysfunction
SPICE Study of Patients Intolerant of Converting Enzyme Inhibitors
STRETCH Symptom, Tolerability, Response to Exercise Trial of Candesartan cilexetil in Heart failure
TRACE Trandolapril Cardiac Evaluation
Val-HeFT Valsartan Heart Failure Trial
V-HeFT Vasodilator Heart Failure Trial
VALIANT Valsartan In Acute myocardial infarction

Table 5.4   ELITE-2 end points

End point	Number of patients		HR (95% CI)	p Value
	Losartan (n=1578)	Captopril (n=1574)		
All cause mortality	280 (17.7%)	250 (15.9%)	1.13 (0.95 to 1.35)	0.16
Sudden death or resuscitated cardiac arrest	142 (9.0%)	115 (7.3)	1.25 (0.98 to 1.60)	0.08
Combined total mortality or hospitalisation for any reason	752 (47.7%)	707 (44.9%)	1.07 (0.97 to 1.19)	0.18
Hospital admissions (all causes)	659 (41.8%)	638 (40.5%)	1.04 (0.94 to 1.16)	0.45

HR, hazard ratio; CI, confidence interval.

nary capillary wedge pressure and systolic blood pressure acutely and after one month's treatment. Valsartan 80 mg and 160 mg twice daily significantly reduced aldosterone at four weeks. Not all studies have supported these findings, however, and there remains the nagging doubt that similar benefits might be obtained by using a bigger dose of ACE inhibitor, rather than adding an ARB.[w17 w18] However, Hamroff and colleagues reported a small but impressive six month randomised trial in which patients with moderately severe CHF were randomised to placebo or losartan 50 mg once daily.[14] All were receiving full conventional treatment including an ACE inhibitor given in an adequate dose (for example, the mean daily dose of enalapril was 32 mg). The primary end points were exercise capacity and New York Heart Association (NYHA) functional class. Both improved significantly and losartan was well tolerated. In the RESOLVD pilot study the combination of enalapril and candesartan had significantly more favourable effects on the left ventricular remodelling than either monotherapy.[9 10] Clinical outcome was not, however, better in the candesartan–enalapril combination group. The hypothesis that combination therapy is the optimum had, therefore, to be tested in a large scale morbidity–mortality trial.

expected to be the first definitive large scale trial, Val-HeFT, exploring this hypothesis.[11]

Small scale studies testing combination therapy

There is conflicting clinical evidence that some of the effect of ACE inhibitors may be caused by the blocking effect these drugs have on bradykinin breakdown. Two recent studies in hypertensive individuals and healthy subjects, using a selective bradykinin inhibitor, supports such an action, though another in heart failure does not.[w13–15] These mechanistic findings are supported by some clinical observations. Dunselman reported that substitution of telmisartan (10–80 mg once daily) for enalapril (10 mg twice daily) in patients with heart failure led to an increase in blood pressure (the REPLACE study), thus supporting the possibility that ACE inhibitors have an additional hypotensive mechanism of action compared to ARBs.[12] Baruch and colleagues studied the immediate and four week haemodynamic and neurohumoral effects of placebo, valsartan 80 mg twice daily or valsartan 160 mg twice daily added to conventional treatment (including an ACE inhibitor) in patients with CHF.[13] Compared to placebo, high dose valsartan reduced pulmo-

Val-HeFT trial

The key features of the design of Val-HeFT trial are shown in tables 5.1 and 5.2.[11] The demographic characteristics and preliminary results of Val-HeFT were presented by J Cohn at the 73rd scientific sessions of the American Heart Association (AHA) in New Orleans, 15 November 2000, and all of the subsequent information reported in this review has been obtained from that presentation. The principal hypothesis tested by Val-HeFT was that adding valsartan to conventional treatment (including an ACE inhibitor and β blocker, where appropriate) would improve clinical outcome. The co-primary end points were: (1) mortality (all cause); and (2) mortality or morbidity (where morbidity included hospitalisation for CHF, resuscitated sudden death, and administration of intravenous inotropic or vasodilator treatment for CHF for ≥ 4 hours). Secondary end points included change in NYHA functional class, signs and symptoms of CHF, left ventricular ejection fraction, and quality of life. Val-HeFT randomised 5010 patients, the clinical characteristics of whom are summarised in table 5.3.[11 15] The average follow up time was approximately 1.9 years.

The principal results of the Val-HeFT trial, as presented at the AHA, are shown in table 5.5. Valsartan did not reduce mortality but did significantly reduce the combined morbidity/mortality end point by approximately 13% (p = 0.009). This effect was principally caused by a substantial 27% reduction in CHF hospitalisation (table 5.5, p = 0.00001). There were similarly impressive and significant improvements in the other secondary outcomes presented. At face value, therefore, Val-HeFT would appear to be a "positive" trial, with significant improvements in pre-specified co-primary and secondary end points. Unfortunately, however, the story may not be that simple. This is because Cohn went on to present detailed subgroup analyses which appeared to raise important questions about the overall findings of Val-HeFT.

Firstly, outcomes in the small minority (7%) of patients not taking on ACE inhibitor at baseline were compared to those in patients taking an ACE inhibitor. The former group had an approximately 45% reduction in mortality/morbidity compared to a 12% reduction in the latter. In other words, this analysis raises the possibility that most of the benefit in the overall trial can be explained by a particularly large effect in patients not receiving an ACE inhibitor. To complicate matters further, patients receiving a β blocker at baseline (about 35%) were compared to those not taking a β blocker. The hazard ratio for the mortality/morbidity end point in patients taking a β blocker was 1.15 (that is, there was a trend for such patients to do worse on valsartan) compared to 0.78 in those not on a β blocker. In other words, this and some further analysis raised the possibility that "triple neurohumoral blockade" (ACE inhibitor, β blocker, ARB) has no advantage over double blockade and may even be disadvantageous. It must be emphasised that subgroup analysis of this type is fraught with danger, can be very misleading, and should only be regarded as hypothesis generating.[w19] Unfortunately, however, the β blocker subgroup analysis has attracted much attention because β blockers, along with ACE inhibitors, are now regarded as mandatory treatment for CHF. The issue is further confounded by an apparently similar β blocker interaction in ELITE-2 (captopril treated patients did better than losartan treated patients if receiving β blocker treatment at baseline).[8]

Where then do we stand with ARBs following both ELITE-2 and Val-HeFT? I would have to conclude that the picture still remains unclear. From a purist perspective

Clinical pharmacology of ARBs versus ACE inhibitors

- Angiotensin II exerts its known biological actions via the angiotensin II type 1 receptor (AT_1R). The angiotensin receptor blockers (ARBs) currently available for clinical use selectively antagonise the action of angiotensin II at the AT_1R

- The role of the angiotensin II type 2 receptor (AT_2R) is uncertain. It may, when stimulated, increase the production of nitric oxide and other vasodilator/anti mitotic substances. The AT_2R is hyperstimulated during selective AT_1R blockade in vivo

- Angiotensin II may be generated through the action of ACE and, probably, chymase on angiotensin I. There may be additional "non-ACE" pathways for angiotensin II production. AT_1R blockers (but not ACE inhibitors) antagonise the effects of angiotensin II generated by "non ACE" pathways

- ACE is also known as kininase II which degrades bradykinin (that is, bradykinin accumulates during ACE inhibition). Bradykinin may, directly or indirectly, cause some of the adverse effects of ACE inhibitors (for example, cough) but may also have beneficial vasodilator, growth, and fibrinolytic actions.

Val-HeFT does suggest that adding an ARB to conventional treatment reduces morbidity (CHF hospitalisation). How much attention one should pay to subgroup analyses is very debatable. Before reaching any firm conclusion we must at least wait for full publication of the Val-HeFT results. It must be reiterated that only preliminary data are available at the time of writing. Analysis of the neurohumoral and left ventricular remodelling data from this study should give additional insight into the issues raised above. We will also have a more complete picture when the CHARM programme completes.[16] This three study programme is now ideally poised to address some of the remaining uncertainty about ARBs.[16] In particular, CHARM includes a study in patients not taking an ACE inhibitor (study 0003 or "alternative CHARM"—see below), and more patients in the ACE-I + ARB combination arm of CHARM (study 0006 or "added CHARM") are receiving a β blocker at baseline than in Val-HeFT (55% v 35%) and all are taking an ACE inhibitor, allowing further exploration of any potential ARB–β blocker interaction.

ARB–placebo comparison studies

Remarkably, it has been generally assumed that ARBs are an effective treatment for CHF (that is, superior to placebo) even though there are very few data to support this assumption.

Table 5.5   Val-HeFT end points (preliminary)

End point	Number of patients		RR (95% CI)	p Value
	Valsartan (n=2511)	Placebo (n=2499)		
All cause mortality	495 (19.7%)	484 (19.4%)	1.02 (0.90 to 1.15)	0.800
Combined all cause mortality + morbidity	723 (28.88%)	801 (32.1%)	0.87 (0.79 to 0.96)	0.009
Heart failure hospitalisations (patients)	349 (13.9%)	463 (18.5%)	0.73 (0.63 to 0.83)	0.00001

Major ARB clinical trials in CHF

- ELITE-2 compared losartan to captopril. The primary end point in this trial was all cause mortality. Mortality was not reduced by losartan compared to captopril

- Val-HeFT compared valsartan to placebo, added to full conventional treatment including, in most patients, an ACE inhibitor. These were two co-primary end points—all cause mortality and morbidity/mortality. While valsartan had no effect on the former, the latter was reduced by 13% (mainly because of a 27% reduction in heart failure hospitalisation). Subgroup analysis suggested a particularly large benefit in the minority of patients not taking ACE inhibitors at baseline. More controversially, there was also the suggestion that adding valsartan to background treatment with both an ACE inhibitor and β blocker *increased* risk

- The CHARM programme is still underway and comprises three component trials. One is comparing candesartan to placebo in patients intolerant of an ACE inhibitor, and the second is making the same comparison in patients taking an ACE inhibitor. The third is comparing these two treatments in patients with heart failure and preserved left ventricular systolic function. The primary end point in each individual trial is cardiovascular death or heart failure hospitalisation and all cause mortality in the overall programme

- I-PRESERVE is a trial still in the planning stage which intends to compare irbesartan to placebo in patients with heart failure, preserved left ventricular systolic function, and an increased plasma BNP concentration.

Clearly, the widely held opinion that ARBs are efficacious in CHF is based on the view that RAAS inhibition is beneficial, a perception based on the belief that ACE inhibitors and spironolactone exert their effect in this way. While almost certainly true, at least in part, even the most apparently obvious hypotheses should be tested in medicine.

Small studies comparing ARBs to placebo in CHF

ARBs, like ACE inhibitors, have favourable acute and chronic neurohumoral and haemodynamic actions in CHF.[10] [13-17] [w17] [w18] [w20] There are, however, remarkably few data showing any clinical benefit of ARBs over placebo. A recent trial, STRETCH, has shown that one of these agents, candesartan cilexetil, can improve exercise tolerance in CHF in a dose dependent manner, compared to placebo.[18] This has not, however, been a consistent finding in all studies (there are two fairly large, unpublished, exercise studies showing no benefit of losartan over placebo).[w21] Meta-analyses of relatively small trials with losartan and candesartan have,

Table 5.6 Angiotensin receptor blocker (ARB) trials in post-myocardial infarction patients: number of patients and main inclusion criteria

	OPTIMAAL	VALIANT
Number of patients	5476	14500*
Entry criteria	≥ 50 years. Anterior Q wave MI or new LBBB or signs of heart failure or LVSD/dilatation	LVSD and/or signs of heart failure
Treatment groups	captopril losartan	captopril valsartan captopril + valsartan

*Target number.
MI, myocardial infarction; LBBB, left bundle branch block; LVSD, left ventricular systolic dysfunction.

however, suggested that ARBs might improve clinical outcomes when compared to placebo, though an imputed placebo analysis of ELITE-2 (using SOLVD-T as the historical control) gives only weak support to these meta-analyses.[19] [w12] [w21] Adding the data from the Val-HeFT subgroup not treated with an ACE inhibitor gives more support to the view that ARBs are more efficacious than placebo (table 5.6). However, no prospective, randomised, placebo controlled trial has, to date, tested the hypothesis that ARBs are superior to placebo in terms of morbidity/mortality or mortality end points in CHF.

One such study is currently underway. This is one of the component trials of the CHARM programme (tables 5.1 and 5.2).[16]

A wider role for RAAS inhibition in CHF?

The emergence of a new class of drug for RAAS inhibition also presents the opportunity to test additional questions not formally tested in previous trials with ACE inhibitors. One pressing issue in clinical cardiology is the treatment of CHF in patients with preserved left ventricular systolic function, who make up perhaps a third of all patients with CHF and who also have an increased morbidity and mortality.[w22] [w23] Though left ventricular ejection fraction (LVEF) measurements were not required for entry into either the CONSENSUS-1 or V-HeFT studies, these trials are generally considered to have recruited patients with left ventricular systolic dysfunction.[1] [w24] [w25]

It is possible that RAAS inhibition might also be of benefit in patients with CHF and preserved left ventricular systolic function. These patients are treated with diuretics which may be expected to cause RAAS activation.[w26] Many are hypertensive, diabetic, and have left ventricular hypertrophy, comorbidities that might be expected to respond favourably to

Table 5.7 Angiotensin receptor blocker (ARB) trials in post-myocardial infarction patients: hypotheses tested

	Non-inferiority	Superiority	
	ARB ≤ ACE-I	ARB > ACE-I	ARB + ACE-I > ACE-I
OPTIMAAL	Yes*	Yes† (20%, P 96%)	No
VALIANT	Yes (2.5%, P 88%) (0%, P 74%)	Yes (17.5%, P 95%) (15%, P 86%)	Yes (17.5%, P 95%) (15%, P 86%)

P, power—that is, power of study to detect that risk reduction.
≤, Not significantly inferior to; *revision of protocol as published[w27]—further details not available; †assuming a captopril group annual mortality of 17%.

RAAS inhibition, especially in the light of the recently reported HOPE study.[w27] [w28] Once more, of course, this is a hypothesis that needs to be tested in an appropriately designed clinical trial. Two trials are underway. One with the ACE inhibitor perindopril (PEP-CHF)[w29] and one which is a component trial of the CHARM programme (study 0007 or "preserved CHARM").[16] Another trial, with irbesartan, is at an advanced stage of planning. This trial, to be known as I-PRESERVE, will enrol patients with current signs/symptoms of heart failure (or an admission to hospital primarily because of heart failure within the last three months), an LVEF ≥ 0.45, and a raised plasma brain natriuretic peptide (BNP) concentration.

ARB myocardial infarction trials

Two trials are underway in patients with acute myocardial infarction. These are OPTIMAAL and VALIANT which are outlined in table 7. OPTIMAAL is similar to the ELITE trials in comparing losartan to captopril.[20 21] The patients randomised are high risk survivors broadly similar, but not identical, to those recruited into the seminal ACE inhibitor post-myocardial infarction trials (SAVE, AIRE, TRACE).[w1–3] OPTIMAAL is sufficiently large to have a 95% power of showing a 20% relative reduction in the risk of death with losartan compared to captopril. VALIANT has a more complex design with three treatment groups (captopril, valsartan, and their combination) and is powered not just to test for superiority but also for non-inferiority (table 5.7).[22]

As a consequence, the patient entry criteria must exactly mirror those of the reference trials SAVE,[w1] AIRE,[w2] and TRACE.[w3] Among the questions VALIANT can address is the one of whether ARBs have similar efficacy to ACE inhibitors (non-inferiority) but are better tolerated. VALIANT will, of course, also show whether combination ACE inhibitor–ARB treatment is superior to ACE inhibitor monotherapy in the post-myocardial infarction setting.

Conclusions and clinical recommendations

It seems reasonable to recommend use of an angiotensin receptor blocker as an alternative to an ACE inhibitor in the patient truly intolerant of the inhibitor. An angiotensin receptor blocker may also be added to an ACE inhibitor to improve symptoms and reduce the risk of hospital admission with worsening heart failure. At present angiotensin receptor blockers are only indicated where there is ACE inhibitor or β blocker intolerance.

- Angiotensin receptor blockers may be used as an *alternative* to an ACE inhibitor in the patient truly intolerant of an ACE inhibitor.
- Angiotensin receptor blockers may also be used in *addition* to an ACE inhibitor when a patient is intolerant of a β blocker.

- "Triple neurohumoral blockade" with an ACE inhibitor, β blocker, and angiotensin receptor blocker is not, presently, recommended.

1. **The CONSENSUS Trial Study Group.** Effects of enalapril on mortality in severe congestive heart failure. Results of the cooperative north Scandinavian enalapril survival study (CONSENSUS). *N Engl J Med* 1987;**316**:1429–35.

2. **The SOLVD Investigators.** Effect of enalapril on survival in patients with reduced left ventricular ejection fractions and congestive heart failure. *N Engl J Med* 1991;**325**:293–302.

3. **Garg R, Yusuf S.** Overview of randomized trials of angiotensin-converting enzyme inhibitors on mortality and morbidity in patients with heart failure. Collaborative group on ACE inhibitor trials. *JAMA* 1995;**273**:1450–6.

4. **Pitt B, Chang P, Timmermans PBM.** Angiotensin-II receptor antagonists in heart failure—rationale and design of the evaluation of losartan in the elderly (ELITE) trial. *Cardiovascular Drugs and Therapy* 1995;**9**:693–700.

5. **Granger B, Ertl G, Kuch J,** *et al.* Randomized trial of candesartan cilexetil in the treatment of patients with congestive heart failure and a history of intolerance to angiotensin-converting enzyme inhibitors. *Am Heart J* 2000;**139**:609–17.
- *SPICE was a three month pilot study for CHARM study 0003 ("alternative CHARM"), comparing placebo to candesartan cilexetil in patients intolerant of an ACE inhibitor. There was no significant difference in the proportion of placebo and candesartan treated patients remaining on treatment for three months.*

6. **Pitt B, Segal R, Martinez FA,** *et al.* Randomised trial of losartan versus captopril in patients over 65 with heart failure (evaluation of losartan in the elderly study, ELITE). *Lancet* 1997;**349**:747–52.
- *ELITE was a relatively small study set up to compare tolerability (as assessed by changes in renal function) of losartan compared to captopril. Unexpected and notably lower mortality was found in the losartan group. This study emphasises how misleading small studies and multiple analyses involving secondary and tertiary end points can be. It actually showed no difference in the primary end point.*

7. **Pitt B, Poole-Wilson P, Segal R,** *et al.* Effects of losartan versus captopril on mortality in patients with symptomatic heart failure: rationale, design and baseline characteristics of patients in the losartan heart failure survival study—ELITE II. *Journal of Cardiac Failure* 1999;**5**:146–54.

8. **Pitt B, Poole-Wilson PA, Segal R,** *et al.* Effect of losartan compared with captopril on mortality in patients with symptomatic heart failure: randomised trial—the losartan heart failure survival study ELITE II. *Lancet* 2000;**355**:1582–7.
- *One of the three "landmark" major ARB mortality or mortality/morbidity trials in heart failure either underway or completed. Essentially a repeat of ELITE, but much larger with longer term follow up and properly powered to examine mortality (the primary end point this time). The study was designed as a "superiority trial" and did **not** show losartan to be better than (superior to) captopril. It was not powered to show "non-inferiority" (losartan no worse than captopril) or equivalence (losartan as good as or equivalent to captopril).*

9. **Tsuyuki RT, Yusuf S, Rouleau JL,** *et al.* Combination neurohormonal blockade with ACE inhibitors, angiotensin II antagonists and beta-blockers in patients with congestive heart failure: design of the randomized evaluation of strategies for left ventricular dysfunction (RESOLVD) pilot study. *Can J Cardiol* 1997;**13**:1166–74.

10. **McKelvie RS, Yusuf S, Pericak D,** *et al.* Comparison of candesartan, enalapril and their combination in congestive heart failure: randomized evaluation of strategies for left ventricular dysfunction (RESOLVD) pilot study. The RESOLVD pilot study investigators. *Circulation* 1999;**100**:1056–64.
- *RESOLVD was a relatively small and complex study designed to compare an ACE inhibitor (enalapril) with a number of doses of an ARB (candesartan) and their combination, with subsequent randomisation to β blocker or placebo. The primary end point was six minute walk distance (no difference between groups). Interesting observations were reported on left ventricular remodelling and neurohumoral measures.*

11. **Cohn JN, Tognoni G, Glazer RD,** *et al.* Rationale and design of the valsartan heart failure trial: a large multinational trial to assess the effects of valsartan, an angiotensin-receptor blocker, on morbidity and mortality in chronic congestive heart failure. *Journal of Cardiac Failure* 1999;**5**:155–60.
- *The design paper for the second of the landmark ARB trials in heart failure. Publication of the results is awaited.*

12. **Dunselman PHJM.** Effects of the replacement of the angiotensin converting enzyme inhibitor enalapril by the angiotensin II receptor blocker telmisartan in patients with

congestive heart failure. The replacement of angiotensin converting enzyme inhibition (REPLACE) investigators. *Int J Cardiol* 2001;**77**:131–8.

13. Baruch L, Anand I, Cohen IS, *et al.* Augmented short and long term hemodynamic and hormonal effects of an angiotensin receptor blocker added to angiotensin converting enzyme inhibitor therapy in patients with heart failure. *Circulation* 1999;**99**:2658–64.

14. Hamroff G, Katz SD, Mancini D, *et al.* Addition of angiotensin II receptor blockade to maximal angiotensin-converting-enzyme inhibition improves exercise capacity in patients with severe congestive heart failure. *Circulation* 1999;**99**:990–2.
- *A small but intriguing study. Very well designed comparison of placebo or ARB (losartan) added to full conventional dose ACE inhibitor treatment in patients with advanced heart failure. Impressive improvements were found in clinical status and exercise time with combination ARB/ACE inhibitor treatment.*

15. Cohn JN, Tognoni G, Glazer R, *et al.* Baseline demographics of the valsartan heart failure trial. *Eur J Heart Failure* 2000;**2**:439–46.

16. Swedberg K, Pfeffer M, Granger C, *et al.* Candesartan in heart failure-assessment of reduction in mortality and morbidity (CHARM): rationale and design. *Journal of Cardiac Failure* 1999;**3**:276–82.
- *The design paper for the third of the landmark ARB trials in heart failure. The CHARM programme consists of three component trials that are currently in their follow up phase:* "alternative CHARM" (in ACE inhibitor intolerant patients), "added CHARM" (in ACE inhibitor treated patients), and "preserved CHARM" (in patients with preserved left ventricular systolic dysfunction).

17. Havranek EP, Thomas I, Smith WB, *et al.* Dose-related beneficial long-term hemodynamic and clinical efficacy of irbesartan in heart failure. *J Am Coll Cardiol* 1999;**33**:117–81.

18. Riegger GAJ, Bouzo H, Petr P, *et al.* Improvement in exercise tolerance and symptoms of congestive heart failure during treatment with candesartan cilexetil. *Circulation* 1999;**100**:2224–30.

19. Erdmann E, George M, Voet B, *et al.* The safety and tolerability of candesartan cilexetil in CHF. *Journal of the Renin Angiotensin Aldosterone System* 2000;**1**:31–6.

20. Dickstein K, Kjekshus J. Comparison of the effects of losartan and captopril on mortality in patients after acute myocardial infarction: the OPTIMAAL trial design. *Am J Cardiol* 1999;**83**:477–81.

21. Dickstein K, Kjekshus J, for the OPTIMAAL Trial Steering Committee and Investigators. Comparison of baseline data, initial course, and management: losartan versus captopril following acute myocardial infarction (the OPTIMAAL trial). *Am J Cardiol* 2001;**87**:766–71.

22. Pfeffer MA, McMurray J, Leizorovicz A, *et al.* Valsartan in acute myocardial infarction trial—VALIANT: rationale and design. *Am Heart J* 2000;**140**:727–50.

website
extra

Additional references appear on the Heart website

www.heartjnl.com

6 What causes the symptoms of heart failure?

Andrew J S Coats

Chronic heart failure (CHF) is a common condition with a poor prognosis. It is associated with debilitating limiting symptoms, even with optimal modern medical management. Foremost among these symptoms is severe exercise intolerance with pronounced fatigue and dyspnoea at low exercise workloads. The UK National Health Service has highlighted it as a key target for improved treatment with the aim of symptom relief and restoration of optimal functional capacity.[1] The severity of symptomatic exercise limitation varies between patients, and this appears to bear little relation to the extent of the left ventricular systolic dysfunction measured at rest, or to markers of central haemodynamic disturbance (fig 6.1).[2] There may be several reasons for this. It may be that measurements of ventricular function at rest bear only a poor relation to changes in central haemodynamic function that occur on exercise,[3] and therefore predict only poorly exercise capacity. It may be that on the background of left ventricular impairment, variability in preservation of right ventricular function and the adequacy of the pulmonary vasculature to dilate and accept a blood flow and to match this flow with ventilation is impaired. Thirdly, it may be that changes, which occur in the periphery as a consequence of the systemic effects of heart failure, may have become the factors limiting exercise more than the heart dysfunction that initiated the syndrome.[4] There is evidence in the literature for all three of these hypotheses.

Exercise capacity in normal subjects

In normal subjects exercise is usually possible until maximal cardiac output is achieved, at which time a further increase in workload will produce extra carbon dioxide (CO_2) but with no commensurate increase in oxygen (O_2) uptake.[5] This is termed maximal oxygen uptake (Vo_2max). At between 85–95% of Vo_2max a point in exercise is reached where there is an excessive release of CO_2 for the rate of O_2 uptake caused by a limitation in the rate of delivery of O_2, leading to the onset of anaerobic muscular metabolism with lactate production. This produces arterial acidosis and directly stimulates the chemoreceptors to produce relative hyperventilation. This point is called the anaerobic threshold. In most normal subjects exercise is limited by cardiac reserve, with lung function rarely being the limiting factor. Training status and genetic factors determine the overall fitness to exercise.

Exercise capacity in CHF

In non-oedematous stable and optimally treated patients with CHF submaximal exercise and the haemodynamic response accompanying it may be remarkably normal, with preservation of muscle blood flow being at the expense of increased vasoconstriction in other vascular beds. Exercise tends to stop abruptly quite frequently with the respiratory exchange ratio (ratio of CO_2 produced to O_2 consumed) being not much above 1.0, indicating true maximal cardiopulmonary reserve has not been reached. Further evidence of this comes from the observation that the addition of arm exercise to maximal leg exercise increased observed peak O_2 uptake in heart failure patients but not in normal controls. This suggest that the heart had the capacity to increase its output and therefore at maximal leg exercise the limiting factor must have been based either on an intolerable symptom, or on the inability of the leg to accept a greater blood supply, or in the muscles of the leg to utilise the oxygen delivered any further.[6] This suggests that the limiting factor in the majority of patients with CHF may be peripheral.[7]

Correlates of exercise capacity in CHF

Much work has recently concentrated on non-cardiac abnormalities in stable CHF. Abnormalities have been described in peripheral blood flow, endothelial function, skeletal muscle, and lung function.[8–11] These changes acting alone, or in combination, may lead to early muscle fatigue and dyspnoea. Better correlations with exercise tolerance are seen with these peripheral abnormalities than for haemodynamic measurements.[12] Patients with heart failure exhibit a subnormal peripheral blood flow response to both exercise and pharmacological vasodilatation, caused by a combination

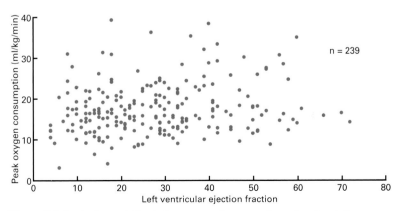

Figure 6.1. Lack of correlation between exercise capacity and resting left ventricular ejection fraction in 239 patients attending the cardiopulmonary exercise laboratory of the Royal Brompton Hospital, London, UK.

of persistent vasoconstrictor drive, a relative paucity of peripheral blood vessels, a deficient nitric oxide vasodilator system, and an enhancement of the vasoconstrictor endothelin system. CHF patients can demonstrate evidence of early muscular lactate release despite normal skeletal muscle blood flow. An inherent defect in skeletal muscle metabolism independent of blood flow has been described in this condition. There are abnormalities in histology, mitochondrial structure and function, oxidative enzymes, and a shift in fibre type distribution with predominance of type IIb over IIa fibres and many of reduced fibre dimension.[13]

Skeletal muscle changes

Skeletal muscle is abnormal in CHF in many ways (fig 6.2). There is impaired gross function, substantial wasting, impaired intrinsic blood flow, and a limited ability to accept a blood flow. This limitation can be seen independent of reduced blood flow, and intrinsic metabolic function is abnormal.[14] Metabolic abnormalities have also been described, including early dependence on anaerobic metabolism, excessive early depletion of high energy phosphate bonds, and excessive early intramuscular acidification. Biopsy studies have confirmed defects in oxidative and lipolytic enzymes, succinate dehydrogenase and citrate synthetase, and β hydroxyacyl dehydrogenase. Muscle is also abnormal in gross function, showing in particular early fatigue, and maximal strength. The changes seen are at least partially similar to those seen in physical deconditioning and are at least partially correctable by exercise training indicating a degree of plasticity.[15]

The abnormalities of muscle and even the degree of wasting show a better correlation with exercise tolerance than do measures of left ventricular function. This is because fatigue is a common symptom interrupting exercise in patients with CHF. Less clear is the aetiology of the muscle changes. Although deconditioning contributes, there are suggestions of a distinct phenotype in CHF muscle not explained by deconditioning.[16] Major abnormalities in catabolic and anabolic function have been described in those CHF patients with substantial wasting of skeletal muscle,[17] and these patients have been identified as having in particular an exaggerated release of catabolic cytokines,[18] and resistance to the effects of growth hormone.[19] The cause, progress, and most appropriate management of these abnormalities in muscle structure and function remain unknown. Physical inactivity is likely to play a role in some cases, along with activation of catabolic processes, and loss of normal anabolic function, such as insulin resistance,[20] raised concentrations of tumour necrosis factor α, and excessive noradrenaline (norepinephrine) concentrations. Anorexia and intestinal malabsorption may also play a role in some patients. When seen, these changes are also markers of an extremely poor prognosis.[21]

> **Abnormalities of skeletal muscle in CHF**
>
> - Loss of bulk
> - Impaired perfusion
> - Increased fatigue
> - Abnormal histology
> - Abnormal metabolism

Endothelial dysfunction

Recent research has demonstrated the importance of the endothelium to the development and progression of a number of cardiovascular conditions, including hypertension, diabetes, heart failure, and atherosclerosis. Endothelial dysfunction is associated with deficiency of the natural endothelial nitric oxide vasodilator system, with exaggerated activity of the vasoconstrictor endothelin system. Both abnormalities are now considered hallmarks of human CHF. When present they lead to a further impairment of nutritive blood flow to already stressed and metabolically abnormal skeletal muscle, and they therefore contribute to exercise intolerance in patients with CHF. Interventions which improve endothelial function, such as exercise training, also increase exercise tolerance and appear to do so by improving the sensation of fatigue within skeletal muscle. All these features make it likely that muscle dysfunction, either intrinsic or caused by impaired blood flow, contributes to exercise intolerance and symptoms in CHF.

Lung and ventilatory abnormalities

It is easy to see how major alterations in skeletal muscle and endothelial function could contribute to fatigue. Major changes have been described within the lung and in two major ventilatory control reflexes (the muscle ergo- or metaboreflexes and the arterial chemoreflexes).[22–24] These appear to be in a better position to explain the dyspnoea which is

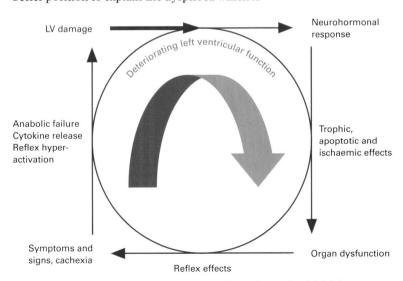

Figure 6.2. The muscle hypothesis of chronic heart failure, in which it is proposed that alterations in skeletal muscle contribute not only to symptom generation but also, via reflex effects, to further neurohormonal activation and progression of the syndrome of CHF.

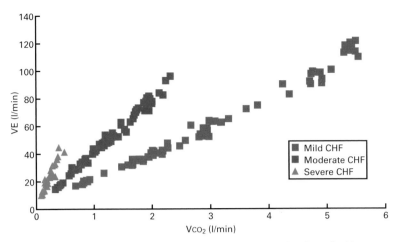

Figure 6.3. Plot of minute ventilation (VE) versus the rate of carbon dioxide production (Vco_2) in three patients with chronic heart failure. You can see that the ventilation needed for the same carbon dioxide elimination rate increases with the increasing severity of heart failure. This is associated with a greater sensation of dyspnoea despite preservation of arterial blood gases in these patients.

so common in CHF even when haemodynamics are relatively well controlled. These may also be important pathophysiological mechanisms as abnormalities of ventilatory control have consistently been shown to predict accurately a poor prognosis in CHF.[25][26] These may be more important in predicting symptomatic limitation than even the underlying cause of the heart failure.[27] More recent research has shown that both exercise tolerance per se, even if measured in simple corridor tests,[28] and the physiological ventilatory response to exercise are important and independent prognostic markers in CHF.[29]

Respiratory muscle is also abnormal in CHF. Early muscle deoxygenation, respiratory muscle fatigue, and histological changes have all been described.[30] These may also contribute to the sensation of dyspnoea. Whether these abnormalities can explain the excessive ventilatory response to exercise seen frequently in CHF remains unknown. The relation between minute ventilation (VE) and CO_2 production (Vco_2) during progressive exercise—the VE/Vco_2 slope—is characteristically raised in patients with non-oedematous CHF (figs 6.3 and 6.4).[31] Possible causes include ventilation–perfusion mismatch within the lung causing excessive, but non-contributory ventilation,[32] along with enhanced sensitivity of ventilatory

control mechanisms described above. The ergoreflex system senses the metabolic state of exercising skeletal muscle and reflexly increases ventilation. It is sensed by small work sensitive afferents and carried by small myelinated or unmyelinated nerve fibres. An overactivity of these fibres and the resultant reflex responses have recently been described in CHF; it was also shown that the overactivity could be partially reduced by localised muscle training, highlighting the possible importance of muscle deconditioning in this abnormal response. The second overactive ventilatory control system in CHF is the chemoreceptor system. We have recently described augmentation of peripheral hypoxic and central CO_2 sensitivity in CHF patients.[33] These alterations could explain the heightened ventilatory responses and also lead to excessive sympathetic excitation. The cause of the heightened chemosensitivity itself remains undetermined, but it is possible that there is a direct interaction between the ergoreflex and chemoreflex systems.

Features of the CHF syndrome

The haemodynamic profile of patients limited by fatigue differs in no substantial measure from those patients limited predominantly by dyspnoea.[34] Ambulatory pulmonary arterial pressure monitoring has shown virtually no correlation between the haemodynamic disturbances and the symptoms noted by the patients at the time of the disturbance. No measure of haemodynamics (with the possible exception of measures of right ventricular performance) has demonstrated a convincing capacity to predict variations in exercise capacity between patients as well as do measures of peripheral function, such as skeletal muscle strength, endothelial function or ventilatory abnormalities. Whatever treatments are used (with a few exceptions in selected patients), there is a delay between haemodynamic effect and any objective change in exercise tolerance.[35] Treatments such as angiotensin converting enzyme (ACE) inhibitors and cardiac transplantation require weeks or months to improve exercise tolerance. The delay may be caused by the need to reverse some of the peripheral pathophysiological changes that have become the weakest link in the chain of oxygen delivery and utilisation necessary for muscular exercise. CHF is, we now realise, a systemic disorder with major neurohormonal,[36] cytokine, metabolic, and inflammatory consequences[37] that affect a myriad of organ systems in the body. The new treatments might come from any of these nontraditional targets for intervention for heart failure sufferers.

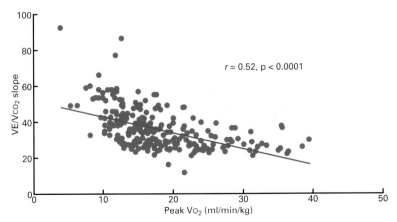

$r = 0.52, p < 0.0001$

Figure 6.4. Relation between the minute ventilation to carbon dioxide production slope and exercise capacity in 248 patients with chronic heart failure.

Exercise training in CHF

Exercise training in carefully selected patients with stable mild to moderate CHF can increase exercise capacity and lessen dyspnoea and fatigue.[38] These improvements have been seen mainly in peripheral pathophysiology, with no consistent effect on left ventricular ejection fraction, either beneficial or detrimental. Most of the beneficial effects seem to depend on training induced adaptations in the periphery, correcting many of the pathophysiological changes described above, and giving further credence to their original importance in mediating symptomatic exercise limitation.

Sullivan and colleagues demonstrated both an increased blood flow to exercising muscle and an increased ability of skeletal muscle to extract oxygen from the nutritive blood flow associated with improved symptoms and exercise tolerance. Ventilatory function was also improved, with a reduction in the respiratory exchange ratio at submaximal exercise and a delay in the anaerobic threshold.[39] The first controlled study was published soon after.[40] After baseline evaluation and familiarisation with laboratory procedures all patients performed eight weeks of exercise training and eight weeks of exercise avoidance in a randomised crossover study. The training regimen led to a 20–25% increase in exercise tolerance and peak oxygen consumption. There was also a significant reduction in questionnaire rated symptoms attributable to heart failure, and a coincident increase in both the extent and ease of performing daily activities. In a study involving 16 women with heart failure, Tyni-Lenne and colleagues[41] showed that eight weeks knee extensor endurance training could increase skeletal muscle citrate synthase activity by 44% (p < 0.0001) and lactate dehydrogenase activity by 23% (p < 0.002). There was an increase in oxidative capacity in relation to the glycolytic capacity of 23% (p < 0.002), showing plasticity of the skeletal muscle abnormalities described as accompanying CHF. In addition peak oxygen uptake increased 14% (p < 0.0005), peak work rate increased 43% (p < 0.0001), and physical (p < 0.05), psychosocial (p < 0.03), and overall (p < 0.01) health related quality of life improved.[41]

Hambrecht and colleagues showed biopsy derived skeletal muscle mitochondrial volume density increased significantly after training in CHF, a finding later shown to correlate well with the training induced improvement in exercise capacity.[42]

Wielanger and associates compared 41 trained and 39 control patients.[43] Training was supervised for 12 weeks. They showed "feelings of being disabled" decreased, while "self-assessment of general well-being" and exercise time increased (+21.4%, p < 0.0001), as did anaerobic threshold (+12.5%, p < 0.05).[43] A summary of trials performed by one collaborative European group[44] and an overview of all trials published to 1998[45] have both shown a consistent increase in exercise capacity across a broad range of heart failure patients of approximately 15–20%. Beneficial changes produced by training have included improvements in haemodynamic responses, myocardial perfusion, diastolic function, skeletal muscle function, histological and biochemical responses, ventilatory control, peri-

> **Symptoms of heart failure: key points**
>
> ● Symptoms are poorly correlated with resting haemodynamics in non-oedematous chronic heart failure (CHF)
>
> ● Fatigue relates to muscle changes in the periphery
>
> ● Dyspnoea in CHF is related to increased ventilation during exercise
>
> ● Ventilatory reflexes are exaggerated in CHF
>
> ● Blood gases remain near normal during exercise in stable CHF
>
> ● Training can improve symptoms in CHF mainly by correcting peripheral non-cardiac pathophysiological changes
>
> ● Conventional treatments—apart from diuretics—poorly control symptoms in CHF
>
> ● Endothelial dysfunction in CHF contributes to fatigue
>
> ● Muscle wasting is associated with a particularly poor prognosis in CHF

pheral vascular and endothelial function, and neurohormonal and autonomic improvements, further reinforcing the close correlation between the systemic pathophysiology of CHF and the symptoms limiting exercise.

Conclusions

In understanding the physiological basis of symptoms of patients with CHF, and in designing optimal strategies to improve these symptoms, we must now begin to unravel the complex physiological processes determining exercise capacity. It appears that the periphery, including muscle endothelium, the lung, and ventilatory control reflexes, play a central role in the factors limiting exercise, in contrast to the more haemodynamic basis of symptom generation in acute heart failure with pulmonary oedema. This introduces a new era in the treatment of heart failure in which antineurohormonal and metabolic[46] treatments might be of increasing importance as we target the pathophysiology limiting our CHF patients.

Professor Coats is supported by the Viscount Royston Trust, the British Heart Foundation, the Clinical Research Committee of the Royal Brompton Hospital, and the Asmarley Trust.

1. **Department of Health.** *National service framework for coronary heart disease.* Heart failure section. http://www.doh.gov.uk/coinh.htm

2. **Franciosa JA, Baker BJ, Seth L.** Pulmonary versus systemic hemodynamics in determining exercise capacity of patients with chronic left ventricular failure. *Am Heart J* 1985;**110**:807–13.

3. **Barletta G, Del Bene MR, Gallini C,** *et al.* The clinical impact of dynamic intraventricular obstruction during dobutamine stress echocardiography. *Int J Cardiol* 1999;**70**:179–89.

4. **Clark AL, Poole-Wilson PA, Coats AJ.** Exercise limitation in chronic heart failure: central role of the periphery. *J Am Coll Cardiol* 1996;**28**:1092–102.

5. **Clausen JP.** Circulatory adjustments to dynamic exercise and effect of physical training in normal subjects and in patients with coronary artery disease. *Prog Cardiovasc Dis* 1976;**18**:459–95.

6. **Jondeau G, Katz SD, Zohman L,** *et al.* Active skeletal muscle mass and cardiopulmonary reserve. Failure to attain peak aerobic capacity during maximal bicycle exercise in patients with severe congestive heart failure. *Circulation* 1992;**86**:1351–6.
- *This study demonstrated that exercise limitation in many heart failure patients is not primarily one of limited cardiac output because even at the point of exercise limitation the addition of more exercising muscle groups increases oxygen consumption and cardiac output further. The limiting factor must therefore reside locally within the exercising limb, being either vascular or muscular in origin.*

7. **Florea VG, Mareyev VY, Achilov AA,** *et al.* Central and peripheral components of chronic heart failure: determinants of exercise tolerance. *Int J Cardiol* 1999;**70**:51–6.

8. **Drexler H, Riede U, Münzel T,** *et al.* Alterations of skeletal muscle in chronic heart failure. *Circulation* 1992;**85**:1751–9.
- *This study showed that there are major ultrastructural changes within the skeletal muscle of patients with chronic heart failure.*

9. **Zelis R, Nellis SH, Longhurst J,** *et al.* Abnormalities in the regional circulations accompanying congestive heart failure. *Prog Cardiovasc Dis* 1975;**18**:181–99.

10. **Clini E, Volterrani M, Pagani M,** *et al.* Endogenous nitric oxide in patients with chronic heart failure (CHF): relation to functional impairment and nitrate-containing therapies. *Int J Cardiol* 2000;**73**:123–30.

11. **Chua TP, Coats AJ.** The lungs in chronic heart failure. *Eur Heart J* 1995;**16**:882–7.
- *Review of major lung and reflex ventilatory control abnormalities in chronic heart failure.*

12. **Volterrani M, Clark AL, Ludman PF,** *et al.* Determinants of exercise capacity in chronic heart failure. *Eur Heart J* 1994;**15**:801–9.

13. **Sullivan MJ, Green HJ, Cobb FR.** Skeletal muscle biochemistry and histology in ambulatory patients with long-term heart failure. *Circulation* 1990;**81**:518–27.

14. **Massie BM, Conway M, Rajagopalan B,** *et al.* Skeletal muscle metabolism during exercise under ischemic conditions in congestive heart failure. Evidence for abnormalities unrelated to blood flow. *Circulation* 1988;**78**:320–6.
- *Important early evidence for an intrinsic metabolic defect in skeletal muscle in heart failure unrelated to abnormalities in muscle blood flow.*

15. **Adamopoulos S, Coats AJ, Brunotte F,** *et al.* Physical training improves skeletal muscle metabolism in patients with chronic heart failure. *J Am Coll Cardiol* 1993;**21**:1101–6.

16. **Vescovo G, Serafini F, Facchin L,** *et al.* Specific changes in skeletal muscle myosin heavy chain composition in cardiac failure: differences compared with disuse atrophy as assessed on microbiopsies by high resolution electrophoresis. *Heart* 1996;**76**:337–43.

17. **Anker SD, Chua TP, Ponikowski P,** *et al.* Hormonal changes and catabolic/anabolic imbalance in chronic heart failure and their importance for cardiac cachexia. *Circulation* 1997;**96**:526–34.
- *This article clearly demonstrated that the major neurohormonal and anabolic and catabolic abnormalities of chronic heart failure are primarily features of the subset of patients with significant weight loss (cachexia).*

18. **Anker SD, Clark AL, Kemp M,** *et al.* Tumor necrosis factor and steroid metabolism in chronic heart failure: possible relation to muscle wasting. *J Am Coll Cardiol* 1997;**30**:997–1001.

19. **Niebauer J, Pflaum CD, Clark AL,** *et al.* Deficient insulin-like growth factor I in chronic heart failure predicts altered body composition, anabolic deficiency, cytokine and neurohormonal activation. *J Am Coll Cardiol* 1998;**32**:393–7.

20. **Swan JW, Walton C, Godsland IF,** *et al.* Insulin resistance in chronic heart failure. *Eur Heart J* 1994;**15**:1528–32.

21. **Anker SD, Ponikowski P, Varney S,** *et al.* Wasting as independent risk factor for mortality in chronic heart failure. *Lancet* 1997;**349**:1050–3.

22. **Chua TP, Clark AL, Amadi AA,** *et al.* Relation between chemosensitivity and the ventilatory response to exercise in chronic heart failure. *J Am Coll Cardiol* 1996;**27**:650–7.

23. **Piepoli M, Clark AL, Volterrani M,** *et al.* Contribution of muscle afferents to the hemodynamic, autonomic, and ventilatory responses to exercise in patients with chronic heart failure: effects of physical training. *Circulation* 1996;**93**:940–52.
- *Study showing the importance of the skeletal muscle ergoreceptors in mediating the increased ventilatory response to exercise in CHF and demonstrating that training can partially reverse this abnormality. This gives an explanation as to why training can reduce ventilation with little if any effect of central haemodynamic function in heart failure patients.*

24. **Grieve DA, Clark AL, McCann GP,** *et al.* The ergoreflex in patients with chronic stable heart failure. *Int J Cardiol* 1999;**68**:157–64.

25. **Ponikowski P, Francis DP, Piepoli MF,** *et al.* Enhanced ventilatory response to exercise in patients with chronic heart failure and preserved exercise tolerance: marker of abnormal cardiorespiratory reflex control and predictor of poor prognosis. *Circulation* 2001;**103**:967–72.

26. **Bol E, de Vries WR, Mosterd WL,** *et al.* Cardiopulmonary exercise parameters in relation to all-cause mortality in patients with chronic heart failure. *Int J Cardiol* 2000;**72**:255–63.

27. **Juilliere Y, Grentzinger A, Houplon P,** *et al.* Role of the etiology of cardiomyopathies on exercise capacity and oxygen consumption in patients with severe congestive heart failure. *Int J Cardiol* 2000;**73**:251–5.

28. **Morales FJ, Montemayor T, Martinez A.** Shuttle versus six-minute walk test in the prediction of outcome in chronic heart failure. *Int J Cardiol* 2000;**76**:101–5.

29. **Francis DP, Shamim W, Davies LC,** *et al.* Cardiopulmonary exercise testing for prognosis in chronic heart failure: continuous and independent prognostic value from VE/VCO$_2$ slope and peak VO$_2$. *Eur Heart J* 2000;**21**:154–61.

30. **Mancini DM, Henson D, LaManca J,** *et al.* Evidence of reduced respiratory muscle endurance in patients with heart failure. *J Am Coll Cardiol* 1994;**24**:972–81.

31. **Chua TP, Ponikowski P, Harrington D,** *et al.* Clinical correlates and prognostic significance of the ventilatory response to exercise in chronic heart failure. *J Am Coll Cardiol* 1997;**29**:1585–90.

32. **Sullivan MJ, Higginbotham MB, Cobb FR.** Increased exercise ventilation in patients with chronic heart failure: intact ventilatory control despite hemodynamic and pulmonary abnormalities. *Circulation* 1988;**77**:552–9.

33. **Chua TP, Ponikowski PP, Harrington D,** *et al.* Contribution of peripheral chemoreceptors to ventilation and the effects of their suppression on exercise tolerance in chronic heart failure. *Heart* 1996;**76**:483–9.

34. **Clark AL, Sparrow JL, Coats AJS.** Muscle fatigue and dyspnoea in chronic heart failure: two sides of the same coin? *Eur Heart J* 1995;**16**:49–52.

35. **Drexler H, Banhardt U, Meinertz T,** *et al.* Contrasting peripheral short-term and long-term effects of converting enzyme inhibition in patients with congestive heart failure. A double-blind, placebo-controlled trial. *Circulation* 1989;**79**:491–502.

36. **Coats AJ.** Inflammation, hormones, the blood and the heart; are cardiologists learning to be internists again? *Int J Cardiol* 2000;**72**:203–5.

37. **Sharma R, Coats AJ, Anker SD.** The role of inflammatory mediators in chronic heart failure: cytokines, nitric oxide, and endothelin-1. *Int J Cardiol* 2000;**72**:175–86.

38. **Coats AJS, Adamopoulos S, Radaelli A,** *et al.* Controlled trial of physical training in chronic heart failure: exercise performance, hemodynamics, ventilation and autonomic function. *Circulation* 1992;**85**:2119–31.
- *First controlled trial of exercise training in CHF demonstrating a variety of non-cardiac benefits.*

39. **Sullivan MJ, Higginbotham MB, Cobb FR.** Exercise training in patients with severe left ventricular dysfunction: hemodynamic and metabolic effects. *Circulation* 1988;**78**:506–15.

40. **Coats AJS, Adamopoulos S, Meyer TE,** *et al.* Effects of physical training in chronic heart failure. *Lancet* 1990;**335**:63–6.

41. **Tyni-Lenne R, Gordon A, Jansson E,** *et al.* Skeletal muscle endurance training improves peripheral oxidative capacity, exercise tolerance, and health-related quality of life in women with chronic congestive heart failure secondary to either ischemic cardiomyopathy or idiopathic dilated cardiomyopathy. *Am J Cardiol* 1997;**80**:1025–9.

42. **Hambrecht R, Niebauer J, Fiehn E,** *et al.* Physical training in patients with stable chronic heart failure: effects on cardiorespiratory fitness and ultrastructural abnormalities of leg muscles. *J Am Coll Cardiol* 1995;**25**:1239–49.

43. **Wielenga RP, Erdman RA, Huisveld IA,** *et al.* Effect of exercise training on quality of life in patients with chronic heart failure. *J Psychosom Res* 1998;**45**:459–64.

44. **European Heart Failure Training Group.** Experience from controlled trials of physical training in chronic heart failure: protocol and patient factors in effectiveness in the improvement in exercise tolerance. *Eur Heart J* 1998;**19**:466–75.

45. **Piepoli MF, Capucci A.** Exercise training in heart failure: effect on morbidity and mortality. *Int J Cardiol* 2000;**73**:3–6.

46. **Harrington D, Chua TP, Coats AJ.** The effect of salbutamol on skeletal muscle in chronic heart failure. *Int J Cardiol* 2000;**73**:257–65.

SECTION III: CARDIOMYOPATHY

7 Differential diagnosis of restrictive cardiomyopathy and constrictive pericarditis

E William Hancock

Varieties of constrictive pericarditis
- Typical forms
  - chronic (calcific, rigid shell)
  - subacute (non-calcific, elastic)
- Effusive-constrictive
- Localised
- Occult

The differentiation of restrictive cardiomyopathy and constrictive pericarditis has been a perennial problem in clinical cardiology. Constrictive pericarditis requires surgical treatment and is usually curable, while restrictive cardiomyopathy, short of cardiac transplantation, is treatable only by medical means and often responds unsatisfactorily. The opinion has often been expressed that there are difficult cases in which only an exploratory operation will allow the two conditions to be distinguished. However, such cases were relatively rare in the past and should be extremely so in the present era. Many differences exist between the two conditions, even though no one diagnostic method can be relied upon to make the distinction by itself.

Constrictive pericarditis

Constrictive pericarditis was recognised in the 19th century and its surgical treatment was developed early in the 20th century. Paul Wood noted in 1961 that only details had been added to the picture presented to the English speaking world by Paul Dudley White in his 1935 St Cyres lecture.[1 2] White described a "chronic fibrous or callous thickening of the wall of the pericardial sac that is so contracted that the normal diastolic filling of the heart is prevented . . . There may or may not be calcification . . . Parietal pericardium or epicardium may be preponderantly involved . . . one area may be involved, other areas free . . . associated heart disease is extremely rare . . . insidious evolution makes diagnosis more difficult than that of active constrictive pericarditis". A history of several years duration and a predominant clinical feature of ascites, simulating liver disease, were notable in White's series.

Haemodynamic features delineated in the 1940s and '50s included the narrow pulse pressure in the right ventricle with normal systolic pressure and greatly increased diastolic pressure, a prominent early diastolic dip and later diastolic plateau in right ventricular pressure waveforms, and an additional prominent systolic dip in the right atrial waveform, giving a "W" atrial waveform. Comments on the difficulty of distinguishing constrictive pericarditis from restrictive cardiomyopathy began to appear in the medical literature only after the pressure recordings from cardiac catheterisation began to be used in the diagnosis of constrictive pericarditis. One may suspect that cardiac catheterisation data in the two conditions were more similar than the clinical features.

Since 1960 the clinical profile of constrictive pericarditis has changed greatly. Tuberculous aetiology has become rare in developed countries, while new aetiologies have appeared. Two of them, previous cardiac surgery and previous radiotherapy, are now responsible for up to one third of cases in some centres.[3] The term "chronic" is often no longer included in the title, because so many cases are now more appropriately considered to be acute or subacute. Subacute constrictive pericarditis differs in several respects from the chronic cases, as Paul Wood noted in his delineation of the differences between active and inactive tuberculous constrictive pericarditis. A distinction between elastic (subacute) and rigid shell (chronic) constriction has been proposed to help to rationalise these differences[4] (table 7.1). Other additions to the clinical profile include the recognition of effusive–constrictive pericarditis,[5] occult constriction,[6] localised constriction,[7] and reversible constriction.[8] These variant forms of constrictive pericarditis each have some features that differ from the classic chronic constrictive pericarditis of the past (table 7.2).

Restrictive cardiomyopathy

As the haemodynamics of constrictive pericarditis became known in the 1940s and '50s it quickly became apparent that amyloid and other forms of myocardial or endocardial disease could have similar haemodynamic features. At the same time, the concept of idiopathic cardiomyopathy was evolving, leading to Goodwin's 1961 classification into three

Table 7.1 Comparison of certain features in subacute (elastic) and chronic (rigid shell) constrictive pericarditis

Subacute (elastic)	Chronic (rigid shell)
Paradoxical pulse usually present, other signs of interdependence usually prominent	Paradoxical pulse usually minimal or absent, other signs of interdependence less prominent
Usually an XY waveform ("M" or "W" waveform)	Y is predominant, X sometimes minimal
Dip–plateau pattern less conspicuous, because early diastolic nadir may not approach zero	Dip–plateau usually conspicuous, because early diastolic nadir often reaches zero
Calcification usually absent	Calcification often present
Pericardial effusion sometimes present, generalised or loculated. Constriction is by the visceral pericardium	Pericardial effusion absent. The two layers of pericardium are fused, and jointly constrict the heart
P waves usually normal	P waves often wide, notched and low in amplitude
Atrial fibrillation or flutter rare	Atrial fibrillation or flutter common

Major forms of restrictive cardiomyopathy

- Amyloid

- Other infiltrative diseases

- Endomyocardial fibrosis

- Idiopathic restrictive cardiomyopathy

Table 7.2   Features of variant forms of constrictive pericarditis

Effusive–constrictive pericarditis	Pericardial effusion is present, sometimes loculated, with constriction by the visceral pericardium
Occult constrictive pericarditis	Haemodynamics are normal at rest, but assume the features of constriction after an acute volume load
Localised constrictive pericarditis	Constriction limited to the right or left ventricle. Ventricular interdependence reduced or absent
Transient constrictive pericarditis	During the resolution of acute pericarditis with effusion, constriction develops, but then resolves spontaneously over a few weeks

types.[9] The hypertrophic and dilated forms quickly became well known, but the third type, "constrictive cardiomyopathy" (later renamed "restrictive cardiomyopathy"), defined as congestive heart failure with neither hypertrophy nor dilatation, was less common and received less attention. The definition of restrictive cardiomyopathy has varied considerably, and the term has usually been used in a broad sense, to include such entities as amyloidosis, tropical endomyocardial fibrosis, endocardial fibroelastosis, haemochromatosis, and eosinophilic endomyocardial disease, as well as the idiopathic cases. Idiopathic restrictive cardiomyopathy, strictly defined to include normal ventricular wall motion as well as normal wall thickness and ventricular chamber dimensions, proved to be relatively rare. Such a strict definition can be carried a step further by defining restrictive cardiomyopathy as those patients who cannot be differentiated from constrictive pericarditis by means of physical examination, chest radiograph, and cardiac catheterisation.[10] No large series of patients with such a condition have been described.

On the other hand, the concept of diastolic heart failure, or diastolic dysfunction, has received a great deal of attention in the past 20 years.[11] When the definition is broadened to permit what is considered to be a lesser degree of systolic dysfunction associated with predominant diastolic dysfunction, diastolic heart failure becomes very common, and perhaps includes about one half of all cases of congestive heart failure. It is particularly common in elderly patients. Such patients may be referred to as having restrictive cardiomyopathy, even though it appears likely that hypertension and increased arterial stiffness are background factors in many of them.[12]

Whatever definition of restrictive cardiomyopathy is used, it is clear that patients who simulate constrictive pericarditis are relatively rare, and that cardiac amyloidosis is the most frequent diagnosis among them. The others have miscellaneous diagnoses, with a small number representing an idiopathic restrictive cardiomyopathy.

Differentiating features

Table 7.3 lists 17 features, obtained by eight different clinical methods, that provide useful

Table 7.3   Features useful in differentiating constrictive pericarditis from restrictive cardiomyopathy

Feature	Constrictive pericarditis	Restrictive cardiomyopathy
Past medical history	Previous pericarditis, cardiac surgery, trauma, radiotherapy, connective tissue disease	These items rare
Jugular venous waveform	X and Y dips brief and "flicking", not conspicuous positive waves	X and Y dips less brief, may have conspicuous A wave or V wave
Extra sounds in diastole	Early S3, high pitched "pericardial knock". No S4	Later S3, low pitched, "triple rhythm". S4 in some cases
Mitral or tricuspid regurgitation	Usually absent	Often present
ECG	P waves reflect intra-atrial conduction delay. Atrioventricular or intraventricular conduction defects rare	P waves reflect right or left atrial hypertrophy or overload. Atrioventricular or intraventricular conduction defects not unusual
Plain chest radiograph	Pericardial calcification in 20–30%	Pericardial calcification rare
Ventricular septal movement in diastole	Abrupt septal movement ("notch") in early diastole in most cases	Abrupt septal movement in early diastole seen only occasionally
Ventricular septal movement with respiration	Notable movement toward left ventricle in inspiration usually seen	Relatively little movement toward left ventricle in most cases
Atrial enlargement	Slight or moderate in most cases	Pronounced in most cases
Respiratory variation in mitral and tricuspid flow velocity	Greater than 25% in most cases	Less than 15% in most cases
Equilibration of diastolic pressures in all cardiac chambers	Within 5 mm Hg in nearly all cases, often essentially the same	Within 5 mm Hg in a small proportion of cases
Dip–plateau waveform in the right ventricular pressure waveform	End diastolic pressure more than one third of systolic pressure in many cases	End diastolic pressure often less than one third of systolic pressure
Peak right ventricular systolic pressure	Nearly always less than 60 mm Hg, often less than 40 mm Hg	Frequently more than 40 and occasionally more than 60 mm Hg
Discordant respiratory variation of ventricular peak systolic pressures	Right and left ventricular peak systolic pressure variations are out-of-phase	Right and left ventricular peak systolic pressure variations are in-phase
Paradoxical pulse	Often present to a moderate degree	Rarely present
MR/CT imaging	Shows thick pericardium in most cases	Shows thick pericardium only rarely
Endomyocardial biopsy	Normal, or non-specific abnormalities	Shows amyloid in some cases, rarely other specific infiltrative disease

clues in differentiating constrictive pericarditis and restrictive cardiomyopathy. The length of the list indicates that no one or two of the features have sufficient sensitivity and specificity to be decisive in all cases. More items could be included, but the list would then become even more unwieldy. The items listed have been selected for having reasonable sensitivity and specificity, and for the most part of being readily and reliably ascertained.

Past medical history
Although many cases of constrictive pericarditis are idiopathic, some have a history of definite or possible acute pericarditis in the past. Factors such as previous cardiac surgery, radiotherapy, connective tissue disease, and thoracic trauma may be the background for the development of constrictive pericarditis, and none of these factors are expected in the past medical history of patients with restrictive cardiomyopathy.

Jugular venous waveform
The typical jugular venous pulse in constrictive pericarditis has two dips per cardiac cycle: the outward movements are less conspicuous. The two dips are the X and Y troughs, in systole and early diastole, respectively. Y is sometimes more prominent than X, especially in chronic (rigid shell) cases, many of whom have atrial fibrillation, a factor that minimises the systolic descent. These features are also common in restrictive cardiomyopathy. What distinguishes constrictive pericarditis is the brief duration of Y, giving a "flicking" appearance in an otherwise continuously distended vein. This is the essential feature of Friedreich's sign, considered by Paul Wood to be the most characteristic physical sign of constrictive pericarditis. Subacute (elastic) cases are more likely to have comparable X and Y dips, giving a "W" or "M" contour, or even a dominant X descent, as in cardiac tamponade. Patients with restrictive cardiomyopathy sometimes have waveforms with conspicuous outward pulsations, caused by large A waves, or obvious tricuspid regurgitation, patterns not seen in constrictive pericarditis.

Examination of the jugular venous pulse is not completely superseded by recording the atrial pressure waveforms at cardiac catheterisation. The jugular veins exhibit dynamic volume changes, which can be more conspicuous than pressure changes in the relatively low pressure atrial–venous system.

Early diastolic sounds
Extra heart sounds in the early diastolic filling period occur in both constrictive pericarditis and in restrictive cardiomyopathy, but can be suspected of being one or the other of two types by the practised auscultator. In restrictive cardiomyopathy, especially when tricuspid regurgitation is prominent, an S3 frequently occurs, falling approximately 0.12–0.18 s after S2, and demonstrating a "thudding" low pitched character. Such sounds result in a "triple rhythm" effect, that needs deciphering as to which members of the trio are S1, S2, and S3.

In constrictive pericarditis an earlier filling sound occurs, usually 0.06–0.12 s after S2, and somewhat high pitched and "snapping" in character. The auscultatory impression tends to be that of a widely split S2 or a mitral opening snap. The term "pericardial knock," although commonly used, is not particularly appropriate. The sound does not resemble a knock on a door, and is not caused by the calcified heart knocking against the chest wall, as students sometimes misconceive.

Late diastolic sounds
Some patients with restrictive cardiomyopathy have S4, resulting from a powerful atrial contraction in response to the increased resistance to ventricular filling. S4 does not occur in constrictive pericarditis, despite similar degrees of resistance to filling, probably because the fibrotic constricting process impairs the atrial contraction.

Mitral/tricuspid regurgitation
The physical examination is also helpful when it indicates pronounced mitral or tricuspid regurgitation. Echo Doppler and cardiac catheterisation are part of this assessment. Mitral and tricuspid regurgitation are rarely prominent in constrictive pericarditis, but are often prominent in restrictive cardiomyopathy.

Electrocardiogram
The P waves in constrictive pericarditis tend to be wide and notched, but low in amplitude, reflecting intra-atrial conduction delay. This is seen in chronic cases more often than in the subacute cases. In restrictive cardiomyopathy the P waves may be wide, but have a particular tendency to be increased in amplitude, reflecting left atrial overload or hypertrophy, as in hypertension or aortic valve disease. The difference probably reflects the invasion of atrial myocardium by fibrosis in constrictive pericarditis. Also, the raised atrial and ventricular diastolic pressure causes less stretch of atrial myofibrils in constrictive pericarditis than in restrictive cardiomyopathy, because of the external compression by the pericardium.

Conduction defects, both atrioventricular and intraventricular, are more often features of restrictive cardiomyopathy than they are of constrictive pericarditis. Bundle branch block occurs in perhaps 20–30% of patients with restrictive cardiomyopathy and is rare in constrictive pericarditis. Low voltage is not critically helpful; it is less common in constrictive pericarditis than it is in cardiac tamponade, and it does occur in some instances of restrictive cardiomyopathy, especially those with amyloid. Left ventricular hypertrophy, however, would be an important factor favouring restrictive cardiomyopathy. Amyloid is notable for showing Q waves simulating infarct in some cases, but this can also occur in constrictive pericarditis, probably on the basis of fibrosis invading the myocardium.

Plain chest radiograph
Pericardial calcification seen in the plain chest radiograph is highly specific for constrictive

pericarditis, in the context of a differential diagnosis between constrictive pericarditis and restrictive cardiomyopathy. Calcification is usually absent in subacute constrictive pericarditis, and is therefore less frequent overall than it was in the past. However, it still occurs in approximately a quarter of cases.[13] It is unclear whether more sensitive methods, such as electron beam computed tomography (CT) or cine fluoroscopy will show pericardial calcification in a higher proportion of patients with constrictive pericarditis, while retaining a similarly high specificity.

Echocardiographic imaging

Echocardiography will have been carried out by the time that a differential diagnosis between constrictive pericarditis and restrictive cardiomyopathy is formulated, because the problem applies only to patients who show normal ventricular chamber dimensions and systolic wall motion. Three further clues from standard echocardiography are particularly important.

The septal notch

In constrictive pericarditis the rate of filling is rapid in early diastole, and the rate of change in ventricular pressure at this time in the cycle is particularly rapid. Slight asymmetry of right and left ventricular filling rate can result in rapid changes in the pressure differential between the two sides of the ventricular septum. The septum may therefore shift in position very abruptly, responding to such rapid changes in pressure. The abnormal septal motion may take several forms, and does not necessarily fit the definition of a "notch".

Ventricular septal shift with respiration

Reciprocal changes in left and right ventricular volumes with respiration are one aspect of the increased degree of ventricular interdependence that is characteristic of constrictive pericarditis. Because the heart is enclosed within a relatively fixed volume, enlargement of one ventricle tends to be associated with a corresponding decrease in volume of the other ventricle. This contrasts with the non-constricted heart, in which enlargement of one ventricle can be associated with a corresponding increase in volume of the two ventricles combined. The volume of the right ventricle increases in inspiration, both normally and in constrictive pericarditis, as a result of lowered intrathoracic pressure drawing in a greater venous return. This aspect of ventricular interdependence is best seen in the two dimensional echocardiogram as a movement of the ventricular septum toward the left ventricle with inspiration and toward the right ventricle in expiration.

Atrial enlargement

Major enlargement of the right and left atrium is a hallmark of restrictive cardiomyopathy. This occurs in response to pronounced chronic elevation of atrial pressure, and is enhanced by mitral and tricuspid regurgitation. Some enlargement of the atria often occurs in constrictive pericarditis, in which the same sustained elevation of atrial pressure is present, but it is rare to see the major enlargement that is characteristic of restrictive cardiomyopathy. Presence of the constricting process around the atria appears to account for this difference.

Thickening of the pericardium in the echocardiogram is a second line feature in differentiating constrictive pericarditis and restrictive cardiomyopathy. The limited resolution of echocardiography lowers the specificity of this finding, although it is sometimes notable in patients with constrictive pericarditis. Transoesophageal echocardiography gives better resolution than the conventional transthoracic study, but chest CT or magnetic resonance imaging (MRI) have better specificity.

Doppler ultrasound studies

Doppler ultrasonic studies for differentiating constrictive pericarditis and restrictive cardiomyopathy were introduced in the late 1980s and have proven considerably valuable.[14 15] In constrictive pericarditis there is an exaggerated variation in the velocity of early diastolic filling of the two ventricles with respiration. The variation is reciprocal, the tricuspid velocity increasing in inspiration and the mitral velocity decreasing. The reciprocal ventricular variation reflects ventricular interdependence, and occurs to a much lesser degree in restrictive cardiomyopathy. It is usually prominent in subacute constriction and less prominent or absent in chronic (rigid shell) cases. It appears that in the chronic (rigid shell) cases the variations in intrathoracic pressure are not transmitted to the interior of the heart.

Further Doppler methods have been added, including the assessment of respiratory variation in pulmonary venous flow velocity, and the study of mitral annular movement ("tissue Doppler").[16] The place of the newer Doppler methods in differential diagnosis remains to be determined.

The sensitivity and specificity of the Doppler respiratory method may be as high as 85–90% in expert hands. However, the studies are difficult to carry out and to interpret. They should ideally incorporate a simultaneous graphic record of the phases of respiration. Irregular patterns of breathing, irregular cardiac rhythm, and short diastolic periods resulting from rapid heart rate cause difficulty in interpretation. Falsely positive results can be seen when intrathoracic pressure variations are exaggerated, as in asthma or chronic obstructive airway disease; in such conditions the flow velocity in the superior vena cava should be recorded, because the superior vena cava has much larger respiratory variation in flow velocity with respiration in pulmonary disease than it does in either constrictive pericarditis or restrictive cardiomyopathy.

Cardiac catheterisation

Cardiac catheterisation studies have perhaps received too much emphasis in the differential diagnosis between constrictive pericarditis and restrictive cardiomyopathy.[17] Indeed, the diagnostic dilemma may almost be defined as existing when the cardiac catheterisation results do not distinguish the two. However, a carefully conducted haemodynamic study is likely to yield important clues.

Equilibration of diastolic pressures
Nearly equal levels of diastolic pressure in all chambers of the heart are a hallmark of constrictive pericarditis, and reflect the usually symmetrical pathological process around the entire heart. Somewhat greater elevation of pressure on the left side than the right is more characteristic of restrictive cardiomyopathy. Comparison of instantaneous end diastolic pressure in the two ventricles is perhaps the most critical way to evaluate this, but in practice a comparison of the mean pressures in the right atrium and the left atrium (or the pulmonary artery wedge position) may be more reliable, because such recordings are less subject to troublesome artefacts. A discrepancy of more than 5 mm Hg is very unusual in constrictive pericarditis, but can be seen when the constriction is relatively or totally localised. The discrepancy is more than 5 mm Hg in many cases with restrictive cardiomyopathy that otherwise resemble constrictive pericarditis rather closely.

Dip–plateau waveform
The dip–plateau, or square root-like, waveform in the right ventricular pressure waveform is a classic hallmark of constrictive pericarditis, but is also the feature of restrictive cardiomyopathy that most commonly simulates constriction. The dip–plateau is most prominent in chronic (rigid shell) cases, where there is initially no limitation of filling and the ventricular diastolic pressure approaches zero before beginning its rapid rise to the elevated plateau level. In the subacute (elastic) constrictive cases, now more common, there is some limitation of filling even in beginning diastole, and the nadir does not approach zero.

Commonly used catheters that are soft, small in calibre, and connected to the transducers by long, fluid filled connectors produce distorted waveforms in right ventricular pressure recordings that obscure the differences in the dip–plateau waveform that occur in constrictive pericarditis and restrictive cardiomyopathy.

Discordant peak systolic pressure variation
Another aspect of ventricular interdependence, characteristic of constrictive pericarditis in contrast to restrictive cardiomyopathy, is the discordant variation of right and left ventricular peak systolic pressure levels with respiration.[18] In restrictive cardiomyopathy the two pressures vary together, while in constrictive pericarditis they vary out-of-phase with one another. Right ventricular peak systolic pressure rises with the onset of inspiration, while the peak pressure falls in the left ventricle. This is a simple observation to make during cardiac catheterisation, but it may not be looked for, most frequently because there is an emphasis on assessing the similarity of diastolic pressures in the two ventricles and the pressure recorder is set at a sensitive calibration that leaves the systolic peaks above the top of the scale. Such recordings must minimise artefacts to be accurately interpreted, and a graphic recording of respiration is also useful.

Paradoxical pulse
Paradoxical pulse is not often mentioned as a distinguishing feature between constrictive pericarditis and restrictive cardiomyopathy. Indeed, some authors state that paradoxical pulse is not a feature of uncomplicated constrictive pericarditis, and some state that it does occur in restrictive cardiomyopathy. Both statements are doubtful. Paradoxical pulse is indeed minimal or absent in the classic chronic (rigid shell) constrictive pericarditis that typified the condition in years past. In the subacute (elastic) cases that are more often seen currently, a moderate paradoxical pulse is often present. This may occur with or without the presence of some pericardial effusion. The respiratory variation is readily seen in direct arterial pressure recordings during cardiac catheterisation, although it is not as pronounced as that typically seen in cardiac tamponade and is often not readily detected by bedside examination. The respiratory variation in restrictive cardiomyopathy is rarely enough to raise a suspicion of constrictive pericarditis, particularly if cases of cor pulmonale are correctly recognised. Since paradoxical pulse is an exaggerated degree of a normal phenomenon, its definition is arbitrary, and it should be treated as a continuous variable, not a categorical one.

Magnetic resonance and computed tomographic imaging
CT and MRI of the thorax have been used since the early 1980s as an improved method of evaluating abnormal thickening of the pericardium. Most cases of constrictive pericarditis do indeed show an apparent pericardial thickness of 3 mm or more, at least in some areas.[19] CT and MRI often appear to show only focal areas of pericardial thickening in cases where the constriction is present around the entire heart. Surgeons often note variable degrees of pericardial thickness in different areas, that do not necessarily correspond to differences in the degree of constriction. It is perhaps insufficiently realised, however, that some patients have constriction with relatively small degrees of thickening. The normal pericardium is less than 1.0 mm thick; a considerable increase may not exceed the threshold of abnormality in a CT or MRI. Indeed, the constricting pericardium can be visually unimpressive, or even appear normal at first glance to the surgeon at the time of operation. Some cases of occult constriction appear to have anatomically normal visceral and parietal pericardium. Thus, the principal limitation of CT and MRI is the occurrence of falsely negative studies. In addition, the finding of thickened pericardium does not necessarily indicate that constriction is present.

CT and MRI have approximately equal value in demonstrating thickening of the pericardium. CT is therefore preferable in

Points frequently helpful in favouring constrictive pericarditis over restrictive cardiomyopathy

- History—active pericarditis

- Examination—Freidreich's sign, paradoxical pulse

- ECG—absence of intraventricular conduction defect

- Chest radiograph—pericardial calcification

- CT/MRI—thickened pericardium

- Echocardiogram—septal notch

- Doppler—ventricular interdependence

- Cardiac catheterisation—close equilibration of diastolic pressures

- Biopsy—absence of amyloid or other infiltrative disease

most cases, with MRI usually reserved for patients with an intolerance of iodinated contrast agent. CT is analogous to a single "snapshot", while MRI represents the average of many heart beats, gated to the cardiac cycle; for this reason, neither method is well adapted to assessing the variations in chamber volumes with respiration.

Endomyocardial biopsy

Endomyocardial biopsy is a nearly certain method of diagnosing cardiac amyloidosis. Therefore, the form of restrictive cardiomyopathy that is the most frequent simulator of constrictive pericarditis should be diagnosable without exploratory thoracotomy, if the diagnosis is considered as a possibility preoperatively. Some other entities such as haemochromatosis and eosinophilic cardiomyopathy can also be diagnosed at biopsy. Cases of idiopathic restrictive cardiomyopathy, however, have only non-specific abnormalities in the endomyocardial biopsy, and such abnormalities may also be found in some cases of essentially uncomplicated constrictive pericarditis. The biopsy is therefore helpful chiefly if it shows a specific infiltrative disease.[20]

Conclusions

Many new diagnostic methods have been introduced since the earliest proposals that only exploratory thoracotomy will differentiate constrictive pericarditis and restrictive cardiomyopathy in all cases. It seems that exploratory thoracotomy should be needed very rarely if ever in the current era. However, a major pitfall is to expect that only one or two diagnostic methods can be regularly decisive in making the differential diagnosis. The apparent urge to rely on one or two methods, to the relative neglect of other methods, may be a disadvantage resulting from the current tendency to

divide cardiology into subspecialities based on the use of specific technologies. A broad clinical viewpoint, in which the results of many diagnostic methods are synthesised, is necessary to achieve the optimal differential diagnosis.

1. **White PD.** Chronic constrictive pericarditis (Pick's disease) treated by pericardial resection. *Lancet* 1935;ii:539–48, 597–603.
- *St Cyres lecture, National Heart Hospital, London, 10 July 1935. Historical review and analysis of 15 cases operated upon at the Massachusetts General Hospital since 1929, defining the disease and its treatment for the English speaking countries. Notable for the great chronicity of the cases and the predominant presentation with ascites.*

2. **Wood P.** Chronic constrictive pericarditis. *Am J Cardiol* 1961;**7**:48–61.
- *Analysis of 40 patients, mostly tuberculous, emphasising clinical differences between active and inactive cases. Long list of features differentiating constrictive pericarditis from restrictive cardiomyopathy, before the introduction of echocardiography, Doppler or CT/MRI.*

3. **Ling LH, Oh JK, Schaff HV,** *et al.* Constrictive pericarditis in the modern era: evolving clinical spectrum and impact on outcome after pericardiectomy. *Circulation* 1999;**100**:1380–6.
- *In 135 patients with constrictive pericarditis seen during 1985 to 1995, the aetiology was previous cardiac surgery in 18%, and radiotherapy in 13%. There was only one proven tuberculous case. Emphasises the role of older age and radiotherapy aetiology in increasing operative mortality and reducing the quality of long term results.*

4. **Hancock EW.** On the elastic and rigid forms of constrictive pericarditis. *Am Heart J* 1980;**100**:917–23.

5. **Hancock EW.** Subacute effusive-constrictive pericarditis. *Circulation* 1971;**43**:183–92.

6. **Bush CA, Stang JM, Wooley CF,** *et al.* Occult constrictive pericardial disease. Diagnosis by rapid volume expansion and correction by pericardiectomy. *Circulation* 1977;**56**:924–30.

7. **Hasuda T, Satoh T, Yamada N,** *et al.* A case of constrictive pericarditis with local thickening of the pericardium without manifest ventricular interdependence. *Cardiology* 1999;**92**:214–6.

8. **Sagrista-Sauleda J G, Permanyer-Miralda G, Caudell-Riera J,** *et al.* Transient cardiac constriction: an unrecognized pattern of evolution in effusive acute idiopathic pericarditis. *Am J Cardiol* 1987;**59**:961–6.
- *In 16 of 177 patients with acute pericarditis with effusion, signs of constriction developed in the next 5–30 days, but resolved within the next few months. The constriction was mostly mild and detected only on careful clinical and haemodynamic evaluation.*

9. **Goodwin JF, Gordon H, Hollman A,** *et al.* Clinical aspects of cardiomyopathy. *BMJ* 1961;i:69–79.

10. **Shabetai R.** Controversial issues in restrictive cardiomyopathy. *Postgrad Med J* 1992;**68**:S47–51.
- *Takes the viewpoint that the term "restrictive cardiomyopathy" should apply only to cases that are indistinguishable from constrictive pericarditis by physical examination, chest x ray, and cardiac catheterisation, and advocates a major role for endomyocardial biopsy.*

11. **Kabbani S, LeWinter MN.** Diastolic heart failure. Constrictive, restrictive, and pericardial. *Cardiol Clin* 2000;**18**:501–9.

12. **Ammash NM, Seward JB, Bailey KR,** *et al.* Clinical profile and outcome of idiopathic restrictive cardiomyopathy. *Circulation* 2000;**101**:2490–6.

13. **Ling LH, Oh JK, Breen JF,** *et al.* Calcific constrictive pericarditis: is it still with us? *Ann Intern Med* 2000;**132**:444–50.
- *135 cases of constrictive pericarditis seen during 1985 to 1995 had calcification in 27% of cases. Calcification was related to chronicity, atrial enlargement, atrial arrhythmia, and higher operative mortality. Ultrafast CT showed calcification in only one of six patients who had no calcification in the plain chest radiograph.*

14. **Hatle L, Appleton C, Popp R.** Differentiation of constrictive pericarditis and restrictive cardiomyopathy by Doppler echocardiography. *Circulation* 1989;**79**:357–70.
- *Echo Doppler studies in seven patients with constrictive pericarditis, all successfully operated, and 12 with restrictive cardiomyopathy, all with either infiltrative disease or extensive myocardial fibrosis in the biopsy. Exaggerated changes in mitral flow velocity with inspiration–expiration separated constrictive pericarditis from restrictive cardiomyopathy. Variation in tricuspid flow velocity with inspiration–expiration overlapped in the two conditions, but averaged greater in constrictive pericarditis. They also noted that the rise and fall in right and left ventricular systolic peaks with inspiration–expiration was out-of-phase in constrictive pericarditis, while they were in-phase in restrictive cardiomyopathy.*

15. **Oh JK, Hatle L, Seward JB,** *et al.* Diagnostic role of Doppler echocardiography in constrictive pericarditis. *J Am Coll Cardiol* 1994;**23**:154–62.

16. **Rajagopaian N, Garcia MJ, Rodriguez L,** *et al.* Comparison of new Doppler echocardiographic methods to differentiate constrictive pericardial heart disease and restrictive cardiomyopathy. *Am J Cardiol* 2001;**87**:86–94.
   * *Studies in 19 patients with constrictive pericarditis (12 operated) and 11 with restrictive cardiomyopathy (8 amyloid). All had pulsed wave Doppler of pulmonary veins and mitral valve with respiration, tissue Doppler of lateral mitral annulus, and colour M mode Doppler flow propagation of left ventricular filling. The two new methods were about equal to the Doppler respiratory methods in differentiating the two conditions. They suggest that the new methods might be useful in cases where exaggerated respiratory variation may be absent in constrictive pericarditis (5/19 in this series).*

17. **Vaitkus PT, Kussmaul WG.** Constrictive pericarditis versus restrictive cardiomyopathy: a reappraisal and update of diagnostic criteria. *Am Heart J* 1991;**122**:1431–41.
   * *Analysis of haemodynamic criteria in 82 cases of constriction and 37 cases of restrictive cardiomyopathy in the literature, concluding that a quarter of cases would be not be correctly classified by haemodynamic criteria. Suggests an algorithm including CT/MR imaging of the pericardium and endomyocardial biopsy.*

18. **Hurrell DG, Nishimura RA, Higano T,** *et al.* Value of dynamic respiratory changes in left and right ventricular pressures for the diagnosis of constrictive pericarditis. *Circulation* 1996;**93**:2007–13.
   * *Catheter tip manometer recordings in 15 patients with constrictive pericarditis and 21 with congestive heart failure of other types, including seven with restrictive cardiomyopathy. Discordant changes in right and left ventricular peak systolic pressure in inspiration separated constrictive pericarditis from the other cases.*

19. **Breen JF.** Imaging of the pericardium. *J Thorac Imaging* 2001;**16**:47–54.

20. **Schoenfeld M, Supple E, Dec W,** *et al.* Restrictive cardiomyopathy versus constrictive pericarditis: role of endomyocardial biopsy in avoiding unnecessary thoracotomy. *Circulation* 1987;**75**:1012–7.
   * *Analysis of 54 biopsies during 1975-85 in patients with congestive heart failure and constrictive/restrictive physiology, showing amyloid in 11. Fourteen cases with constrictive pericarditis showed normal biopsy in three patients, non-specific abnormality in nine, and myocarditis in two. They consider that biopsy is essential if thoracotomy for constriction is contemplated.*

57

8 The diagnosis of hypertrophic cardiomyopathy

E Douglas Wigle

Table 8.2 *Types of HCM and approximate incidence*[*]

Types of HCM	Incidence (%)
Left ventricular involvement	
Asymmetrical hypertrophy	95
Ventricular septal hypertrophy	80
Apical hypertrophy	9
Midventricular hypertrophy	4
Rare types	2
Symmetrical (concentric) hypertrophy	5
Right ventricular involvement	–

[*]At the Toronto General Hospital where approximately 1300 patients are registered in the HCM clinic. The incidence of the different types of HCM varies considerably among different centres.

Although the pathology of hypertrophic cardiomyopathy (HCM) was first described by French pathologists in the mid 19th century, it remained for the virtually simultaneous reports of Brock and Teare in England some 43 years ago to bring modern attention to this fascinating entity.[1] [2] Subsequent to these surgical[1] and pathological[2] observations, there has been an almost exponential growth in the number of research reports and in our knowledge of HCM, and a number of extensive reviews have been published.[3–9] HCM was initially thought to be relatively rare, but it is now recognised to be an important cause of morbidity and mortality in people of all ages. In tertiary referral populations the annual mortality is 3–4% per annum (higher in the young) and 1–2% per annum in non-referred populations. It occurs in 1 in 500 live births, making it as common as cystic fibrosis, and is the most common cause of sudden death during athletic endeavour in young people. The diagnosis of HCM is therefore of great importance, particularly in the young where sudden death is such a risk.

More recently, the results of molecular genetic studies have resulted in a quantum leap in our basic knowledge and understanding of the Mendelian dominant inheritance of HCM and have far reaching prognostic and clinical implications. HCM is now described as a heterogeneous disease of the sarcomere in that more than 150 different mutations in 10 different sarcomeric proteins have been shown to cause HCM[8] (table 8.1). These molecular genetic studies are already having important clinical implications in that some mutations carry a benign prognosis, whereas others, possibly interacting with various growth factors, have increased penetrance, early onset of manifestations, and a bad prognosis, thus explaining the malignant family history noted in some instances. Because of the time

Table 8.1 *Genetics of hypertrophic cardiomyopathy (HCM)*

Mendelian dominance: variable penetrance
A disease of sarcomeric proteins
α and β myosin heavy chain
Troponin T and I
α Tropomyosin
Myosin binding protein C
α Cardiac actin
Myosin (essential and regulatory) light chain
Titin

A genetically heterogeneous disease.
Mutations in the 10 listed sarcomeric proteins have been shown to account for the Mendelian dominant inheritance of HCM.

consuming nature of these molecular genetic studies, they are only currently available in research centres. However, within five years it is expected techniques for genetic diagnosis will become more generally available and hence more generally applicable.

In addition to the genetically determined form of the disease, HCM may also occur in older patients (HCM in the elderly), where it is often related to hypertensive left ventricular hypertrophy and/or age related changes of the heart (sigmoid septum).[10] It is important to realise, however, that a certain percentage of cases of HCM in the elderly will be genetically determined in that certain mutations, such as those in myosin binding protein C, have delayed penetrance and late onset of disease (up to age 60 years).[11]

Just as the inheritance of HCM is heterogeneous, so are the phenotypic manifestations, even in a single family cohort, with the same molecular genetic defect. HCM may be defined as left and/or right ventricular hypertrophy of unknown cause that is usually, but not always, asymmetrical, and associated with microscopic evidence of myocardial fibre disarray. Ventricular septal hypertrophy is by far the most common type of asymmetrical hypertrophy, with apical, midventricular, and rarer types of asymmetrical hypertrophy being far less common (table 8.2). The extent of hypertrophy at any given site can vary greatly and bears importantly on the manifestations of the disease.[5]

From a clinical standpoint, it is very important to classify HCM haemodynamically (table 8.3). The subaortic obstruction is by far the most common form of obstructive HCM and may be latent (provocable), labile (variable), or there may be a persistent obstruction at rest (resting obstruction). Figure 8.1 demonstrates the pathophysiology of the subaortic obstruction and the concomitant mitral regurgitation, both of which are caused by systolic anterior motion of the anterior and/or posterior mitral leaflet.[7] The two forms of obstructive HCM may co-exist in the same patient. Non-obstructive HCM may be defined as a patient having no obstruction at rest or on provocation.

Clinical diagnosis

Family history
A detailed and accurate family history is of obvious importance in dealing with patients in

Table 8.3 Haemodynamic classification of HCM

Obstructive HCM
   Subaortic obstruction
   Midventricular obstruction
Non-obstructive HCM
   Normal (supranormal) systolic function
   Impaired systolic function (end-stage HCM)

See text for more detail

whom HCM is a diagnostic possibility. In families in whom several family members have heart disease at a relatively young age, HCM is a distinct possibility. That possibility is increased significantly if there are sudden deaths at a young age in a family. Once the diagnosis is established in a member of a family, other family members should be screened with ECGs and echocardiograms in keeping with the known Mendelian dominant inheritance of the condition.

Symptoms

Patients with obstructive HCM typically complain of dyspnoea, angina, and presyncope and/or syncope on exertion. At times syncope may occur on truly minimal exertion. The severity of symptoms on upright exertion do not necessarily correlate with the magnitude of the obstructive pressure gradient measured in the supine position, which is understandable particularly when the lability of the obstruction is taken into account. The severity of symptoms is often variable from day to day, as is the

> **Obstructive versus non-obstructive HCM**
>
> ● Extremely important to determine whether HCM is obstructive or non-obstructive
>
> ● If obstructive, is the obstruction subaortic or midventricular, or both?
>
> ● If non-obstructive, is ventricular systolic function normal or impaired?
>
> ● Non-obstructive HCM should be provoked to determine if latent (provocable) obstruction is present
>
> ● There are important clinical signs that distinguish obstructive from non-obstructive HCM

severity of the obstruction, which varies according to ventricular afterload (systolic blood pressure), preload, and contractility. The symptoms are often worse after a large meal or alcohol ingestion, when the obstruction is more severe. Many patients will also note presyncope on standing suddenly for the same reason. In our experience, patients with non-obstructive HCM present with these symptoms less frequently and usually the symptoms are milder,[5] but in some there is very severe disability resulting from left ventricular systolic and/or diastolic dysfunction. Congestive heart failure is rarely seen in HCM in normal sinus rhythm, but it may be seen with severe obstruction to outflow or severe systolic and/or diastolic dysfunction and is common in the presence of atrial fibrillation.

Although presyncope and syncope on exertion are common in obstructive HCM, it is extremely important to recognise that these symptoms may also result from atrial and ventricular arrhythmias at rest or on exertion, or from failure of blood pressure to rise normally on exertion, even in non-obstructive HCM.[12] Thus, a history of palpitations, particularly rapid heart action when associated with presyncope/syncope, is an integral part of history taking.

Physical examination

Right ventricular involvement in HCM may be detected by a prominent A wave in the jugular venous pulse, that rises on inspiration and rarely by a right sided fourth heart sound, reflecting right ventricular diastolic dysfunction. A systolic ejection murmur along the high left sternal border often indicates subpulmonic or midventricular obstruction to right ventricular outflow.[5 7]

Left ventricular involvement is reflected by a variably displaced and forceful left ventricular impulse and a left sided fourth heart sound that is often palpable, reflecting impaired left ventricular relaxation. Patients with non-obstructive HCM either have no murmur or a faint grade 1/6 systolic murmur at the cardiac apex, that does not increase significantly with provocation. In patients with latent subaortic obstruction, the murmur at the apex is usually

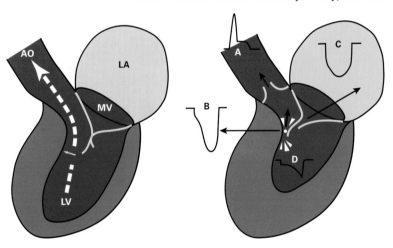

Early systole   Mitral leaflet – septal contact

Figure 8.1. Diagram of the pathophysiology of the obstruction to outflow and mitral regurgitation in subaortic obstructive hypertrophic cardiomyopathy (HCM). Early systole (left): The left ventricular outflow tract is narrowed by the ventricular septal hypertrophy and the anterior displacement of the papillary muscles and the mitral leaflets. The point of coaptation of the elongated mitral leaflets occurs in the body of the leaflets, rather than at the tips, as is normal. That part of the anterior leaflet beyond the coaptation point is carried anteriorly and superiorly (systolic anterior motion, arrow) by venturi and/or drag forces and results in mitral leaflet–septal contact, causing the subaortic obstruction (indicated by the converging and diverging lines, right). Mitral leaflet–septal contact (right): The systolic anterior motion of the anterior leaflet results in a failure of coaptation of the mitral leaflets and the onset of mitral regurgitation, which is directed posteriorly into the left atrium, through the funnel shaped interleaflet gap. The length and mobility of the posterior leaflet may also affect the size of this gap, and hence the degree of mitral regurgitation. A, B, C, and D indicate Doppler velocity recordings throughout systole in the ascending aorta (A) (flow toward transducer), at the level of mitral leaflet–septal contact (B), in the left atrium (C), and near the apex of the left ventricle (D). In B, C, and D, flow is away from the transducer. Reduced forward flow in the presence of the obstruction is indicated by the shape of the aortic velocity waveform (A) and the smaller aortic arrow. Peak velocities recorded at B correlate accurately with the simultaneously measured pressure gradient, whereas late peaking velocities at D do not. AO, aorta; LA, left atrium, LV, left ventricle, MV, mitral valve. Adapted from Wigle et al.[7]

Familial HCM

● Inherited as Mendelian dominant characteristic

● Related to mutations in sarcomeric proteins (a disease of the sarcomere)

● Taking a family history is important, particularly with regard to the occurrence of sudden cardiac death

● Screening family members is also important

● De novo mutations also cause HCM

● HCM in the elderly may be familial, or non-familial and related to hypertensive hypertrophy and/or age related changes (sigmoid septum)

grade 1/6 to grade 2/6 in intensity, and increases to grade 3/6 with appropriate provocation such as amyl nitrite inhalation, assuming the upright posture from the squatting position or during the Valsalva manoeuvre. In patients with subaortic obstructive HCM at rest, the murmur at or just medial to the apex is grade 3/6 to 4/6 in intensity, and begins after the first heart sound. It is harsh and crescendo/decrescendo in character with radiation to the base of the heart, reflecting the obstruction, and to the axilla, reflecting the concomitant mitral regurgitation[7] (figs 8.1 and 8.2). In 20% of patients with subaortic obstructive HCM there may be independent abnormalities of the mitral valve (other than systolic anterior motion) that cause mitral regurgitation such as abnormal papillary muscle insertions, mitral valve prolapse or excessive fibrotic thickening of the anterior mitral leaflet, resulting from repeated mitral leaflet–septal contact.[5] In such cases there may also be a pansystolic murmur at the apex.

In addition to the louder apical murmur, there is an intriguing constellation of physical signs in subaortic obstructive HCM that are not seen in the non-obstructive form of the disease.[7] On palpation there is often a bifid (spike and dome) arterial pulse, which at times has been referred to as a bisferiens pulse incorrectly. A bisferiens pulse is seen in dominant aortic regurgitation. On palpation at the left ventricular apex, there is often a double systolic impulse, the first impulse coming before the onset of the obstruction, the second after. Frequently, there is a triple apex beat, resulting from a palpable left atrial gallop sound, plus a double systolic impulse. To appreciate the abnormalities on palpation over the left ventricular apex, it is extremely important that the patient be examined in the left lateral position (fig 8.2).

On auscultation in subaortic obstructive HCM, there may be a reversed or paradoxically split second heart sound when the obstruction is severe or in the presence of left bundle branch block. When the mitral regurgitation is

significant, it is often accompanied by a mitral diastolic inflow murmur. Rarely a mitral leaflet–septal contact sound may also be heard (fig 8.2).

Patients with midventricular obstruction also have an apical systolic murmur, although it is usually softer, grade 2/6 to 3/6, than with subaortic obstruction. A bifid arterial pulse, double systolic apex beat or triple apex beat are not characteristic of midventricular obstruction and a mitral leaflet–septal contact sound is never found. If the obstruction is severe, there may be reversed splitting of the second heart sound. In midventricular obstruction, there is at times a very distinctive long mitral diastolic murmur, caused by the midventricular narrowing and asynchronous relaxation.[7]

In midventricular obstruction, the size of the obstructed apical cavity varies considerably. It may be quite large and haemodynamically significant or very small and more a manifestation of cavity obliteration with a small non-obliterated pocket of blood remaining at the apex. The syndrome of midventricular obstruction with apical infarction and aneurysm formation most often results from apical infarction in a patient with apical HCM in whom the non-infarcted hypertrophy at the midventricular level results in midventricular obstruction.[13]

Laboratory investigation

Patients referred with suspected HCM should have an ECG, a chest x ray, and a transthoracic echo Doppler examination on the initial visit.

The ECG in HCM may be normal with mild degrees of hypertrophy or show left ventricular hypertrophy and strain in the presence of extensive hypertrophy. Abnormal Q waves, which may mimic myocardial infarction, and which at times reflect septal hypertrophy, are a feature of the ECG in HCM, as are sharply negative T waves, particularly in precordial leads V3–V5 (giant T negativity syndrome)

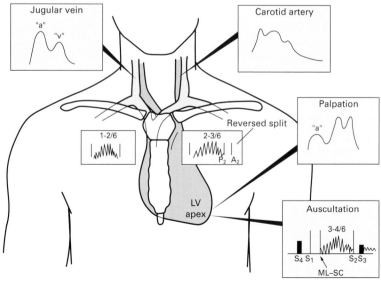

Figure 8.2. Diagram showing the seven findings on physical examination that are found in subaortic obstructive HCM and are not present in non-obstructive HCM (see text). ML–SC, mitral leaflet-septal contact sound.

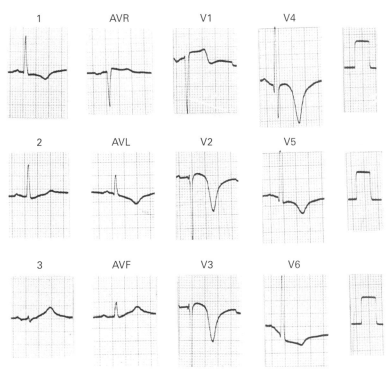

Figure 8.3. ECG from a patient with apical HCM showing the "giant T negativity syndrome"[14] (T waves more negative than 10 mm) in the precordial leads, usually maximal in V4. There is also voltage evidence of left ventricular hypertrophy.

typical of apical HCM[14] (fig 8.3). Apical infarction may also be reflected in the ECG, and it is important to recognise that the ECG may be abnormal in HCM when echocardiography reveals no evidence of left ventricular hypertrophy.

The chest x ray may be normal or show left ventricular and/or left or right atrial enlargement, with or without vascular redistribution in the lungs. The aorta is typically small. A bulge on the left heart border, between the left atrial appendage and left ventricular apex, may reflect anterolateral wall extension of anteroseptal hypertrophy.

Transthoracic echo Doppler examination in HCM is undoubtedly the most important form of laboratory investigation. These combined techniques can determine the location and extent of hypertrophy, systolic and diastolic function, the presence and degree of systolic anterior motion, the severity of the subaortic and/or midventricular obstruction, the direction and degree of mitral regurgitation, the presence of additional mitral valve abnormalities, and left atrial size. The mitral regurgitation that results from systolic anterior motion of the anterior mitral leaflet is directed posteriorly into the left atrium (fig 1). If the mitral regurgitation is directed anteriorly or centrally, then additional abnormalities of the mitral valve such as abnormal papillary muscles or mitral valve prolapse should be suspected. Transoesophageal echo Doppler studies are particularly valuable in defining these additional mitral valve abnormalities and in distinguishing which type of obstruction is present in the left ventricle.[15 16] Patients who have no evidence of outflow obstruction at rest should routinely undergo appropriate provocation to determine whether there is echo Doppler evidence of latent or provocable obstruction.[5]

Previously, certain criteria of septal, apical, or free wall thickness were used to establish the diagnosis of HCM.[5] It is now recognised, as the result of molecular genetic–clinical correlations, that milder degrees of hypertrophy may also indicate HCM.

Ambulatory rhythm monitoring for detection of atrial and/or ventricular arrhythmias or conduction disturbances is of extreme importance in HCM once the diagnosis is established.

Nuclear angiography is very valuable in HCM to assess both systolic and diastolic ventricular function. Stress perfusion studies and positron emission tomography are important for detecting evidence of myocardial ischaemia or infarction.

Magnetic resonance imaging is of particular value in HCM when two dimensional echocardiography is unable to document the site and extent of hypertrophy, especially in apical HCM.

Heart catheterisation and angiography in HCM are usually reserved for diagnostic problems or when septal alcohol ablation or surgery are being considered in either type of obstructive HCM; they are also of value in the investigation of HCM with impaired systolic function with regard to the possibility of cardiac transplantation. The diagnostic accuracy of echo Doppler studies has dramatically lessened the need for invasive investigation in HCM. The precise role of electrophysiologic testing in the assessment of arrhythmia risk is as yet to be defined.

Genetic screening for HCM is prognostically important and undoubtedly will become more common once all the molecular genetic defects are defined and screening procedures simplified.

Assessment of risk

Assessment of risk of sudden cardiac death is an integral part of the work up of patients with HCM,[5 12 17 18] and will be addressed in a subsequent article in this series.

Investigation of HCM

- Echo Doppler examination is the most important diagnostic test in HCM and for determining the haemodynamic abnormalities present

- ECG may be abnormal when echo is normal, especially in the young

- Apical HCM most commonly suspected by an abnormal ECG (giant T negativity syndrome)

- Echo may fail to detect apical HCM in 10% of cases unless specifically looked for. Even then, magnetic resonance imaging may be required for definitive diagnosis

61

Special situations

Apical HCM

This form of HCM was originally described in Japan in the 1970s and is being recognised with increasing frequency in western populations.[14] Currently, we are following 120 patients with apical HCM, which represents a 9% incidence in our HCM clinic population of approximately 1300 patients (table 8.1). In approximately 50% of patients with apical HCM, the diagnosis will be first suspected or suggested by the abnormal ECG, with sharply inverted T waves in the lateral precordial leads (fig 8.3). A significant percentage of patients with apical HCM will present with atypical chest pain and the ECG abnormalities suggest ischaemia. These patients are often admitted to a coronary care unit if the admitting physician is not familiar with the ECG of apical HCM, which of course has voltage evidence of left ventricular hypertrophy, in addition to the sharply inverted T waves (fig 8.3). A second diagnostic characteristic of apical HCM is the spade shape of the left ventricle at end-diastole, which can be detected by echocardiography, angiography, or magnetic resonance imaging.[19 20] It is important to realise that apical hypertrophy can easily be missed on echocardiography unless great care is taken in the examination. Even then, magnetic resonance imaging is sometimes required to be definite about the diagnosis.

The prognosis in apical HCM is generally more favourable than in other forms of HCM, but these patients may suffer from apical ischaemia and/or infarction, which is often associated with ventricular arrhythmias, or atrial fibrillation, caused by left atrial enlargement resulting from left ventricular diastolic dysfunction.

Impaired systolic and/or diastolic dysfunction in HCM (end-stage HCM)

Progressive myocardial fibrosis from ischaemia and/or from fibrous transformation of the often abundant loose intercellular connective tissue in the myocardium[2 5 7] results in impaired systolic and/or diastolic function. In this stage of the disease, the left and right ventricular walls become thinner, the ventricles dilate, systolic function decreases, there is no longer evidence of outflow obstruction, and often mitral and tricuspid regurgitation in the presence of atrial fibrillation and congestive heart failure dominate the clinical picture. It is important to recognise this late stage of HCM because the negative inotropic drug therapy used for the treatment of obstructive HCM is now contraindicated, whereas treatments that would be contraindicated in obstructive HCM are now indicated—that is, afterload reduction, digitalis glycosides, and diuretics.[7] Patients with end-stage HCM are candidates for cardiac transplantation.

Atrial fibrillation

Atrial fibrillation in HCM is usually related to an enlarged left atrium, which most frequently

> **Atrial fibrillation**
>
> - An important cause of morbidity: congestive heart failure, risk of systemic emboli, rarely syncope
>
> - Almost always related to left atrial enlargement, which is most frequently seen in subaortic obstructive HCM (caused by concomitant mitral regurgitation) or in the presence of systolic and/or diastolic dysfunction
>
> - In the presence of subaortic obstructive HCM, atrial fibrillation may lead to a mistaken diagnosis of mitral regurgitation because of the apical murmur
>
> - Every attempt should be made to restore sinus rhythm pharmacologically or by cardioversion

occurs in subaortic obstructive HCM caused by the concomitant mitral regurgitation; it may also be seen in non-obstructive HCM as the result of left atrial enlargement caused by diastolic dysfunction, particularly impaired left ventricular relaxation.[5 7] The onset of atrial fibrillation often precipitates left and right heart failure. When patients with subaortic obstructive HCM are seen in the emergency department with this arrhythmia, they are often misdiagnosed as mitral regurgitation because of the loud apical murmur. An incorrect diagnosis under these circumstances is to be avoided.

Conclusion

HCM is a heterogeneous disease, both genotypically and phenotypically, and is often a diagnostic challenge. Being aware of the diverse clinical and laboratory manifestations of HCM should avoid mistaken diagnoses in a disease that has been termed "The Great Masquerader".

1. **Brock RC.** Functional obstruction of the left ventricle. *Guys Hosp Report* 1957;**106**:221–38.
- *Initial surgical observations in obstructive HCM.*

2. **Teare RD.** Asymmetrical hypertrophy of the heart in young adults. *Br Heart J* 1958;**20**:1–8.
- *Excellent gross and microscopic description of the pathology of HCM, including a description of myocardial fibre disarray and the abundant loose intercellular connective tissue that may undergo fibrous transformation in the late stages of the disease.*

3. **Braunwald E, Lambrew C, Rockoff SD,** et al. Idiopathic hypertrophic subaortic stenosis, I: description of the disease based upon an analysis of 64 patients. *Circulation* 1964;**29**:IV-3–119.
- *An early review of obstructive HCM.*

4. **Goodwin JF.** The frontiers of cardiomyopathy. *Br Heart J* 1982;**48**:1–18.
- *An early review of HCM.*

5. **Wigle ED, Sasson Z, Henderson MA,** et al. Hypertrophic cardiomyopathy: the importance of the site and the extent of hypertrophy: a review. *Prog Cardiovasc Dis* 1985;**28**:1–83.
- *An extensive review of all aspects of HCM focusing on the Toronto experience. One of the earlier papers to point out the importance of the site and extent of hypertrophy as indicated in the title.*

6. **Maron BJ, Bonow RO, Cannon RO,** et al. Hypertrophic cardiomyopathy: interrelations of clinical manifestations, pathophysiology, and therapy. *N Engl J Med* 1987;**316**:780–9, 884–52.

• *This review updates the experience of the National Institutes of Health in the USA with the diagnosis and management of HCM.*

7. **Wigle ED, Rakowski H, Kimball BP,** *et al*. Hypertrophic cardiomyopathy. Clinical spectrum and treatment. *Circulation* 1995;**92**:1680–92.
• *Another review of the pathophysiology, diagnosis, and management of HCM from the Toronto group.*

8. **Spirito P, Seidman CE, McKenna WJ,** *et al*. The management of hypertrophic cardiomyopathy. *N Engl J Med* 1997;**336**:775–85.
• *A review of the molecular genetics, manifestations, and management of HCM.*

9. **Maron B.** Hypertrophic cardiomyopathy. *Lancet* 1997;**350**:127–33.
• *A recent review emphasising the better prognosis in non-referred patient populations.*

10. **Lever HM, Karam RF, Currie PJ,** *et al*. Hypertrophic cardiomyopathy in the elderly: distinctions from the young based on cardiac shape. *Circulation* 1989;**79**:580–9.
• *One of several papers published on "HCM in the elderly" attempting to distinguish it from the inherited form of the disease.*

11. **Nimura H, Bachinski LL, Sangwatanaroj S,** *et al*. Mutations in the gene for cardiac myosin-binding protein C and late-onset familial hypertrophic cardiomyopathy. *N Engl J Med* 1998;**338**:1248–56.
• *The first of several papers on HCM caused by mutations in myosin binding protein C, which results in delayed penetrance and late onset of the disease.*

12. **Elliott PM, Gimeno Blanes JR, Mahon NG,** *et al*. Relation between severity of left-ventricular hypertrophy and prognosis in patients with hypertrophic cardiomyopathy. *Lancet* 2000;**357**:420–4.
• *An authoritative paper on risk stratification in HCM indicating that risk factors other than the degree of left ventricular hypertrophy should be taken into account in prescribing prophylactic treatment.*

13. **Ishiwata S, Nishyama S, Nakanishi S,** *et al*. Two types of left ventricular wall motion abnormalities with distinct clinical features in patients with hypertrophic cardiomyopathy. *Eur Heart J* 1993;**14**:1629–39.
• *A clear description of apical infarction in apical HCM evolving to the syndrome of midventricular obstruction with apical infarction ± aneurysm formation.*

14. **Sakamoto T, Tei C, Murayama M,** *et al*. Giant negative T-wave inversion as a manifestation of asymmetric apical hypertrophy (AAH) of the left ventricle: echocardiographic and ultrasono-cardiotomographic study. *Jpn Heart J* 1976;**17**:611–29.

• *The first description of the "giant T negativity syndrome" in apical HCM.*

15. **Grigg LE, Wigle ED, Williams WG,** *et al*. Transesophageal Doppler echocardiography in obstructive hypertrophic cardiomyopathy: clarification of pathophysiology and importance in intraoperative decision making. *J Am Coll Cardiol* 1992;**20**:42–52.
• *A description of the pathophysiology of the subaortic obstruction and concomitant mitral regurgitation in HCM based on transoesophageal echo Doppler observations.*

16. **Yu EHC, Omran AS, Wigle ED,** *et al*. Mitral regurgitation in hypertrophic obstructive cardiomyopathy: Relationship to obstruction and relief with myectomy. *J Am Coll Cardiol* 2000;**36**:2219–24.
• *A description of the direct relation between the degree of mitral regurgitation and the magnitude of the pressure gradient in subaortic obstructive HCM and the relief of both by myectomy.*

17. **Maron BJ, Shen WK, Link MS,** *et al*. Efficacy of implantable cardioverter-defibrillators for the prevention of sudden death in patients with hypertrophic cardiomyopathy. *N Engl J Med* 2000;**342**:365–72.
• *A description of the rate of appropriate defibrillator discharge in the primary and secondary prevention of sudden death in patients at risk of sudden cardiac death in HCM.*

18. **Spirito P, Bellone P, Harris KM,** *et al*. Magnitude of left ventricular hypertrophy and risk of sudden death in hypertrophic cardiomyopathy. *N Engl J Med* 2000;**342**:1778–85.
• *Evidence is presented to the effect that the magnitude of left ventricular hypertrophy in HCM is a strong and independent risk factor for sudden cardiac death, a conclusion that differs from the conclusions in reference 12.*

19. **Yamaguchi H, Ishimura T, Nishiyama S,** *et al*. Hypertrophic nonobstructive cardiomyopathy with giant negative T-waves (apical hypertrophy): ventriculographic and echocardiographic features in 30 patients. *Am J Cardiol* 1979;**44**:401–11.
• *A description of the spade shape of the left ventricle at end diastole in patients with apical HCM.*

20. **Webb JG, Sasson Z, Rakowski H,** *et al*. Apical hypertrophic cardiomyopathy: clinical follow-up and diagnostic correlates. *J Am Coll Cardiol* 1990;**15**:83–90.
• *This paper indicates that the characteristics of apical HCM in western populations are exactly as described by Japanese authors (references 14 and 19).*

SECTION IV: VALVE DISEASE

9 Balloon valvuloplasty

Alec Vahanian

Until the early 1980s surgery was the only possible treatment for severe valvar stenosis. Then a new alternative appeared—percutaneous balloon valvuloplasty.

I will deal here with percutaneous valvuloplasty for acquired valvar stenoses in the fields of mitral stenosis, aortic stenosis, and, although it occurs far less frequently, tricuspid or bioprosthetic stenoses.

Percutaneous mitral commissurotomy

Rheumatic mitral stenosis continues to be endemic in developing countries where mitral stenosis is the most frequent valve disease.[1] Although the prevalence of rheumatic fever has greatly decreased in western countries, it continues to represent an important clinical entity because of immigration from developing countries.

The first to perform percutaneous mitral commissurotomy (PMC) as an alternative to surgery was Inoue in 1982.[2] The good results obtained with the technique have led to its increasing worldwide use and its positioning as the second most important technique in the field of interventional cardiology.

Evaluation before PMC

Clinical evaluation is the first step when deciding whether to operate or intervene. Under particular scrutiny here are functional disability and any possible risks with surgery.

The assessment of anatomy aims to eliminate contraindications and define prognostic considerations. Echographic assessment allows the classification of patients into anatomic groups with a view to predicting the results. Most authors use the Wilkins score (table 9.1) while others, like Cormier (table 9.2), use a more general assessment of valve anatomy.[3] More recently, scores which take into account the uneven distribution of anatomic abnormalities, particularly in regard to commissural areas, have been developed. In fact, none of the scores available has been shown to be superior to any of the others, and we can only recommend the use of the score with which one is most familiar and at ease.

Technique

The transvenous, or antegrade, approach, is the most widely used. Transseptal catheterisation,[3] which allows access to the left atrium, is the first step of the procedure and one of the most crucial. The transarterial, or retrograde approach, could represent an alternative in the rare cases where the transeptal approach is contraindicated.[4]

There are currently two main techniques—balloon commissurotomy, and metallic commissurotomy.

Balloon commissurotomy

In balloon commissurotomy the two major techniques are the *double balloon technique* and the *Inoue technique*.

The double balloon technique requires the use of a floating balloon catheter to cross the mitral valve and then the positioning of two guidewires in the apex of the left ventricle. It is effective but demanding, and carries the risk of left ventricular perforation by the guidewires or the tip of the balloons (fig 9.1). The multi-track system is a recent variant of the double balloon technique and aims to make the procedure easier, as it only requires the presence of a single guide wire (fig 9.2).

The design of the Inoue balloon allows safe and fast positioning across the valve. In addition, it is pressure extensible, allowing for the performance of a stepwise dilatation (fig 9.3). The data available comparing the Inoue and the double balloon techniques suggest that the Inoue technique makes the procedure easier and has equivalent efficacy, but with lower risk. In fact the Inoue technique has become the most popular worldwide.

Table 9.1 *Anatomic classification of the mitral valve (Wilkins' score, Massachusetts General Hospital)*

Leaflet mobility
- Highly mobile valve with restriction of only the leaflet tips
- Mid portion and base of leaflets have reduced mobility
- Valve leaflets move forward in diastole mainly at the base
- No or minimal forward movement of the leaflets in diastole

Valvar thickening
- Leaflets near normal (4–5 mm)
- Mid leaflet thickening, pronounced thickening of the margins
- Thickening extends through the entire leaflets (5–8 mm)
- Pronounced thickening of all leaflet tissue (> 8–10 mm)

Subvalvar thickening
- Minimal thickening of chordal structures just below the valve
- Thickening of chordae extending up to one third of chordal length
- Thickening extending to the distal third of the chordae
- Extensive thickening and shortening of all chordae extending down to the papillary muscle

Valvar calcification
- A single area of increased echo brightness
- Scattered areas of brightness confined to leaflet margins
- Brightness extending into the mid portion of leaflets
- Extensive brightness through most of the leaflet tissue

Table 9.2 *Anatomic classification of the mitral valve (Cormier's score, Tenon and Bichat Hospitals, Paris)*

Echocardiographic group	Mitral valve anatomy
Group 1	Pliable non-calcified anterior mitral leaflet and mild subvalvar disease—that is, thin chordae ⩾ 10 mm long
Group 2	Pliable non-calcified anterior mitral leaflet and severe subvalvar disease—that is, thickened chordae < 10 mm long
Group 3	Calcification of mitral valve of any extent, as assessed by fluoroscopy, whatever the subvalvar apparatus

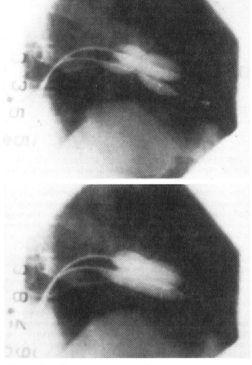

Figure 9.1. Transvenous technique using the combination of a trefoil and a conventional balloon.

Metallic commissurotomy

Recently Cribier introduced the metallic commissurotomy (fig 9.4), which uses a device similar to the Tubb's dilator used during closed surgical commissurotomy.[5] The experience with this device is only preliminary and exclusively reported by the promoter of the method. These initial results suggest that its efficacy is similar to balloon commissurotomy, but the risk of haemopericardium seems higher because of the device and the presence of a guide wire in the left ventricle. In addition, this technique is more demanding for the operator than the Inoue technique. The potential advantage of metallic commissurotomy is that the dilator is reusable, which will reduce the cost of the procedure. This is of interest in developing countries, where high rates of rheumatic disease often co-exist with low financial means, limiting the use of percutaneous dilatation.

The definite comparison of the respective merits of the two methods requires further data concerning metallic commissurotomy and randomised comparisons of the two techniques.

The results of PMC in the catheterisation laboratory can be assessed haemodynamically or by echocardiography. Although echocardiography may be difficult to perform in the catheterisation laboratory for logistical reasons, it is very important as it enables the detection of early complications and provides essential information on the course of the mitral opening; this is crucial when using a stepwise Inoue technique. The following criteria have been proposed for the desired end point of the procedure: valve area > 1 cm^2/m^2 body surface area (BSA); complete opening of at least one commissure; appearance or increment of regurgitation greater than grade 1 in the Sellers 0 to 4 classification. These are of course only

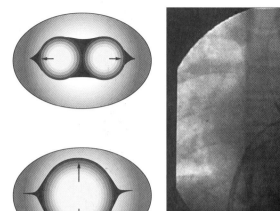

Figure 9.2. Multi-track technique: inflation of two balloons across the mitral valve—note the presence of one guidewire in the apex. Courtesy of Dr P Bonhoeffer.

indications and it is necessary to tailor the strategy according to individual circumstances.

After the procedure, the most accurate evaluation of valve area is provided by echocardiography using planimetry whenever possible. The final assessment of the degree of regurgitation may be made by angiography and by Doppler colour flow. Transoesophageal examination is recommended after the procedure to determine the mechanisms involved in case of severe regurgitation.

Results

The technique has now been evaluated in several thousand patients with different clinical circumstances.[6 7]

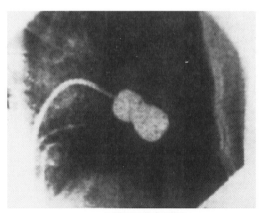

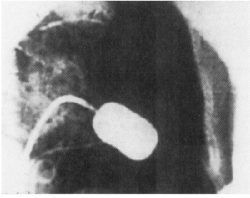

Figure 9.3. The Inoue balloon technique with the balloon at full inflation. The balloon's "waist" located at its mid-portion disappears.

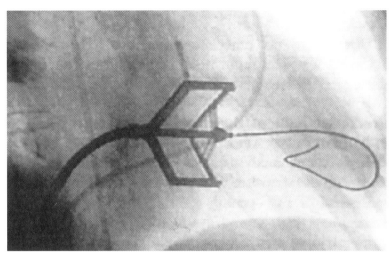

Figure 9.4. Metallic commissurotomy: opening of the metallic commissurotome across the mitral valve. Courtesy of Dr A Cribier.

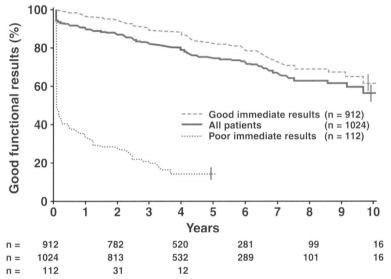

n =	912	782	520	281	99	16
n =	1024	813	532	289	101	16
n =	112	31	12			

Figure 9.5. Percutaneous mitral commissurotomy: good functional results (survival considering cardiovascular related deaths with no need for mitral surgery or repeat dilatation and in New York Heart Association functional class I or II). Reproduced with permission from Iung B, et al. Circulation 1999;3272–8, with permission of the publisher.

dium intractable by pericardiocentesis or, less frequently, for severe mitral regurgitation, leading to haemodynamic collapse or refractory pulmonary oedema. Immediately after PMC colour Doppler echo shows small intra-atrial shunts in 40–80% of cases. However, oximetry shows that the QP:QS ratio is seldom over 1.5.

The complication rate of the procedure is clearly related to the experience of the team. PMC should probably be restricted to groups whose experience of transseptal catheterisation has been positive and who have been able to carry out an adequate number of procedures, thus improving their technical performance and ability to select patients. This recommendation carries even more weight in western countries, where mitral stenosis is infrequent.

Predictors of immediate results
The prediction of the immediate results is multifactorial. Besides morphological factors, pre-operative variables such as age, history of commissurotomy, functional class, small mitral valve area, presence of tricuspid regurgitation, as well as procedural factors such as the non-use of the Inoue technique, are all independent predictors of poor immediate results.[7]

Long term results
We are now able to analyse follow up data up to 10 years. In clinical terms, several large single centre series confirm the late efficacy of PMC in a large population comprising a variety of patient subsets (fig 9.5).[9] As shown with surgical commissurotomy, late outcome after PMC differs according to the quality of the immediate results.

When the immediate results are unsatisfactory, patients experience only transient or no functional improvement. The prognosis for patients with severe mitral regurgitation is usually poor and surgical treatment is usually required in the months following. In cases of insufficient initial opening, delayed surgery is usually performed when the clinical conditions allow it. However, in some patients moderate improvement in valve function provides functional improvement for several years, although they must be carefully followed to allow for a timely operation.

Conversely, if PMC is initially successful survival rates are excellent, the need for subsequent surgery is infrequent, and functional improvement occurs in the majority of cases. When functional deterioration occurs in these patients it is late and mainly related to mitral restenosis. The incidence of restenosis is around 40% after seven years.[10] The possibility of repeating PMC in cases of recurrent mitral stenosis is one of the potentials of this non-surgical procedure. Repeat PMC can be proposed if recurrent stenosis leads to symptoms, occurs several years after an initially successful procedure, and if the predominant mechanism of restenosis is commissural refusion. At the moment, we have available only a very small number of series on re-PMC, showing encouraging results in selected patients, but

PMC usually provides over 100% increase in valve area, with a final valve area of 2 cm^2 on average. The improvement in valve function results in an immediate decrease in left atrial and pulmonary pressures, both at rest and on exercise.

Risks
The failure rates range from 1–15% and they mostly occur soon after the procedure, in the investigators' experience. Procedural mortality ranges from 0–3%. The incidence of haemopericardium varies from 0.5–12%, and embolism is encountered in 0.5–5% of cases. Severe mitral regurgitation is the most worrying complication.[8] It occurs in 2–10% of patients, and results from non-commissural leaflet tearing, mostly in cases with unfavourable anatomy, and even more so if there is a heterogeneous distribution of the morphologic abnormalities. Surgery is often necessary later and can be conservative in cases with less severe valve deformity. Although urgent surgery (within 24 hours) is seldom needed for complications, it may be required for massive haemopericar-

Contraindications for percutaneous mitral commissurotomy

- Left atrial thrombosis

- Mitral regurgitation > 2/4

- Massive or bicommissural calcification

- Severe aortic valve disease, or severe tricuspid stenosis + regurgitation, associated with mitral stenosis

- Severe concomitant coronary artery disease requiring bypass surgery

the exact role of re-PMC can only be defined when we have larger series with longer follow up.

Follow up studies using sequential trans-oesophageal echocardiographic examinations have shown that the degree of mitral regurgitation remains on the whole stable or slightly decreases during follow up. Atrial defects are likely to close later in the majority of cases. Successful PMC decreases the intensity of spontaneous left atrial contrast, reduces the size of the left atrium, and improves left atrial function. Even if these findings do not constitute proof of the efficacy of PMC on thromboembolism or atrial fibrillation, they consistently show the beneficial effect of the procedure on their causes.

Predictors of long term results

Prediction of the long term results is multifactorial, based on clinical variables such as age, valve anatomy, factors related to the stage of the disease (such as functional class), atrial fibrillation, history of previous commissurotomy, severe tricuspid regurgitation, cardiomegaly, and high pulmonary pressure.[9] [10] Finally, the long term outcome is closely related to the quality of the immediate results, as assessed by final gradient, valve area, and degree of regurgitation.

Selection of the candidates

Contraindications to PMC are summarised in the box below. The most important is the presence of left atrial thrombosis which can be detected by the systematic performance of transoesophageal echocardiography a few days before PMC. A contraindication is self-evident if the thrombus is floating, localised in the cavity or on the interatrial septum. However, no consensus has been reached in cases with thrombosis localised in the left atrial appendage. In our opinion, in such cases the indications for PMC should be limited to patients with contraindications to surgery, or those without urgent need for intervention when oral anticoagulation can been given for at least one month before PMC, and a new transoesophageal echocardiographic examination shows the disappearance of the thrombus.

It has been suggested that PMC should be performed in patients with moderate stenosis in the hope of delaying the natural course of the disease. However, these patients are usually candidates for medical treatment, and the risks of PMC outweigh the benefits.

Indications for percutaneous mitral commissurotomy

PMC is the procedure of choice when surgery is contraindicated[11] or for patients with favourable characteristics—that is, young patients with favourable anatomy. In this latter population several randomised studies comparing PMC and surgical commissurotomy are now available.[12] They show that PMC is at least comparable to surgical commissurotomy as regards immediate and long term results, and is no doubt more comfortable for the patient. In addition, if restenosis occurs, these patients could undergo repeat PMC or surgery without the difficulties and inherent risks resulting from pericardial adhesion and chest wall scarring.

On the other hand, much remains to be done in refining indications for the other patients, especially those with minimal symptoms and those with unfavourable anatomy.

In cases of symptomatic patients, the indications for PMC are perfectly clear. Because of the small but definite risk inherent in the technique, however, truly asymptomatic patients are not usually candidates for the procedure, except in the following cases: increased risk of thromboembolism—for example a previous history of embolism, dense spontaneous contrast in the left atrium, or recurrent atrial fibrillation; need for major extracardiac surgery; or finally to allow pregnancy. In such patients, PMC should only be performed by experienced interventionists and if valve anatomy is favourable, in which case a safe and successful procedure can be expected.

Patients with unfavourable anatomy are common in western countries. Unfortunately, no randomised study is available for these patients and a comparison of the results of PMC with those of surgical series is difficult because of the differences in the patients involved. For this group of patients some favour immediate surgery because of the less satisfying results of PMC, whereas others prefer PMC as an initial treatment for selected patients, resorting to surgery in the event of failure. In such cases the decision must be individualised and one should take into account the multifactorial nature of the prediction of the results for patient selection.[9] Data available suggest that continuing good long term results may be obtained and PMC may be useful to defer surgery in selected patients with mild to moderate calcification or severe impairment of the subvalvar apparatus, but with otherwise favourable characteristics.[13]

The same strategy can also be proposed when the risk of surgery is high—in the elderly[11] [14] where PMC can be considered as a palliative treatment, in patients with a previous history of surgical commissurotomy[15] or aortic valve replacement, and during pregnancy if symptoms persist despite medical treatment.[16]

Percutaneous mitral commissurotomy (PMC)

- PMC has been used in the treatment of severe mitral stenosis for over 10 years

- PMC is usually performed after transeptal catheterisation of the left atrium using the Inoue balloon technique

- The treatment is effective, with valve area doubling on average following the procedure

- The risk with PMC is low when performed by an experienced interventionist team

- 10 year follow ups have shown good results

- Prediction of immediate and mid term results is multifactorial, based on clinical and anatomic variables

- Quality of the immediate results is an important predictor of long term outcome

- In patients with favourable characteristics, PMC has become the technique of choice, replacing surgical commissurotomy

- In other patients a decision to use PMC should be taken on an individual basis, and the percutaneous technique could be considered as complementary to valve replacement

Percutaneous aortic valvuloplasty

Severe degenerative calcified aortic stenosis is the most frequent valve disease in western countries, which accounts for the initial interest in its potential treatment by interventional cardiology. The percutaneous aortic valvuloplasty (PAV) technique was described by Cribier in 1985.[17]

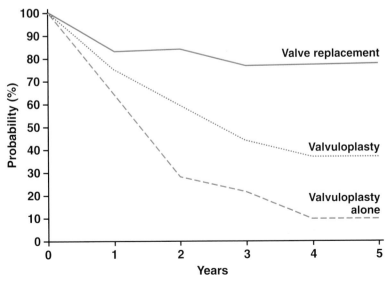

Figure 9.6. Long term survival rate after aortic valve replacement or balloon valvuloplasty. Reproduced with permission from the American College of Cardiology, J Am Coll Cardiol 1992;20:796-801.

Technique
The femoral approach is the most frequently used. The alternative is the antegrade approach which necessitates a transseptal catheterisation and results in a difficult procedure. Valvuloplasty is performed with balloons from 15–25 mm in diameter.

The most viable method for assessing the results is measuring the valve area by echo Doppler in the days following the procedure. Aortography before and after the procedure evaluates any changes in the degree of aortic incompetence.

Results
As could be expected from the anatomic lesions in severe degenerative aortic stenosis—that is, absence of commissural fusion and extensive calcification—PAV has only a limited efficacy. Overall it reduces tight stenosis to moderate stenosis with a final valve area between 0.7–1.1 cm^2. This is clearly inferior to the valve area obtained with a valvar prosthesis, which usually provides a valve area over 1.5 cm^2.

Risks
Mortality and morbidity of the procedure are high. Hospital mortality varies from 3.5–13.5%, and within 24 hours 20–25% of the patients have at least one serious complication, in particular vascular complications at the puncture site.[18]

Long term results
Despite a relatively modest improvement in valve function, it is common to note a degree of functional improvement during the first months; this functional improvement is, however, of short duration. It seems that PAV improves survival rates at one year and especially the quality of life; beyond one year, however, the benefit decreases and finally disappears after two years.[19] With selected patients, an aortic valve replacement has been subsequently performed with good results, but on the other hand the prognosis for the other patients is particularly poor (fig 9.6).[20] Overall it is now admitted that PAV alone does not change the natural course of the disease. The poor mid-term results are mainly due to the clinical status of the patients and to the moderate and transient improvement in valve function obtained by PAV.

Patient selection
There are no randomised comparisons available between PAV and surgery. Therefore the indications should take into account the excellent results of aortic valve replacement when it is possible, and the poor results of PAV.

The question today is whether or not there is still really a place for PAV. Most groups have abandoned the technique, while for others it would appear that there is a very limited role in the following circumstances:

- critically ill patients with cardiogenic shock and multiorgan failure—good mid-term results can be obtained if secondary operation is possible;

72

Percutaneous aortic valvuloplasty (PAV) and other percutaneous valve dilatation applications

- PAV for degenerative calcified aortic stenosis is of limited efficacy and provides only short term alleviation of symptoms at the cost of high procedural risk

- The role of PAV should be restricted to very rare cases, if any

- Percutaneous triscuspid or polyvalvar dilatation are very seldom used

- Percutaneous dilatation of bioprosthesis probably has no future

---

- necessity of significant emergency non-cardiac surgery in patients with severe and poorly tolerated aortic stenosis;
- cases with absolute but non-life threatening short term contraindications to surgery when a significant disability exists;
- in patients who refuse surgery.

It would appear important, however, to evaluate PAV better in rheumatic aortic stenosis because it might ultimately be an attractive application of the technique.

Other applications of percutaneous valve dilatation

Other applications of percutaneous valve dilatation are used very sparingly. The few procedures performed show that these interventions are feasible, but they are insufficient in number to allow us to evaluate results and establish indications.

At the present time it seems that indications for *tricuspid valvuloplasty* are rare and reserved for patients presenting a tight tricuspid stenosis, either pure or associated with mild regurgitation.

Percutaneous dilatation of bioprostheses may give rise to severe immediate complications at the level of the left heart and give poor mid term results in the tricuspid position. Therefore percutaneous dilatation may in certain rare cases be performed as a palliative for stenotic degeneration of a bioprosthesis in the tricuspid position.

Conclusion

After nearly 15 years of extensive clinical evaluation, the technique of percutaneous valvuloplasty, which for practical purposes can be summed up as percutaneous mitral commissurotomy, is now here to stay. This is because of its proven efficacy in the treatment of mitral stenosis, as a substitute for surgical commissurotomy, and a complement to valve replacement.

1. **Carroll JD, Feldman T.** Percutaneous mitral balloon valvotomy and the new demographics of mitral stenosis. *JAMA* 1993;**270**:1731–6.

- This articled describes the features of mitral stenosis in different parts of the world with a special emphasis on western countries.

2. **Inoue K, Owaki T, Nakamura T,** et al. Clinical application of transvenous mitral commissurotomy by a new balloon catheter. *J Thorac Cardiovasc Surg* 1984;**87**:394–402.

3. **Vahanian A, Iung B, Cormier B.** Mitral valvuloplasty. In: Topol EJ, ed. *Textbook of interventional cardiology*. Philadelphia: WB Saunders, 1994:821.
- This chapter reviews the current techniques of percutaneous balloon commissurotomy, and the results obtained in the different subgroups.

4. **Stefanadis C, Toutoutzas P.** Retrograde non-transseptal mitral valvuloplasty. In: Topol EJ, ed. *Textbook of interventional cardiology*. Philadelphia: WB Saunders,1994:1253.

5. **Cribier A, Eltchaninoff H, Koning R,** et al. Percutaneous mechanical mitral commissurotomy with a newly designed metallic valvulotome. *Circulation* 1999;**99**:793–9.

6. **Chen CR, Cheng TO.** Percutaneous balloon mitral valvuloplasty by the Inoue technique: a multicenter study of 4832 patients in China. *Am Heart J* 1995;**129**:1197–202.

7. **Iung B, Cormier B, Ducimetiere P,** et al. Immediate results of percutaneous mitral commissurotomy. *Circulation* 1996;**94**:2124–30.
- The immediate results of the PMC technique are presented and the multifactorial aspects of the predictors described.

8. **Herrmann HC, Lima JAC, Feldman T,** et al. Mechanisms and outcome of severe mitral regurgitation after Inoue balloon valvuloplasty. *J Am Coll Cardiol* 1993;**27**:783–9.
- This article provides an overview of the incidence, mechanisms, and predictors of traumatic mitral regurgitation.

9. **Iung B, Garbarz E, Michaud P,** et al. Late results of clinical deterioration: frequency, anatomic findings, and predictive factors. *Circulation* 1999;**99**:3272–8.
- The longest, currently available follow up following PMC is presented, together with a description of the mechanisms of late deterioration after successful PMC and an analysis of the predictors of results.

10. **Hernandez R, Bañuelos C, Alfonso F,** et al. Long-term clinical and echocardiographic follow-up after percutaneous mitral valvuloplasty with the Inoue balloon. *Circulation* 1999;**99**:1580–6.

11. **Shaw TRD, Mc Areavey D, Essop AR,** et al. Percutaneous balloon dilatation of mitral valve in patients who were unsuitable for surgical treatment. *Br Heart J* 1992;**67**:454–9.
- The results of PMC in the elderly and other patients with contraindications for surgery are reported.

12. **Ben Fahrat M, Ayari M, Maatouk F.** Percutaneous balloon versus surgical closed and open mitral commissurotomy. *Circulation* 1998;**97**:245–50.
- This article reports on the largest randomised comparison between PMC, closed, and open chest commissurotomy with a follow up of up to seven years.

13. **Iung B, Garbarz E, Doutrelant L,** et al. Late results of percutaneous mitral commissurotomy for calcific mitral stenosis. *Am J Cardiol* 2000;**85**:1308–14.
- The long term results of PMC in patients with valve calcification are presented, with a special emphasis on the multifactorial nature of prediction in this subgroup.

14. **Tuzcu EM, Block PC, Griffin BP,** et al. Immediate and long-term outcome of percutaneous mitral valvotomy in patients 65 years and older. *Circulation* 1992;**85**:963–71.

15. **Iung B, Garbarz E, Michaud P,** et al. Percutaneous mitral commissurotomy for restenosis after surgical commissurotomy: late efficacy and implications for patient selection. *J Am Coll Cardiol* 2000;**35**:1295–302.

16. **Presbitero P, Prever SB, Brusca A.** Interventional cardiology in pregnancy. *Eur Heart J* 1996;**17**:182–8.

17. **Cribier A, Savin T, Saoudi N,** et al. Percutaneous transluminal valvuloplasty of acquired aortic stenosis in elderly patients: an alternative to valve replacement? *Lancet* 1986;**11**:63–7.

18. **National Heart, Lung, and Blood Institute Balloon Registry Participants.** Percutaneous balloon aortic valvuloplasty. Acute and 30-day follow-up results in 674 patients from the NHLBI balloon valvuloplasty registry. *Circulation* 1991;**84**:2383–7.
- The immediate results using the PAV technique from a large multicentre study are presented in terms of efficacy and risk.

19. **Otto CM, Mickel MC, Kennedy W,** et al. Three-year outcome after balloon aortic valvuloplasty: insights into prognosis of valvular aortic stenosis. *Circulation* 1994;**89**:642–50.

20. **Bernard Y, Etievent J, Mourand JL** et al. Long-term results of percutaneous aortic valvuloplasty compared with aortic replacement in patients more than 75 years old. *J Am Coll Cardiol* 1992;**92**:1439–46.

10 Should patients with asymptomatic mild or moderate aortic stenosis undergoing coronary artery bypass surgery also have valve replacement for their aortic stenosis?

Shahbudin H Rahimtoola

The older you get, the closer you are to death
—an old Asian saying

In 1994-96, three studies described patients who had previously undergone coronary artery bypass graft surgery (CABG) and then had subsequent aortic valve replacement (AVR) (the aortic stenosis was "mild to moderate" at time of initial CABG); these patients were subsequently associated with a "high" operative mortality of 14–19%.[1–3]

From these studies arose the rationale that patients who have mild to moderate aortic stenosis at the time of CABG will develop severe aortic stenosis within 10 years; such patients should therefore have combined CABG+AVR at time of initial bypass surgery.[1–3]

There were several problems with this rationale, which have been previously described in detail and are summarised below.[4]

- Two subsequent studies showed that the operative mortality for later AVR, if necessary, was not significantly different from those undergoing CABG+AVR (0% and 7.7%).[5][6]
- Most importantly, these studies provided no information on the numbers of patients during the same time period who had mild to moderate aortic stenosis but did not require AVR during subsequent follow up.[4][7]
- There was little or no documentation to show that the aortic stenosis was mild to moderate at the time of the initial CABG. Moreover, some patients already had severe aortic stenosis at the time of initial CABG which was misdiagnosed.[4]
- At time of subsequent AVR, the documentation showing that aortic stenosis was severe was sketchy. Many patients had angina as their symptom and 46–75% of these patients also needed repeat CABG at the time of late AVR.[4]
- There was very little or no documentation of the patients' clinical condition at time of initial CABG and at the time of late AVR. At the time of late AVR some of the studies stated that many patients were in heart failure and New York Heart Association (NYHA) functional classes III and IV.[4]

- The rate of progression of aortic stenosis, the manner of progression and whether it was linear or not, and factors determining more rapid progression were not fully known, especially in patients who had undergone CABG.[4]

Severity of aortic stenosis

Aortic stenosis is considered to be mild when the calculated aortic valve area (AVA) is > 1.5 cm² (table 10.1).[8–12] An AVA ≤ 1.0 cm² or an AVA index ≤ 0.6 cm²/m² signify severe aortic stenosis. Reliance on gradients alone poses problems which have been previously described in detail.[4]

The gradient across an aortic valve is related to flow across the valve in systole and is a "per beat", and not a "per minute", function.[4][10][12] Thus, aortic valve gradient (AVG) is dependent on forward stroke volume from the left ventricle and systolic ejection time, both of which are a function of heart rate, and of left ventricular preload, afterload and myocardial contractility.[4][10][12] AVG is also dependent on the distal obstruction (systemic vascular resistance), and thus, on the pressure in the ascending aorta.[12] Therefore, AVGs can change from one minute to the next.

Measurement of gradients by Doppler ultrasound is clinically useful. However, their limitations must be kept in mind. Feigenbaum stated: "None of the echocardiographic techniques measures intravascular pressures directly."[13] The modified Bernoulli equation used to estimate gradients from Doppler velocities makes many assumptions, ignores several factors, and has been shown to be inaccurate in several subgroups.[4]

Peak AVG by Doppler poses particular problems[4] and it is better to calculate mean AVG. In 636 patients studied by cardiac catheterisation over a 10 year period, no AVG (peak or mean) was found that was both sensitive and specific for severe aortic stenosis.[14] A mean gradient of ≥ 50 mm Hg or a peak gradient of ≥ 60 mm Hg were "specific" with a 90% or more positive predictive value. However, it was not possible to find a lower limit with 90% negative predictive value. The authors emphasised the importance of measuring AVA[14] in all patients with suspicion of severe aortic stenosis with a cardiac catheterisation mean AVG < 50 mm Hg (present in 50% of patients in their study) and a peak of < 60 mm Hg (present in 47% of patients in their study).

Patients with low mean AVG and reduced left ventricular ejection fraction (< 0.35) may have severe aortic stenosis and frequently have

Table 10.1 Criteria for severity of aortic stenosis

Aortic stenosis	AVA[8] (cm²)	AVA[9] (cm²)	AVA[10] (cm²)	AVA index[11] (cm²/m²)
Mild	> 1.5	> 1.5	> 1.5	> 0.9
Moderate	0.95–1.4	0.8–1.5	> 1.0–1.5	> 0.6–0.9
Severe	< 0.9	< 0.8	≤ 1.0	≤ 0.6

Superscripts denote reference source.
AVA, aortic valve area.

Results of CABG alone

- An operative (30 day) mortality of ≤ 3% in those aged < 80 years and of ≥8.1% in those aged ≥80 years (table 10.2)[16–19]

- Many patients who undergo this operation will die from coronary artery disease, graft disease, graft occlusion, left ventricular dysfunction, and other comorbid conditions; approximately 30% at 10 years (table 10.3)[16 17 19 20]

- A certain percentage will need repeat revascularisation for graft disease, graft occlusion, and progression of coronary artery disease—approximately 16% at 10 years.[16]

Results of CABG+AVR initially

- An average operative mortality of 7.9% in those aged < 80 years and of 10.6% in those ≥ 80 years (table 10.2)

- Many patients will die from coronary artery disease, graft disease, graft occlusion, left ventricular dysfunction, and other comorbid conditions, and the survivors will be subject to prosthesis related deaths—approximately 60% at 10 years (table 10.3)

- A certain percentage will need repeat revascularisation for graft disease, graft occlusion, and progression of coronary artery disease—approximately 16% at 10 years.[16]

- A significant percentage will have prosthesis related complications, including reoperation for prosthetic valve malfunction—up to approximately 2–6% per year.[21 22]

Table 10.2   Operative mortality

	Years	Age	Number of patients	Operative mortality (%)
CABG				
Rahimtoola et al[16]	1974–88		7026	2.1
Davis et al[17]	1974–79		8213	2.9
Alexander et al[18]	1994–97	< 80 years	60161	3.0
		≥ 80 years	4306	8.1
CABG+AVR				
Alexander et al[18]	1994–97	< 80 years	1690	7.9
		≥ 80 years	345	10.6
Cohn et al[19]	1972–97		365	6.0

AVR, aortic valve replacement; CABG, coronary artery bypass surgery.

Mild aortic stenosis

Of two studies on the natural history of mild aortic stenosis (AVA > 1.5 cm^2) documented by cardiac catheterisation, one showed that by 10 years 8% of patients had developed severe aortic stenosis,[9] and in the other the event rate (which includes AVR plus mortality before and after AVR) was 15%.[8] Thus, it is likely that, at most, ≤ 12% of survivors who initially did not have AVR will develop severe aortic stenosis; even if one assumes that the operative mortality of late AVR in these patients may be up to 15% (probably too high an estimate of mortality rate with modern surgical technique), the total

Table 10.3   Ten year mortality

	Years	Mean age (years)	Number of patients	10 year mortality (%)
CABG				
Rahimtoola et al[16]	1974–88	61	7026	26
Davis et al[17]	1974–79	56	8213	33
			(15239)	(30)
CABG+AVR				
Cohn et al[19]	1974–97	69	365	55*
Peterseim et al[20]	1976–96	63	347	65
			(712)	(60)

*Excludes operative mortality of 6%

Table 10.4   Expected outcome of patients with severe coronary artery disease and mild aortic stenosis

	Initial CABG + AVR	Initial CABG + later AVR if necessary	Initial CABG + AVR is associated with:	
			Unnecessary AVR	Excess mortality
Total number of patients	100	100		
1. At 30 days				
(a) Mortality	8	3	100	5
2. At 3 years				
(a) Mortality	18†	9*		
(b) Late AVR in survivors	0	0	100	9
3. At 5 years				
(a) Mortality	30†	15*		
(b) Late AVR/reop AVR in survivors	0	5		
(c) 15% 30 day mortality of late AVR	0	1		
(d) Total deaths	30	16	95	14
4. At 10 years				
(a) Mortality	60†	30*		
(b) Late AVR/reop AVR in survivors	6	9‡		
(c) 15% 30 day mortality of late AVR	1	2		
(d) Total deaths	61	32	91	29

*Mortality after CABG
†Mortality after CABG+AVR
‡No late deaths from mild aortic stenosis other than mortality after late AVR for late severe aortic stenosis.
Repeat revascularisation should be similar in both groups; its incidence and associated mortality are not included.
Ten year complications after revascularisation and with prosthetic heart valves are not included.
Mortality at time of reoperation are included in the 5 and 10 year data. The assumed 15% mortality for reoperation is probably too high.

associated coronary artery disease; these patients therefore pose a more difficult clinical problem.[12] However, they benefit from CABG+AVR, and thus there is a need for early diagnosis and surgery in such patients.[12 15]

Resolution of the problem

This clinical situation is more common in older patients (average age at time of initial CABG ≥ 60 years)[4] and their mortality with or without surgery can be expected to be greater than in younger patients, especially if they have associated comorbid conditions. In the cited studies, late AVR was performed on average 8–9 years after the initial CABG.[4]

Since there are no good prospective studies or trials addressing this clinical circumstance, one way to proceed is to: (1) determine the 10 year results of CABG+AVR; and (2) determine the 10 year results of isolated CABG and add to this the outcome of patients with mild to moderate aortic stenosis.

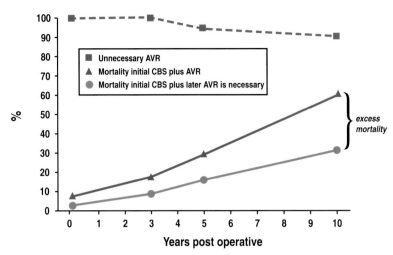

Figure 10.1. Projected patient outcomes in those with severe coronary artery disease who are to undergo coronary bypass surgery and also have mild aortic stenosis. AVR, aortic valve replacement; CBS, coronary bypass surgery.

number of deaths from late AVR will be very small. Moreover, at the end of five years only 5% will need AVR.

If initially 100 patients had CABG+AVR, then at the end of 30 days, three years, and five years, the expected number of unnecessary AVRs would be 100, 100, and 95 and the number of excess deaths would be five, nine, and 14, respectively (table 10.4).

At 10 years, to reduce one death from late AVR by a policy of AVR for mild aortic stenosis at time of initial CABG in 100 patients (table 10.4), the projected cumulative incidence of unnecessary AVR would be 91 and that of excess deaths would be 29, when compared to a policy of initial isolated CABG and later AVR if necessary (fig 10.1). It should be noted that figures for reoperation, and mortality associated with reoperation, are included in the 10 year estimated outcome data in table 10.4 and fig 10.1.

Summary

- The results after 10 years of a policy of initial CABG+AVR for mild and for moderate aortic stenosis are summarised in table 10.6

- A uniform policy of initial CABG for severe CAD plus AVR cannot be supported at this time for:
  - mild aortic stenosis (AVA > 1.5 cm^2, AVA index > 0.9cm^2/m^2)
  - moderate aortic stenosis (AVA > 1.0–1.5 cm^2, AVA index > 0.6–0.9 cm^2/m^2)

- In view of the uncertainty of rate of progression of calcific aortic stenosis in older patients, at this time, CABG for severe coronary artery disease plus AVR may be reasonable for moderate aortic stenosis (AVA ⩽ 1.2 cm^2, AVA index ⩽ 0.8 cm^2/m^2) in patients ⩾ 60–65 years of age, provided the patients are not at high risk for thromboembolism, and thus can receive a biological valve (bioprosthesis)

- In patients with severe coronary artery disease and low mean AVG great care should be taken to ensure that severe aortic stenosis is not being misdiagnosed, especially in those in whom the left ventricular ejection fraction is reduced

- All patients with severe aortic stenosis (AVA ⩽ 1.0 cm^2, AVA index ⩽ 0.6cm^2/m^2) and severe coronary artery disease should have AVR at the time of CABG.

- Properly designed and carefully performed prospective studies are needed.

Table 10.5   Expected outcome of patients with severe coronary artery disease and moderate aortic stenosis

	Initial CABG + AVR	Initial CABG + later AVR if necessary	Initial CABG + AVR is associated with:	
			Unnecessary AVR	Excess mortality
Total number of patients	100	100		
1. At 30 days				
(a) Mortality	8	3	100	5
2. At 3 years				
(a) Mortality	18†	9*		
(b) Late AVR in survivors	0	0	100	9
3. At 5 years				
(a) Mortality	30†	15*		
(b) Late AVR/reop AVR in survivors	0	15		
(c) 15% 30 day mortality of late AVR	0	2		
(d) Total deaths	30	17	85	13
4. At 10 years				
(a) Mortality	60†	30*		
(b) Late AVR/reop AVR in survivors	6	46‡		
(c) 15% 30 day mortality of late AVR	1	7		
(d) Total deaths	61	37	54	24

*Mortality after CABG
†Mortality after CABG+AVR
‡Events (death+AVR) at 10 years is 65%; for this analysis it was considered 65% of 70 survivors (that is, 46) would need late AVR which is most likely an overestimate.
Repeat revascularisation similar in both groups; its incidence and associated mortality are not included.
Ten year complications after revascularisation and with prosthetic heart valves are not included.
Mortality at time of reoperation are included in the 5 and 10 year data. The assumed 15% mortality for reoperation is probably too high.

Moderate aortic stenosis

The natural history of moderate aortic stenosis is more difficult to estimate for a number of reasons. One study[8] provided information only on event-free survival which was 100% at the end of three years and 35% at the end of 10 years. Since all the events occurred in the intervening years, the event-free survival at five years can be expected to be about 81%. The event-free survival includes AVR plus mortality before and after AVR; the need for late AVR is not given separately.[8]

A further study classified moderate aortic stenosis as an AVA of 0.8–1.5cm^2.[9] However, another study has shown that the incidence of death and AVR in patients with "moderate" aortic stenosis (AVA of 0.7–1.2 cm^2) is 10% per year[23]; many of these patients in fact had severe aortic stenosis,[9 23]—that is, AVA ⩽ 1.0 cm^2 (table 10.1).

Other issues include the problem of assessing aortic stenosis progression, which has been extensively reviewed,[4] and the conflicting data over whether aortic stenosis in older patients progresses more rapidly than in younger

75

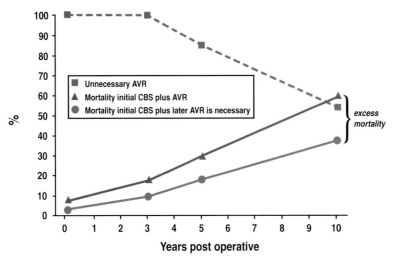

Figure 10.2. Projected patient outcomes in those with severe coronary artery disease who are to undergo coronary bypass surgery and also have moderate aortic stenosis. AVR, aortic valve replacement; CBS, coronary bypass surgery.

patients.[24][25] Thus, even if one assumes that 65% of the survivors who initially did not have AVR will develop severe aortic stenosis (an overestimate) and will need late AVR, and that the operative mortality of late AVR in these patients may be up to 15% (probably too high), the total number of deaths from late AVR will be quite small.

If initially, 100 patients had CABG+AVR, then at the end of 30 days, three years, and five years, the expected number of unnecessary AVRs would be 100, 100, and 85, and the number of excess deaths would be five, nine, and 13, respectively (table 10.5). It should be noted that the figures for reoperation, and mortality associated with reoperation, are included in the 10 year estimated outcome data in table 10.5 and fig 10.2.

At 10 years, to reduce six deaths from late AVR by a policy of AVR for moderate aortic stenosis at time of initial CABG in 100 patients (table 10.5), the projected cumulative incidence of unnecessary AVR would be 54 and that of excess deaths would be 24 when compared to a policy of initial isolated CABG and later AVR if necessary (fig 10.2).

In view of the uncertainty of the rate of progression of calcific aortic stenosis in older patients, at this time CABG for severe coronary artery disease plus AVR may be reasonable for moderate aortic stenosis with an AVA ≤ 1.2 cm^2 and an AVA index ≤ 0.8 cm^2/m^2 in patients ≥ 60–65 years of age, provided the patients are not at high risk for thromboembo-

lism,[11] and thus can receive a biological valve (bioprosthesis).[11][22]

In patients who initially had only CABG, at the time of subsequent AVR there is a risk of damage to internal mammary and vein grafts. Although this risk is small with appropriate care, and with skilled and experienced surgeons, it must be recognised this risk applies to reoperation in both subgroups (CABG and CABG+AVR).

1. **Collins JJ, Aranki SF.** Management of mild aortic stenosis during coronary artery bypass graft surgery. *J Cardiovasc Surg* 1994;**9**(suppl):145–7.

2. **Odell JA, Mullany CJ, Schaff HV,** *et al.* Aortic valve replacement after previous coronary artery bypass grafting. *Ann Thorac Surg* 1996;**62**:1424–30.

3. **Fighali SF, Avendaño A, Elayda MA,** *et al.* Early and late mortality of patients undergoing aortic valve replacement after previous coronary artery bypass graft surgery. *Circulation* 1995;**92**(suppl II):II-163–68.

4. **Rahimtoola SH.** "Prophylactic" valve replacement for mild aortic valve disease at time of surgery for other cardiovascular disease? . . .No. *J Am Coll Cardiol* 1999;**33**:2009–15.
• *A review detailing problems of the relevant studies, and assessment of severity and progression of aortic stenosis. Also presents suggested management of such patients.*

5. **Hoff SJ, Merrill WH, Stewart JR,** *et al.* Safety of remote aortic valve replacement after prior coronary artery bypass grafting. *Ann Thorac Surg* 1996;**61**:1689–92.

6. **Sundt TM, III, Murphy SF, Barzilai B,** *et al.* Previous coronary artery bypass grafting is not a risk factor for aortic valve replacement. *Ann Thorac Surg* 1997;**64**:651–8.

7. **Spodick DH.** Revascularization of the heart numerators in search of denominators. *Am Heart J* 1971;**81**:149–57.
• *An early article describing the problem of assessing patient outcome after treatment when the outcome of the total number of patients with that disorder is not known.*

8. **Turina J, Hess O, Sepulcri F,** *et al.* Spontaneous course of aortic valve disease. *Eur Heart J* 1987;**8**:471–83.
• *A study that details the natural history of all grades of aortic valve disease.*

9. **Horstkotte D, Loogen F.** The natural history of aortic valve stenosis. *Eur Heart J* 1988;**9**(suppl E):57–64.
• *A further study detailing the natural history of aortic stenosis.*

10. **Rahimtoola SH.** Perspective on valvular heart disease: an update. *J Am Coll Cardiol* 1989;**14**:1–23.
• *A review of several aspects of valvar heart disease including that of the natural history of aortic stenosis and grading its severity (155 cited references).*

11. **Bonow RO, Carabello B, de Leon AC Jr,** *et al.* ACC/AHA guidelines for the management of patients with valvular heart disease. *J Am Coll Cardiol* 1998;**32**:1486–8.
• *An exhaustive review of valvar heart disease with guidelines on diagnosis and management (102 pages, 737 cited references).*

Table 10.6 *Results after 10 years of a policy of initial CABG+AVR for mild and moderate aortic stenosis*

	Severe CAD and mild AS: 100 patients	Severe CAD and moderate AS: 100 patients
• To eliminate:		
– late AVR	9	46*
– deaths from late AVR	2	7
• Results in		
– unnecessary AVR	91	54
– excess deaths	29	24

*An overestimate—see text.
AS, aortic stenosis; CAD, coronary artery disease.

12. **Rahimtoola SH.** Severe aortic stenosis with low systolic gradient: the good and bad news. *Circulation* 2000;**101**:1892–4.
• *A review of severe aortic stenosis with low ejection fraction and low aortic valve gradient, emphasising the importance of early diagnosis and management.*

13. **Feigenbaum H.** *Echocardiography*, 5th ed. Philadelphia: Lea & Febiger, 1993:195–6.

14. **Griffith MJ, Carey C, Coltart DJ,** *et al.* Inaccuracies of using aortic valve gradients alone to grade severity of aortic stenosis. *Br Heart J* 1989;**62**:372–8.
• *A large study documenting the need to obtain aortic valve areas to assess severity of aortic stenosis.*

15. **Connolly HM, Oh JK, Schaff HV,** *et al.* Severe aortic stenosis with low transvalvar gradient and severe left ventricular dysfunction: result of aortic valve replacement in 52 patients. *Circulation* 2000;**101**:1940–6.

16. **Rahimtoola SH, Fessler CL, Grunkemeier GL,** *et al.* Survival 15 to 20 years after coronary bypass surgery for angina. *J Am Coll Cardiol* 1993;**21**:151–7.

17. **Davis KB, Chaitman B, Ryan T,** *et al.* Comparison of 15-year survival for men and women after initial medical or surgical treatment for coronary artery disease: a CASS registry study. *J Am Coll Cardiol* 1995;**25**:1000–9.

18. **Alexander KP, Anstrom KJ, Muhlbaier LH,** *et al.* Outcomes of cardiac surgery in patients age ≥80 years: results from the national cardiovascular network. *J Am Coll Cardiol* 2000;**35**:731–8.

• *A study of over 67 000 patients describing the operative mortality of isolated aortic and mitral valve replacement and when combined with associated coronary bypass surgery.*

19. **Cohn LH, Collins Jr JJ, Rizzo RJ,** *et al.* Twenty-year follow-up of the Hancock modified orifice porcine aortic valve. *Ann Thorac Surg* 1998;**66**:S30–4.

20. **Peterseim DS, Cen Y-Y, Cheruvu S,** *et al.* Long-term outcome after biologic versus mechanical aortic valve replacement in 841 patients. *J Thorac Cardiovasc Surg* 1999;**117**:890–7.

21. **Kirklin JW, Barrat-Boyles BG.** Aortic valve disease. In: *Cardiac surgery*, 2nd ed. New York: Churchill Livingstone, 1992:491–57.

22. **Hammermeister KE, Sethi GK, Henderson WG,** *et al.* Outcomes 15 years after valve replacement with a mechanical versus a bioprosthetic valve: final report of the VA randomized trial. *J Am Coll Cardiol* 2000;**36**:1152–8.

23. **Kennedy KD, Nishimura RA, Holmes DR,** *et al.* Natural history of moderate aortic stenosis. *J Am Coll Cardiol* 1991;**17**:313–19.

24. **Wagner S, Selzer A.** Patterns of progression of aortic stenosis: a longitudinal hemodynamic study. *Circulation* 1982;**65**:709–12.

25. **Nestico PF, DePace NL, Kimbris D,** *et al.* Progression of isolated aortic stenosis: analysis of 29 patients having more than 1 cardiac catheterization. *Am J Cardiol* 1983;**52**:1054–8.

77

11 Endocarditis: problems—patients being treated for endocarditis and not doing well

Celia M Oakley, Roger J C Hall

Most patients with infective endocarditis respond to appropriate antibiotic treatment within 72 hours, with a definitive loss of fever and improvement in general well being. Patients who show such prompt improvement will usually do well, but those who remain febrile and septic despite optimal antibiotics usually need surgery.[1] Late recurrence of fever is frequently the result of antibiotic sensitivity or an infected central line, and is less often caused by the development of bacterial resistance, infection by multiple organisms or a second infection by fungus or staphylococcus. Lack of success in treating endocarditis frequently comes from failure to observe recognised guidelines,[2 3] and from lack of a team approach involving both the clinical microbiologist and the cardiac surgeon from an early stage.

Persistent or recurrent fever

Microbiological issues
From the outset the clinical microbiologist needs to be involved closely. The treatment regimen needs to be matched to both the clinical and microbiological circumstances. When there is a continuing clinical problem, despite appropriate initial treatment, then the microbiologist must be consulted again.

Infection elsewhere
The possibility of infection occurring elsewhere—intracardiac or extracardiac—must be the first thought of the clinician faced with this situation.

Line infection
A common cause of recurrence of fever is the central line. This should be removed and the tip sent for culture. Often the culture is sterile but the fever resolves rapidly after removal of the line. Recolonisation of the infected valve by staphylococcus or fungus derived from the line is rare but can occur. It is usually caused by poor sterile technique and line care. Such additional infection is a serious problem. It needs appropriate antibiotic treatment and frequently requires urgent surgery.

Paravalvar/intracardiac abscess
The patient not doing well despite being infected by an antibiotic sensitive organism probably has a paravalvar abscess until proved otherwise. This must be sought vigorously and usually requires surgery to effect a cure.[4] Most patients with paravalvar abscesses also have severe valvar regurgitation and heart failure with evidence of uncontrolled infection.[5] Therefore there is usually little or no difficulty in arriving at the decision to advise urgent surgery both to remove the infected tissue and to replace the leaking valve.

If there is a proven abscess plus evidence of persistent sepsis but without severe valvar regurgitation, the clinician is often slow to recommend surgery because he or she believes that the antibiotics will eventually produce a cure. This is nearly always a mistaken belief and surgery should be carried out sooner rather than later. Occasionally abscesses will discharge into the heart leaving a cavity with a wide entrance that the antibiotics can sterilise, but this is rare. It is not an event which should be anticipated thereby delaying the needed surgical cure.

In a small percentage of patients the infection appears to be under control and there is no haemodynamic requirement for surgery, but abscess is detected on echocardiography (usually transoesophageal echocardiography (TOE)) (fig 11.1). On cessation of the antibiotics the infection nearly always returns unless the very rare occurrence of internal discharge of the abscess has occurred. In this respect some abscesses appear to be functionally inaccessible to circulating antibiotics, and in such circumstances patients will usually need to undergo surgery.[6]

Coxiella produces an indolent illness but often with extensive local abscess formation.[7] Diagnosis depends on a high index of suspicion in patients in whom no infecting organism has been found immediately. Such patients should routinely have serology for Q fever even if there is no known contact with animals. These

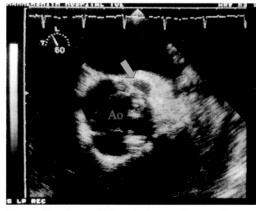

Figure 11.1. Aortic (Ao) root abscess (arrowed) shown in short axis of transoesophageal study. Figure reproduced courtesy of Dr Petros Nihoyannopoulos.

patients often have only intermittent fever. Constitutional symptoms also are sometimes intermittent and clinical examination can be unrevealing in the early stages. Later on hepatosplenomegaly may dominate the clinical scene, deflecting attention away from the heart.[8]

Although echocardiography via the transoesophageal route, particularly with a multiplane transducer, has greatly improved the detection of abscesses, not all are visible. Most abscesses are para-aortic. In a French study nearly 90% of aortic abscesses subsequently confirmed at surgery had been seen by transoesophageal study compared with less than 50% via the transthoracic route.[5] They may be missed if they are in the aortic wall. Mitral ring abscesses were less common, were only rarely detected by the transthoracic route, and more than half had still been missed by TOE in this study.[5] Echocardiography can only detect abscesses which show a difference in acoustic properties compared to the surrounding tissue or when there is Doppler evidence of flow through a defect or communication caused by the abscess. If no such difference or abnormal flow exists, echocardiography will miss the diagnosis—no technique is 100% sensitive. If the clinical picture points to an abscess but none is detected this is an unusual but a good reason to repeat the TOE in a few days.

Extracardiac
Metastatic infection or mycotic aneurysm may cause fever. Any remote pain or focal symptoms should raise suspicion. Headache, particularly if lateralised, may suggest cerebral abscess or a mycotic aneurysm of a cerebral vessel. Mycotic aneurysms can present during the course of treatment or even after a satisfactory microbiological cure has been achieved and the antibiotic treatment has been completed. Adjacent aseptic meningitis is common. Focal signs in the nervous system may be absent but a computed tomographic scan of the brain may bring surprises. Abscesses in the frontal lobes may cause no more than a change in personality or there may be multiple infarcts in relatively silent areas.

Acute low back pain may be caused by spinal abscess formation and vertebral osteomyelitis or discitis should be suspected, particularly when there is evidence of a radiculopathy.[9]

Antibiotic problems
The development of drug sensitivity may lead to recurrence of fever with or without a rash but usually with a blood eosinophilia and a rise in C reactive protein in a patient who had been previously doing well. The patient is often not clinically ill or septic, but occasionally such patients feel and look very unwell. This is usually a reaction to a penicillin, most often in the third week of treatment. Sometimes, it may be appropriate to stop antibiotic treatment or it may be considered wise to continue with a different combination chosen on the advice of the bacteriologist.

Surgical goals
• Restoration of haemodynamic competence
• Removal of all infected tissue

Wrong diagnosis or more than one diagnosis
It is possible that the patient being treated for infective endocarditis and not doing well may have been given a wrong or incomplete diagnosis. The patient may have been regarded as having culture negative infective endocarditis or the positive cultures may have been misleading or not have grown a typical organism. If vegetations are seen, they may not be caused by infective endocarditis and in reality may be sterile thrombotic vegetations in a patient with adenocarcinoma or systemic lupus. The fever and rise in acute phase reactants may be caused by lymphoma, tuberculosis, opportunistic infection in AIDS or active autoimmune disease or, rarely, the patient may have a fever producing portal of entry such as ulcerative colitis, or carcinoma or Hodgkin's disease in addition to infective endocarditis.

It is obvious that whereas patients with any of these conditions are not harmed by administration of unnecessary antibiotics, steroid treatment of a patient with infective endocarditis on a false diagnosis of polyarteritis may be lethal.

Major immune activation
Immune activation, particularly with progressive renal failure, may be another cause for a patient failing to improve despite antibiotic treatment. In these patients blood cultures may have been negative (even if there has been no previous antibiotic treatment) and negative serology and microbiology will have excluded infection by cell dependent organisms. There may be doubt about the diagnosis but flamboyant vegetations are usually seen on echocardiography and the patient may have had emboli. Changing the antibiotics fails to help. In these rare patients deterioration will continue until removal and replacement of the valve. No organisms may be grown from it or stain microscopically, but the rapid improvement that follows surgical intervention clearly shows that the bacterial antigen had persisted in the valve. There is a danger of such patients being falsely diagnosed as having Libmann-Sacks (in association with systemic lupus erythematosus) or marantic endocarditis but, unlike such patients, they have an erosive destructive endocarditis with positive rheumatoid factor but no lupus specific antibodies. Renal biopsy shows a focal crescentic glomerulitis and a "lumpy bumpy" deposit of polyclonal immunoglobulins on the basement membrane shown on immunofluorescence microscopy.[10 11]

Multiple organisms
Infection by multiple organisms is unusual and is most often seen in intravenous drug abusers. Again the advice of the microbiologist on

appropriate treatment should be sought and consideration given to surgery.

Acute myocardial and valvar problems, disappearing murmur or insignificant murmurs

---

MYOCARDIAL PROBLEMS

These are important although not very common. The patient may be unwell because of a low cardiac output which may be caused by coronary embolism with myocardial infarction or intramyocardial abscess formation (fig 11.2). Infectious myocardial infiltration or toxic myocardial depression may also be responsible, but this is rare.

VALVAR PROBLEMS

A low cardiac output leading to cardiogenic shock and/or pulmonary oedema more commonly results from a sudden increase in mitral or aortic regurgitation. Chordal rupture and a flail, or perforated mitral valve or perforation/prolapse of an aortic cusp, may lead to free regurgitation. In both situations the very severe regurgitation alters the haemodynamics in such a way that the physical signs of the valve lesion and particularly the murmur may become insignificant and the clinical picture is dominated by the low cardiac output and a loud gallop rhythm.

Mitral valve

Reduction in gradient between a low left ventricular systolic pressure and a high left atrial systolic V wave in severe mitral regurgitation results in a softer or even disappearing murmur and a plummeting forward stroke output.

Aortic valve

Tachycardia and rapid diastolic equilibration of central aortic and left ventricular diastolic pressures in acute aortic regurgitation may obliterate the murmur and, by closing the mitral valve prematurely (an important sign on the M mode echocardiogram), severely limit forward flow.

In both situations urgent transthoracic echocardiography and Doppler usually confirm the cause of the clinical problem; if there is any doubt TOE should be done without delay. Such patients need immediate surgery, and

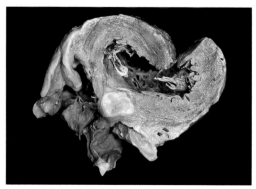

Figure 11.2. Myocardial abscess. These are usually inoperable.

Indications for surgery

- Haemodynamic
  – acute aortic or mitral regurgitation

- Staphylococcal infection
  – often urgently

- Infective endocarditis which is difficult to cure medically
  – fungus: always
  – coxiella: usually
  – chlamydia: usually
  – *Staphylococcus epidermidis*

- Persistent fever
  – abscess: paravalvar or extracardiac

- Major immune activation
  – persistent fever despite appropriate antibiotics

- Emboli
  –remove very large vegetations (early or not at all)

---

cardiac catheterisation before surgery usually causes dangerous delay and a fluid load when time is of the essence.[6 12–14]

Role of surgery in the problem patient

When a patient is not doing well the possible benefits that might come from surgery should be considered. The goals of surgery are to remove all infected tissue and to restore haemodynamic competence. In the majority of patients who are not doing well while being treated for infective endocarditis, the problem is either uncontrolled infection, a haemodynamic problem, or a combination of both; surgery is therefore frequently essential. This is the most compelling reason for involving a surgeon at an early stage in the management of most patients with infective endocarditis. Surgeons are far happier to act quickly and appropriately when needed if they already know the patient or are at least familiar with the details through discussion.

The benefits of surgery are often enormous and usually almost immediate. It reverses a deteriorating haemodynamic situation, which uncorrected will often lead to death, and has the added advantage of removing infection which was "hidden" from the antibiotics—for example, in an abscess. Removal of infected tissue also leads to a rapid overall constitutional improvement as the infected burden is drastically reduced.

Staphylococcal infection

Staphylococcal endocarditis may cause rapid tissue destruction and embolism, although vegetations may be difficult or impossible to detect. Surgical treatment is needed at once in patients who are toxic despite adequate antibiotics or who have evidence of abscess formation either on echocardiography or deduced

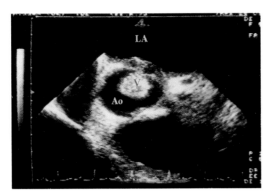

Figure 11.3. Huge pedunculated vegetation (V) on the aortic valve caused by secondary candida infection in a young women with a variable course after treatment for enterococcal infection on a floppy mitral valve. Transoesophageal view—LA, left atrium; Ao, aorta. Figure reproduced courtesy of Dr Petros Nihoyannopoulos.

from ECG conduction system delay (prolonged PR interval). Failure to act quickly in this situation often leads to a fatal outcome. Emergency surgery in these situations is the only treatment which provides any chance of averting a fatal outcome and preventing spread of infection despite full antibiotic treatment.

Nosocomial staphylococcal endocarditis (caused by coagulase negative staphylococci originating from the patient) carries a particularly high mortality because it is often not suspected in patients being treated for other diseases (particularly renal failure) and who are not known to have valve disease. It is diagnosed late and tends not to be operated on because of co-morbidity. The portal of entry is usually an indwelling intravenous line.[15]

FUNGI AND OTHER ORGANISMS
Infection by certain organisms usually requires surgical excision because although they are technically sensitive to antimicrobial agents (albeit often very toxic in the case of fungi), they rarely if ever are cured without surgery. This always applies to fungus infection (fig 11.3), which usually occurs following antibiotic treatment or parenteral feeding in a patient who has had major abdominal surgery; alternatively the fungal infection may have gained entry at or just after cardiac surgery, especially in patients with wound infections or mediastinitis.

Similarly in patients with infective endocarditis caused by coxiella (Q fever) or chlamydia, the infection may appear to respond to antibiotics only to recur when they are stopped; in general, the patient needs either surgical excision of the infection or lifelong antibiotics, or sometimes both.[14]

PREVENTION OF EMBOLISM
Surgery to prevent embolism is a contentious area. The patient may have had previous emboli or have large vegetations when first examined. Since the risk of embolism diminishes rapidly after the onset of antibiotic treatment, the decision for surgery to prevent embolism or further embolism in a patient with large vegetations when first seen should be made immediately and the surgery carried out urgently or not at all.[16] Vegetations over 10 mm

in diameter are associated with an increased risk of embolism but this risk has never been quantified accurately, nor has it been proved to be higher than risk posed by an operation to remove the vegetation. Often the decision is made easier because the large vegetation is associated with a degree of valve regurgitation that merits surgery in its own right, and the vegetation is removed with the valve. Vegetations, which are viewed anxiously day after day, will probably not become emboli.

In the past it was taught that anticoagulant treatment was contraindicated in infective endocarditis. However, since it will not influence the risk or result of rupture of a mycotic aneurysm the usual indications for anticoagulant treatment apply. Control of the international normalised ratio (INR) needs to be meticulous and is often difficult because of the interplay of other factors such as changes in diet, the influence of antibiotics on the INR, and pro-coagulant states induced by the infection. Patients who are sufficiently ill to be in bed should receive prophylactic heparin, but most patients should be encouraged to be up and about. There is some evidence that low dose aspirin may reduce the size of vegetations and lower the risk of embolism.[17]

ANTIBIOTIC TREATMENT AND SURGERY
The management of antibiotic treatment in the immediate preoperative period and following surgery needs careful planning. In general it is a serious mistake to delay urgently needed surgery in an attempt to give more antibiotics before surgery. This issue will be addressed in a separate article.

RESULTS OF SURGERY
Comparisons between the results of medical and surgical treatment have been made in many publications but are flawed from the scientific point of view mainly because of case selection. No randomised prospective trials of medical versus surgical treatment have ever been done or are ever likely to be done because they could include only patients suitable for medical treatment alone and thus would be neither ethical nor informative.

In certain circumstances, surgery may not be an option. For example, fig 2 shows an abscess in the wall of the left ventricle remote from an infected aortic valve. Sometimes detected by echocardiography, such abscesses are fortunately rare because they usually present the surgeon with an impossible task.

Because of the lack of an evidence base, decision making regarding surgery in infective endocarditis must be based on common sense and clinical experience. On this basis aggressive early surgery appears to reduce the mortality of this disease greatly. The threshold for surgical intervention is still too high in many centres, but despite this surgery must be reserved for patients with a definite indication.[11 12 15 17] Early surgery is rarely regretted and very close observation with frequent clinical examination, and ECGs and echocardiograms repeated from time to time, will allow the timing to be decided appropriately. Undue

Failure to respond: summary

- Abscess formation
  - paravalvar
  - metastatic

- Low cardiac output
  - flail mitral valve or perforation
  - free aortic regurgitation
  - toxic myocardial depression or infectious infiltration
  - coronary embolism

- Wrong diagnosis
  - lymphoma
  - sarcoidosis
  - autoimmune disease—for example, systemic lupus erythematosus
  - AIDS
  - tuberculosis

- Major immune activation
  - progressive renal failure
  - vasculitis
  - emboli

delay is fraught with hazard, increasing the technical difficulties for the surgeon, extending the length of time spent in hospital, reducing the patient's chance of an uncomplicated recovery, and increasing future morbidity and the need for further surgery. It is of particular importance not to delay surgery in order to give more preoperative antibiotics in a patient with a strong indication for surgery

1. **Weinstein L.** Infective endocarditis. In: Braunwald E, ed. *Heart disease. A textbook of cardiovascular medicine*, 3rd ed. Philadelphia: WB Saunders Co, 1988:1093–134.

2. **Delahaye F, Rial M-O, de Gevigney G,** *et al.* A critical appraisal of the quality of the management of infective endocarditis. *J Am Coll Cardiol* 1999;**33**:788–93.
- *This report from leaders in the field testifies to the frequent neglect of established principles and publicised guidelines revealed in a French regional survey.*

3. **Littler WA, Simmons NA, Ball AP,** *et al.* Antibiotic treatment of streptococcal, enterococcal and staphylococcal endocarditis. *Heart* 1998;**79**:207–10.

4. **Brecker SJD, Pepper JR, Eykyn SJ.** Aortic root abscess [editorial]. *Heart* 1999;**82**:260–2.

5. **Choussat Thomas D, Isnard R, Michel PL,** *et al.* Perivalvular abscesses associated with endocarditis. Clinical features and prognostic factors of overall survival in a series of 233 cases. *Eur Heart J* 1999;**20**:232–41.

6. **Colombo T, Lanfranchi M, Passini L,** *et al.* Active infective endocarditis: surgical approach. *Eur J Cardiovasc Surg* 1994;**8**:15–24.

7. **Palmer WR, Young SEJ.** Q fever endocarditis in England and Wales 1975-81. Lancet 1982;ii:1448–9.
- *Chronic coxiella (Q fever) infection means endocarditis in any patient who has structural heart disease whether or not echocardiography is positive, and this review indicates that the disease is not a great rarity.*

8. **Turck WPG, Howitt G, Turnberg,** *et al.* Chronic Q fever. *QJM* 1976;**178**:192–217.

9. **Buchman A.** Streptococcus viridans osteomyelitis with endocarditis presenting as acute onset lower back pain. *J Emerg Med* 1989;**8**:21.
- *The first referral is often to a rheumatologist, with symptoms attributed to collagen vascular disease rather than infection; acute low back pain is also a frequent early manifestation.*

10. **Phair JP, Clarke J.** Immunology of infective endocarditis. *Prog Cardiovasc Dis* 1979;**22**:137–44.

11. **Bayer AS, Theofilopoulos AN.** Immunopathogenetic aspects of infective endocarditis. *Chest* 1990;**97**:204.

12. **Stulz P, Pfisterer M, Jenzer HR,** *et al.* Emergency valve replacement for active infective endocarditis. *J Cardiovasc Surg* 1989;**30**:20–6.

13. **Danchin N, Retournay G, Stchepinsky S,** *et al.* Comparison of long term outcome in patients with or without aortic ring abscess treated surgically for aortic valve endocarditis. *Heart* 1999;**81**:177–81.

14. **Chaturredi R, de Leval M, Sullivan ID.** Urgent homograft aortic root replacement for aortic root abscess in infants and children. *Heart* 1999;**81**:62–6.

15. **Lamas CC, Eykyn SJ.** Hospital acquired native valve disease endocarditis: analysis of 22 cases presenting over 11 years. *Heart* 1998;**442**:7.
- *A high mortality because heart disease is not known and the patients are already sick. Meticulous care of intravenous lines and their earliest possible removal are obvious imperatives.*

16. **Steckelberg JM, Murphy JG, Ballard D** *et al.* Emboli in infective endocarditis: the prognostic value of echocardiography. *Ann Intern Med* 1991;**114**:635–40.

17. **Taha TH, Darrant S, Crick C,** *et al.* Haemostatic studies in patients with infective endocarditis: a report of nine consecutive cases with evidence of coagulopathy. *Heart and Vessels* 1991;**6**:102–6.

12 Prosthetic valve endocarditis

C Piper, R Körfer, D Horstkotte

After 40 years of continuous improvements in the design and materials used for prosthetic heart valves, valve replacement surgery is now performed with low morbidity and mortality. These advantages have been hampered by a few but severe adverse effects; in particular, infections of the prosthetic material continue to be an extremely serious complication occurring with a relatively low but increasing frequency ranging from 0.1–2.3% per patient year.[1–3] The prosthesis obviously predisposes to device related infections, especially those caused by novobiocin susceptible, coagulase negative staphylococci, which are able to adhere to a variety of surfaces[4] and produce an antibiotic resistant biofilm.[5] [6]

Definition and frequency

Prosthetic valve endocarditis (PVE) is an endovascular, microbial infection occurring on parts of a valve prosthesis or on reconstructed native heart valves.[7] It is recommended to determine whether (a) a mechanical prosthesis, (b) a bioprosthetic xenograft, stented or unstented, (c) an allograft, (d) a homograft, or (e) a repaired native valve with or without implantation of an annular ring is involved.[8] Although clinical relevance and therapeutic considerations may be similar, infections of devices or lines placed inside the heart but not connected to the endocardial structures should be classified as "polymer associated infections" rather than PVE.

PVE should be classified as either being acquired perioperatively, and thus nosocomial (early PVE), or as community acquired (late PVE).[8] Because of significant differences in microbiology of PVE observed within the first year of operation and later on, the time cut off point between early and late PVE should be regarded as one year.[9]

The risk for early PVE is higher (approximately 5%) in patients with replacement surgery during active infective endocarditis, especially if the causal organism is unknown or the antibiotic treatment is insufficient. The incidence of late PVE is lower for mechanical prostheses than for bioprostheses. The weighted mean incidence for infections of bioprostheses calculated from published series is 0.49% per patient year for mitral valves and 0.91% per patient year for aortic valves. For mechanical prostheses, the incidence is 0.18% per patient year for mitral, 0.27% per patient year for aortic, and 0.29% per patient year for multiple implants.[10]

Comparing different periods of implantation, hazard functions reveal a significant decline in early PVE cases in recent years, contrasting with a slight increase in the hazard for late PVE (fig 12.1).

Pathogenesis

Prostheses made from metal, pyrolyte or other materials do not allow adherence of microorganisms as long as they are free from thrombotic material. Infections of mechanical prostheses generally originate from the sewing cuff or from thrombi located near the sewing ring downstream in recirculation areas. Inflammatory periprosthetic leaks, ring abscesses, and invasion of the infective process into the adjacent tissue are common findings. The pathogenesis of bioprosthetic infections may be similar to that of native valves. In these cases, the infection is restricted to the cusps, eventually initiating secondary bioprosthetic failure but with only a low tendency to invade the sewing cuff or to result in periprosthetic abscesses.[10] If the sewing cuff, however, is involved, the pathogenesis and clinical course are more or less the same as in PVE involving mechanical prostheses.

Microbiology

The microbiology of PVE is very different from that of native valve endocarditis (NVE). Streptococci and enterococci occur less frequently, while staphylococci, bacteria of the HACEK group (*Haemophilus, Actinobacillus, Cardiobacterium, Eikinella*, and *Kingella*), and fungi are found more frequently in cases of PVE. Novobiocin susceptible, coagulase negative staphylococci have a particularly high affinity for implanted or indwelling foreign surfaces, especially polymers.[4] They are the most frequent

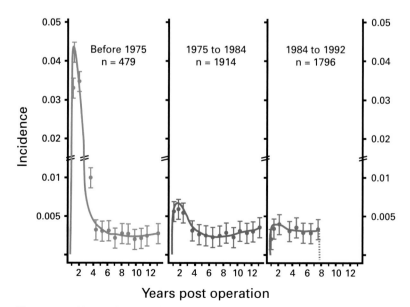

Figure 12.1. Hazard functions for prosthetic valve endocarditis in 4189 consecutive patients during three successive follow up periods.

Definition, pathogenesis, and microbiology of prosthetic valve endocarditis (PVE)

- Microbial infection of parts of a prosthetic valve or reconstructed native heart valve

- Early PVE is usually acquired perioperatively (nosocomial)

- Late PVE is mostly community acquired

- Time cut off point between early and late PVE should be one year (notable differences in microbiology)

- The risk of early PVE is higher (approximately 5%) in patients with replacement surgery during active infective endocarditis

- Mechanical prosthesis infections originate from the sewing cuff or from nearby located thrombi → periprosthetic leaks, ring abscesses, invasion of adjacent tissue

- Bioprosthesis infections mostly are restricted to the cusps → secondary bioprosthetic failure

- Staphylococci (especially novobiocin susceptible, coagulase negative staphylococci), bacteria of the HACEK group, and fungi occur more frequently in PVE

- Streptococci and enterococci are found more frequently in native valve endocarditis

pathogens causing PVE. The usual spectrum for Europe is given in table 12.1.

Diagnostic approach

The diagnostic approach in PVE does not differ from that in NVE, as both are systemic infections maintaining a continuous bacteraemia. Hence, the diagnosis is established if in addition to typical clinical signs and symptoms and positive blood cultures, the device can be shown to be affected by echocardiography, preferably using multiplane transoesophageal (TOE) probes. TOE should be performed without delay in all patients with suspicion of PVE.[11] For the diagnosis of PVE, TOE is of such immense importance that institutions without this facility are best advised to ask for assistance from a specialised centre. With TOE the size of vegetation can be defined more precisely than with transthoracic echocardiography (TTE), and periannular complications indicating a locally uncontrolled infection (for example, abscesses, dehiscence, fistulas) may be detected earlier. Both size of vegetations and infection morphology significantly influence therapeutic decisions (namely duration of antimicrobial treatment and the need for urgent surgical intervention).

In otherwise unproven cases, gallium-67 scans or indium-111 leucocyte scintigraphy have been reported to be useful in detecting myocardial abscesses or diffuse tissue infiltrations. Their diagnostic impact has not been established so far.[12]

Treatment

ANTIMICROBIAL TREATMENT

The basic principles of antimicrobial treatment in PVE do not differ from those for NVE. Some special aspects need to be considered, however.

PVE is usually associated with vegetations larger than those found in NVE. Consequently, antibiotics have to be used in dosages which result in maximum, non-toxic serum concentrations in order to penetrate the total vegetation. The duration of treatment usually has to be longer than for the treatment of NVE and should consider vegetation size as determined by TOE as well as the minimal inhibitory concentration (MIC) of the most efficient combination of antibiotics (table 12.2). Antibiotic sterilisation of large vegetations is unlikely with an MIC ⩾ 4 µg/ml.

In PVE caused by coagulase negative staphylococci, complex interactions between the microorganism and the synthetic material—for example, irreversible adhesion and production of a biofilm, which inhibit the host defence mechanisms—protects against antimicrobial treatment and makes antibiotic sterilisation extremely difficult.[5 6]

The presence of (micro-) abscesses is likely in PVE caused by coagulase negative staphylococci, and triple therapy including rifampicin

Table 12.1   Microbiology of early and late PVE. Authors' own findings compared to a recent European literature review[3]

	Early PVE (%)		Late PVE (%)	
	Own experience (n=34)	Europe (n=68)	Own experience (n=132)	Europe (n=194)
Staphylococcus epidermidis	29	43	21	28
Staphylococcus aureus	18	13	19	13
Streptococci	6	3	15*	20
Enterococci	6	2	18	7.5
HACEK	18	17	8	7
Fungi	9	6	5	4
Mixed infections	6	–	3	–
Others	6	12	7	9
Culture negative	3	4	4	12

*Viridans group n=13 (10%), β haemolytic streptococci n=3 (2%), and *Streptococcus bovis* n=4 (3%).
HACEK, *Haemophilus, Actinobacillus, Cardiobacterium, Eikinella, Kingella.*

Table 12.2   Duration of antimicrobial treatment in prosthetic valve endocarditis with respect to vegetation size and minimal inhibitory concentration (MIC)

	Vegetation size*		
	< 4 mm	5–9 mm	> 10 mm
MIC ⩾ 4 µg/l	Antibiotic cure unlikely		
4 µg/ml > MIC ⩾ 2 µg/ml	> 6 weeks	Antibiotic cure unlikely	
2 µg/ml > MIC ⩾ 0.5 µg/ml	6 weeks	> 6 weeks	Antibiotic cure unlikely
0.5 µg/ml > MIC ⩾ 0.1 µg/ml	6 weeks	6 weeks	> 6 weeks
MIC < 0.1 µg/ml	4 weeks	4 weeks	> 6 weeks

*Actual size of vegetation during treatment; MIC, minimal inhibitory concentration of the most effective antibiotic combination.

(900 mg/day divided into three doses) is recommended.[13] Rifampicin is actively taken up by granulocytes and becomes effective against intracellular staphylococci and staphylococci inside abscesses.[4]

When PVE is clinically apparent and blood cultures are not yet positive, empiric treatment should be initiated with vancomycin and gentamicin.[8] For PVE caused by penicillin sensitive streptococci ($MIC_{PEN} < 0.1$ μg/ml), it is advisable to combine penicillin (20–24 million units/24 hours intravenously (iv) divided into 4–6 doses) with an aminoglycoside (preferably gentamicin, 3 mg/kg/24 hours iv, divided into 2–3 doses), treating for at least two weeks with this combination and at least a further two weeks with penicillin alone. In the case of penicillin allergy, vancomycin as a single drug treatment (30 mg/kg/24 hours iv divided into two doses) or ceftriaxone (2 g/24 hours iv as single dose) in combination with gentamicin should be given. PVE caused by streptococci less sensitive to penicillin ($MIC_{PEN} \geqslant 0.5$ μg/ml) or enterococci ($MIC_{PEN} \leqslant 8$ μg/ml) are best treated with a combination of penicillin and gentamicin for at least four weeks. Vancomycin can replace penicillin, if the patient is allergic to penicillin or if $MIC_{PEN} > 8$ μg/ml. Vancomycin resistant strains susceptible to teicoplanin ($MIC_{TEICOPL} \leqslant 4$ μg/ml) may be treated with teicoplanin (10 mg/kg iv divided into two doses) plus gentamicin. If the isolates are highly resistant to gentamicin or multiresistant to the standard antimicrobial agents, alternative combinations of drugs (for example, quinolones) must be considered in consultation with an expert in clinical microbiology. Enterococcal PVE is often complicated by periprosthetic dehiscence, annular abscesses or fistulas. In these cases, if antibiotic treatment fails an early surgical intervention should be considered.

If the pathogen is an oxacillin susceptible staphylococcus ($MIC \leqslant 0.1$ μg/ml), gentamicin should be combined with dicloxacillin/flucloxacillin (12 g/24 hours iv, divided into six doses) for two weeks; thereafter dicloxacillin/flucloxacillin should be given for an additional four weeks. In oxacillin resistant strains, vancomycin (see above for doses) should replace oxacillin derivates. There is no valid evidence to prove that teicoplanin is superior to the established antistaphylococcal drugs. Early surgery in most cases is indicated to prevent secondary complications.[8 13]

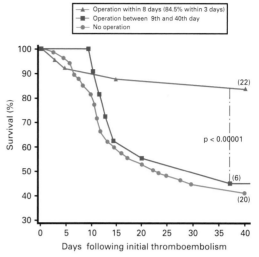

Figure 12.2. Influence of the timing of surgery on the prognosis of patients with cerebral thromboembolism complicating prosthetic valve endocarditis.

ANTITHROMBOTIC TREATMENT

Antithrombotic management in patients with PVE has been discussed widely.[14] There seems to be a consensus that oral anticoagulation treatment should be suspended and replaced by intravenous heparin. The dosage of heparin depends on the presence and nature of secondary complications (for example, thrombocytopenia) and varies between 7–30 U/kg body weight. Low molecular weight heparins may be advantageous, as side effects (especially thrombocytopenia) are less frequent.

Surgical reintervention

If PVE is complicated, it has to be decided whether medical treatment should be continued or urgent surgical intervention is required. The indications for surgery in PVE are similar to those in NVE: large (> 10 mm), mobile vegetations, thromboembolic events with vegetations still demonstrable, sepsis persisting for more than 48 hours despite effective antibiotic treatment (guided by blood cultures and MICs), and acute renal failure. A cerebral embolic event is not a contraindication for open heart surgery provided that there is no cerebral haemorrhage and the time between embolic event and surgery is short (preferably < 72 hours) so that the blood–brain barrier can be expected not to be significantly disturbed (fig 12.2).[15] Periprosthetic dehiscence with or without myocardial failure has a poor prognosis. If congestion is not promptly removed by

Table 12.3 Guidelines for endocarditis prophylaxis in patients with biological or prosthetic heart valves, categorised according to the patient population at high risk of acquiring endocarditis

	Oropharynx, gastrointestinal tract, urogenital tract		Skin, heart catheterisation
	No penicillin allergy	In case of penicillin allergy	
1 hour before the procedure	• Outpatient: 2 g (3 g > 70 kg bodyweight) amoxicillin orally • Hospitalised: 2 g amoxicillin iv + 1.5 mg/kg gentamicin	• Outpatient: 600 mg clindamycin orally or 1 g vancomycin iv for 1 hour or 800 mg teicoplanin • Hospitalised: vancomycin 1 g iv for 1 hour + 1.5 mg/kg gentamicin	• 600 mg clindamycin orally or 1 g vancomycin iv for 1 hour or 800 mg teicoplanin
6 hours after the procedure	• Outpatient: 1 g amoxicillin orally • Hospitalised: 1 g amoxicillin + 1.5 mg/kg gentamicin	• Outpatient: 300 mg clindamycin orally • Hospitalised: vancomycin 1 g iv for 1 hour + 1.5 mg/kg gentamicin	• 300 mg clindamycin

iv, intravenous.

> **Treatment and prophylaxis of prosthetic valve endocarditis (PVE)**
>
> ● Duration of treatment for PVE is usually longer than for native valve endocarditis
>
> ● Antibiotic sterilisation of coagulase negative staphylococci or enterococci PVE is extremely difficult
>
> ● Early surgical intervention is necessary in most cases to prevent secondary complications
>
> ● Oral anticoagulation should be replaced by intravenous heparin or low molecular weight heparin
>
> ● For PVE prophylaxis, antibiotics should be taken one hour before and six hours after the interventional procedure
>
> ● In hospitalised patients, antibiotics may be administered intravenously in combination with aminoglycosides

medical treatment, surgical intervention is mandatory. Allograft aortic root replacement is a valuable technique in the complex setting of PVE with involvement of the periannular region.[16]

Prophylaxis

As the risk for an infection is much higher in patients with prosthetic heart valves than in patients with valvar heart disease, more intensive prophylaxis is needed in these patients. In patients with prosthetic valves, the antibiotics should be taken one hour before the interventional procedure and a repeat but reduced dosage administered six hours after the procedure. If patients are hospitalised, the antibiotics may be applied intravenously in combination with aminoglycosides one hour before and six hours after the procedure (table 12.3).

1. **Blackstone EH, Kirklin JW.** Death and other time-related events after valve replacement. *Circulation* 1985;**72**:753–67.
   • *Experience with 1533 patients undergoing valve surgery between 1975 and 1979 revealed that PVE occurs uncommonly after original valve replacement surgery (4.4% in five years) but with a high mortality of 63%.*

2. **Kloster FE.** Complications of artificial heart valves. *JAMA* 1979;**241**:2201–3.

3. **Vlessis AA, Khaki A, Grunkemeier GL,** et al. Risk, diagnosis and management of prosthetic valve endocarditis: a review. *J Heart Valve Dis* 1997;**6**:443–65.
   • *This article reviews the current understanding of PVE and provides an outline for diagnosis and treatment based on the published literature and on the authors' personal clinical experiences.*

4. **Zimmerli W.** Experimental models in the investigation of device-related infections. *J Antimicrob Chemother* 1993;**31** (suppl D):97–102.

5. **Horstkotte D, Weist K, Rueden H.** Better understanding of the pathogenesis of prosthetic valve endocarditis—recent perspectives for prevention strategies. *J Heart Valve Dis* 1998;**7**:313–15.
   • *Editorial on the recent perspectives for prevention of PVE.*

6. **Hyde JAJ, Darouiche RO, Costeron JW.** Strategies for prophylaxis against prosthetic valve endocarditis. A review article. *J Heart Valve Dis* 1998;**7**:316–26.
   • *This article gives the historic background to the prevention of PVE and discusses the current state of research in this area.*

7. **Edmunds LH, Clark RE, Cohn LH,** et al. Guidelines for reporting morbidity and mortality after cardiac valvular operation. *Ann Thorac Surg* 1988;**46**:257–9.

8. **Horstkotte D, Follath F, v Graevenitz A,** et al. Recommendations for prevention, diagnosis and treatment of infective endocarditis. The task force on infective endocarditis of the European Society of Cardiology. *Eur Heart J* (in press)
   • *A European consensus status giving the latest guidelines for prevention, diagnosis, and treatment of infective endocarditis.*

9. **Karchmer AW, Gibbons GW.** Infections of prosthetic heart valves and vascular grafts. In: Bisno AL, Waldvogel FA, eds. *Infections associated with indwelling medical devices.* Washington: ASM Press, 1994:213–49.

10. **Horstkotte D, Piper C, Niehues R,** et al. Late prosthetic valve endocarditis. *Eur Heart J* 1995;**16**(suppl B):39–47.
    • *Prevalence, sources of infection, microbiology, diagnostic approach, and medical as well as surgical treatment of 140 patients with PVE from 4182 consecutive patients operated on in Düsseldorf between 1970 and 1992.*

11. **Pedersen WR, Walker M, Olseon JD,** et al. Value of transesophageal echocardiography in evaluation of native and prosthetic valve endocarditis. *Chest* 1991;**100**:351–6.
    • *This study reported better visualisation of valvar vegetations in native as well as in prosthetic valve endocarditis with transoesophageal (TOE) than with transthoracic (TTE) echocardiography. TTE was positive in only 5 of 10 patients with infective endocarditis, while TOE not only yielded abnormal findings in all 10 patients but also revealed additional information in 4 of 5 patients.*

12. **O'Brien K, Barnes D, Martin RH,** et al. Gallium-SPECT in the detection of prosthetic valve endocarditis and aortic ring abscess. *J Nucl Med* 1991;**32**:1791–3.

13. **Wilson WR, Geraci JE, Danielson GU,** et al. Anticoagulant therapy and central nervous system complications in patients with prosthetic valve endocarditis. *Circulation* 1978;**57**:1004–7.
    • *Adequate anticoagulant treatment in patients with PVE resulted in fewer central nervous system complications than inadequate anticoagulation.*

14. **Wilson WR, Karchmer AW, Dajani AS,** et al. Antibiotic treatment of adults with infective endocarditis due to streptococci, enterococci, staphylococci, and HACEK microorganisms. *JAMA* 1995;**274**:1706–13.
    • *Consensus opinion regarding management of PVE caused by commonly encountered microorganisms and those cases resulting from infrequent causes of PVE.*

15. **Horstkotte D, Piper C, Wiemer M,** et al. Dringlicher Herzklappenersatz nach akuter Hirnembolie während florider Endokarditis. *Med Klinik* 1998;**93**:284-93.
    • *The analysis of an urgent surgical intervention after embolic cerebral infarction in 22 patients compared to 27 medically treated patients revealed that removing the source of infection and embolic hazard seems to be beneficial and that surgery should be performed within 72 hours to prevent secondary cerebral haemorrhage.*

16. **Dossche KM, Defauw JJ, Ernst SM,** et al. Allograft aortic root replacement in prosthetic aortic valve endocarditis: a review of 32 patients. *Ann Thorac Surg* 1997;**63**:1644–9.
    • *This review of 32 patients showed that allograft aortic root replacement is a valuable technique in the complex setting of PVE with involvement of the periannular region with low perioperative mortality and morbidity.*

13 Endocarditis: basics

S J Eykyn

Microbiological expertise is essential in the diagnosis, management, and prevention of infective endocarditis (IE). Unfortunately old habits die hard and there are still doctors who persist in referring to this infection as "SBE" (subacute bacterial endocarditis) whether the patient has been ill for days, weeks or months, and think that it is generally caused by a microbe they know as "*Strep viridans*" and can often be blamed on dentists. IE cannot be considered as a homogeneous infection. It may arise in the community or, increasingly, in hospital or as a result of procedures undertaken in hospital; it may affect native valves (previously normal or abnormal) or prosthetic valves and may occur in intravenous drug users (IVDU) as well as those who do not use drugs. Although overall most cases of IE are caused by staphylococci, streptococci, and enterococci, the incidence of each group of organisms differs in the various types of IE. A wide variety of organisms account for the infections not caused by these three genera, and virtually every organism known to microbiologists has been reported to cause IE, albeit very rarely. At St Thomas' Hospital, in some 650 cases of IE seen over 30 years we have encountered infections caused by *Erysipelothrix rhusiopathiae*, *Listeria monocytogenes*, *Campylobacter fetus*, *Lactobacillus rhamnosus*, and *Histoplasma capsulatum!*

Native valve endocarditis

Native valve endocarditis (NVE) is the most common type of IE. The affected valve may be previously normal or abnormal, and the infection is usually acquired in the community but increasingly is also acquired in hospital.

Community acquired NVE

Community acquired NVE is now as likely to be caused by staphylococci, usually *Staphylococcus aureus* but sometimes by coagulase negative staphylococci, as it is to be caused by oral ("viridans") streptococci (fig 13.1), most commonly those of the *sanguis* and *oralis* groups. Enterococci (until quite recently known as streptococci) are less common but their incidence is increasing; most are *Enterococcus faecalis*. A trivial predisposing skin lesion is occasionally detected in staphylococcal IE and there may be poor dentition in oral streptococcal IE, but seldom relevant preceding dentistry. Staphylococci, even some coagulase negative strains such *Staphylococcus lugdunensis*, are virulent bacteria and are as likely to attack a previously normal valve as an abnormal one, whereas oral streptococci and enterococci are much less virulent and seem only to infect previously abnormal valves.

Hospital acquired or hospital associated NVE

These infections are almost always caused by staphylococci, usually *S aureus* but occasionally coagulase-negative staphylococci, most often *Staphylococcus epidermidis*. The inexorable rise in methicillin resistant *S aureus* (MRSA) in UK hospitals over the last decade has been paralleled by an increase in hospital acquired MRSA endocarditis. Most cases of hospital acquired NVE result from intravascular access site infections, even those used for peripheral venous access. Intravascular access site infection is especially common in patients on haemodialysis. Pacemaker associated NVE is also increasingly encountered.

Prosthetic valve endocarditis

Any prosthetic valve—whether mechanical or bioprosthetic—can become infected and the risk of infection is life long, with some infections occurring over 20 years after valve replacement. Although for many years it has been conventional to classify prosthetic valve endocarditis (PVE) as *early* (occurring within 60 days of valve surgery and acquired in the theatre or soon thereafter perhaps on the intensive care unit) or *late* (occurring more than 60 days after valve surgery and presumed to have been acquired in the community), these definitions are unsatisfactory. Infections acquired in the theatre, and particularly those caused by relatively avirulent bacteria such as *S epidermidis* and corynebacteria, may present many months or even a year or more after surgery, and as with native valves, prosthetic valves can become infected from intravascular access sites at any time after implantation. Thus it may be preferable to classify PVE, as with NVE, as hospital acquired or community acquired. PVE acquired in hospital is predominantly caused by staphylococci, often coagulase negative strains, whereas infections acquired in the community have a similar range of pathogens as community acquired NVE but a higher incidence of unusual organisms.

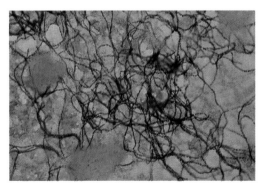

Figure 13.1. Gram stained smear from blood culture bottle showing viridans streptococci from patient with native valve endocarditis.

Infective endocarditis in intravenous drug users

This infection, which usually involves the tricuspid valve, is frequently misdiagnosed as pneumonia by those unfamiliar with the respiratory presentation of right sided IE. Most cases are caused by *S aureus* (fig 13.2).

Microbiological diagnosis and monitoring of IE

The mainstay of the microbiological diagnosis of IE is the blood culture. Not surprisingly, persistent positive blood cultures constitute a major diagnostic criterion on the Duke classification system[1] now universally recognised as a means of confirming a definite case of IE. For some organisms their very presence in both bottles of a single blood culture more or less equates with a diagnosis of IE, and examples of this include many oral streptococci, *Streptococcus bovis*, and community acquired enterococci, but for others the demonstration of a persistent bacteraemia is required for diagnostic reassurance. Hence the convention is for several sets of blood cultures to be taken if IE is suspected. However, in practice in many cases of IE caused by virulent bacteria, especially *S aureus*, the patient is recognised to be septic and unwell (fig 13.3) when first seen though IE is rarely suspected, and only a single set of blood cultures is done before broad spectrum antibiotics are started. There is no point in waiting for a spike of temperature before taking blood for culture, or taking cultures at specific time intervals or from different sites. Previous antibiotics will rarely prevent recovery of *S aureus* from the blood but are very likely to prevent recovery of oral streptococci. It is seldom worth waiting 24–48 hours after stopping antibiotics before doing blood cultures. In most cases of IE the causative pathogen will be recovered from blood cultures within about 48 hours and most if not all bottles are positive. Recovery of an organism may take longer if antibiotics have been given or if fastidious organisms such as those known as the HACEK group (this includes *Haemophilus* species (though not *Haemophilus influenzae*), *Actinobacillus actinomycetemcomitans*, *Cardiobacterium hominis*, *Eikenella corrodens*, and *Kingella kingae*) are involved.

Although not strictly microbiological and not specific to IE, it is worth mentioning here that C-reactive protein (CRP) and the erythrocyte sedimentation rate (ESR) will usually be raised in IE and these have been proposed as additional minor criteria to the Duke classification of IE.[2] The peripheral white blood cell count is usually very high in infections caused by virulent organisms but often normal in those caused by oral streptococci; the haemoglobin is usually low in the latter though not in the former. There may be microscopic haematuria and when this is not associated with a urethral catheter, urinary infection, end stage

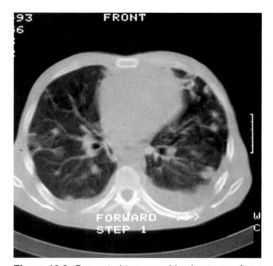

Figure 13.2. Computed tomographic chest scan from intravenous drug user with *Staphylococcus aureus* endocarditis on the tricuspid valve. Multiple cavitating lesions are evident.

renal disease or menstruation has been proposed as an additional minor criterion to the Duke classification.[2]

It is only worth taking blood cultures during treatment of IE if the patient is febrile or unwell; "check" cultures to see if the blood has been sterilised when the patient is doing well are pointless. Serial CRP estimations can give laboratory reassurance that the infection is under control but the ESR often falls so slowly that it is much less useful in monitoring response to treatment than the CRP. Titrations of the serum bactericidal activity against the infecting organism ("back titrations") are of very limited value in monitoring antibiotic treatment, and at worst can produce false reassurance of bacteriological efficacy which may be accompanied by clinical deterioration. They should be abandoned.

Blood culture negative IE

In a variable percentage of cases where there is convincing clinical and echocardiographic evidence of IE the blood cultures are negative. In such cases it is essential to send blood for antibodies to bacteria that cannot be cultured by routine blood culture methods, specifically *Coxiella burnettii* (Q fever), *Chlamydia* species, and *Bartonella* species. A detailed history may reveal possible clues to these infections and it is worth noting that *Bartonella* species cross react with *Chlamydia* species. Also important in blood culture negative cases is a careful history of previous antibiotic administration which may necessitate a call to the general practitioner, because if antibiotics have been given and blood culturees are negative the pathogen is likely to be an oral streptococcus. Occasionally in blood culture negative IE the pathogen can be isolated from an excised valve or embolus, or sometimes detected on microscopy of such material even if this is sterile on culture. Blood cultures are seldom negative in intravenous drug users with IE, but if they are the pathogen can usually be isolated from respiratory specimens. When all these con-

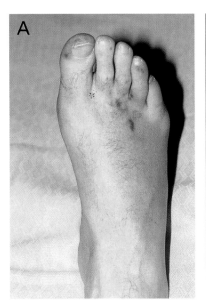 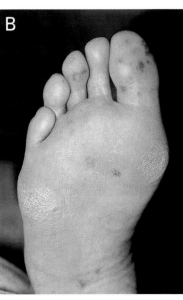

Figure 13.3. Embolic lesions on the feet of a patient with *Staphylococcus aureus* endocarditis.

siderations have been taken into account, there really is no clue to the pathogen in less than 5% of patients with blood culture negative IE.

When should antibiotic treatment be started in suspected IE, and what with?

When a patient with suspected IE has been unwell for many weeks or months it is reasonable to wait 48–72 hours to see if the blood cultures are positive before starting antibiotics, and then appropriate treatment can be given from the outset for the organism isolated. If the blood cultures are negative then the investigations outlined above should be done without delay and their results will determine treatment. The UK guidelines devised by the working party on endocarditis of the British Society for Antimicrobial Chemotherapy (BSAC) should be used.[3] In those patients who are very unwell with suspected IE then obviously treatment should not be delayed after blood cultures have been taken and a combination such as vancomycin and gentamicin given. In reality endocarditis caused by virulent organisms is seldom diagnosed on admission and the initial broad spectrum antibiotic can be modified in light of culture results. Much mystique is attached to the value of in vitro tests on the pathogen by many microbiologists and the MIC (minimum inhibitory concentration) has long been the sacred cow of laboratory management. Not only are routine (disc) sensitivity tests quite adequate in almost all cases but treatment is generally well under way by the time in vitro tests are available. At least the MBC (minimum bactericidal concentration) has now been deemed of no value and with luck abandoned even by enthusiasts with time to spare.

Length of treatment

Many doctors are still convinced of the need for six weeks antibiotic treatment in all cases of IE, yet 20 years ago successful short course (two weeks) therapy for sensitive streptococcal infection was reported.[4] Bacteriological failure—that is, recurrence of the infection—in IE generally means that surgery, not more antibiotics, is needed. There are distinct benefits for the patient from shorter courses of antibiotics as toxicity and intravenous access infection are less likely and usually the hospital admission shorter. There are no trials of short course treatment for IE caused by organisms other than oral streptococci; here the treatment is often complicated by the need for surgery and this may occur soon after the start of antibiotics. It is remarkable that surgery, even in the face of persistent infection and sometimes positive blood cultures, can be so dramatically curative. The length of treatment in most cases who have emergency surgery can be determined by microscopy and culture of the excised valve. If the pathogen is isolated from the valve (and this may happen with *S aureus* IE even after more than a week of appropriate antibiotics) then two weeks of intravenous antibiotics should be given after surgery. If the valve culture is sterile but organisms are detected on a Gram stained smear then the bacteria are dead; the intravenous antibiotics should be continued until the valve culture has been incubated for five days then they can be stopped. If no bacteria are detected on the Gram stained smear and the culture is sterile (cultures are likely to be sterile if no bacteria are seen on the smear) then there is no need for further antibiotic treatment.

Choice of antibiotic for specific pathogens and the need for two agents

The BSAC guidelines have already been mentioned. However they are only *guidelines* and in the individual case other regimens may be appropriate. It is quite possible, for example, to treat sensitive oral streptococcal IE in patients who are haemodynamically stable entirely by oral amoxicillin, provided the drug is taken reliably and absorbed. Likewise outpatient regimens have been used, though not I suspect in the UK. The long acting cephalosporin ceftriaxone has been successfully used in this way, usually given with an aminoglycoside. As has previously been mentioned, recurrence in IE is very seldom attributable to inadequate antibiotic treatment.

Most oral streptococci can be treated with a single agent (penicillin or amoxicillin), but there are no trials to show that a two week regimen with a single agent is appropriate and so it should be given for four weeks. The combination of an aminoglycoside (gentamicin but previously streptomycin) was originally devised to achieve bactericidal synergy against enterococci, as these bacteria cannot be eradicated with a penicillin alone. The combination is also recommended for oral streptococci on the basis of the reports of its successful use in two week regimens, even though for most oral streptococci there is no in vitro evidence of synergy. It is possible that two weeks of penicillin alone might be as effective, but this is unproven and thus cannot be recommended. There are unfortunately increasing numbers of enterococci with high level resistance to gentamicin and often also to streptomycin; therefore, the addition of the aminoglycoside to penicillin or amoxicillin will not result in synergy. For these strains there is currently no bactericidal regimen and prolonged courses of high dose amoxicillin are used, though in many cases surgery will be curative. Vancomycin resistant enterococci also occasionally cause IE; if these also show high level gentamicin resistance they pose a formidable therapeutic problem in patients allergic to penicillin.

It is conventional to treat staphylococcal IE with two antibiotics though there is very little evidence that this is beneficial. Trials of different treatment regimens in staphylococcal IE are almost impossible to assess because so many patients come to emergency surgery and it is this, not the antibiotics, that cures them. The addition of gentamicin to the β lactam for two weeks in staphylococcal IE reduced the duration of fever and bacteraemia by about 24 hours in both IVDU and non-IVDU, but had no effect on morbidity or mortality.[5] Fusidic acid is sometimes given in combination with flucloxacillin for staphylococcal IE, but benefit over the single agent is anecdotal. Rifampicin is often recommended in combination with vancomycin for MRSA or coagulase negative staphylococcal IE, especially PVE, but again convincing evidence of efficacy is lacking.

Persistence or recurrence of fever during appropriate antibiotic treatment of IE

While many patients with IE, particularly that caused by oral streptococci, respond within about 48 hours to antibiotic treatment with rapid resolution of fever, amelioration of many systemic symptoms and a decrease in the markers of bacterial infection, specifically CRP, some do not and this is cause for concern.[6] Unless the symptoms can be attributed to drug hypersensitivity the antibiotic regimen should not be changed. The last thing such patients need, but often get, is an increased dose of antibiotic, an additional agent or a different regimen. Further blood cultures should be done and if the original pathogen is isolated then this in itself means that surgery is indicated. In practice only virulent bacteria such as *S aureus* are likely to be recovered from blood cultures during antibiotic treatment—oral streptococci never will. Infected intravenous access sites are rarely responsible for persistent fever but should be carefully inspected nonetheless. By far the most common

cause of fever is an abscess of the valve ring and surrounding structures or widespread tissue destruction without abscess formation. Although abscess formation and extensive tissue destruction are more likely to occur in IE caused by virulent bacteria, it may also occur in IE caused by oral streptococci especially when the diagnosis has been delayed.

Antibiotic prophylaxis of IE

The rationale for antibiotic prophylaxis to prevent the acquisition of IE depends on two premises—firstly, certain procedures, especially dental procedures, result in bacteraemia with organisms that commonly cause IE; and secondly, that certain cardiac conditions, both congenital and acquired, predispose to IE. Hence, the need to cover at risk procedures in at risk patients has been accepted clinical dogma for half a century. There are numerous national guidelines, including those from the UK devised by the BSAC working party; they differ mainly in detail not in principle.[7] Overall, compliance with the guidelines is generally known to be poor for dental procedures, ranging from 15–35%, and there are no data on compliance for the other procedures for which prophylaxis is recommended. The value of such prophylaxis in the prevention of IE has been questioned for some years as there is little or no objective evidence that it is effective in preventing IE; it is likely that spontaneous bacteraemias from chewing and various oral hygiene practices may be more significant in the pathogenesis of IE than certain dental procedures. Four studies of patients with IE during the last 16 years either fail to show a dental connection or can only show a small one, though the study designs are open to criticism.[8] More recently a report from the USA suggested that the risk of IE after dental treatment is virtually nil.[9]

Some have argued that the danger of an anaphylactic reaction from penicillin/amoxicillin is much greater than the risk of IE, and it has been suggested that patients receiving penicillin/amoxicillin prophylaxis to prevent IE are five times more likely to die from an anaphylactic reaction to the drug than to die from contracting IE. There is also the potential for the selection of antibiotic resistance by the continued and repeated use of antibiotic prophylaxis. It has been estimated that a randomised placebo controlled study to assess the efficacy of antibiotic prophylaxis in dentistry would require at least 6000 at risk patients and would understandably encounter ethical objections, not least because of the ever present spectre of litigation. Perhaps, as David Durack has suggested, it is "time to scale back" and re-think the recommendations for dental prophylaxis though this would require a re-think of titanic proportions. It will be clear from the foregoing that there are cogent reasons for questioning dental prophylaxis; this applies even more so to non-dental prophylaxis such as that for many urological procedures. There is no evidence of efficacy and the antibiotics recommended for prophylaxis are parenteral and potentially toxic (for example, gentamicin and vancomycin in patients allergic to penicillin). It would thus seem reasonable to cease to recommend prophylaxis for these indications until there is a trial demonstrating efficacy, a formidable undertaking.

1. **Durack DT, Lukes AS, Bright DK, and the Duke Endocarditis Service.** New criteria for the diagnosis of infective endocarditis: utilization of specific echocardiographic findings. *Am J Med* 1994;**96**:200–9.
- *The Duke criteria have been accepted internationally and no paper on IE would be acceptable without this assessment. The Duke criteria replaced the earlier case definitions introduced by von Reyn and colleagues in 1981.*

2. **Lamas CC, Eykyn SJ.** Suggested modifications to the Duke criteria for the clinical diagnosis of native valve and prosthetic valve endocarditis: analysis of 118 pathologically proven cases. *Clin Inf Dis* 1997;**25**:713–9.
- *Assessment of the Duke criteria in a large number of pathologically proven cases with suggestions for additional minor criteria that improved diagnostic sensitivity while retaining specificity.*

3. **Working Party of the British Society for Antimicrobial Chemotherapy.** Antibiotic treatment of streptococcal, enterococcal and staphylococcal endocarditis. *Heart* 1998;**79**:207–10.
- *The most recent UK guidelines on treatment. They cover treatment of the organisms that cause most cases of IE. Treatment of infections caused by unusual organisms cannot be expected from general guidelines. These guidelines, in contrast to the earlier ones (1985), no longer recommend either the MBC or serum bactericidal titrations.*

4. **Wilson WR, Thompson RL, Wilkowske CJ,** *et al.* Short-term therapy for streptococcal infective endocarditis. Combined intramuscular administration of penicillin and streptomycin. *JAMA* 1981;**245**:360–3.
- *Although there are earlier studies of short course regimens this study found no relapses after two weeks of treatment in 91 patients. Its results seem to have been largely ignored in the UK.*

5. **Korzeniowski O, Sande MA and the National Collaborative Endocarditis Study Group.** Combination antimicrobial therapy for *Staphylococcus aureus* endocarditis in patients addicted to parenteral drugs and in nonadddicts. A prospective study. *Ann Intern Med* 1982;**97**:496–503.
- *One of the few studies to try and assess the efficacy of combination therapy in IE both in IVDU and non-IVDU and showing only a marginal benefit from the addition of gentamicin and more renal toxicity.*

6. **Douglas A, Moore-Gillon J, Eykyn S.** Fever during treatment of infective endocarditis. *Lancet* 1986; i:1341–3.
- *A study of 83 cases of culture positive NVE with persistent or recurrent fever during treatment that emphasises that the most common cause for this is extensive infection of the valve ring requiring surgery.*

7. **Working Party of the British Society for Antimicrobial Chemotherapy.** Recommendations for endocarditis prophylaxis. *J Antimicrob Chemother* 1993;**31**:437–8.
- *These are the most recently published UK guidelines and feature in the British National Formulary and the Dental Formulary. They need updating and revising but are they are used in all litigation concerning prophylaxis.*

8. **Seymour RA, Lowry R, Whitworth JM,** *et al.* Infective endocarditis, dentistry and antibiotic prophylaxis; time for a rethink? *Br Dent J* 2000;**189**:610–6.
- *A useful and stimulating review of the current evidence that links dental treatment to IE and an appraisal of the risks of antibiotic prophylaxis.*

9. **Strom BL, Abrutyn E, Berlin JA,** *et al.* Dental and cardiac risk factors for endocarditis. A population-based, case-control study. *Ann Intern Med* 1998;**139**:761-9.
- *A major multicentre study that showed that dental treatment did not seem to be a risk factor for IE even in patients with valvar abnormalities whereas cardiac abnormalities are a strong risk factor.*

14 Surgery of valve disease: late results and late complications

Peter Groves

Valve surgery remains the treatment of choice for most significant valve lesions. Symptomatic improvement has been well demonstrated in a number of studies and is usually sustained into the late postoperative period, especially when valve replacement is undertaken for stenotic lesions. Invasive studies have shown that symptomatic relief is consistently accompanied by haemodynamic improvement, and the overall superiority of surgical intervention over conservative medical treatment for most patients with advanced valve disease has been firmly established.

Late results after valve surgery

The analysis of survival rates of patients following valve replacement relative to age and sex matched populations have shown an impaired prognosis in all but a minority.[1] In patients older than 65 years undergoing aortic valve replacement for aortic stenosis, relative survival is "normalised" after the first postoperative year, but in all other indications an excess late mortality has been observed in surgical patients. Long term follow up studies consistently report better survival rates in patients undergoing aortic rather than mitral valve replacement, with 10 year actuarial survival rates of approximately 65% for aortic valve replacement, 55% for mitral valve replacement, and 55% for double (aortic and mitral) valve replacement. Late mortality is greater when surgery is undertaken for regurgitant as opposed to stenotic lesions, while long term survival is better in the context of degenerative as opposed to ischaemic or rheumatic valve pathologies. These observations illustrate the fact that long term mortality following valve replacement is most reflective of the nature of the original disease process, the pre- and postoperative state of the myocardium and coronary circulation, as well as the general wellbeing of the patient with valve related deaths being relatively infrequent. Approximately 60% of late mortality is attributable to cardiac causes that are independent of the valve surgery (namely, cardiac failure, myocardial infarction, arrhythmia or sudden death), approximately 20% is caused by valve related complications, and 20% is from non-cardiac causes. Independent predictors for death in the late postoperative period include advanced age (> 65 years), left ventricular impairment, New York Heart Association functional class IV symptoms at the time of surgery, coincident coronary artery disease, and documented ventricular arrhythmias.[2] The presence or absence of these negative factors at the time of aortic valve replacement, for example, gives rise to a predicted 10 year survival rate varying between 16–90%.[3] In the presence of three vessel or left main stem coronary artery disease nine year survival is as low as 29%[4] and the negative influence of coronary disease is not completely ameliorated by grafting at the time of initial surgery. Favourable and rather similar survival rates have been reported with a variety of mechanical and bioprostheses. While the specific selection of a mechanical or bioprosthesis is usually dependent on factors such as age, valve position, risk of anticoagulation, and patient preference, the presence or absence of these negative predictors of clinical outcome should also be considered in order to minimise valve related complications and maximise quality of life within the life span expected. While attention to the medical treatment of additional cardiac comorbidities is important, improvements in long term survival after valve surgery will most likely be achieved through the earlier recognition and correction of significant valve lesions.

Late complications after valve surgery

Left ventricular failure

Following the successful surgical correction of left sided valve defects, residual left ventricular impairment may be present in some patients, exposing them to the risks of progressive cardiac failure and sudden death. Left ventricular dysfunction is usually the consequence of longstanding pathological changes that are secondary to sustained preoperative pressure and/or volume overload, but may also be related to the influence of other cardiac diseases including coronary artery disease, poorly controlled hypertension, and coincident cardiomyopathy.

The pathophysiology of late left ventricular dysfunction is greatly dependent on the preoperative left ventricular load, and therefore the specific valve lesion corrected. When aortic valve replacement is undertaken for aortic stenosis, postoperative improvement in systolic and diastolic left ventricular function may occur over a period of years but is by no means inevitable. In aortic stenosis, severe left ventricular systolic dysfunction may be caused by "afterload mismatch" with an increase in left ventricular systolic pressure and wall stress leading to a reduction in stroke volume and ejection fraction. Under these circumstances, systolic function improves once left ventricular pressure is normalised. Alternatively, systolic dysfunction may be caused by reduced contractility as a result of hypertrophy and fibrosis or by the additional insult of scarring following myocardial infarction. When this is the case, postoperative improvement in left ventricular systolic function often does not occur and long term clinical outcome may be severely compromised. Factors associated with residual postoperative left ventricular systolic impairment following the correction of aortic stenosis include low preoperative ejection fraction and aortic valve gradient, presence of coronary artery disease, and previous myocardial infarction. The combination of severe preoperative left ventricular dysfunction and previous myocardial infarction is particularly ominous, with a high operative risk and only 30% of patients alive two years after surgery.

Improvement in left ventricular diastolic function following aortic valve replacement for aortic stenosis is equally important in determining clinical outcome and is critically dependent on regression of left ventricular hypertrophy.[5] While this occurs predictably in most patients over a period of years[6] it rarely does so to normal ventricular mass; it may also be impaired by the presence of irreversible myocardial disease, and if only partial may be accompanied by persistent diastolic dysfunction and associated with excess mortality.

The long term results of surgery to correct mitral and aortic regurgitation are not as good as when aortic stenosis is the dominant lesion. The main reason for this is the more commonly encountered problem of postoperative left ventricular dysfunction and the impact that this has on clinical outcome. Impaired left ventricular function following successful correction of valvar regurgitation is thought to be attributable to a variable degree of irreversible damage to the dilating left ventricle, which is often subtle and difficult to identify preoperatively. Symptoms are delayed in chronic aortic and mitral regurgitation so that surgery is often offered too late. Once present, symptoms may indicate the presence of an irremediable degree of left ventricular dysfunction and are associated with an unfavourable long term prognosis. In mitral regurgitation, a deterioration in postoperative left ventricular function is to be expected anyway, with the presence of a competent valve leading to an increase in afterload and decrease in preload; thus in the presence of already depressed contractile function, left ventricular failure is likely to hinder long term recovery. In order to minimise the degree of postoperative left ventricular impairment following surgery for mitral and aortic regurgitation, surgery should be considered at an early stage and often before symptoms develop. Careful surveillance of left ventricular function in asymptomatic patients is essential. A reduced ejection fraction is predictive of a postoperative left ventricular impairment and in itself is an indication for early surgical intervention.[7] In mitral regurgitation, measurement of left ventricular end systolic volume is useful, being independent of preload, correlating well with measurements of myocardial contractility, and when elevated (> 50 ml/m^2) being predictive of postoperative left ventricular impairment.[8] In aortic regurgitation, subtle degrees of left ventricular dysfunction may only be apparent during haemodynamic stress, but once discovered may serve as an indication for surgical intervention.

When surgery is undertaken, surgical technique is an important factor in determining postoperative left ventricular function and therefore early and late clinical outcome. For pure mitral regurgitation, the benefits of mitral repair and reconstruction as opposed to replacement are well established.[9] There is a lower rate of perioperative mortality and improved long term survival. Left ventricular function is better preserved, thromboembolic complications and the risk of future infective endocarditis are reduced, while the need for long term anticoagulation is obviated in most patients. These advantages in anatomically suitable patients and with appropriate surgical expertise are achieved at lower cost both in the short and long term[10] such that the weight of medical and economic evidence in favour of valve repair is compelling. When patients with mitral regurgitation are unsuitable for valve repair and replacement is undertaken, evidence suggests that overall left ventricular function may be best preserved through the retention of the subvalvar apparatus.

Right ventricular failure and tricuspid regurgitation

The late appearance of tricuspid regurgitation accompanied by symptoms and signs of right heart failure is an important cause of late morbidity and mortality in patients undergoing mitral and aortic valve surgery. Recent studies have shown that significant tricuspid regurgitation is detectable by echocardiography in up to two thirds of patients late after mitral valve replacement, and that it is clinically apparent in more than one third.[11] These patients have a pronounced reduction in exercise capacity and a poor functional outcome attributable to an impaired cardiac output response to exercise.[12] The pathophysiology of this interesting clinical syndrome is variable and complex. In patients with rheumatic valve disease, the development of progressive organic tricuspid valve pathology may occur and accounts for about 25% of patients presenting with late tricuspid regurgitation. The persistence or late development of left heart pathology and the presence of unresolved pulmonary hypertension (see below) are important causes of increased afterload on the right ventricle which predisposes to progressive right ventricular dilatation. In many patients, however, persistent right ventricular and tricuspid annular dilatation may be present despite a postoperative reduction in pulmonary artery pressure. In some, this may reflect longstanding preoperative pressure overload since it is often apparent in those in whom mitral surgery was delayed for many years, while in others, right ventricular impairment may be caused by perioperative ischaemia. In many patients, however, the presence of uncorrected tricuspid regurgitation at the time of initial surgery is likely to be important since this may lead to a vicious cycle developing over subsequent years comprising right ventricular enlargement, further annular dilatation, and gradual worsening of tricuspid regurgitation and right ventricular function.

A number of studies have shown that correcting the mitral lesion without intervening on the tricuspid valve is associated in many patients with persistence and often worsening in the severity of tricuspid regurgitation postoperatively. Since reoperation to correct severe tricuspid regurgitation at a later stage is associated with a high mortality,[13] an emphasis should be placed on prevention rather than cure. In this regard, a strategy of earlier surgical intervention combined with the accurate detection and liberal correction of tricuspid regurgitation at the time of the initial operation seems prudent. Pre- and intraoperative echocardiography allows for the assessment of the severity of tricuspid regurgitation and its relation to abnormalities of right ventricular and tricuspid annular function before and after correction of the left heart lesion. Tricuspid annuloplasty should be contemplated when tricuspid regurgitation is moderate or severe and accompanied by tricuspid annular dilatation (> 21 mm/m^2) since spontaneous regression of tricuspid regurgitation postoperatively is rare under these circumstances.

Pulmonary hypertension

Pulmonary hypertension is commonly present in patients with left sided valve disease and is usually most pronounced in those with long-standing rheumatic mitral valve involvement. Pulmonary hypertension reflects not only passive transmitted back pressure from left atrial hypertension but also an active increase in pulmonary vascular resistance caused by a combination of pulmonary vasoconstriction and obliterative changes in the pulmonary vascular bed. Following the correction of left sided valve defects, an early fall in pulmonary artery pressure is expected and reflects normalisation of left atrial pressure as well as vasomotor changes including relief of vasoconstriction. The most dramatic haemodynamic changes in the pulmonary circulation therefore occur within the first few days after surgery and certainly within the first six months. Thereafter, any further fall in pulmonary vascular resistance is unpredictable and dependent upon structural changes within the hypertrophied pulmonary arteries, arterioles, and veins, a process which is slow, variable, and often incomplete. While a dramatic early reduction in pulmonary pressure is expected in most patients with even extreme pulmonary hypertension undergoing mitral or aortic valve surgery, full normalisation is rarely if ever achieved. Even when pulmonary pressures are apparently normal at rest, a hypertensive pulmonary response to exercise is often seen, with a rapid rise in pulmonary artery pressure at relatively low workload.[14] This irreversible component of increased pulmonary vascular resistance probably reflects residual morphological changes within the pulmonary vasculature and leads to a continued and chronic increase in afterload on the right heart. The more complete the correction of the left sided lesion the more likely it is that pulmonary vascular resistance will fall, while conversely the late emergence of pulmonary hypertension and right heart failure may sometimes reflect left sided prosthetic dysfunction or new left heart pathology. While a temporary reduction in pulmonary pressures has been described with the use of nitrates or inhaled nitric oxide in the early postoperative period following mitral valve replacement, no specific treatment is available for persistent pulmonary hypertension; however, earlier diagnosis and surgical intervention may prevent the development of irreversible structural changes in the pulmonary circulation.

Sudden death, arrhythmias, and conduction abnormalities

Overall rates of sudden death in patients with prosthetic valves vary considerably and generally range from 15–30% with an estimated annual risk of 0.2–0.9%. Sudden death is defined as death within one hour of an event of abrupt onset and accounts for approximately 25% of all late deaths following valve replacement. Broadly speaking, sudden deaths may be stratified into three categories: those caused by natural disease processes, those relating to the prosthesis itself, and those resulting from management failure. Necropsy studies[15] have shown that the majority of sudden deaths fall into the first category with the most common cause being ventricular arrhythmias, which are seen more often after aortic than mitral valve replacement and are sometimes a manifestation of coincident underlying ischaemic heart disease. Although the rate of sudden death decreases after aortic valve replacement, it is still a common cause of death with an incidence of 10–40%. Relating to this, the incidence of ventricular arrhythmia remains relatively high especially in those with cardiomegaly, residual cardiac hypertrophy, and left ventricular impairment. Causes of valve related sudden death include valve thrombosis, thromboembolism, endocarditis, paravalvar leak, and mechanical failure (see below), while sudden deaths relating to management failure include those caused by intracerebral haemorrhage occurring as a complication of anticoagulation treatment.

Because of the close anatomical relation between the aortic valve and conducting tissue, conduction defects are commonly found in association with aortic valve disease and are frequently encountered in the early postoperative period following aortic valve replacement. In those who develop complete atrioventricular (AV) block immediately after aortic valve replacement and who require pacing for more than six hours, permanent pacemaker implantation is usually required before discharge, while even when spontaneous recovery of AV conduction occurs, pacemaker implantation is required at a later date in 50% of cases. Patients with no change in the perioperative ECG after aortic valve replacement are also at risk, with an incidence of almost 14% of progressive conducting tissue disease emerging over the first six postoperative years.[16] Although late pacemaker implantation rates are relatively low, this natural progression in conducting tissue disease combined with the known association between sudden death and the development of left bundle branch block (LBBB) after aortic valve replacement means that careful outpatient surveillance is critical and a low threshold for permanent pacemaker implantation should be set, especially in patients with a history of syncope or presyncope.

THROMBOSIS, THROMBOEMBOLISM, AND COMPLICATIONS FROM ANTICOAGULATION

Thrombotic and haemorrhagic complications are a major cause of morbidity and mortality and therefore are important determinants of long term outcome following valve surgery. Thrombosis on prosthetic valves (fig 14.1) can give rise to local mechanical problems including valve obstruction, but can also lead to thromboembolism and peripheral ischaemic complications including stroke. Overall, the risk of bleeding is greater than that of thromboembolism.[17] For every 100 patient-years, the risk of valve thrombosis is reported to be 1 to 3, of thromboembolism 0.71, and of bleeding 2.68. Mortality is greater with haemorrhagic than with thromboembolic complications, being 0.3 versus 0.03 per 100 patient-years, reflecting the likelihood of death associated with intracranial bleeding. The development of these complications, however, cannot always be attributed to previous valve surgery and it is easy to forget that there is a background risk of stroke, transient cerebral ischaemia, and intracranial bleed that rises with age to approximately 2% per year by the age of 75 years.

Numerous factors may influence the rate of valve thrombosis and thromboembolism, many of which are not specifically related to the surgical intervention. For valve thrombosis, the most important risk factors are periods of under-anticoagulation, low cardiac output, and the presence of hypercoagulable states including pregnancy.[18] The lowest thrombosis rates have been reported with unstented homografts and pericardial heterografts in the aortic

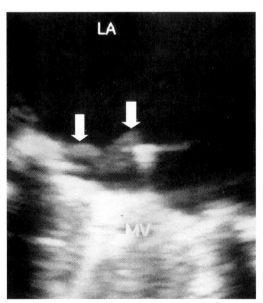

Figure 14.1. Transoesophageal echocardiographic image showing multiple mobile thrombi (arrows) on the left atrial (LA) aspect of a prosthetic mitral valve (MV) in a patient who presented with transient cerebral ischaemia.

position. Comparison between mechanical prostheses is difficult since a fair assessment would have to assume equivalent levels of anticoagulation during the time of surveillance. The large variation in valve thrombosis rates reported for mechanical prostheses in the literature is at least partly caused by the fact that anticoagulation levels have varied substantially in published studies. Patients are at particular risk of valve thrombosis when anticoagulation is interrupted, even temporarily, during non-cardiac surgery at a time when the thrombotic substrate is often increased as a result of systemic illness. For thromboembolism, the constellation of risk factors is more numerous and their interactions more complex, but the quality of anticoagulation control and cardiac rhythm are by far the most important.[19] Increasing age (> 50 years), ethnicity, associated hypertension, diabetes, and cigarette smoking are important, while the presence of chronic disease and intercurrent illness, especially infection, intermittently and substantially increases thromboembolic risk. During the advancement of chronic valve disease, many of the adaptive changes to pressure and volume overload will expose patients to chronic and irreversible changes in cardiac anatomy and physiology despite corrective surgery. Thus, atrial and ventricular dilatation, impaired ventricular function, chronic atrial fibrillation, atrial thrombus, and previous systemic embolisation increase the risk of thromboembolism. Valve type and position are also important. The incidence of events with ball and cage, tilting disc, and bileaflet valves is estimated at 2.5, 0.7, and 0.5 per 100 patient-years, respectively, with valves in the mitral position or more than one valve replacement being associated with double the risk of aortic valves.

Increased risk of bleeding is associated with age (> 70 years), erratic anticoagulation control, and recent initiation of warfarin. The latter is probably related both to fluctuations that often occur in the early stages of anticoagulation but also to the ability of this form of treatment to unmask underlying pathology. Even though clinical events do occur during periods of apparently excellent anticoagulation control, bleeding complications can be minimised through a combination of patient education and careful monitoring of anticoagulation with appropriate dose adjustment. Studies in anticoagulation clinics have shown that only approximately 50% of patients will be within their target range at any given moment of time so that improvements can be made by aiming to achieve narrower and more specific target INRs (international normalised ratios) with a greater proportion of time spent "in range".

Research continues to improve surgical technique and to reduce the thrombogenicity of replacement heart valves, but the risk of thrombosis, thromboembolism, and bleeding will never be abolished. Improved patient safety will be achieved by the careful selection of the most appropriate and least thrombogenic replacement valve in each patient, through the careful achievement of tight

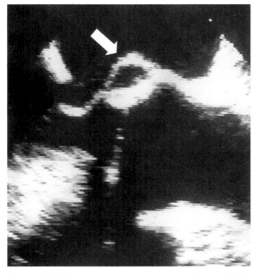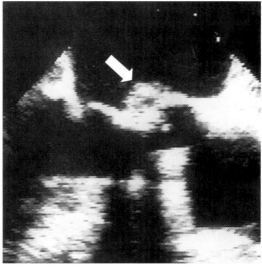

Figure 14.2. Transoesophageal echocardiographic image showing systolic (right panel) and diastolic (left panel) frames of a peri-aortic cavity (arrow) in a patient with infective endocarditis on a prosthetic aortic valve. The systolic expansion of the cavity is caused by its communication with the left ventricular outflow tract.

anticoagulation control, and through the close surveillance of patients in the outpatient clinic looking for symptoms and signs of impending valve thrombosis and degeneration, especially during systemic illness or at the time of non-cardiac surgery.

A previous article in this series provides a detailed review of the role of anticoagulation in valvar heart disease.[20]

Infective endocarditis

Infective endocarditis is a dreaded late complication following valve surgery, with infection usually located on the replacement device (prosthetic valve endocarditis; PVE) but sometimes developing on other diseased valves. PVE is traditionally classified as either "early", when it develops within 60 days of initial surgery, or "late" when it presents at a later stage. Early PVE is caused by contamination of the valve during or immediately after implantation, with the culprit organisms therefore reflecting those likely to be acquired in a hospital setting, including resistant strains of *Staphylococcal epidermidis*, Gram-negative bacilli, and fungi. The likelihood of early PVE is less with porcine than with mechanical valves and is least with homografts.[21] Late PVE results from the infection of a previously sterile implant so that the spectrum of bacteria and their portal of entry is more analogous to that of native valve endocarditis, with the streptococci most common. There are conflicting reports regarding the relative likelihood of late PVE with bioprostheses and mechanical prostheses, but the lower risk of PVE seen in the early postoperative period with homografts seems to be largely nullified at later time points.

PVE is a grave condition, being associated with a reported mortality of 25–60% which is highest for early infections when the degree of valve destruction tends to be greatest. With mechanical prostheses, the infection tends to colonise the sewing ring of the valve while in bioprostheses the infection can, in addition, involve the valve cusps. Vegetations may develop around the valve and give rise to systemic embolisation, while local periannular tissue destruction may lead to paravalvar leak, abscess, and fistula formation (fig 14.2). Clinical presentation is similar to that of native infective endocarditis but there should be a higher level of suspicion in patients with prosthetic valves in whom the presence of fever or a new or changing murmur should be regarded as PVE until proven otherwise. Diagnostic criteria are also similar but transoesophageal echocardiography is of particular importance in PVE, with a diagnostic sensitivity rate of up to 95% as compared with up to 65% for transthoracic echocardiography, reflecting the superior clarity and breadth of unimpeded visualisation of both the prosthetic valve and the perivalvar complications.

Prompt treatment with broad spectrum antibiotics is critical once the diagnosis is suspected. It is advisable to begin treatment before culture results are available because the incidence of systemic embolisation diminishes rapidly once effective treatment is commenced.[22] Treatment strategies for PVE usually combine prolonged appropriate antibiotic treatment (at least six weeks after reoperation) with timely surgical intervention. Medical treatment alone may occasionally be successful—for example, when late PVE develops because of infection with a highly sensitive streptococcus or when there is localised colonisation of the leaflets of a bioprosthesis—but reoperation is usually required. Indications for surgery include prosthetic valve dysfunction, abscess or fistula formation, systemic embolisation, persistent bacteraemia despite appropriate antibiotic treatment, cardiac failure, and progressive multiorgan dysfunction. Operative mortality rates are high (up to 50%) but improving with the primary aim being to excise and remove all infected tissue before replacing the culprit valve.

For detailed reviews of endocarditis in valvar heart disease see earlier articles in this series.[23 24]

MECHANICAL COMPLICATIONS

Paravalvar leak may occur with both mechanical and biological valves and, in the absence of infection, usually reflects a technical problem relating to suture failure. Subclinical levels of haemolysis can be biochemically detectable with all types of mechanical prosthesis, but clinically significant levels of haemolysis are rarely found in the absence of paravalvar leak.

In mechanical valves, sudden failure of the components of the valve is exceedingly rare but usually fatal. More common is a gradual deterioration in valve performance that is seen with the slow in-growth of fibrous tissue (pannus) over the sewing ring, a phenomenon also observed with bioprostheses. This overexuberant fibrous reaction usually develops over years and is likely to be multifactorial in aetiology, relating to local flow conditions, periods of under-anticoagulation, foreign body reaction, and fibroblast activity as well as sewing ring damage and implantation technique. In-growth of fibrous tissue narrows the valve orifice (fig 14.3), may interfere with occluder movement, and act as a platform for thromboembolism. Reoperation is the only effective treatment.

In biological valves, late degeneration is the major late complication. Pathological changes range from thinning, atrophy, and perforation seen particularly in allografts, through to leaflet calcification, thickening, and tearing seen with porcine and pericardial bioprostheses. Age is the most important determinant of failure with valve degeneration accelerated by youth. Rates of aortic valve failure of 42% are reported at 10 years after implantation of a porcine bioprosthesis in patients aged 21–30 years as compared with 0% in those aged 61–70 years.[25] Careful outpatient surveillance is important since presentation is usually gradual, with progressive symptomatic limitation and development of new murmurs.

Follow up after valve surgery

There is an absence of consensus over optimal patient follow up after valve surgery, and the paucity of published clinical studies mandates that clinical practice is usually determined by physician preference and experience. The American Heart Association/American College of Cardiology guidelines[26] suggest that a detailed first follow up visit should be undertaken with clinical assessment, ECG, and chest *x* ray in all patients. Echocardiography is helpful at this stage to document the presence or absence of satisfactory early prosthetic function, to detect residual ventricular dysfunction or pulmonary hypertension, and to serve as a baseline for future examinations should complications or deterioration develop at a later stage. Thereafter, controversy exists as to the necessity, frequency, and optimal location for further outpatient visits in patients who have enjoyed a good result from surgery and who are free of complications. For patients with prosthetic valves, annual hospital follow up has been proposed by some to enable a review of anticoagulation control, to screen for mechanical or haemodynamic problems, and to reinforce advice concerning endocarditis prophylaxis.[26] On the other hand, complications from prosthetic valves are rare and usually catastrophic with no definitive evidence existing to suggest that routine screening enhances their detection over and above a strategy of dealing with problems when symptoms develop. Mahy and colleagues[27] found routine hospital follow up of limited benefit in detecting or averting complications in asymptomatic patients with prosthetic valves, and reasonably concluded that in the present era of well developed primary care and effective community based anticoagulation clinics, such care could be safely devolved away from the surgical centre provided rapid access was offered to patients with new symptoms. The situation is somewhat

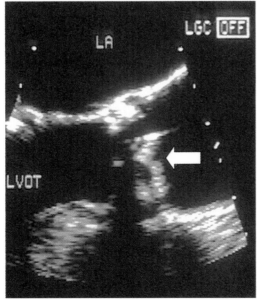
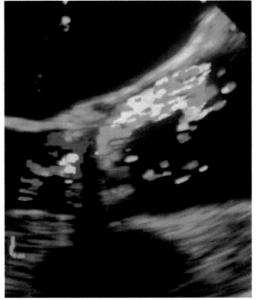

Figure 14.3. Transoesophageal echocardiographic image of an aortic prosthetic valve partly obstructed by pannus. Grey scale (left) and colour flow (right) images show that the movement of the occluder is limited in systole (arrow). LA, left atrium; LVOT, left ventricular outflow tract.

different in patients with bioprosthetic valves since valve degeneration is often more insidious, with the development of new murmurs that may be detected and investigated by echocardiography during routine outpatient surveillance.

1. **Lindblom D, Lindblom U, Qvist J,** *et al.* Long-term survival rates after heart valve replacement. *J Am Coll Cardiol* 1990;**15**:566–73.
• *A large study of survival rates in consecutive patients after heart valve replacement. Through adjustments in background mortality relative survival rates are presented and thereby identify important variables that impact on survival in different valve lesions.*

2. **Cohen G, David TE, Ivanov J,** *et al.* The impact of age, coronary artery disease and cardiac co-morbidity on late survival after bioprosthetic aortic valve replacement. *J Thorac Cardiovasc Surg* 1999;**117**:273–84.

3. **Lund O.** Pre-operative risk evaluation and stratification of long-term survival after valve replacement for aortic stenosis. *Circulation* 1990;**82**:124–39.

4. **Czer LSC, Chaux A, Matloff JM,** *et al.* Ten year experience with the St Jude medical valve for primary valve replacement. *J Thorac Cardiovasc Surg* 1990;**100**:44–55.

5. **Lund O, Erlandsen M.** Changes in left ventricular function and mass during serial investigations after valve replacement for aortic stenosis. *J Heart Valve Dis* 2000;**9**:583–93.

6. **Villari B, Vassalli G, Monrad ES,** *et al.* Normalization of diastolic dysfunction in aortic stenosis late after valve replacement. *Circulation* 1995;**91**:2353–8.
• *A detailed invasive study documenting left ventricular function before, early, and late after aortic valve replacement. The results document the possibility of normalisation of diastolic dysfunction and the time course over which this can be achieved.*

7. **Bonow RO.** Radionuclide angiography in the management of asymptomatic aortic regurgitation. *Circulation* 1991;**84**:(suppl I):296–302.

8. **Nakano S, Sakai K, Taniguchi K,** *et al.* Relation of impaired left ventricular function in mitral regurgitation to left ventricular contractile state after mitral valve replacement. *Am J Cardiol* 1994;**73**:70–4.

9. **Enriquez-Sarano M, Schaff HV, Orszulak TA,** *et al.* Valve repair improves the outcome of surgery for mitral regurgitation: a multivariate analysis. *Circulation* 1995;**91**:1022–8.

10. **Pagani FD, Benedict MB, Marshall BL,** *et al.* The economics of uncomplicated mitral valve surgery. *J Heart Valve Dis* 1997;**6**:466–9.

11. **Porter A, Shapira Y, Wurzel M,** *et al.* Tricuspid regurgitation late after mitral valve replacement: clinical and echocardiographic evaluation. *J Heart Valve Dis* 1999;**8**:57–62.

12. **Groves PH, Lewis NP, Ikram S,** *et al.* Reduced exercise capacity in patients with tricuspid regurgitation after successful mitral valve replacement for rheumatic mitral valve disease. *Br Heart J* 1991;**66**:295–301.
• *In this study the use of objective parameters of exercise performance defines the functional impact of severe tricuspid regurgitation while echocardiography provides clues to the pathophysiology of this late complication of mitral valve replacement.*

13. **King MR, Schaff HF, Danielson GK,** *et al.* Surgery for tricuspid regurgitation late after mitral valve replacement. *Circulation* 1984;**70**(suppl I):193–7.

14. **Zielinski T, Pogorzelska H, Rajecka A,** *et al.* Pulmonary haemodynamics at rest and effort 6 and 12 months after mitral valve replacement: a slow regression of effort pulmonary hypertension. *Int J Cardiol* 1993;**42**:57–62.
• *A detailed study of pulmonary haemodynamics at rest and on exercise at 6 and 12 months after mitral valve replacement. The results define the greatest changes in pulmonary pressures in the early stages and the presence of exercise related abnormalities in pulmonary pressures that may persist at later follow up.*

15. **Burke PA, Farb A, Sessums L,** *et al.* Causes of sudden cardiac death in patients with replacement valves: an autopsy study. *J Heart Valve Dis* 1994;**3**:10–16.

16. **Habicht JM, Scherr P, Zerkowski H-R,** *et al.* Late conduction defects following aortic valve replacement. *J Heart Valve Dis* 2000;**9**:629–32.
• *A prospective analysis of 100 consecutive patients after aortic valve replacement which defines the incidence, time course, and clinical significance of late cardiac conduction defects.*

17. **Cannegeiter SC, Rosendaal FR, Wintzen AR,** *et al.* Optimal oral anticoagulant therapy in patients with mechanical heart valves. *N Engl J Med* 1995;**333**:11–17.

18. **Ryder SJ, Bradley H, Brannan JJ,** *et al.* Thrombotic obstruction of the Bjork-Shiley valve: the Glasgow experience. *Thorax* 1984;**39**:487–92.

19. **Butchart EG, Lewis PA, Bethel JA,** *et al.* Adjusting anticoagulation to prosthesis thrombogenicity and patient risk factors: recommendations for the Medtronic Hall valve. *Circulation* 1991;**84**(suppl IV):61–9.

20. **Gohlke-Bärwolf C.** Anticoagulation in valvar heart disease: new aspects and management during non-cardiac surgery. *Heart* 2000;**84**:567–72.

21. **Calderwood SB, Swinski LA, Waternaux CM,** *et al.* Risk factors for the development of prosthetic valve endocarditis. *Circulation* 1985;**72**:31–7.

22. **Davenport J, Hart RG.** Prosthetic valve endocarditis 1976-1987. Antibiotics, anticoagulation and stroke. *Stroke* 1990;**21**:993–9.

23. **Eykyn SJ.** Endocarditis: basics. *Heart* 2001;**86**:476–80.

24. **Oakley CN, Hall RH.** Endocarditis: problems—patients being treated for endocarditis and not doing well. *Heart* 2001;**85**:47–4.

25. **Gallo I, Nistal F, Artinano E.** Six to ten year follow-up of patients with the Hancock cardiac bioprosthesis. Incidence of primary tissue failure. *J Thorac Cardiovasc Surg* 1986;**92**:14–20.

26. **American College of Cardiology/American Heart Association.** ACC/AHA practice guidelines. Guidelines for the management of patients with valvular heart disease. *Circulation* 1998;**98**:1949–84.

27. **Mahy IR, Dougall H, Buckley A,** *et al.* Routine hospital based follow up for patients with mechanical valve prostheses: is it worthwhile? *Heart* 1999;**82**:520–2.
• *An interesting study defining the rather poor return from outpatient clinic follow up in 100 consecutive patients after valve replacement. Clinic attendance contributed little to the detection of complications and the conclusions raise the question as to whether or not routine hospital follow up is required in most patients.*

SECTION V: ELECTROPHYSIOLOGY

15 Radiofrequency catheter ablation of supraventricular arrhythmias

Hugh Calkins

For most types of supraventricular arrhythmias medical treatment with antiarrythmic drugs is not completely effective. In addition to poor or sporadic efficacy, such drugs can be associated with a number of bothersome and even fatal side effects (although rarely), proarrhythmia, cost, and inconvenience. It is for these reasons that non-pharmacologic interventions, initially using a surgical approach and more recently utilising catheter ablation, have played an increasingly important role in the management of cardiac arrhythmias. Catheter ablation can be defined as the use of an electrode catheter to destroy small areas of myocardial tissue or conduction system, or both, that are critical to the initiation or maintenance of cardiac arrhythmias. Arrhythmias most likely to be amenable to cure with catheter ablation are those which have a focal origin or involve a narrow, anatomically defined isthmus.

Over the past two decades, catheter ablation has evolved from a highly experimental technique to first line treatment for many cardiac arrhythmias. Before 1989, catheter ablation was performed primarily with high energy direct current (DC) shocks. More recently, DC energy has been replaced with radiofrequency energy as the preferred energy source during catheter ablation procedures.

This article reviews the current state of knowledge about the technique, indications, and results of radiofrequency catheter ablation for the treatment of supraventricular cardiac arrhythmias.

Technical considerations

Catheter ablation procedures are performed in a specially equipped catheterisation laboratory, on either an inpatient or outpatient basis. Patients receive conscious sedation before and during the procedure. Two to five multipolar electrode catheters are inserted percutaneously under local anaesthesia into a femoral, brachial, subclavian, or internal jugular vein and positioned in the heart under fluoroscopic guidance. Each electrode catheter has four or more electrodes. Typically, the most distal electrode pair is used for pacing and the delivery of critically timed extra stimuli, while the proximal electrodes are used to record electrograms from localised regions within the heart. Catheter ablation is now performed primarily using radiofrequency energy. Up to 50 W of radiofrequency energy is delivered for 30–60 seconds as a continuous, unmodulated, sinusoidal waveform with a frequency of approximately 500 000 cycles per second, between the 4 mm tip of a deflectable ablation catheter and a ground plate positioned on the patient's back or chest. The majority of catheter ablation systems in use today monitor the temperature of the ablation electrode and automatically adjust power output to achieve a targeted electrode temperature of between 60–70°C. Knowledge of the electrode temperature at a particular ablation site is useful in determining whether an unsuccessful application of radiofrequency energy failed because of inaccurate mapping or inadequate heating.[1] In the event of inadequate heating, additional applications of energy at the same site with improved catheter stability may result in success. Automatic adjustment of power output using closed loop temperature control has been shown to reduce the incidence of coagulum development, which may also facilitate catheter ablation by reducing the number of times the catheter has to be withdrawn from the body to have a coagulum removed from the electrode tip.

During radiofrequency ablation, current flows into the tissue underlying the active electrode in alternating direction at high frequency. Resistive heating as a result of ionic agitation in the tissue then ensues. Thus the tissue underlying the ablation electrode, rather than the electrode itself, is the source of heat generation. The heating of tissue during radiofrequency catheter ablation may be thought of as a two step process; resistive heating followed by conductive heat transfer from the area of resistive heating to surrounding tissue. Because direct resistive heating falls precipitously with increasing distance from the ablation electrode, resistive heating is responsible for heating only a very narrow rim of tissue extending approximately 1 mm beyond the ablation electrode.[1] The majority of lesion volume is determined by the relative contributions of conductive heat exchange into surrounding tissue and convective heat loss towards the relatively cooler moving blood.

Thermal injury is the principal mechanism of tissue destruction during radiofrequency catheter ablation procedures. Elevation of tissue temperature results in desiccation and the denaturation of proteins, and coagulation of tissue and blood. Irreversible tissue injury occurs at temperatures above 50°C.[1] When the temperature at the electrode tissue interface exceeds 100°C, tissue immediately adjacent to the electrode desiccates and plasma proteins denature to form a coagulum. The development of a coagulum results in a rapid increase in impedance which leads to a dramatic decrease in current density, thereby limiting further lesion growth. As a result of the need to achieve a tissue temperature of 50°C for irreversible tissue injury, the 100°C temperature ceiling for tissue heating, and the rapid decrease in tissue temperature with increasing distance from the ablation electrode, the lesions created during radiofrequency catheter ablation procedures are small (5 mm) and have well demarcated borders (fig 15.1). Recently, methods for improved cooling of the electrode have been developed to allow delivery of higher radiofrequency power. These include the use of larger (8 mm) electrodes, which receive greater convective cooling by the blood, and saline irrigated electrode tips, in which the electrode is actively cooled.

As the range of ablatable arrhythmias has broadened, the ablation procedures have, in some cases, become more technically challenging. In such cases, particularly when targeting atrial tachycardias, visualisation of the catheter tip in relation to the cardiac anatomy is crucial. Since a single fluoroscopic view displays the catheter only against the cardiac silhouette, biplane fluoroscopy is a useful addition to the electrophysiology laboratory. When the two fluoroscopic planes are placed orthogonal to each other, the position of the catheter in three dimensional space can be inferred. Several new technologies have provided a means for non-fluoroscopic tracking of catheter tip position and orientation in three dimensional space using either magnetic fields or ultrasound ranging technology. Intracardiac ultrasound is another technique which may allow better imaging of the anatomic substrate relative to the ablation catheter.

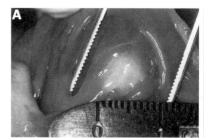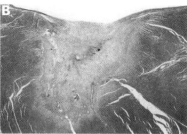

Figure 15.1. (A) Lesion created with radiofrequency energy one month previously in a canine ventricle. The lesion is pale, about 5 mm in diameter, and has smooth borders. (B) Histologic section of the same lesion. The lesion has a distinct border surrounded by normal myocardium, is hemispherical, and shows extensive fibrosis. The lesion depth is 6 mm.

Atrial tachycardia

The term atrial tachycardia refers to a group of arrhythmias confined to the atrium which have a rate < 240 beats per minute. Atrial tachycardias, which have a focal site of origin or result from macroreentry involving a critical isthmus of atrial tissue, are amenable to cure with radiofrequency catheter ablation. From an ablation perspective, two major types of atrial tachycardia can be considered: focal (or ectopic) atrial tachycardia, and scar mediated (or incisional) atrial tachycardia.

Focal atrial tachycardia may present as either a paroxysmal or a sustained arrhythmia. The mechanism of the tachycardia may be elucidated by pharmacologic and pacing manoeuvres, and may be classified as automatic, triggered, or re-entrant.[2] The origin of these arrhythmias may be located in either the right or left atrium, usually near the pulmonary vein orifices, right atrial appendage, or crista terminalis. In the automatic and triggered tachycardias, catheter ablation is performed by manipulating one or more steerable electrode catheters in the right or left atrium to identify the site of earliest atrial activation, usually at least 30 ms before onset of the P wave. The atrial activation sequence with pacing at that site should match the activation sequence during the clinical tachycardia. In the re-entrant atrial tachycardias, appropriate ablation sites are identified using the entrainment techniques described above. Once the site is identified, 25–50 W of radiofrequency energy is delivered for 30–60 seconds. Results of radiofrequency catheter ablation of focal atrial tachycardias have recently been reviewed by Chen and colleagues.[3] The success rate for ablation among a collective total of 252 patients included in their review was 93%. The collective recurrence rate was 7%.

Catheter ablation of supraventricular arrhythmias

The therapeutic options for patients with supraventricular arrhythmias include pharmacologic treatment, arrhythmia surgery, and catheter ablation. The optimal management of an individual patient depends on many factors, including the type of arrhythmia, asscociated symptoms, frequency and duration of episodes, concomitant disease, and patient preference. With the exception of the Wolff-Parkinson-White syndrome, supraventricular arrhythmias are generally not life threatening. Thus, the inherent attractiveness of catheter ablation as a curative approach is tempered by the cost and potential complications associated with an invasive procedure. From the perspective of catheter ablation, supraventricular arrhythmias can be classified into atrial tachycardia, atrial flutter, atrial fibrillation, accessory pathways/Wolff-Parkinson-White syndrome, and atrioventricular nodal re-entrant tachycardia (AVNRT). Catheter ablation of the atrioventricular junction is also used to control the ventricular response in some patients with supraventricular arrhythmias (mainly atrial fibrillation) which cannot be cured with catheter ablation and which are associated with a rapid ventricular response despite the use of pharmacologic treatment. The technique, results, and complications associated with ablation of atrial tachycardia, accessory pathways/Wolff-Parkinson-White syndrome, AVNRT, and the atrioventricular junction are discussed below.

"Inappropriate" sinus tachycardia (IST) is an ill-defined and uncommon clinical syndrome characterised by an increased resting heart rate and an exaggerated response to stress or exercise.[4] The mechanism of this tachycardia is unknown, although it may involve a primary abnormality of the sinus node demonstrating enhanced automaticity or a primary autonomic disturbance with increased sympathetic activity and enhanced sinus node β adrenergic sensitivity. The diagnosis of IST is one of exclusion. It most commonly occurs in young women, particularly those employed in the health care field. It is important to distinguish IST from the postural orthostatic tachycardia syndrome (POTS). POTS is a type of dysautonomia that typically occurs in young women.[5] It is defined as a > 28 beats per minute increase in heart rate on standing with associated symptoms of orthostatic intolerance such as lightheadedness and palpitations.

Patients with POTS are treated primarily with increased salt intake, fludrocortisone, and midodrine. Catheter ablation does not have a role in the management of these patients. The recognition that the sinus node region is a distributed complex exhibiting rate dependent site differentiation allows for targeted ablation to eliminate the fastest sinus rates while maintaining some degree of sinus node function. This may require some fairly extensive ablation along 3–4 cm of the crista terminalis. The goal may be to either modify sinus node function to prevent the fastest rates, or to ablate the sinus node completely and implant a dual chamber or atrial pacemaker. Unfortunately, only about half of affected patients receive symptomatic relief from sinus node modification. Some patients remain symptomatic even after complete sinus node ablation and pacemaker implantation, despite the absence of severe tachycardia.

There are no specific guidelines to decide which patients with IST should undergo modification of the sinus node. However, this infrequently performed procedure should be reserved for the most highly symptomatic of patients (in whom POTS has been excluded), who have failed attempts at pharmacologic treatment and are willing to undergo a procedure with considerable risk of recurrence or the need for a pacemaker, and without assurance that their symptoms will be improved.

Incisional atrial tachycardia is mediated by macroreentry around the scar of a prior surgical atriotomy. These tachycardias are frequently seen as late sequelae after surgical repair of congenital heart disease.[6] Optimal ablation sites are those which occur within a protected isthmus of slow conduction that typically develops between one end of an atriotomy scar and a nearby anatomical barrier, such as the inferior or superior vena cava, or the tricuspid annulus. The extent of the atriotomy scar may be mapped by identifying sites with distinct double potentials. The two deflections are widely separated near the middle of the scar and coalesce at the ends. Entrainment techniques are used to identify optimal ablation sites within the critical isthmus. The published clinical experience with catheter ablation is small. The acute success rate has been reported to be approximately 85%.[7] However, recurrences are frequent with one series reporting a recurrence rate of nearly 50%.[7]

Pre-excitation syndromes, Wolff-Parkinson-White syndrome, concealed pathways

Accessory pathways are anomalous extra nodal connections which connect the epicardial surface of the atrium and ventricle along the atrioventricular groove. Accessory pathways can be classified based on their location along the mitral or tricuspid annulus, type of conduction (decremental or nondecremental), and whether they are capable of antegrade conduction, retrograde conduction, or both. Accessory pathways which are capable only of retrograde conduction are concealed whereas those capable of antegrade conduction are manifest, demonstrating pre-excitation on a standard ECG. The term "Wolff-Parkinson-White syndrome" is reserved for patients who have both pre-excitation and symptomatic tachyarrhythmias. Among patients with the Wolff-Parkinson-White syndrome, atrioventricular reciprocating tachycardia (AVRT) is the most common arrhythmia, occurring in 75% of patients. AVRT is further subclassified into orthodromic and antidromic AVRT. During orthodromic AVRT the re-entrant impulse utilises the atrioventricular node and specialised conduction system for conduction from the atrium to the ventricle, and utilises the accessory pathway for conduction from the ventricle to the atrium. During antidromic AVRT the re-entrant impulse travels in the reverse direction with conduction from the atrium to the ventricle occurring via the accessory pathway. Atrial fibrillation is a less common but potentially more serious arrhythmia in patients with the Wolff-Parkinson-White syndrome as it can result in a very rapid ventricular response, and rarely ventricular fibrillation. The incidence of sudden cardiac death in patients with the Wolff-Parkinson-White syndrome has been estimated to be 0.15% per patient year.

Catheter ablation of accessory pathways is performed in conjunction with a diagnostic electrophysiology test. The purpose of the electrophysiology test is to confirm the presence of an accessory pathway, determine its conduction characteristics, and define the role of the accessory pathway in the patient's clinical arrhythmia. Accurate localisation of an accessory pathway is critical to the success of catheter ablation procedures. Among patients with pre-excitation, preliminary localisation of the accessory pathway can be determined based on the delta wave and QRS morphology. Mapping of concealed accessory pathways and more accurate localisation of manifest accessory pathways require analysis of the retrograde atrial activation sequence and/or antegrade ventricular activation sequence.

Right sided and posteroseptal accessory pathways are typically localised and ablated using a steerable electrode catheter with a 4 mm distal electrode positioned along the tricuspid annulus or in the coronary sinus os from the inferior vena cava. The location of left sided accessory pathways can be determined using a multipolar electrode catheter positioned in the coronary sinus, which runs parallel to the left atrioventricular groove, or with a steerable catheter positioned in the left atrium or ventricle. Once localised to a region of the heart, precise mapping and ablation is performed using a steerable 4 mm tipped electrode catheter positioned along the mitral annulus using either the transseptal or retrograde aortic approach. These

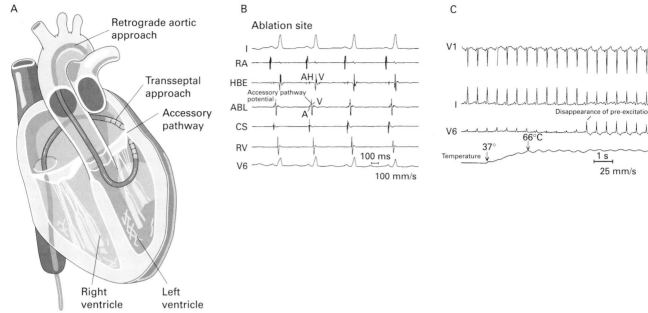

Figure 15.2. (A) Schematic drawing of the two approaches which are available to ablate left sided accessory pathways. The retrograde aortic approach involves inserting the ablation catheter into the femoral artery and crossing the aortic valve to enter the left ventricle. The ablation catheter is positioned against the ventricular aspect of the mitral annulus. The transseptal approach involves crossing the interatrial septum and positioning a long transeptal sheath into the left atrium. The ablation catheter is then passed through the sheath and positioned against the atrial aspect of the mitral annulus at the site of the location of the accessory pathway. (B) The electrogram characteristics of a typical successful ablation site of an accessory pathway (ABL) are shown. Also shown are the surface leads I and V6 and intracardiac recordings obtained from the high right atrium (RA), the right ventricle apex (RV), the electrode catheter positioned to record a His bundle (HBE), and an electrode catheter positioned in the coronary sinus os (CS). The surface leads show a short PR interval and slurring of the upstroke of the QRS complex, which are characteristic of the pre-excitation pattern observed in patients with the Wolff-Parkinson-White syndrome. The interval from the His bundle recording (H) to onset of the QRS complex is less than 50 ms, confirming the presence of pre-excitation. At the successful ablation site, the ventricular electrogram (V) occurs very early relative to the onset of the QRS complex. Also observed is a discrete deflection between the atrial (A) and the ventricular components of the electrogram recorded at the ablation site, which is suggestive of an accessory pathway potential. (C) The disappearance of pre-excitation several seconds after onset of radiofrequency energy delivery during catheter ablation of an accessory pathway. Shown are the surface leads V1, I, V6, and the temperature recorded from the ablation catheter. The temperature recorded from the ablation electrode increases from 37°C to 66°C within two seconds of radiofrequency energy delivery. Pre-excitation resolves several seconds thereafter.

two approaches for ablation of left sided accessory pathways are associated with a similar rate of success and incidence of complications.[8] The decision over which approach to employ is usually based on physician preference, although the transeptal approach may be preferable in the elderly and in young children. In rare instances, left sided accessory pathways can only be ablated via the coronary sinus.

Appropriate sites for radiofrequency energy delivery during ablation of manifest accessory pathways are characterised by early ventricular activation, the presence of an accessory pathway potential, and stability of the local electrogram[9] (fig 15.2). Appropriate sites for energy delivery in patients with retrograde conduction accessory pathways mapped during ventricular pacing or orthodromic AVRT are characterised by continuous electrical activity, the presence of accessory pathway potential, and electrogram stability. Once an appropriate target site is identified, radiofrequency energy is delivered for 30–60 seconds with a target electrode temperature of 60–70°C. At successful ablation sites, interruption of conduction through the accessory pathway usually occurs within 10 seconds, and often within two seconds of the onset of radiofrequency energy delivery (fig 2).

The reported efficacy of catheter ablation of accessory pathways varies from 89–99% with an overall success rate of approximately 93–95%.[10–13] The success rate for catheter ablation of accessory pathways is highest for left free wall accessory pathways and lowest for posteroseptal and right free wall accessory pathways (table 15.1).[10–13] Following an initially successful procedure, recurrence of accessory pathway conduction occurs in approximately 7% of patients (fig 15.3).[10–13] Recurrence of conduction is more common following ablation of posteroseptal and right free wall pathways. Accessory pathways which recur can usually be successfully reablated. Complications associated with catheter ablation of accessory pathways may result from obtaining vascular access (haematomas, deep venous thrombosis, perforation of the aorta, arteriovenous fistula, pneumothorax), catheter manipulation (valvar damage, microemboli, perforation of the coronary sinus or myocardial wall, coronary dissection and/or thrombosis), or delivery of radiofrequency energy (atrioventricular block, myocardial perforation, coronary artery spasm or occlusion, transient ischaemic attacks or cerebrovascular accidents). Complete heart block during ablation of an accessory pathway occurs in approximately 1% of patients, observed most commonly after ablation of septal and posteroseptal accessory pathways. The overall incidence of complications varies between 1–4%. The incidence of procedure related death is estimated to be less than 0.2%.[12]

Atrioventricular nodal re-entrant tachycardia

AVNRT is a common arrhythmia which occurs in patients with two functionally distinct conduction pathways through the atrioven-

Table 15.1   Results of catheter ablation of the atrioventricular junction, accessory pathways, and atrioventricular nodal re-entrant tachycardia from a multicentre prospective clinical trial

Arrhythmia	Number of patients	Medium number (range) of RF applications	Number of patients requiring second procedure for success	Success with investigational system	Overall success	Recurrence*
Atrioventricular junction	121	4 (1–57)	3 (3%)	108 (89%)	121 (100%)	2 (2%)
AVNRT	373	6 (1–73)	3 (1%)	348 (93%)	362 (97%)	16 (5%)
Accessory pathway	500	6 (1–98)	24 (5%)	398 (80%)	465 (93%)	31 (8%)
LFW	270	5 (1–77)	9 (3%)	224 (82%)	257 (95%)	7 (3%)
RFW	92	9 (1–98)	6 (7%)	66 (72%)	83 (90%)	9 (14%)
Posteroseptal	98	6 (1–46)	8 (8%)	73 (74%)	86 (88%)	9 (12%)
Septal	40	6 (1–31)	1 (3%)	35 (88%)	39 (98%)	6 (17%)
Multiple accessory pathways	36	16 (1–54)	8 (22%)	24 (67%)	31 (86%)	5 (21%)
Multiple targets	20	16 (2–58)	4 (20%)	11 (55%)	17 (85%)	2 (17%)
Total	1050	6 (1–98)	42 (4%)	889 (85%)	996 (95%)	56 (6%)

*Analysis of arrhythmia recurrence was confined to those patients in whom success was achieved with the investigational ablation system.
AVNRT, atrioventricular nodal re-entrant tachycardia; LFW, left free wall; RFW, right free wall; RF, radiofrequency.
Reproduced from Calkins et al, *Circulation* 1999;**99**:262–70, with permission of the publisher.

105

tricular node, referred to as the fast and slow pathways. The slow pathway has a shorter refractory period than the fast pathway. Both the fast and slow pathways are necessary to maintain AVNRT. The common form of AVNRT is typically initiated when an atrial premature beat blocks the fast pathway, conducts down the slow pathway, and returns via the fast pathway to depolarise the atrium. During the uncommon form of AVNRT the wave front propagates in the opposite direction, conducting down the fast pathway and returning via the slow pathway. The fast pathway is located anteriorly along the septal portion of the tricuspid annulus, near the compact atrioventricular node, whereas the atrial insertion of the slow pathway is located more posteriorly along the tricuspid annulus, closer to the coronary sinus os.

AVNRT may be cured by ablation of either the fast or the slow pathway. These alternative approaches are referred to as the "anterior" and the "posterior" approaches respectively. The anterior approach targets the fast pathway. Catheter ablation is performed by locating an electrogram with a large His potential and then withdrawing the ablation catheter into the right atrium until the atrial signal is at least twice that of the ventricular signal (A:V ratio > 2) with a His potential no larger than 50 μV. Radiofrequency energy is then applied during sinus rhythm for 30–60 seconds while watching for prolongation in the PR interval. Energy delivery is immediately terminated if atrioventricular block occurs.

Successful ablation of AVNRT using the anterior approach is characterised by lengthening of the PR interval and the inability to induce the tachycardia. Typically, there is elimination or pronounced attenuation of retrograde conduction during ventricular pacing. The atrioventricular block cycle length and the atrioventricular node effective refractory period are not usually altered during ablation of AVNRT using the anterior approach. Catheter ablation of AVNRT using the anterior approach is successful in approximately 90% of patients. Major limitations of the technique are the creation of inadvertent atrioventricular block in approximately 7% of patients and a 9% incidence of recurrence.

The posterior approach to ablation of AVNRT targets the slow pathway. The ablation catheter is directed into the right ventricle low near the posterior septum and is then withdrawn until an electrogram is recorded with a small atrial electrogram and a large ventricular electrogram (A:V ratio < 0.5). Specific ablation sites along the posterior portion of the tricuspid annulus can be selected based either on the appearance of the local atrial electrogram or based strictly on anatomic factors. When using the electrogram guided approach, fractionated atrial electrograms with a late "slow potential" are targeted (fig 15.4). When using the anatomic approach, the initial appli-

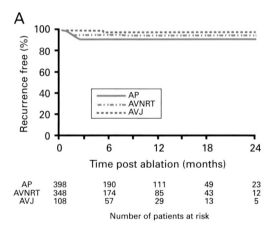

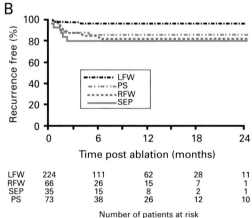

Figure 15.3. (A) Kaplan-Meier curve showing freedom from arrhythmia recurrence among patients who underwent successful ablation of an accessory pathway (AP), atrioventricular nodal re-entrant tachycardia (AVNRT), or atrioventricular junction (AVJ). (B) Kaplan-Meier curve showing freedom from arrhythmia recurrence among patients who underwent successful ablation of an accessory pathway subclassified by its location. LFW, left free wall; RFW, right free wall; PS, posteroseptal; SEP, septal. Reproduced from Calkins et al, Circulation 1999;99:262–70, with permission of the publisher.

A

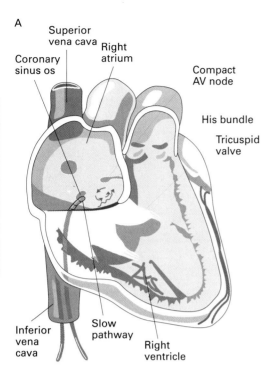

Superior
vena cava
Right
atrium
Coronary
sinus os
Compact
AV node
His bundle
Tricuspid
valve
Inferior
vena
cava
Slow
pathway
Right
ventricle

B

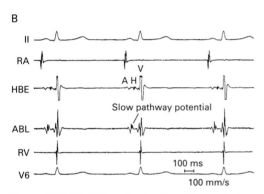

II

RA

HBE

V

A H

Slow pathway potential

ABL

RV

100 ms

V6

100 mm/s

Figure 15.4. (A) Schematic drawing of the posterior or "slow pathway" approach to catheter ablation of atrioventricular nodal re-entrant tachycardia (AVNRT). The ablation catheter is positioned anterior to the coronary sinus os. A schematic drawing of the hypothesised re-entrant circuit for AVNRT is also shown. (B) The electrogram of a successful slow pathway ablation site. Also shown are surface leads 1 and V6 and intracardiac recordings obtained from the right atrium, the right ventricle, and the electrode catheter positioned to record a His bundle. The intracardiac electrogram at the ablation site reveals a ventricular electrogram substantially larger than the atrial electrogram, and a distinct deflection consistent with a slow pathway potential immediately after the atrial electrogram. The arrow points to a slow pathway potential.

cations are delivered at the level of the coronary sinus os with subsequent applications of energy delivered to more superior sites.

With either approach, junctional beats occurring during the application of radiofrequency energy are a marker for successful ablation. Successful ablation of AVNRT using the posterior approach is characterised by an increase in the atrioventricular block cycle length and in the atrioventricular node effective refractory period and elimination of inducible AVNRT. The posterior approach for ablation of AVNRT is effective in greater than 95–97% of patients (table 15.1).[12 14 15]

Atrioventricular block is the most common complication, occurring in 0.5–1% of patients. The incidence of recurrence following successful ablation of AVNRT using the posterior approach is approximately 3% (fig 3). Because of the higher efficacy, lower incidence of atrioventricular block and arrhythmia recurrence, and the greater likelihood of maintaining a normal PR interval during sinus rhythm, the posterior approach is now considered the preferred approach to ablation of AVNRT.

Atrioventricular junction

Theoretically, catheter ablation of the atrioventricular junction can eliminate any type of supraventricular arrhythmia which utilises the atrioventricular node as part of the re-entrant circuit, and can slow the ventricular response to supraventricular arrhythmias confined to the atrium. In practice, catheter ablation of the atrioventricular junction is reserved for atrial arrhythmias which cannot be controlled with pharmacologic treatment and which result in a rapid ventricular response.

The procedure is performed by positioning a steerable ablation catheter across the tricuspid annulus to record the largest His bundle electrogram associated with the largest atrial electrogram. A second electrode catheter is placed at the apex of the right ventricle for temporary pacing. Once an appropriate target site is identified, radiofrequency energy is delivered for 30–60 seconds. If atrioventricular conduction remains unchanged, the catheter is repositioned and a repeat attempt is made. If unsuccessful, a left sided approach can be used.[16] The ablation catheter is passed retrogradely across the aortic valve into the left ventricle and positioned immediately below the aortic valve to record a His bundle electrogram. Radiofrequency energy is then delivered in a standard fashion. The overall efficacy of catheter ablation of the atrioventricular junction using these two approaches is 100% (table 15.1).[12 16–18]

Following ablation of the atrioventricular junction a permanent rate responsive pacemaker is inserted. Complication rates are generally less than 2% with an estimated incidence of procedure related death of 0.2%.[12] Late sudden death has been reported following DC or radiofrequency ablation of the atrioventricular junction. Because many of these patients have severe underlying heart disease, it is difficult to attribute these late sudden deaths directly to the ablation procedure.

Economic considerations

The cost of catheter ablation procedures compares favourably with that of arrhythmia surgery or lifelong antiarrhythmic treatment. In one US study, the cost of surgery in patients with Wolff-Parkinson-White syndrome was estimated to be $53 000, compared with $15 000 for catheter ablation.[19] Another study, which compared the cost of medical management before catheter ablation with the cost of the procedure in patients with AVNRT, found total costs of

Key points

- Catheter ablation is now considered as a first line alternative to pharmacologic therapy for the treatment of focal atrial tachycardia, atrioventricular nodal re-entrant tachycardia, and atrioventricular reciprocating tachycardia associated with an accessory pathway

- Catheter ablation of the atrioventricular junction is also commonly used to control the ventricular response in patients with atrial fibrillation

- Arrhythmias recur following 3–5% of successful catheter ablation procedures

- Recurrences generally present within the first three months following an ablation procedure

- A repeat ablation procedure is associated with a very high likelihood of long term success

$7600 and $16 000, respectively.[20] The investigators estimated that the annual medical costs, including medications and an annual office visit, for a patient whose tachycardia is effectively controlled with verapamil, for example, would equal the cost of catheter ablation in approximately 15 years. These cost effective ratios are within the range generally thought to warrant adoption of the procedures. Thus, from an economic perspective, the expense of catheter ablation appears justifiable.

Conclusion

The safety and efficacy of radiofrequency catheter ablation for treatment of most types of supraventricular arrhythmias is well established. These arrhythmias/arrhythmia substrates include AVNRT, accessory pathways, and focal atrial tachycardia. Because of this catheter ablation is considered as an alternative to pharmacologic therapy in the treatment of these cardiac arrhythmias. The technique, safety, and efficacy of catheter ablation for treatment of atrial fibrillation remains an area of active research. Although the potential for catheter ablation of atrial fibrillation has been demonstrated, further research is needed to approach the remarkably high safety, efficacy, and ultimately clinical acceptance which has been seen with catheter ablation of most other types of supraventricular arrhythmias.

1. **Dinerman J, Berger RD, Calkins H.** Temperature monitoring during radiofrequency ablation. *J Cardiovasc Electrophysiol* 1996;**7**:163–73.
   - *This is a recent and comprehensive review of the literature concerning the biophysics of radiofrequency catheter ablation and the clinical role of temperature monitoring.*

2. **Chen SA, Chiang CE, Yang CJ,** *et al.* Sustained atrial tachycardia in adult patients. Electrophysiological characteristics, pharmacological response, possible mechanisms, and effects of radiofrequency ablation. *Circulation* 1994;**90**:1262–78.
   - *A description is provided of the technique, results, and complications associated with catheter ablation of atrial tachycardias.*

3. **Chen SA, Tai CT, Chiang CE,** *et al.* Focal atrial tachycardia: reanalysis of the clinical and electrophysiologic characteristics and prediction of successful radiofrequency ablation. *J Cardiovasc Electrophysiol* 1998;**9**:355–65.

4. **Lee, RJ, Kalman JM, Fitzpatrick AP,** *et al.* Radiofrequency catheter modification of the sinus node for "inappropriate" sinus tachycardia. *Circulation* 1995;**92**:2919–28.

5. **Low PA, Opfer-Gehrking TL, Textor SC,** *et al.* Postural tachycardia syndrome (POTS). *Neurology* 1995;**45**(suppl 5):S19–25.

6. **Lesh MD, Kalman JM, Saxon LA,** *et al.* Electrophysiology of "reentrant" reentrant atrial tachycardia complicating surgery for congenital heart disease. *PACE* 1997;**20**:2107–11.

7. **Baker BM, Lindsay BD, Bromberg BI,** *et al.* Catheter ablation of clinical intraatrial reentrant tachycardias resulting from previous atrial surgery: localizing and transecting the critical isthmus. *J Am Coll Cardiol* 1996;**28**:411–17.

8. **Lesh MD, Van Hare G, Scheinman MM,** *et al.* Comparison of the retrograde and transseptal methods for ablation of left free-wall accessory pathways. *J Am Coll Cardiol* 1993;**22**:542–9.
   - *This article describes, and prospectively compares, the retrograde aortic and the transeptal approach to catheter ablation of left sided accessory pathways.*

9. **Calkins H, Kim YN, Schmaltz S,** *et al.* Electrogram criteria for identification of appropriate target sites for radiofrequency catheter ablation of accessory atrioventricular connections. *Circulation* 1992;**85**:565–73.

10. **Jackman WM, Wang X, Friday KJ,** *et al.* Catheter ablation of accessory atrioventricular pathways (Wolff-Parkinson-White syndrome) by radiofrequency current. *N Engl J Med* 1991;**324**:1605–11.
    - *This landmark article describes the technique and results of radiofrequency catheter ablation of accessory pathways.*

11. **Calkins H, Sousa J, El-Atassi R,** *et al.* Diagnosis and cure of the Wolff-Parkinson-White syndrome or paroxysmal supraventricular tachycardias during a single electrophysiology test. *N Engl J Med* 1991;**324**:1612–18.
    - *A further landmark article describing the technique and results of radiofrequency catheter ablation of atrioventricular nodal re-entrant tachycardia and accessory pathways. This study was also the first to demonstrate the clinical utility of performing both a diagnostic electrophysiology test and catheter ablation in a single setting.*

12. **Calkins H, Yong P, Miller JM,** *et al,* **for the Atakr Multicenter Investigators Group.** Catheter ablation of accessory pathways, atrioventricular nodal reentrant tachycardia, and the atrioventricular junction: final results of a prospective, multicenter clinical trial. *Circulation* 1999;**99**:262–70.
    - *This describes the results of the only prospective multicentre clinical trial of radiofrequency catheter ablation of accessory pathways, atrioventricular nodal re-entrant tachycardia, and the atrioventricular junction.*

13. **Calkins H, Prystowsky E, Berger RD,** *et al,* **and the Atakr Multicenter Investigators Group.** Recurrence of conduction following radiofrequency catheter ablation procedures: relationship to ablation target and electrode temperature. *J Cardiovasc Electrophysiol* 1996;**7**:704–12.

14. **Haissaguerre M, Gaita F, Fischer B,** *et al.* Elimination of atrioventricular nodal reentrant tachycardia using discrete slow potentials to guide application of radiofrequency energy. *Circulation* 1992;**85**:2162–75.

15. **Jackman WM, Beckman KJ, McClelland JH,** *et al.* Treatment of supraventricular tachycardia due to atrioventricular nodal reentry by radiofrequency catheter ablation of slow-pathway conduction. *N Engl J Med* 1992;**327**:313–18.
    - *This is the first article to report the technique, results, and complications associated with catheter ablation of atrioventricular nodal re-entrant tachycardia using the posterior or "slow pathway" approach. This approach is now considered the standard approach.*

16. **Sousa J, El-Atassi R, Rosenheck S,** *et al.* Radiofrequency catheter ablation of the atrioventricular junction from the left ventricle. *Circulation* 1991;**84**:567–71.

17. **Curtis AB, Kutalek SP, Prior M,** *et al.* Prevalence and characteristics of escape rhythms after radiofrequency ablation of the atrioventricular junction: results from the registry for atrioventricular junction ablation and pacing in atrial fibrillation. *Am Heart J* 2000;**139**:122–5.

18. **Scheinman MM, Huang S.** The 1998 NASPE prospective catheter ablation registry. *Pacing Clin Electrophysiol* 2000;**23**:1020–8.

19. **De Buitleir M, Sousa J, Bolling SF,** *et al.* Reduction in medical care cost associated with radiofrequency catheter ablation of accessory pathways. *Am J Cardiol* 1991;**68**:1656–61.

20. **Kalbfleisch SJ, El-Atassi R, Calkins H,** *et al.* Safety, feasibility and cost of outpatient radiofrequency catheter ablation of accessory atrioventricular connections. *J Am Coll Cardiol* 1993;**21**:567–70.

16 Implantable cardioverter-defibrillators

Derek T Connelly

Sudden cardiac death is a common problem, and increasing numbers of patients are surviving a first episode of a life threatening ventricular arrhythmia. In the absence of an acute myocardial infarction, patients who survive either ventricular fibrillation or sustained ventricular tachycardia have a high risk of further episodes, which may be fatal.[1] Until recently, class I and class III antiarrhythmic drugs have been the standard treatment for patients with malignant ventricular arrhythmias. Amiodarone[2] and sotalol[3] have been shown to be superior to class I drugs, but despite using the best appropriate medical treatment, arrhythmia recurrence rates are still 40–50% at five years.

There is now growing evidence to support the wider use of implantable cardioverter-defibrillators (ICDs) as primary treatment in certain patients with serious ventricular arrhythmias. These devices were developed in the 1970s, with the first human implant in 1980.[4] Original devices had a single therapy option of defibrillation only; the generator was implanted in the abdomen, and thoracotomy was required for electrode placement. With advances in technology the units have become smaller (current ICDs are little bigger than a pacemaker) and can be implanted pectorally. With improvements in sensing, the latest devices offer graded therapeutic responses to a sensed ventricular arrhythmia. Antitachycardia pacing, low energy synchronised cardioversion, and high energy defibrillation shocks can be given via a single transvenous lead.

Implant procedure

Implantation of an ICD is now technically very straightforward, and only a little more complicated than pacemaker implantation. As with pacemaker implantation, strict attention to asepsis is necessary, and prophylactic antibiotics are generally used. In the past, ICD implants were performed under general anaesthesia; however, many centres now implant these devices using a combination of local anaesthesia and intravenous sedation. Usually an incision 5–8 cm in length is made in the left infraclavicular region, and a pocket is fashioned for the generator either subcutaneously or deep to the pectoralis major muscle. A ventricular lead (for sensing, pacing, and defibrillation) is inserted via the cephalic or subclavian vein, and if appropriate an atrial lead is also inserted. Standard tests of pacing and sensing are performed, as for pacemaker implantation. It is then important to induce ventricular fibrillation, in order to test that the device can detect the arrhythmia and defibrillate effectively with an adequate safety margin. Ventricular fibrillation is usually induced either by delivering a small shock (via the device) synchronous with the T wave, or less commonly by alternating current at 50 Hz or by rapid ventricular pacing. It is customary to test efficacy of defibrillation at an output energy at least 10 J less than the maximum stored energy of the device (that is—if the device can deliver a maximum of 30 J, defibrillation testing is performed at 20 J or less). If defibrillation is successful at this energy level on two consecutive occasions, the implant is completed; if not, an additional intravascular or subcutaneous lead may be required.

Programming and follow up

Before hospital discharge, the pacing and sensing functions of the device are tested, and chest radiographs (posteroanterior and lateral) are obtained (fig 16.1). The device is programmed to detect and treat episodes of ventricular tachycardia and fibrillation, the precise programmed values being governed by the patient's clinical history, maximum sinus rate, and rates of any documented ventricular (and supraventricular) arrhythmias. Separate "zones" can be programmed for detection of ventricular fibrillation (for example, rate > 200–220/min) and ventricular tachycardia, and some devices allow for two separate ventricular tachycardia detection zones. Additional discriminatory features, such as sudden onset, beat-to-beat variability, QRS width and/or morphology, and (if available) atrial rate can also be programmed in order to help discriminate between atrial and ventricular arrhythmias. Even if the patient only has a history of ventricular fibrillation, it is customary to program the device for detection and treatment of ventricular tachycardia, as many patients will present with new onset ventricular tachycardia after the implant. Ventricular fibrillation is usually treated with shocks at the

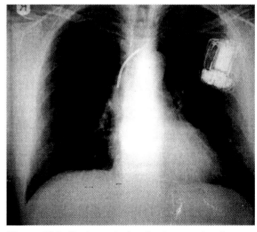

Figure 16.1. Posteroanterior chest *x* ray showing positioning of ICD generator and lead.

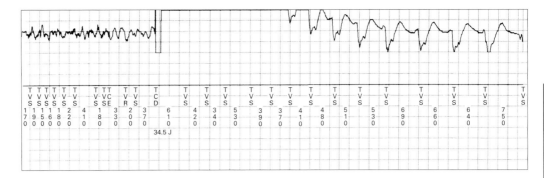

Figure 16.2. Stored intracardiac electrograms from an ICD which treated a spontaneous episode of ventricular fibrillation with a 34 J shock.

maximum energy of the device (fig 16.2), but the ICD can be programmed to treat ventricular tachycardia by a variety of modalities of antitachycardia pacing (fig 16.3) or if necessary by low energy cardioversion shocks. Some centres routinely test the efficacy of antitachycardia pacing modalities at a post-implant electrophysiological study. However, many implanters now consider this unnecessary, since spontaneous episodes of ventricular tachycardia are often easier to terminate than tachycardias induced in the laboratory, and a standardised antitachycardia pacing algorithm appears to be effective in the majority of patients.

Most patients can be discharged home 24–48 hours after implantation. Patients are usually followed up 4–6 weeks post-implant, then at 3–6 monthly intervals. At each follow up visit, the device is interrogated, standard pacing and sensing tests are performed, and the device memory is interrogated. Details of any stored arrhythmic events are downloaded and printed, and correlated with the patient's symptoms. If necessary, appropriate programming changes (either in arrhythmia detection or treatment) can be made, or alterations in the patient's medication can be instigated.

Complications of ICDs

ICDs are much simpler to implant now than they were five years ago, and the complication rate is diminishing. Nevertheless, all the complications of cardiac pacing (for example,

infection, erosion, conductor/insulation fracture, over- and undersensing) can occur with ICDs, and many of these complications may require operative revision or even replacement of the system, which can be a major undertaking. Additional problems may occur, the most common being inappropriate shocks, usually for atrial fibrillation or (less commonly) sinus tachycardia. Such complications can usually be treated or circumvented either by additional antiarrhythmic medication or by further programming of the tachycardia detection parameters. Rarely, when rapid uncontrolled atrial fibrillation leads to inappropriate shocks (or when atrial fibrillation induces ventricular tachycardia) it may be necessary to perform radiofrequency ablation of atrioventricular conduction and pace the patient permanently (either via the ICD or using a separate permanent pacemaker).

Clinical trials of ICDs

ICDs are effective at treating ventricular arrhythmias but until recently there has not been clear evidence that they reduce mortality. Recently, the results of three large randomised controlled trials of ICD treatment have been published.[5–7] Their results are summarised in table 16.1.

A meta-analysis of these three trials has been published recently.[8] In the three studies, 934 patients were treated with an ICD and 932 with amiodarone. In over 2000 patient years of follow

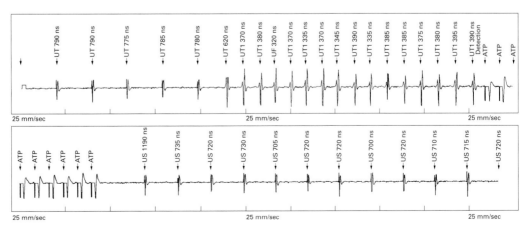

Figure 16.3. Stored intracardiac electrograms from an ICD showing spontaneous onset of ventricular tachycardia with a cycle length of 380 ms (rate 158/min) treated by a burst of antitachycardia pacing (ATP), which restored sinus rhythm.

Table 16.1   Trials of ICDs in patients with ventricular tachycardia/ventricular fibrillation

	Number in trial	Control treatment	Mean follow up	ICD mortality	Control mortality	p Value
AVID[5]	1016	Amiodarone or sotalol	18 months	25% at 3 years	36% at 3 years	< 0.02
CIDS[6]	659	Amiodarone	36 months	8.3% per year	10.2% per year	0.142
CASH[7]	288	Amiodarone or metoprolol	57 months	36%	44%	0.081

up in each group, there were 200 deaths in patients treated with an ICD and 255 deaths in patients treated with amiodarone. This equates to a 28% reduction in mortality in the ICD group (95% confidence intervals (CI) 60% to 87%, p = 0.0006). Importantly, the meta-analysis showed that patients who presented with ventricular tachycardia had as much to gain from a defibrillator as those whose index arrhythmia was ventricular fibrillation, and patients in all functional classes appeared to benefit. There did not appear to be any benefit from epicardial ICDs (mainly implanted before 1991). Patients with left ventricular ejection fraction of 35% or below had more to gain (34% reduction in mortality compared to amiodarone) than those with preserved ventricular function (no significant difference in mortality compared to amiodarone).

Several studies have also assessed the efficacy of defibrillator treatment for "primary prevention" in patients at high risk for sudden death who have not yet had a clinical event. The MADIT study[9] studied 196 high risk survivors of myocardial infarction with impaired left ventricular function and non-sustained ventricular tachycardia on ECG monitoring. Patients recruited to this trial had to have an inducible sustained ventricular arrhythmia at electrophysiological study which could not be suppressed by an antiarrhythmic drug. These patients were randomly allocated to treatment with an ICD or an antiarrhythmic drug (amiodarone in 80% of the cases). The trial was terminated in 1996 after demonstrating a 54% reduction in mortality with defibrillator therapy compared to antiarrhythmic drug treatment.

More recently, the MUSTT study[10] recruited patients who had prior myocardial infarction, impaired left ventricular function, spontaneous episodes of non-sustained ventricular tachycardia, and inducible sustained ventricular tachycardia at electrophysiological study. Patients were randomly allocated to a "control" group, who received no specific antiarrhythmic treatment (353 patients), and an electrophysiologically guided treatment group, who received antiarrhythmic drugs if the tachycardia could be suppressed by drugs (158 patients), or an ICD if drugs were ineffective at electrophysiological study (161 patients). The five year mortality in this study was 48% in those not treated with antiarrhythmic medication; patients on antiarrhythmic drugs fared marginally worse, but those treated with an implantable defibrillator had a five year mortality rate of 24% (p < 0.001). These results from the MUSTT study support the data from the MADIT study, and show that patients with prior myocardial infarction, impaired left ventricular function, and non-sustained ventricular tachycardia can be strati-fied by electrophysiological study. Patients with inducible sustained ventricular arrhythmias are highly likely to benefit from prophylactic ICD implantation, even though they have not yet had a major spontaneous arrhythmic event.

The CABG Patch trial[11] was a trial of prophylactic ICD treatment in patients undergoing surgical revascularisation. Patients recruited to the CABG Patch trial had ejection fractions of less than 36% and an abnormal signal averaged ECG, but there was no necessity for either spontaneous or inducible ventricular arrhythmias. In this study of 900 patients, there was no benefit for prophylactic ICD implantation.

There are several other ongoing trials which are comparing the efficacy of ICD therapy with either no specific antiarrhythmic treatment or drugs such as amiodarone in high risk patients with heart failure or with poor left ventricular function postmyocardial infarction (see box on next page).

Cost effectiveness of ICDs

There is no doubt that the ICD is an expensive piece of medical technology, the total cost of the hardware for an implant approaching £20 000 (nearly US$30 000). Although the cost has not come down in recent years, the battery life has been extended considerably: devices implanted 10 years ago had a battery life of only two years, whereas modern devices are expected to last seven to nine years.

Several studies in the early 1990s attempted to estimate the cost of implantable defibrillators per life year saved. These studies were conducted before the publication of the major trials documenting the efficacy of the ICD in reducing mortality, and therefore involved estimates of the likely improvement in mortality and the likely lifetime costs of treatment by antiarrhythmic drugs or by ICD. More recently, data based on true costs and actual longevity have begun to emerge from the randomised trials. The cost analysis of the MADIT study[12] showed that the average survival for the group treated with a defibrillator over four years was 3.66 years, compared with 2.80 years for conventionally treated patients. The accumulated net costs in the ICD and conventional groups were $97 560 and $75 980 respectively. This equates to a cost of $27 000 (£18 500) per life year saved for the ICD group. If all the ICDs were modern transvenous systems, the costs would be lower at $23 000 (£16 000) per life year saved. This figure is not excessive, and is comparable with the cost effectiveness of several other accepted medical procedures.

Ongoing trials of ICD versus medical treatment

- SCD-HeFT

    –New York Heart Association functional class II/III, left ventricular ejection fraction < 35%

    –randomised to ICD, amiodarone, or control

    –primary end point is total mortality

    –secondary end points: quality of life, cost effectiveness, incidence of ventricular tachycardia/ventricular fibrillation

- MADIT-2

    –patients > 1 month post-myocardial infarction, left ventricular ejection fraction < 30%

    –randomised to ICD or control

    –post-randomisation: non-invasive markers, electrophysiological study

    –primary end point is total mortality

    –secondary end points: quality of life, cost effectiveness

- DINAMIT

    –patients 6–40 days post-myocardial infarction, left ventricular ejection fraction < 35%

    –decreased heart rate variability or mean 24 hour heart rate > 80/min

    –randomised to ICD or control

    –primary end point is total mortality

Similar cost effectiveness analyses have been performed on the data from the AVID and CIDS[13] studies, and the estimated costs per life year saved in those analysis were considerably higher. The AVID trial was stopped prematurely after a mean follow up period of only 18 months (compared to 27 months in the MADIT study). Any studies such as these which are terminated early will tend to overestimate the costs in the group treated with defibrillators (which are paid for at implantation) compared with those treated with drugs (the costs of which continue to accumulate throughout the follow up period). Further data on cost effectiveness is likely to be produced from the meta-analysis of the AVID, CASH, and CIDS studies.

Quality of life in patients with ICDs

An ICD is not a cure. Patients are still considered to be at risk of an arrhythmia, which might cause syncope or cardiac arrest, if only for a few seconds before treatment is delivered. Inevitably many patients face significant lifestyle restrictions, and a minority of patients have severe psychological problems. Although the implant procedure is similar to pacemaker implantation, follow up of patients with ICDs tends to be more complex. Many of the patients have coronary artery disease and poor left ventricular function, and are likely to require ongoing medical treatment for heart failure, ischaemia, and hyperlipidaemia.

Although some patients may develop an adverse psychological reaction to ICD implantation, it is important to be aware that these patients often improve with the passage of time as they become accustomed to having the device and adapt to their physical limitations. There is no doubt, however, that many patients tolerate defibrillation shocks very poorly, particularly if they experience multiple shocks (appropriate or inappropriate). For this reason, antiarrhythmic drugs may have a role in reducing the incidence of both ventricular and supraventricular arrhythmias in patients with ICDs. In one recent study,[14] 302 patients were randomised to treatment with sotalol (160–320 mg/day) or placebo. Sotalol treatment reduced the mean (SD) frequency of shocks (both appropriate and inappropriate) compared to placebo (1.43 (3.53) shocks per year in the sotalol group *v* 3.89 (10.65) shocks per year on placebo).

The issue of fitness to drive in patients with ICDs is a contentious one. Up until five years ago, patients with ICDs in the UK faced a lifetime ban from driving. Since then the regulations in the UK have been gradually relaxed. Currently, ICD recipients may be allowed to drive provided that the device has been implanted for at least six months and has not delivered shock therapy or symptomatic antitachycardia pacing therapy for six months (except during formal clinical testing), and if previous discharges have not been accompanied by incapacity. Patients must stop driving for one month if the device (lead or generator) is revised, or if any change is made in antiarrhythmic treatment. Patients who have an ICD implanted for "primary prevention" need only refrain from driving for one month, unless they subsequently receive shocks from the device. Licences are subject to annual review. Patients with ICDs are permanently disqualified from driving lorries and buses. These recommendations are similar to the current North American[15] and European guidelines on driving for patients with arrhythmias.

ICD indications

In the UK, the National Institute for Clinical Excellence (NICE) has recently published guidance on the use of ICDs.[16] The institute has stated that ICDs should be routinely considered for both primary and secondary prevention of life threatening arrhythmias. Their guidance is summarised in table 16.2. These indications are similar to those published by the American College of Cardiology and the American Heart Association,[17] and by the North American Society of Pacing and Electrophysiology.[18]

Trial acronyms

AVID Antiarrhythmics Versus Implantable Defibrillators

CASH Cardiac Arrest Study Hamburg

CASCADE Cardiac Arrest in Seattle: Conventional versus Amiodarone Drug Evaluation

CIDS Canadian Implantable Defibrillator Study

DINAMIT Defibrillator In Acute Myocardial Infarction Trial

MADIT Multicenter Automatic Defibrillator Implantation Trial

MUSTT Multicenter Unsustained Tachycardia Trial

SCD-HeFT Sudden Cardiac Death in Heart Failure Trial

The NICE guidance in the UK also recommends that protocols for ICD implantation be developed, to include:

- early referral of appropriate patients;
- rapid decision making and implantation;
- conscious sedation rather than general anaesthesia;
- rehabilitation, including psychological preparation for living with an ICD;
- early discharge;
- efficient and comprehensive follow up;
- screening of high risk survivors of myocardial infarction.

Conclusions

The ICD implant rate in the UK is approximately 17 devices per million population per year. Although the rate has doubled over the past three years, the implant rate in the UK is still little more than half that for western Europe, and less than 10% of the rate in the USA. It is now clear from several randomised controlled trials that, in selected high risk patients, ICDs are more effective than antiarrhythmic drugs in prolonging life. When faced with a patient who has had sustained ventricular tachycardia or successful resuscitation from ventricular fibrillation, physicians should now consider an ICD as first line treatment.[16–18] Furthermore, when we are faced with post-myocardial infarction patients who have significant impairment of left ventricular function, it is now our duty to perform ambulatory ECG monitoring in order to detect those patients with asymptomatic non-sustained ventricular tachycardia. Such patients should be referred for electrophysiological study, as about 30% of them will have inducible sustained ventricular arrhythmias and will be likely to benefit from prophylactic ICD implantation.

Table 16.2 Indications for ICD implantation[16–18]

"Secondary prevention"
For patients who present, in the absence of a treatable cause, with:
- Cardiac arrest caused by either VT or VF
- Spontaneous sustained VT causing syncope or significant haemodynamic compromise
- Sustained VT without syncope/cardiac arrest, and who have an associated reduction in ejection fraction (< 35%) but are no worse than NYHA functional class III heart failure

"Primary prevention"
For patients with:
- A history of previous myocardial infarction and *all* of the following:
  - non-sustained VT on Holter monitoring
  - inducible VT on electrophysiological testing
  - left ventricular dysfunction with an ejection fraction < 35% and no worse than NYHA functional class III heart failure
- A familial cardiac condition with a high risk of sudden death, including:
  - long QT syndrome
  - hypertrophic cardiomyopathy
  - Brugada syndrome
  - arrhythmogenic right ventricular dysplasia
  - following repair of tetralogy of Fallot

Patient groups in whom an ICD is usually *not* indicated
- Syncope of undetermined aetiology, VT/VF not inducible
- Incessant VT
- VT amenable to surgical or catheter ablation
- VT/VF due to transient or reversible cause
- Significant psychiatric illness that might be aggravated by device implant or may preclude systematic follow up
- Terminal illness with life expectancy < 6 months
- Patients with impaired left ventricular function undergoing coronary artery bypass graft surgery, without spontaneous or inducible VT
- Patients with NYHA functional class IV heart failure who are not candidates for heart transplantation

NYHA, New York Heart Association; VF, ventricular fibrillation; VT, ventricular tachycardia.

1. **Cobb LA, Baum RS, Alvarez H III,** *et al.* Resuscitation from out-of-hospital ventricular fibrillation: 4 years follow-up. *Circulation* 1975;**52**(suppl III):223–35.

2. **The CASCADE Investigators.** Randomized antiarrhythmic drug therapy in survivors of cardiac arrest (the CASCADE study). *Am J Cardiol* 1993;**72**:280–7.

3. **Mason JW.** A comparison of seven antiarrhythmic drugs in patients with ventricular tachyarrhythmias. *N Engl J Med* 1993;**329**:452–8.

4. **Mirowski M, Reid PR, Mower MM,** *et al.* Termination of malignant ventricular arrhythmias with an implanted automatic defibrillator in human beings. *N Engl J Med* 1980;**303**:322–4.

5. **The AVID Investigators.** A comparison of antiarrhythmic drug therapy with implantable defibrillators in patients resuscitated from near-fatal ventricular arrhythmias. *N Engl J Med* 1997;**337**:1576–83.
   - *This was the first major "secondary prevention" trial comparing ICDs to amiodarone in patients with a history of ventricular tachycardia or ventricular fibrillation.*

6. **Connolly SJ, Gent M, Roberts RS,** *et al.* Canadian implantable defibrillator study (CIDS): a randomized trial of the implantable cardioverter defibrillator against amiodarone. *Circulation* 2000;**101**:1297–302.

7. **Kuck KH, Cappato R, Siebels J,** *et al.* Randomized comparison of antiarrhythmic drug therapy with implantable defibrillators in patients resuscitated from cardiac arrest: the cardiac arrest study Hamburg (CASH). *Circulation* 2000;**102**:748–54.

8. **Connolly SJ, Hallstrom AP, Cappato R,** *et al.* Meta-analysis of the implantable cardioverter defibrillator secondary prevention trials. *Eur Heart J* 2000;**21**:2071–8.
   - *This is a meta-analysis of the above three trials (refs 5–7), comparing the outcome in patients treated with a defibrillator to those treated with amiodarone. There was a significant reduction in all cause mortality of 28% in the defibrillator group.*

9. **Moss AJ, Hall WJ, Cannom DS,** *et al.* Improved survival with an implanted defibrillator in patients with coronary disease at high risk for ventricular arrhythmia. *N Engl J Med* 1996;**335**:2933–40.
   - *The MADIT study was the first "primary prevention" trial, showing a 54% reduction in mortality with the ICD in high risk post-myocardial infarction patients.*

10. **Buxton AE, Lee KL, Fisher JD,** *et al*, **for the MUSTT Investigators.** A randomized study of the prevention of sudden death in patients with coronary artery disease. *N Engl J Med* 1999;**341**:1882–90.
    - *The MUSTT study confirmed the benefits of the MADIT study in a larger patient population. There was a 60% reduction in mortality with the ICD, and no evidence of benefit for antiarrhythmic drugs.*

11. **Biggar JT, for the CABG Patch Trial Investigators.** Prophylactic use of implanted cardiac defibrillators in patients at high risk for ventricular arrhythmias after coronary artery bypass graft surgery. *N Engl J Med* 1997;**337**:1569–75.

12. **Mushlin AI, Hall WJ, Zwanziger J,** *et al.* The cost-effectiveness of automatic implantable cardiac defibrillators: results from MADIT. *Circulation* 1998;**97**:2129–35.

13. **O'Brien BJ, Connolly SJ, Goeree R,** *et al.* Cost-effectiveness of the implantable cardioverter-defibrillator: results from the Canadian implantable defibrillator study (CIDS). *Circulation* 2001;**103**:1416–21.

14. **Pacifico A, Hohnloser SH, Williams JH,** *et al.* Prevention of implantable-defibrillator shocks by treatment with sotalol. *N Engl J Med* 1999;**340**:1855–62.

15. **Epstein AE, Miles WM, Benditt DG,** *et al.* AHA/NASPE medical/scientific statement. Personal and public safety issues related to arrhythmias that may affect consciousness: implications for regulation and physician recommendations. *Circulation* 1996;**94**:1147–66.

16. **National Institute for Clinical Excellence.** Guidance on the use of implantable cardioverter defibrillators for arrhythmias, September 2000. http://www.nice.org.uk

17. **Gregoratos G, Cheitlin MD, Conill A,** *et al.* ACC/AHA guidelines for implantation of cardiac pacemakers and antiarrhythmia devices: a report of the ACC/AHA task force on practice guidelines (committee on pacemaker implantation). *J Am Coll Cardiol* 1998;**31**:1175–206.

18. **Winters SL, Packer DL, Marchlinski FE,** *et al.* Consensus statement on indications, guidelines for use, and recommendations for follow-up of implantable cardioverter defibrillators. *PACE* 2001;**24**:262–9.
• *The most recent statement of guidance for ICD implantation, from the North American Society of Pacing and Electrophysiology.*

113

17 Permanent pacing: new indications

Michael R Gold

Over the past 40 years, permanent pacemakers have become standard treatment for patients with symptomatic sinus node disease and documented, or suspected, high grade atrioventricular (AV) block. Permanent pacemakers were first developed for the treatment of heart block, often in young patients following surgical repair of congenital heart defects. These early pacemakers were primitive devices, allowing only for fixed rate asynchronous pacing in the ventricle (that is, VOO mode). Subsequently, sensing circuits were developed to permit inhibited modes of pacing (that is, VVI mode). Permanent pacemakers were designed primarily to prevent mortality, which was inevitable and often occurred early in patients with complete heart block.

The development of dual chamber pacing and rate responsiveness allowed pacemaker therapy to progress from simply maintaining a minimal heart rate to allowing for restoration of physiologic chronotropy and normal atrioventricular activation. This led to the expansion of this technology from immediate life saving treatment to use aimed at improving haemodynamic function and quality of life, and reducing morbidity. While it is clear that modern dual chamber pacemakers can increase exercise capacity in subjects with chronotropic incompetence and prevent pacemaker syndrome caused by ventricular pacing, the effects on other end points including mortality and arrhythmia prevention remain controversial. With the development of more physiologic pacing, attempts have been made to apply pacemaker technology to the treatment of problems other than symptomatic bradycardia. These problems include pacing to prevent atrial arrhythmias, to improve haemodynamic function and symptoms in patients with hypertrophic or dilated cardiomyopathy, and to prevent neurocardiogenic syncope. Thus, much of the interest in modern pacemakers is for indications other than primary bradycardia. It is these new indications that are the subject of this review.

Sick sinus syndrome

Atrial arrhythmias, and in particular atrial fibrillation, are common in patients with sinus node dysfunction. This tachy-brady variant of sick sinus syndrome is one of the most common indications for permanent pacing. Early retrospective studies showed a major reduction in the incidence of atrial fibrillation with atrial based pacing (AAI or DDD modes) compared with ventricular pacing alone (VVI mode).[1] These reports also suggested that the rates of congestive heart failure, strokes, and mortality were all reduced with atrial based pacing. This led to the common practice of implanting dual chamber devices in all patients with sinus node dysfunction, despite the lack of prospective data supporting this strategy.

Recently, several large studies comparing atrial based pacing with ventricular pacing have been completed. In a single centre study from Denmark, Anderson and colleagues compared single chamber atrial pacing with ventricular pacing in 225 patients with sinus node dysfunction.[2] They showed a significant reduction in the development of atrial fibrillation with atrial pacing. This study also established the relative safety of atrial pacing with no ventricular back up, as the rate of heart block requiring pacemaker revision to a dual chamber system was low (0.6%/year). In addition to reducing the incidence of atrial fibrillation, long term follow up of these patients revealed reductions in mortality, stroke, and congestive heart failure in the atrial pacing group. In the pacemaker selection in the elderly (PASE) study, 407 patients were implanted with dual chamber devices and were then randomised to pacing in DDDR or VVIR modes.[3] There was a reduction in the incidence of atrial fibrillation from 28% to 19% with DDDR pacing (p = 0.06) in the subgroup of patients with sick sinus syndrome, but no difference was noted in those patients with heart block. No mortality reduction was noted with DDDR pacing in this study. One possible explanation for the failure to observe benefit with dual chamber pacing in this study was the relatively high crossover rate (26%) from VVIR to DDDR mode. The much higher crossover rate was likely due to the study design, where randomisation was by "software" (by programming the device mode), in contrast to randomisation by "hardware" (the positioning of the leads) in the Danish study. Since it is much easier to reprogram a device than to revise a pacing system to implant an atrial lead, the crossover rate was higher. In the pacemaker atrial tachycardia (PAC-a-TACH) trial, 198 patients with sick sinus syndrome were randomised to ventricular or dual chamber pacing. No effect on the incidence of atrial fibrillation was noted, but there was a significant reduction in mortality with dual chamber pacing.

The largest study to date evaluating the role of pacing mode on atrial fibrillation was the Canadian trial of physiologic pacing (CTOPP).[4] In this study, 2568 subjects were randomised to atrial based pacing (atrial or dual chamber) or ventricular pacing. There was an 18% reduction of atrial fibrillation with atrial based pacing in this trial, but no effects on mortality or stroke were observed. It is noteworthy that the mean duration of follow up in this trial was three years, while a mortality benefit of atrial pacing was only observed in the study of Andersen and colleagues[2] when the mean follow up was extended to 5.5 years.

The results of these studies, in general, support the use of atrial based pacing for the prevention of atrial fibrillation, at least in subjects with symptomatic sinus node dysfunction. The benefit of such pacing in reducing mortality in less clear. The choice of pacing mode (AAI *v* DDDR) and the relative benefit of single chamber atrial and dual chamber pacemakers remains unknown, because there have been no controlled studies addressing this issue. Atrial pacemakers have the advantages of lower costs and increased longevity. The disadvantages of these systems include the inability to optimise AV delay, and the absence of ventricular pacing if complete heart block or a lead malfunction develop. Although the optimisation of AV delay may be important in certain patients, in general ventricular activation through the native conduction system is superior haemodynamically to right ventricular pacing.[5] The risks of developing heart block can be minimised by avoiding atrial pacemakers in subjects with bundle branch block or other severe intraventricular conduction delays, in patients who show atrioventricular block (Mobitz I or II) at pace rates of 130 beats per minute or less, or in patients where it is anticipated that potent AV nodal blocking drugs such a amiodarone will be needed in the future. If a dual chamber pacemaker is implanted in the absence of heart block, then it is reasonable to program a prolonged AV delay or use one of the new features in pacemakers that automatically prolongs the AV delay to minimise ventricular pacing.

In addition to the effect of pacing mode on the incidence of atrial fibrillation, atrial rate and pacing site can also have an important impact on atrial arrhythmias. Overdrive pacing is routinely used following cardiac surgery to prevent postoperative atrial fibrillation. Similarly, higher base pacing rates are often employed in patients with paroxysmal atrial fibrillation to inhibit tachyarrhythmias, although the utility of this strategy is not well documented. In fact a recent study comparing maintaining atrioventricular synchrony with no atrial pacing (VDD mode) and frequent dual chamber pacing (DDDR mode) showed no difference in the frequency of atrial fibrillation.[6] The potential disadvantages of atrial overdrive pacing include decreased pulse generator longevity and the development of palpitations and insomnia if constant rapid rates are used. In an effort to avoid rapid overdrive pacing, several algorithms are being tested that periodically sample the intrinsic heart rate and pace at a programmable increment above the sinus rate to maintain atrial pacing. This strat-

Issues in multisite pacing

- Is pacing in the distal coronary sinus superior to pacing at the ostium?

- Where is the optimal right atrial pacing site?

- How much overdrive is needed to optimise the pacing benefit?

- Can intra-atrial septal pacing (Bachmann's bundle) achieve the same benefit as dual site pacing?

egy preserves the normal fluctuations in heart rate, although the ability to suppress atrial fibrillation with this degree of overdrive pacing is not yet established. It is likely that sufficient overdrive to achieve almost continual atrial pacing will be necessary to reduce the incidence of atrial fibrillation.

Multisite atrial pacing

In addition to overdrive pacing, there has been increasing interest in the evaluation of atrial activation as a means to prevent tachyarrhythmias. Traditionally, atrial leads were positioned in the right atrial appendage for stability. However, with the development of active fixation mechanisms, leads can now be positioned virtually anywhere in the atrium. Saksena and his colleagues studied the role of multisite pacing in a group of patients with frequent, drug refractory paroxysmal atrial fibrillation; they showed that overdrive pacing with simultaneous stimulation of the ostium of the coronary sinus and the high right atrium significantly reduced the frequency of arrhythmia compared with single site pacing or no pacing.[7] Presumably, the mechanism of benefit of this approach is a reduction of the dispersion of activation with dual site pacing. Prospective, randomised, multicentre trials are underway to evaluate the benefit of dual site pacing in more detail in patients with sick sinus syndrome. In support of this concept, following open heart surgery, biatrial pacing with temporary epicardial leads positioned on the right and left atria reduces postoperative atrial fibrillation.[8] Another approach to reducing the dispersion of atrial activation is to pace the interatrial septum either near the coronary sinus ostium or near Bachmann's bundle. This is an attractive option because it does not require additional leads. A preliminary report of this technique demonstrated a decrease of atrial fibrillation compared with pacing at traditional right atrial sites.

Pacing issues in sick sinus syndrome patients

- What is the optimal pacing mode (AAIR or DDDR)?

- Do antiarrhythmic drugs enhance the effect of pacing?

- What is the role of atrial or ventricular lead position?

- What is the optimal pacing rate?

Congestive heart failure

Over the past decade the use of pacing to improve haemodynamic function in patients with congestive heart failure and left ventricular systolic dysfunction has been the focus of intense interest. In subjects with advanced heart failure a surprising proportion of sudden deaths are reportedly caused by bradyarrhythmias.[9] Moreover, medications with negative chronotropic properties, such as β blockers and amiodarone, are commonly used in this population. In addition, the incidence of bundle branch block and intraventricular conduction delays is high in the presence of dilated cardiomyopathy. Therefore, permanent pacing is frequently indicated in subjects with congestive heart failure. However, approximately half of the deaths in this population are caused by progressive haemodynamic deterioration, so if pacing could prevent bradyarrhythmic death and favourably affect heart failure symptoms, then it would be a very useful treatment modality.

Initially, standard dual chamber pacemaker implantation with pacing from the right ventricular apex was investigated. The initial studies evaluated pacing with an AV delay of 100 ms; striking improvements in left ventricular ejection fraction and pulmonary congestive symptoms were observed. Unfortunately, controlled studies have failed to confirm the benefit of short AV delay pacing in this patient population. We were unable to demonstrate any benefit, either acutely or chronically, in a double blind, randomised, crossover trial in patients with advanced heart failure.[10] Similarly, Innes and colleagues found that dual chamber pacing with a short AV delay did not acutely improve haemodynamic function in 12 patients with heart failure despite a significant increase in left ventricular filling time.[11] Finally, Linde and associates were unable to demonstrate significant clinical improvement over a three month follow up period in a group of 10 patients with New York Heart Association (NYHA) functional class III or IV heart failure paced with an optimised AV delay.[12]

Atrial pacing with intact AV conduction is usually associated with a higher cardiac output than DDD pacing,[5] suggesting that the pattern of ventricular activation may be important for optimising haemodynamic function. For this reason, alternative pacing sites in the right ventricle have been evaluated. VVI pacing from the right ventricular outflow tract was reported to improve cardiac output compared with pacing from the right ventricular apex in patients with sinus node dysfunction. However, more recently we and others have shown no difference in acute haemodynamic function with DDD pacing from either the right ventricular apex or outflow tract. Compared with AAI pacing at the same rate, there is haemodynamic deterioration with VVI pacing from either right ventricular site.[13] In a well designed chronic study, Victor and colleagues compared apical and outflow tract pacing in patients with complete heart block and chronic atrial fibrillation.[14] Each patient received a dual chamber pacemaker with one lead in the right ventricular apex and the other in the outflow tract. No effect on exercise tolerance, ejection fraction or haemodynamic parameters was observed in this prospective randomised evaluation.

In summary, pacing mode, but not right ventricular pacing site, affects haemodynamic parameters in the setting of congestive heart failure. However, all of the studies have been small, so it remains possible that there are subsets of patients or unique approaches to selecting pacing sites, such as activation mapping, that would benefit from right ventricular pacing in the absence of bradycardic indications.

In contrast to the generally disappointing results with right ventricular pacing, left ventricular based pacing has emerged as an exciting new approach. The first controlled study of biventricular pacing involved the use of temporary epicardial electrodes to pace simultaneously the right atrium and paraseptal locations on the right and left ventricles early after coronary artery bypass surgery.[15] Atriobiventricular pacing was associated with a significantly higher cardiac output compared with univentricular pacing. Subsequently, this technique was applied to patients with congestive heart failure. Initially, left ventricular pacing was achieved with epicardial leads placed by thoracotomy. The morbidity of this procedure limited the systematic evaluation of the chronic effects of biventricular pacing, although promising results were noted in several uncontrolled series of patients.[16 17] More recent acute studies have shed important insights into the benefit of biventricular pacing.

Blanc and colleagues performed acute haemodynamic studies in 23 patients with severe heart failure and raised pulmonary capillary wedge pressures. Haemodynamic parameters were unchanged with pacing performed from either the right ventricular apex or outflow tract, but were greatly improved by biventricular or left ventricular endocardial pacing.[18] Similar results were obtained in a separate group of subjects in chronic atrial fibrillation, suggesting that left ventricular activation and not optimisation of AV timing was primarily responsible for the benefits observed.[19] Kass and colleagues found a significant improvement in systolic function with left ventricular pacing (via the coronary sinus) in 14 patients with severe dilated cardiomyopathy.[20] Results with biventricular pacing were worse than with single site left ventricular pacing.

These acute studies have established that left ventricular based pacing can improve haemodynamic function. Moreover, they have helped define the patient population likely to benefit from this treatment. Haemodynamic improvement has been observed both in subjects with ischaemic and non-ischaemic cardiomyopathies, but is primarily observed in those with left bundle branch block and pronounced QRS prolongation. Recently, two prospective studies of the long term effects of biventricular pacing were completed. In the pacing therapies in congestive heart failure (PATH-CHF) study, an epicardial left ventricular lead was used and two pacemakers synchronised to achieve biventricular pacing. Haemodynamic and functional improvement was noted during paced periods. In the multisite stimulation in cardiomyopathy (MUSTIC)

Pacing issues in congestive heart failure

- What is the optimal stimulation site for right and left ventricular leads?

- Is biatrial (that is, four chamber) pacing necessary with biventricular pacing?

- What are the optimal atrioventricular and intraventricular pacing delays?

- Does a single left ventricular lead provide sufficient haemodynamic benefit or is it necessary to employ simultaneous right ventricular (that is, biventricular) stimulation?

- Does the aetiology (that is, ischemic v dilated) or severity of heart failure predict clinical benefit?

- What is the role of pacing in systolic versus diastolic dysfunction?

- Does biventricular pacing favourably affect mortality?

study, a coronary sinus lead was used to achieve left ventricular activation. Using a randomised, crossover design, exercise capacity and functional status were shown to improve significantly with cardiac resynchronisation.

Despite these encouraging results, many questions remain unanswered with regard to the benefit of left ventricular based pacing to achieve cardiac resynchronisation. For instance, is biventricular pacing necessary or can left ventricular pacing alone achieve the same long term benefit? The patient population that benefits most is not well defined. Most attention has been directed towards evaluating subjects with severe congestive heart failure (NYHA class III or IV) and left bundle branch block. Typically a QRS duration of at least 150 ms is necessary to show an acute haemodynamic improvement with biventricular pacing. This obviously will limit the number of patients who could benefit from this technology if such conduction system disease is necessary for long term functional benefit. The optimal position of left ventricular leads is not well studied in part because of the limitations of positioning leads in the tortuous coronary venous system, although many investigators feel that posterior and lateral sites are best. New leads and delivery systems have been designed to allow for better access to the coronary venous system. Finally, the effect of biventricular pacing on mortality is unknown. All studies to date have continued to observe sudden cardiac death in paced patients with congestive heart failure. Hopefully, this is not caused by an increased mortality or proarrhythmic effect of this treatment, as was noted for many positive inotropic agents. It is reassuring that recent studies have reported that left ventricular or biventricular pacing improves myocardial energetics in contrast with a dobutamine infusion.[21] Regardless of the mechanism of sudden death in paced patients, combined biventricular pacemakers and implantable defibrillators are being developed to treat patients with life threatening arrhythmias, in case prospective trials show that this

combined technology is needed to reduce mortality in this high risk population.

Hypertrophic cardiomyopathy

Patients with obstructive hypertrophic cardiomyopathy often are highly symptomatic with dyspnoea, chest pain, and fatigue. In those patients who remain symptomatic despite standard medical treatment with β blockers and calcium channel blockers, non-pharmacologic approaches are often employed. Such approaches include surgical myotomy and myomectomy, often with mitral valve replacement, chemical septal ablation with ethanol, and dual chamber pacing. Interest in permanent pacing for the treatment of hypertrophic cardiomyopathy began in the 1970s following several case reports and small series demonstrating symptomatic improvement in those subjects with outflow tract obstruction. Subsequent small studies provided objective evidence for a reduction of outflow tract gradient and increased exercise duration with pacing. The haemodynamic benefit occurs only with pacing with a short AV delay from the right ventricular apex causing full pre-excitation. This results in paradoxical septal movement reducing the outflow tract gradient.

The largest single centre series of patients paced with hypertrophic cardiomyopathy was from the National Institutes of Health. Fananapazir and colleagues reported observations on 84 patients.[22] Over a mean follow up of more than two years, symptoms were eliminated or diminished in 89% of patients. In 23% of their patients, there was regional regression of left ventricular hypertrophy, suggesting that myocardial remodelling may occur with chronic pacing.

More recently, several double blind randomised trials of pacing in hypertrophic cardiomyopathy have been completed. Unfortunately, the results of these trials have been largely disappointing. Nishimura and colleagues evaluated 19 subjects.[23] Although quality of life improved in 63% of patients during DDD pacing, 42% improved during the control mode (AAI pacing). There were no significant differences in the functional parameters measured, although the outflow tract gradient improved with dual chamber pacing. In a multicentre European study, Kappenberger and associates showed a significant improvement in angina and dyspnoea in the majority of subjects along with a major reduction in left ventricular outflow gradient, although there was no change in left ventricular function or septal wall thickness.[24] Finally, a report by Maron and colleagues of a multicentre North American study showed no significant effect of pacing on quality of life parameters, although again the outflow tract gradient was reduced with right ventricular apical pacing.[25] A subset of elderly patients was identified who benefited from pacing.

Thus, despite promising early reports, the symptomatic benefit of dual chamber pacing in hypertrophic cardiomyopathy has not been documented conclusively in randomised double blind studies. No effect on mortality has been noted, so implantable defibrillators are being used with increasing frequency in high risk patients. It is clear that pacing can reduce the outflow tract gradient, but this does not result in long term functional benefit in many individuals. One explanation for the discrepancy between the results of randomised and observational studies is elucidated by the analysis of Linde and colleagues, who evaluated the effect of pacemaker implantation in this population.[26] They studied patients who underwent dual chamber pacemaker placement but were programmed to a non-pacing mode. Despite the lack of pacing, most quality of life parameters improved. Such effects of the administration of inactive drugs are well described and is why placebo control groups are typically included in studies. Similarly, a potent placebo effect occurs with device implantation in this population. At present, the widespread enthusiasm for the use of pacing as primary treatment for hypertrophic cardiomyopathy is decreasing. All studies suggest that there may be some patients who benefit, but this subgroup is not well defined.

Neurocardiogenic syncope

Syncope is a common cause of emergency room visits and hospital admissions. Bradycardia is one of the well described mechanisms of syncope, and pacemaker implantation for the treatment of syncope in the setting of sick sinus syndrome or high grade heart block is well established. Probably the most common cause of the transient loss of consciousness is neurocardiogenic syncope. Often there are both vasodepressor (that is, hypotension caused by vasodilation) and cardioinhibitory (that is, bradycardia from sinus slowing or arrest) components to these episodes which can be reproduced with head-up tilt table testing. Despite early anecdotal reports of the benefit of pacing in patients with neurocardiogenic or vasovagal syncope, this treatment strategy did not gain widespread acceptance. That was caused in part by the observation that hypotension frequently precedes bradycardia with upright tilt.[27] Therefore, it was argued that a pacemaker will not prevent syncope which is caused by the hypotension.

Despite the pessimism about the potential role of pacing to prevent neurocardiogenic syncope, several recent studies have demonstrated dramatic reductions in the frequency of syncope in selected groups with frequent episodes and an abnormal tilt table response. In the North American vasovagal pacemaker study, 54 patients were evaluated during the pilot phase of the study.[28] Subjects were randomised to receive a pacemaker with the rate drop response activated or to not receive a pacemaker. With the rate drop response, high rate dual chamber pacing is activated when there is a sudden rate drop. There was an 85% reduction in the risk of syncope in those

> ### Pacing issues in hypertrophic cardiomyopathy
>
> - Is there a subgroup of patients that can be identified clinically who benefit consistently from pacing?
>
> - Does an "optimum" AV delay need to be identified for each individual?
>
> - Does the magnitude of the reduction of the outflow tract gradient predict symptomatic improvement?
>
> - Does pacing lead to permanent structural or biochemical changes in the ventricular septum?
>
> - What is the role of pacing in symptomatic patients with non-obstructive cardiomyopathy?

implanted with a pacemaker, so this trial was terminated before the larger full study was begun. In a multicentre European study of neurocardiogenic syncope (VASIS trial), 42 patients were randomised again to pacemaker implantation with the pulse generator programmed to DDI mode with hysteresis or no pacemaker.[29] Recurrent syncope developed in 61% of paced patients and only 5% of unpaced patients. Of note, fewer than 5% of screened patients met the strict criteria of frequent syncope with a tilt table response showing pronounced bradycardia. Accordingly, this study evaluated the most severely affected patients with neurocardiogenic syncope and identified a very selected subgroup who benefit from pacing. In addition, the control groups in these studies did not have a device implanted, so a placebo effect of pacemaker implantation cannot be excluded as a cause of the benefit observed. Other studies are ongoing to evaluate pacemaker patients randomised to pacing on or off to address this issue directly.

Conclusions

In summary, pacemaker indications are expanding as this technology is being applied to the prevention of arrhythmias and to the optimisation of haemodynamic function. The incidence of atrial fibrillation is decreased with atrial based pacing compared to ventricular

> ### Pacing issues for neurocardiogenic syncope
>
> - Does the haemodynamic response to head-up tilt predict pacemaker responders?
>
> - What pharmacologic agents are most effective when used with pacemakers?
>
> - What is the optimal dual chamber pacing rate to prevent syncope?
>
> - What is the role of advanced pacing features such as sudden rate drop in preventing syncope?
>
> - Can clinical criteria be used to identify subgroups that benefit from pacing?

pacing. However, it remains unclear if standard dual chamber or atrial pacing prevents atrial fibrillation in the absence of bradycardia, although dual site pacing is a promising approach for this problem. Multiple studies have now shown a haemodynamic benefit from biventricular pacing in patients with dilated cardiomyopathy and pronounced conduction system disease. Ongoing studies will help identify better the patient population that benefits most from this treatment, the optimal lead positions for pacing, and the effect of long term pacing on ventricular arrhythmias and mortality. The role of pacing in obstructive hypertrophic cardiomyopathy is less clear, as much of the benefit previously observed was likely caused by factors other than pacing. Although some patients with obstructive physiology likely benefit from pacing, this population is not well defined. Finally, randomised studies have established the role of dual chamber pacing to prevent neurocardiogenic syncope, at least in the subset of patients with frequent episodes and a prominent cardioinhibitory component to their haemodynamic response. As pacemaker technology is combined with other devices such as defibrillators, drug pumps, haemodynamic monitors, and non-invasive measures of arrhythmia vulnerability (for example, heart rate variability and T wave alternans), this therapy will likely expand to help in the prevention and treatment of other haemodynamic and arrhythmic problems.

1. **Connolly SJ, Kerr C, Gent M,** *et al.* Dual chamber versus ventricular pacing. Critical appraisal of current data. *Circulation* 1996;**94**:578–83.

2. **Andersen HR, Nielsen JC, Thomsen PEB,** *et al.* Long-term follow-up of patients from a randomized trial of atrial versus ventricular pacing for sick-sinus syndrome. *Lancet* 1997;**350**:1210–6.
   • *A randomised evaluation of single chamber atrial pacing (n = 110) or single chamber ventricular pacing (n = 115) in patients with sick sinus syndrome. With long term follow up, there were significant reductions of mortality (39 v 57 subjects), thromboembolic events (13 v 26 subjects), and atrial fibrillation (44% v 65%) with atrial pacing.*

3. **Lamas GA, Orav EF, Stambler BS,** *et al.* Quality of life and clinical outcomes in elderly patients treated with ventricular pacing as compared with dual-chamber pacing. Pacemaker selection in the elderly investigators. *N Engl J Med* 1998;**338**:1097–104.

4. **Connolly SJ, Kerr CR, Gent M,** *et al.* Comparison of the effects of physiologic pacing versus ventricular pacing on cardiovascular death and stroke. *N Engl J Med* 2000;**342**:1385–91.

5. **Rosenqvist M, Isaaz K, Botvinick EH,** *et al.* Relative importance of activation sequence compared to atrioventricular synchrony in left ventricular function. *Am J Cardiol* 1991;**67**:148.

6. **Gillis AM, Connolly SJ, Lacombe P,** *et al.* Randomized crossover comparison of DDDR versus VDD pacing after atrioventricular junction ablation for prevention of atrial fibrillation. *Circulation* 2000;**102**:736–41.
   • *A randomised comparison of DDDR and VDD pacing in 67 patients following AV node ablation. No effects on atrial fibrillation burden or frequency were noted with frequent atrial pacing. Specialised algorithms that achieve almost 100% atrial pacing may be necessary to show any effect of atrial pacing on arrhythmias.*

7. **Saksena S, Prakash A, Hill M,** *et al.* Prevention of recurrent atrial fibrillation with chronic dual-site right atrial pacing. *J Am Coll Cardiol* 1996;**28**:687–94.
   • *A small study of 12 patients evaluating the role of dual right atrial pacing to prevent atrial fibrillation in highly symptomatic and drug refractory patients. Although these were provocative results, larger, randomised studies are needed to confirm this benefit.*

8. **Levy T, Fotopoulos G, Walker S,** *et al.* Randomized controlled study investigating the effect of biatrial pacing in prevention of atrial fibrillation after coronary artery bypass grafting. *Circulation* 2000;**102**:1382–7.

9. **Luu M, Stevenson WG, Stevenson LW,** *et al.* Ventricular tachycardia is not the predominant cause of monitored sudden death in heart failure. *Circulation* 1989;**80**:1675–80.

10. **Gold MR, Feliciano Z, Gottlieb SS,** *et al.* Dual-chamber pacing with a short atrioventricular delay in congestive heart failure: a randomized study. *J Am Coll Cardiol* 1995;**26**:967–73.

11. **Innes D, Leitch JW, Fletcher PJ.** VDD pacing at short atrioventricular intervals does not improve cardiac output in patients with dilated heart failure. *PACE* 1994;**17**:959–65.

12. **Linde C, Gadler F, Edner M.** Results of atrioventricular synchronous pacing with severe congestive heart failure. *Am J Cardiol* 1995;**75**:919–23.

13. **Gold MR, Brockman R, Peters RW,** *et al.* Acute hemodynamic effects of right ventricular pacing site and pacing mode in patients with congestive heart failure secondary to either ischemic or idiopathic dilated cardiomyopathy. *Am J Cardiol* 2000;**85**:1106–9.

14. **Victor F, Leclerq C, Mabo P,** *et al.* Optimal right ventricular pacing site in chronically implanted patients: a prospective randomized cross-over comparison of apical and outflow tract pacing. *J Am Coll Cardiol* 1999;**33**:311–16.

15. **Foster AH, Gold MR, McLaughlin JS.** Acute hemodynamic effects of atrio-biventricular pacing in humans. *Ann Thorac Surg* 1995;**59**:294–300.

16. **Bakker PF, Meijurg HW, de Vries JW,** *et al.* Biventricular pacing in end-stage heart failure improves functional capacity and left ventricular function. *J Intervent Cardiol Electrophysiol* 2000;**4**:395–404.

17. **Cazeau S, Ritter P, Lazarus A,** *et al.* Multisite pacing for end-stage heart failure: early experience. *PACE* 1996;**19**:1748–57.

18. **Blanc J-J, Etienne Y, Mansourati J,** *et al.* Evaluation of different ventricular pacing sites in patients with severe heart failure: results of an acute hemodynamic study. *Circulation* 1997;**96**:3273–7.

19. **Etienne Y, Mansourati J, Gilard M,** *et al.* Evaluation of left ventricular based pacing in patients with congestive heart failure and atrial fibrillation. *Am J Cardiol* 1999;**83**:1138–40.

20. **Kass DA, Chen C-H, Curry C,** *et al.* Improved left ventricular mechanics from acute VDD pacing in patients with dilated cardiomyopathy and ventricular conduction delay. *Circulation* 1999;**99**:1567–73.
   • *An elegant acute haemodynamic study demonstrating the benefit of left ventricular based pacing in subjects with dilated cardiomyopathy, congestive heart failure, and ventricular conduction delay, primarily left bundle branch block. Left ventricular (or biventricular) pacing, but not right ventricular pacing, improved measures of systolic function. This was largely independent of AV delay over a large physiologic range.*

21. **Nelson GS, Berger RD, Fetics BJ,** *et al.* Left ventricular or biventricular pacing improves cardiac function at diminished energy cost in patients with dilated cardiomyopathy and left bundle-branch block. *Circulation* 2000;**102**:3053–9.

22. **Fananapazir L, Epstein ND, Curiel RV,** *et al.* Long-term results of dual-chamber (DDD) pacing in obstructive hypertrophic cardiomyopathy. *Circulation* 1994;**90**:2731–42.

23. **Nishimura RA, Trusty JM, Hayes DL,** *et al.* Dual-chamber pacing for hypertrophic cardiomyopathy; a randomized, double-blind, crossover trial. *J Am Coll Cardiol* 1997;**29**:435–41.

24. **Kappenberger L, Linde C, Daubert C,** *et al.* Pacing in hypertrophic obstructive cardiomyopathy (PIC). A randomised crossover study. *Eur Heart J* 1997;**18**:1249–56.

25. **Maron BJ, Nishimura RA, McKenna WJ,** *et al.* Assessment of permanent dual-chamber pacing as a treatment for drug-refractory symptomatic patients with obstructive hypertrophic cardiomyopathy: a randomized, double-blind, crossover study (M-PATHY) *Circulation* 1999;**99**:2927–33.

26. **Linde C, Gadler F, Kappenberger L,** *et al.* Placebo effect of pacemaker implantation in obstructive hypertrophic cardiomyopathy. *Am J Cardiol* 1999;**83**:903–7.

27. **Sra JS, Jazayeri MR, Avitall B,** *et al.* Comparisons of cardiac pacing with drug therapy in the treatment of neurocardiogenic (vasovagal) syncope with bradycardia or asystole. *N Engl J Med* 1993;**328**:1085–90.

28. **Connolly SJ, Sheldon R, Roberts RS,** *et al* for the **North American Vasovagal Pacemaker Study.** A randomized trial of permanent cardiac pacing for the prevention of vasovagal syncope. *J Am Coll Cardiol* 1999;**33**:16–20.
   • *A randomised study of 54 patients with vasovagal syncope. This was the pilot study of a much larger planned study, but it was stopped because of a major reduction (relative risk reduction 85%) in syncope with dual chamber pacing. A follow up study is now underway to control for the placebo effect of pacemaker implantation.*

29. **Sutton R, Brignole M, Menozzi C,** *et al.* Dual-chamber pacing in the treatment of neurally mediated tilt-positive cardioinhibitory syncope. Pacemaker versus no therapy: a multicentre randomized study. *Circulation* 2000;**102**:294–9.

18 Ventricular tachycardia: diagnosis of broad QRS complex tachycardia

Hein JJ Wellens

When confronted with a tachycardia having a broad QRS complex, it is important to be able to differentiate between a supraventricular and a ventricular tachycardia. Medication given for the treatment of a supraventricular tachycardia (SVT) may be harmful to a patient with a ventricular tachycardia (VT).[1][2] A reasonable haemodynamic condition during a tachycardia may erroneously lead to the wrong diagnosis of SVT.[3] Familiarity with the ECG signs allowing the diagnosis of a VT is therefore essential. But as will be discussed here, the ECG should not only tell you how to distinguish VT from other tachycardias with a broad QRS complex, but also to suspect its aetiology and its site of origin in the ventricle. Both aspects are important in decision making about the prognostic significance of VT and correct treatment.

Classification of tachycardias with a broad QRS complex

As shown in fig 18.1, broad QRS tachycardia can be divided in three groups.

- SVT with bundle branch block—Bundle branch block (BBB) may be pre-existing or can occur when the refractory period of one of the bundle branches is reached because of the heart rate of the SVT (so called tachycardia related or phase 3 block). BBB can also occur because of retrograde invasion in one of the bundle branches.[4] These causes of BBB can be found in patients with atrial tachycardia, atrial flutter, atrial fibrillation, atrioventricular (AV) nodal tachycardia, and also during orthodromic circus movement tachycardia (with AV conduction over the AV node and ventriculo-atrial (VA) conduction over an accessory AV pathway).

- SVT with AV conduction over an accessory AV pathway—This may occur during atrial tachycardia, atrial flutter, atrial fibrillation, AV nodal tachycardia, and during antidromic circus movement tachycardia (with AV conduction over an accessory AV pathway and VA conduction over the AV node or a second accessory AV pathway). It is also the case in the so called Mahaim tachycardia where AV conduction goes by way of a slowly conducting right sided accessory AV pathway or a nodo-ventricular fibre inserting into the right ventricle.

- Ventricular tachycardia.

A

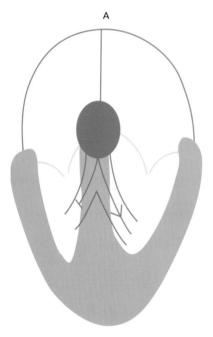

B

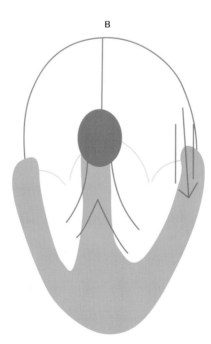

C

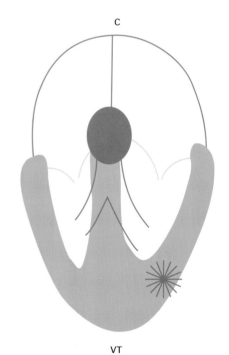

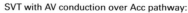

SVT with BBB:
- atrial tachy
- atrial flutter
- atrial fibrillation
- AV nodal tachy
- CMT with AV conduction over AV node and VA conduction over Acc pathway

SVT with AV conduction over Acc pathway:
- atrial tachy
- atrial flutter
- atrial fibrillation
- AV nodal tachy
- CMT with AV conduction over Acc pathway and VA conduction over AV node or second Acc pathway

VT

Figure 18.1. Different types of SVT with BBB (diagram A), SVT with AV conduction over an accessory pathway (diagram B), and VT (diagram C) resulting in a broad QRS tachycardia. Acc, accessory; AV, atrioventricular; BBB, bundle branch block; CMT, circus movement tachycardia; SVT, supraventricular tachycardia; VA, ventriculo-atrial; VT, ventricular tachycardia.

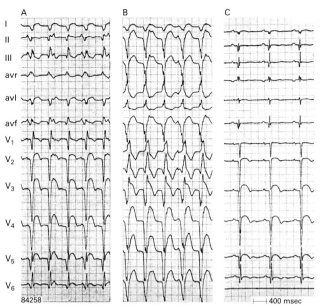

Figure 18.2. Two types of VT (panel A and B) in the same patient (panel C during sinus rhythm). Atrioventricular dissociation is present during both VTs. Note the effect of the frontal plane axis on the R:S ratio in lead V6 in RBBB shaped VT. R:S < 1 is present in case of a superior axis (panel B), but R:S > 1 with an inferior axis (panel A).

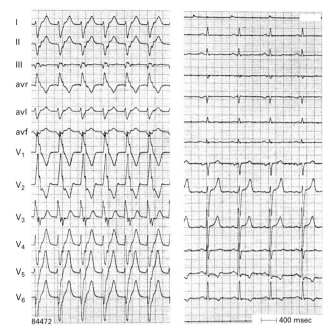

Figure 18.3. One to one ventriculo-atrial conduction during VT. The p waves are negative in leads II, III, and avf and follow each QRS complex. Left panel—VT; right panel—same patient during sinus rhythm.

The ECG diagnosis

Importance of AV dissociation

Although dissociation between atrial and ventricular activity during tachycardia is a hallmark of VT (fig 18.2), some form of VA conduction can be present during VT, especially at slow VT rates (fig 18.3).[4] P waves can be difficult to recognise during a broad QRS tachycardia and it is always useful to look for non-electrocardiographic signs such as variations in jugular pulsations, the loudness of the first heart sound, and changes in systolic blood pressure.[5]

In patients with slow VT rates occasional conduction from atrium to ventricle over the AV node–bundle branch system may happen resulting in "capture" or "fusion" beats (fig 18.4). Sudden narrowing of a QRS complex during VT may also be the result of a premature ventricular depolarisation arising in the ventricle in which the tachycardia originates, or it may occur when retrograde conduction during VT produces a ventricular echo beat leading to fusion with the VT QRS

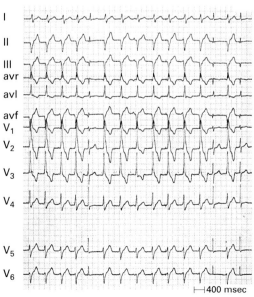

Figure 18.4. "Capture" (QRS complexes: 5, 13, and 15) and "fusion" beats (QRS complex number 8) during VT.

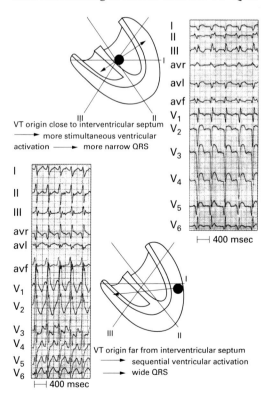

Figure 18.5. VT origin and QRS width. Upper panel: an origin close to the interventricular septum results in more simultaneous right and left ventricular activation and therefore a more narrow QRS complex. In contrast (lower panel) a VT origin in the lateral ventricular wall results in sequential ventricular activation and a wider QRS complex.

complex.[5] Very rarely, AV dissociation is present in tachycardias other than VT. It may occur in AV junctional tachycardia with BBB after cardiac surgery or during digitalis intoxication.

Width of the QRS complex

As depicted in fig 18.5, the site of origin of the VT plays a role in the width of the QRS complex. When the arrhythmia arises in the lateral free wall of the ventricle sequential activation of the ventricles occurs resulting in a very wide QRS. The QRS complex will be smaller when the VT has its origin in or close to the interventricular septum. Of course other factors also play a role in the QRS width during VT, such as scar tissue (after myocardial infarction), ventricular hypertrophy, and muscular disarray (as in hypertrophic cardiomyopathy). It is of interest that a QRS width of more than 0.14 seconds in right BBB (RBBB) tachycardias and 0.16 seconds during left BBB (LBBB) argues for a VT.[4] But a QRS width below such values may occur in VTs having their origin in or close to the interventricular septum. Of course, QRS width is not helpful in differentiating VT from a tachycardia with AV conduction over an accessory AV pathway because such a pathway inserts into the ventricle leading to eccentric ventricular activation and a wide QRS complex (fig 18.6).

An SVT can have a QRS width of more than 0.14 (RBBB) or 0.16 (LBBB) seconds under three circumstances: (1) in the presence of pre-existent BBB in the elderly with fibrosis in the bundle branch system and ventricular myocar-

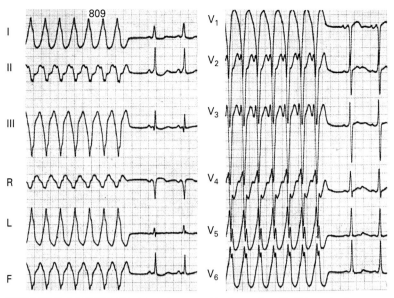

Figure 18.6. An antidromic circus movement tachycardia with AV conduction over a right sided accessory pathway. The insertion of the accessory pathway in the free wall of the right ventricle results in sequential (right to left) ventricular activation and a wide QRS complex.

dium; (2) when during SVT AV conduction occurs over an accessory AV pathway; (3) when class IC drugs (especially flecainide) are present during SVT.

QRS axis in the frontal plane

The QRS axis is not only important for the differentiation of the broad QRS tachycardia but also to identify its site of origin and aetiology. As shown in fig 18.7, a VT origin in the apical part of the ventricle has a superior axis (to the left of −30). An inferior axis is present when the VT has an origin in the basal area of the ventricle. Previous work[4] showed that the presence of a superior axis in patients with RBBB shaped QRS very strongly suggests VT. This does not hold for an LBBB shaped tachycardia. On the contrary, presence of an inferior axis in LBBB shaped QRS tachycardia argues for a VT arising in the outflow tract of the right ventricle.

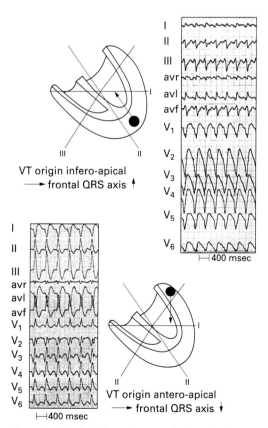

Figure 18.7. VT origin and QRS axis. An apical origin results in a superiorly directed axis in the frontal plane. In contrast, a basal origin leads to an inferior QRS axis (lower panel).

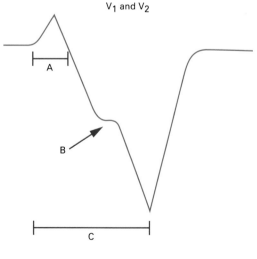

A: > 30 ms FAVOURS VT
B: NOTCHING, SLURRING FAVOURS VT
C: > 70 ms FAVOURS VT

Figure 18.8. Findings in lead V1 and V2 during LBBB shaped tachycardia pointing to a ventricular origin (see text).

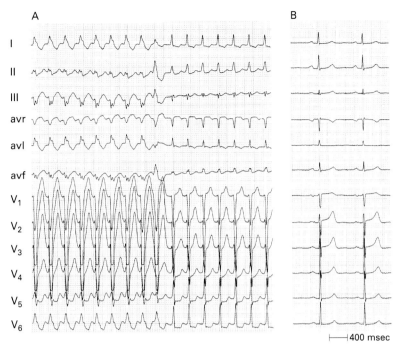

Figure 18.9. SVT with LBBB. In panel A LBBB changes during tachycardia into a narrow QRS following a ventricular premature beat. As described in the text, lead V1 during LBBB clearly shows signs pointing to a supraventricular origin of the tachycardia.

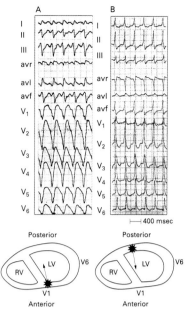

Figure 18.10. Concordant pattern. The left panel shows a VT arising in the apical area of the left ventricle resulting in negative concordancy of all precordial leads. In the right panel ventricular activation starts in the left posterior area, resulting in positive concordancy of all precordial leads. The latter can be found in left posterior VT but also in SVT with AV conduction over a left posterior accessory pathway.

Configurational characteristics of the QRS complex

Leads V1 and V6

Marriott[6] described that in RBBB shaped tachycardia, presence of a qR or R complex in lead V1 strongly argued for a ventricular origin of the tachycardia, while a three phasic (RSR) pattern suggested a supraventricular origin. Apart from lead V1, lead V6 can also be very helpful in correctly differentiating RBBB shaped tachycardia. When in V6 the R:S ratio is < 1, a VT is very likely.[4] As shown in fig 2B an R:S ratio < 1 in V6 is typically found when there is left axis deviation in the frontal plane.

If the axis is inferiorly directed, lead V6 often shows an R:S ratio > 1 (fig 18.2A). In LBBB shaped VT, lead V1 (and also V2) (fig 18.8) shows: an initially positive QRS with positivity measuring more than 0:03 seconds; slurring or notching of the downstroke of the S wave; and an interval between the beginning of the QRS and the nadir of the S wave of 0.07 seconds or more.[7] When lead V6 shows a qR pattern during LBBB shaped tachycardia, VT is very likely. In SVT with LBBB, lead V1 shows no or minimal initial positivity, a very rapid downstroke of the S wave, and a short interval between the beginning of the QRS and the nadir of the S wave (fig 18.9).

Interval onset QRS to nadir of S wave in precordial leads

Brugada and colleagues[8] suggested that an RS interval > 100 ms in one or more precordial leads is highly suggestive for VT. One should be careful, however, because such a duration may occur in SVT with AV conduction over an accessory pathway, SVT during administration of drugs that slow intraventricular conduction (in particular, flecainide), and in SVT with pre-existent BBB, especially LBBB.

Concordant pattern

When all precordial leads show either negative or positive QRS complexes this is called negative or positive concordancy. Negative concordancy is diagnostic for a VT arising in the apical area of the heart (fig 18.10). Positive concordancy means that in the horizontal plane ventricular activation starts left posteriorly. This can be found either in VT originating in the left posterior wall or during tachycardias using a left posterior accessory AV pathway for AV conduction (fig 18.10).

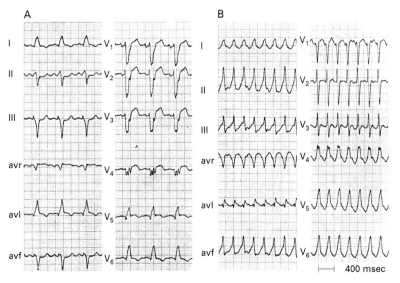

Figure 18.11. Tachycardia QRS smaller than QRS during sinus rhythm. On the left sinus rhythm is present with a very wide QRS because of anterolateral myocardial infarction and pronounced delay in left ventricular activation. On the right a VT arising on the right side of the interventricular septum results in more simultaneous activation of the right and left ventricle than during sinus rhythm and therefore a smaller QRS complex.

Tachycardia QRS more narrow than sinus QRS

When during tachycardia the QRS is more narrow than during sinus rhythm a VT should be diagnosed. As shown in fig 18.11, a very wide QRS is present during sinus rhythm because of sequential activation of first the right and then the left ventricle. During tachycardia the QRS is more narrow. This can only be explained by a ventricular origin close to the intraventricular septum, resulting in more simultaneous activation of the right and left ventricle than during sinus rhythm.

Presence of QR complexes

Coumel and colleagues[9] called attention to the significance of a QR (but not a QS) complex during a broad QRS tachycardia, showing that their presence indicates a scar in the myocardium usually caused by myocardial infarction. Figure 18.12 gives an example of QR complexes during VT in patients with an anterior (panel A) and an old inferior myocardial infarction (panel B). QR complexes during VT are present in approximately 40% of VTs after myocardial infarction.[10]

Aetiology of VT

Most VTs have a previous myocardial infarction as their aetiology and, as pointed out, a QR complex during VT can be very helpful to make that diagnosis. However, characteristic ECG patterns can also be found in idiopathic VT[11] and VT in patients with arrhythmogenic right ventricular dysplasia (ARVD).[12] Figure 18.13 shows three patterns of idiopathic VT arising in or close to the outflow tract of the right ventricle. All three have an LBBB-like QRS complex indicating a right ventricular origin. In panel A the frontal QRS axis is +70 and lead 1 shows a positive QRS complex,

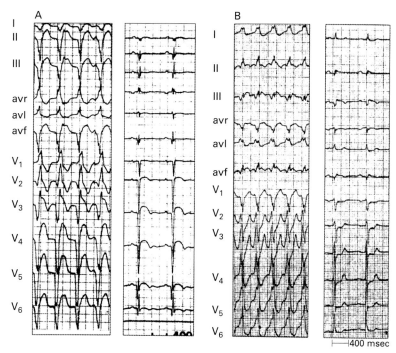

Figure 18.12. QRS complexes during VT indicating a myocardial scar. As shown by the accompanying tracing, during sinus rhythm anterior wall myocardial infarction is present in the left panel and inferior wall myocardial infarction in the right one.

indicating an origin of the tachycardia in the lateral part of the outflow tract of the right ventricle. In panel B the frontal QRS axis is inferior and the QRS is negative in lead 1, pointing to an origin on the septal side in the right ventricular outflow tract. In panel C an inferior frontal QRS axis and QRS negativity in lead 1 are also present, but leads V1 and V2 clearly show initial positivity of the QRS complex. This is a tachycardia not arising on the endocardial surface of the right ventricular outflow tract but epicardially in between the root of the aorta and the posterior part of the

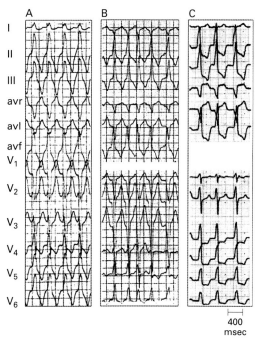

Figure 18.13. Three types of idiopathic VT arising in or close to the outflow tract of the right ventricle (see text).

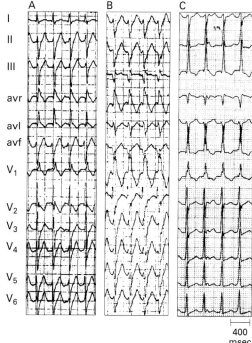

Figure 18.14. Three types of left ventricular idiopathic VT (see text).

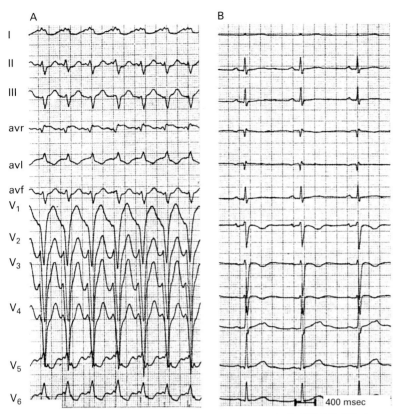

Figure 18.15. VT in arrhythmogenic right ventricular dysplasia (ARVD). VT shows LBBB shape and left axis deviation indicating an origin in the apex of the right ventricle. Note also the negative T waves in V1–V3 during sinus rhythm, which is often found in ARVD.

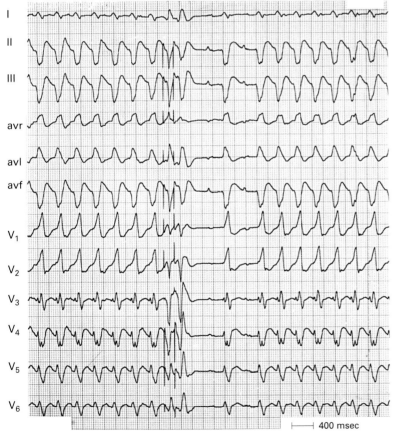

Figure 18.16. Bundle branch re-entry VT. Following two electrically induced premature beats the tachycardia terminates in the middle of the recording. However, tachycardia resumes after two conducted sinus beats. The QRS is identical during sinus rhythm and tachycardia. Note the presence of AV dissociation during tachycardia indicating a ventricular origin.

outflow tract of the right ventricle. It is important to recognise this pattern because this site of origin of the VT cannot be treated with catheter ablation in contrast to the tachycardias depicted in panel A and B.

The QRS configuration in idiopathic left VT is shown in fig 14. They all have an RBBB shape because of an origin in the left ventricle. The most common type is shown in panel A. The frontal QRS axis shows left axis deviation. The site of origin of the VT is in or close to the posterior fascicle of the LBB. In panel B the frontal QRS axis is further leftward (a so called north-west axis). This tachycardia arises more anteriorly close to the interventricular septum. The least common idiopathic left VT is the one shown in panel C. Now the frontal QRS axis is inferiorly directed. This VT originates in the anterior fascicle of the LBB. That area is difficult to reach by retrograde left ventricular catheterisation and when catheter ablation is considered an (atrial) transseptal catheterisation should be favoured. In ARVD there are three predilection sites in the right ventricle: the inflow and outflow tracts, and the apex. While the first two sites have a QRS configuration during tachycardia which is difficult to differentiate from right ventricular idiopathic VT, left axis deviation in a young person with an LBBB shaped VT should immediately lead to the suspicion of ARVD. In fact, there is an important rule in LBBB shaped VT with left axis deviation that cardiac disease should be suspected and that idiopathic right ventricular VT is extremely unlikely.

Figure 18.15 gives an example of an LBBB shaped VT in a patient with ARVD. When the broad QRS is identical during tachycardia and sinus rhythm, one has to differentiate SVT with pre-existent BBB from bundle branch re-entrant tachycardia.[13] In diseased hearts, especially when the bundle branches and the interventricular septum are involved, a tachycardia may occur based upon a circuit with anterograde conduction down one bundle branch or one of the left sided fascicles and after septal activation retrograde conduction over another branch of the bundle branch system (fig 18.16).

This type of re-entry may occur in patients with anteroseptal myocardial infarction, idiopathic dilated cardiomyopathy, myotonic dystrophy, after aortic valve surgery, and after severe frontal chest trauma.

Value of the ECG during sinus rhythm

The ECG during sinus rhythm may show changes such as pre-existent BBB, ventricular pre-excitation, or an old myocardial infarction which are very helpful in correctly interpreting the ECG during broad QRS tachycardia. Also the presence of AV conduction disturbances during sinus rhythm make it very unlikely that a broad QRS tachycardia in that patient has a supraventricular origin and, as already shown in fig 18.11, a QRS width during tachycardia more narrow that during sinus rhythm points to a VT.

Value and limitations of ECG findings in diagnosing broad QRS tachycardia

- AV dissociation suggests VT, but VA conduction may be present during VT

- A QRS width of > 160 ms suggests VT, but need to rule out:
  - pre-existent BBB (especially LBBB)
  - SVT with AV conduction over an AP
  - use of drugs slowing intraventricular conduction (flecainide).

Keep in mind—VT arising close to or in the intraventricular conduction system may have a width of < 140 ms

- Left axis deviation (to the left of −30) suggests VT, but is not helpful in:
  - LBBB shaped QRS
  - SVT with conduction over a right sided or posteroseptal AP
  - SVT during use of class 1 C drugs

- Right axis deviation (to the right of +90) suggests VT in LBBB shaped QRS

- Concordant pattern in precordial leads suggests VT, but positive concordancy may occur during SVT with AV conduction over a left posterior AP

- R nadir S > 100 ms in one or more precordial leads suggests VT, but may be found in:
  - SVT on drugs slowing intraventricular conduction
  - SVT with AV conduction over an AP
  - pre-existent BBB (especially LBBB)

- QR complexes during VT suggest previous myocardial infarction as aetiology

AP, accessory pathway; AV, atrioventricular; BBB, bundle branch block; LBBB, left bundle branch block; SVT, supraventricular tachycardia; VA, ventriculo-atrial; VT, ventricular tachycardia

---

Conclusion

Do not panic when confronted with a broad QRS tachycardia. Look for clinical signs of AV dissociation and evaluate the 12 lead ECG systematically (see box above). Also, when available, look at the 12 lead ECG during sinus rhythm. This approach usually gives the correct diagnosis of VT versus SVT. Keep in mind that statistically VT is much more common than SVT in the broad QRS tachycardia. Never make the mistake of rejecting VT because the broad QRS tachycardia is haemodynamically well tolerated. When in doubt, do not give verapamil or adenosine; procainamide should be used instead.

1. **Stewart RB, Bardy GH, Greene HL.** Wide complex tachycardia: misdiagnosis and outcome after emergent therapy. *Ann Intern Med* 1986;**104**:766–71.

2. **Buxton AE, Marchlinski FE, Doherty JU.** Hazards of intravenous verapamil for sustained ventricular tachycardia. *Am J Cardiol* 1987;**59**:1107–10.

3. **Dancy M, Camm AJ, Ward D.** Misdiagnosis of chronic recurrent ventricular tachycardia. *Lancet* 1985;ii:320–3.
   • *Three articles (refs 1–3) illustrating the dangers of giving calcium antagonists to patients with a broad QRS tachycardia erroneously interpreting a reasonable haemodynamic condition as pointing to an SVT.*

4. **Wellens HJJ, Bar FWHM, Lie KI.** The value of the electrocardiogram in the differential diagnosis of a tachycardia with a widened QRS complex. *Am J Med* 1978;**64**:27–33.
   • *First article systematically evaluating ECG findings in broad QRS tachycardia indicating value and limitations of AV dissociation, QRS width, QRS axis, and QRS characteristics in leads V1 and V6 to differentiate between VT and SVT.*

5. **Harvey WP, Ronan JA.** Bedside diagnosis of arrhythmias. *Prog Cardiovasc Dis* 1966;**8**:419–45.
   • *Physical examination is still of great value in the correct diagnosis of the patient with a tachycardia.*

6. **Marriott HJL.** Differential diagnosis of supraventricular and ventricular tachycardia. *Geriatrics* 1970;**25**:91–101.
   • *The first systematic approach to use the ECG for differentiating tachycardias.*

7. **Kindwall E, Brown J, Josephson ME.** Electrocardiographic criteria for ventricular tachycardia in wide QRS complex left bundle-branch block morphology tachycardia. *Am J Cardiol* 1988;**61**:1279–83.
   • *Basic information for the correct interpretation of LBBB shaped tachycardias.*

8. **Brugada P, Brugada J, Mont L,** *et al.* A new approach to the differential diagnosis of a regular tachycardia with a wide QRS complex. *Circulation* 1991;**83**:1649–59.
   • *A useful approach to the ECG diagnosis of the broad QRS tachycardia.*

9. **Coumel P, Leclerq JF, Attuel P,** *et al.* The QRS morphology in postmyocardial infarction ventricular tachycardia: a study of 100 tracings compared with 70 cases of idiopathic ventricular tachycardia. *Eur Heart J* 1984;**5**:792–805.
   • *Important article indicating that the ECG contains information about the aetiology of the broad QRS tachycardia.*

10. **Wellens HJJ.** The electrocardiographic diagnosis of arrhythmias. In: Topol E, ed. *Textbook of cardiovascular medicine.* Philadelphia: Lippincott, Raven, 1998:1591–609.
    • *This chapter includes an analysis of the incidence of QR complexes in a large series of patients with VT after myocardial infarction.*

11. **Wellens HJJ, Rodriguez LM, Smeets JL.** Ventricular tachycardia in structurally normal hearts. In: Zipes DP, Jalife J, eds. *Cardiac electrophysiology—from cell to bedside,* 2nd ed. Philadelphia: WB Saunders, 1995:780–8.
    • *A review of the ECG characteristics of patients with right and left sided idiopathic ventricular tachycardia.*

12. **Leclercq JF, Coumel PH.** Characteristics, prognosis and treatment of the ventricular arrhythmias of right ventricular dysplasia. *Eur Heart J* 1989;**10** (suppl D):61–70.
    • *ECG findings in patients with ARVD.*

13. **Touboul P, Kirkorian G, Atallah G, et al.** Bundle branch reentrant tachycardia treated by electrical ablation of the right bundle branch. *J Am Coll Cardiol* 1986;**7**:1404–9.
    • *A careful analysis of the bundle branch system as circuit for a re-entry tachycardia.*

SECTION VI: CONGENITAL HEART DISEASE

19 Haemodynamic calculations in the catheter laboratory

James L Wilkinson

Many of the calculations used in the evaluation of haemodynamic abnormalities are relatively simple and can be performed rapidly with a hand held calculator or (for the mentally agile) "in the head". Others are more complex and require a more time consuming process of analysis of the recorded data, often performed some time after the actual procedure.

Currently available catheter laboratory equipment for physiological monitoring and analysis will often provide a range of semi automatic calculations which will save time and allow the production of a comprehensive report at the conclusion of the procedure. It is vital, however, that cardiologists continue to have a clear understanding of the basis of such calculations and the limitations/pitfalls intrinsic to them and to some of the data on which they are based. Some of the calculations that can be made are of limited clinical utility while others are potentially misleading unless the data from which they are derived are carefully checked for accuracy and have been obtained using rigorous methodology.

When, as is all too often the case, the data have been acquired largely automatically and have not been carefully scrutinised by someone familiar with the potential errors, the figures for pulmonary and systemic blood flow, shunt flows and resistances may be almost meaningless and can readily lead to inappropriate and potentially dangerous decisions.

In practice most of the important calculations—shunt ratio (Qp:Qs), pulmonary blood flow, and pulmonary vascular resistance—can be estimated, albeit imprecisely, on the basis of straightforward and quick "guesstimates" which provide a rapid and generally useful "cross check" of the figures produced by the computer (or by a more time consuming and comprehensive manual method). While such rapid calculations are not a substitute for a careful and detailed analysis of the data, they are an effective way of understanding how the data relate to the haemodynamic disturbance; they also allow the trainee (or the established cardiologist) to demonstrate his or her mastery of the concepts involved and to avoid being over dependent on the "computer generated" report.

This article will focus on the usefulness of the different calculations in clinical practice and on a number of simple (short cut) methods of performing some of them, in an effort to "cross check" the more complete data obtained by the computer or by more laborious manual methods.

Shunts

In patients with congenital heart disease in whom there is a communication between the two sides of the heart, or between the aorta and the pulmonary artery, allowing a shunt to exist, a number of calculations may be made. These include:
(1) left to right shunt;
(2) right to left shunt;
(3) effective pulmonary blood flow;
(4) pulmonary to systemic flow ratio (Qp:Qs).

Of these calculations the only one that is of practical value is probably the pulmonary to systemic flow ratio (Qp:Qs). This provides a simple and reliable estimate of the extent to which pulmonary flow is increased or reduced and provides a useful insight into the severity of the haemodynamic disturbance in most cases. It is also very simple to perform, employing solely the oxygen saturation data from systemic arterial blood, left atrial/pulmonary venous blood, pulmonary artery, and vena caval/right heart samples.

The samples need to be acquired with the patient breathing (or being ventilated with) air or a gas mixture containing no more than a maximum of 30% oxygen. If oxygen enriched gas is being given (> 30% oxygen) then the saturation data may not provide accurate information regarding pulmonary blood flow, as a significant amount of oxygen may be present in dissolved form in the pulmonary venous sample (which will not be factored into the calculation if saturations alone are used). Under such circumstances pulmonary flow will tend to be overestimated and the Qp:Qs ratio will be correspondingly exaggerated.

The calculations to determine left to right shunt, right to left shunt, and effective pulmonary blood flow are all fairly simple. They do not provide particularly useful information, however, and will not be discussed further here.

Pulmonary to systemic flow ratio (Qp:Qs)

The calculation is based on the Fick principle, by which both pulmonary and systemic flow may be estimated. As such factors as oxygen carrying capacity and oxygen consumption are used for each individual calculation (for pulmonary and for systemic flow), they cancel out when only the ratio of the two flows is being estimated. This is very convenient as it removes the more difficult and time consuming parts of the calculation. The resulting equation (after removing the factors which cancel out) is pleasingly simple:

$$Q_p{:}Q_s = \frac{\text{Sat Ao} - \text{Sat MV}}{\text{Sat PV} - \text{Sat PA}} \qquad (1)$$

where: Sat Ao is aortic saturation, Sat MV is mixed venous saturation, Sat PV is pulmonary vein saturation, and Sat PA is pulmonary artery saturation.

As the arterial saturation (Sat Ao) and the pulmonary artery saturation (Sat PA) are routinely estimated, the only components of this set of data that may present any problem are the pulmonary vein saturation (Sat PV) and the "mixed venous" saturation (Sat MV). If a pulmonary vein has not been entered an assumed value of 98% may be employed for Sat PV. The left atrial saturation can be substituted provided that there is no right to left shunt at atrial level. Similarly left ventricular or arterial saturation may be substituted, provided that there is no right to left shunt.

For "mixed venous" (Sat MV) the tradition is to use the most distal right heart chamber or site where there is no left to right shunt. Thus, right atrium may be used in the absence of an atrial septal defect or right ventricle if there is no shunt at atrial or ventricular level. In practice superior vena cava (SVC) saturation is often used but a value intermediate between SVC and inferior vena cava (IVC) may be preferable as the two may be significantly different. It has been demonstrated that the mixed venous saturation more closely approximates to the SVC than to the IVC. Hence the following formula is often used[1]:

$$\text{Sat MV} = \frac{3 \times \text{Sat SVC} + 1 \times \text{Sat IVC}}{4} \quad (2)$$

It is noteworthy that IVC saturation varies depending on where the sample is obtained, and the sampling site should be at the level of the diaphragm to ensure that hepatic venous blood is taken into account.

A very simple way of calculating this ("in the head") is to use the formula:

$$\text{MV} = \text{Sat SVC} - \frac{\text{Sat SVC} - \text{Sat IVC}}{4} \quad (3)$$

Thus if SVC saturation (Sat SVC) is 78% and IVC saturation (Sat IVC) is 70%, mixed venous (MV) should be 76% (78 − 70 = 8; 8/4 = 2; 78 − 2 = 76).

As mentioned above, it is important that the samples used for this calculation are acquired with the patient breathing air or an oxygen enriched mixture not exceeding 30%. If higher concentrations of oxygen (50% or greater) are to be used (to test for pulmonary vascular reactivity, for example) then the calculation of pulmonary blood flow (and Qp:Qs ratio) should involve measurement of pO_2 on at least the pulmonary vein sample (preferably also the pulmonary artery sample). This allows inclusion of dissolved oxygen in the calculation (a more complex calculation, which necessitates calculation of the oxygen content of the samples—see below).

Usefulness of shunt ratio in practice

Qp:Qs ratio is very useful in many situations—such as in making decisions about surgery for a child with a ventricular septal defect where, in

a child beyond infancy, a shunt producing a Qp:Qs ≥ 1.8:1 is likely to require intervention, while one of ≤ 1.5:1 may be regarded as insignificant. Qp:Qs is also helpful in assessing the haemodynamics of many more complex defects but it should be recognised that under some circumstances it is of limited practical help. For instance, with an atrial septal defect, if there is evidence of a significant shunt on clinical grounds and non-invasive testing (for example, right ventricular dilatation on echocardiography, with paradoxical movement of the ventricular septum; cardiomegaly on *x* ray; well developed right ventricular volume load pattern on ECG (incomplete right bundle branch block)), the shunt ratio at catheter should not be used to decide about treatment. This is because of the fact that atrial shunts, which depend on right ventricular filling characteristics, can vary depending on conditions (for example, sympathetic tone, catecholamine concentrations). It is not uncommon for the measured shunt, at the time of catheter, to be small (for example, < 1.5:1) despite other evidence of a significant atrial septal defect/shunt.

Cardiac output and pulmonary blood flow

Assessment of cardiac output and of pulmonary blood flow is important in several situations. In the absence of any shunt pulmonary flow and systemic cardiac output are the same and may be measured as part of the investigation of patients with impaired cardiac function for a variety of reasons—notably as part of transplant assessment (for example, in patients with cardiomyopathy). In such patients the simplest methods of measuring cardiac output are by thermodilution or using the Fick method. The latter requires estimation of oxygen consumption, which presents considerable practical difficulties, and assumed values based on age, sex, and heart rate are often substituted (see below).

Thermodilution provides a straightforward and useful alternative,[2] but will only provide meaningful data when no shunt is present. The principle is similar to that of indicator (dye) dilution methods for measuring cardiac output.

The latter (dye dilution) is now seldom used but involves the injection of a bolus of indicator (dye) into the circulation, which is diluted in the blood stream[3]. Sampling is done at a site some distance "downstream" and the concentration of indicator is measured continuously, using a cuvette, during its first pass through the circulation, producing a time/concentration curve. The down slope of the primary curve is projected to the baseline, in order to exclude recirculation of the indicator. The mean concentration of the indicator during this first passage is then used, with the duration (in seconds) of the extrapolated curve (from the time of first detection of indicator) and an estimate of cardiac output can be obtained using the "Stewart-Hamilton" formula:

$$Cardiac\ output(l/min) = \frac{I \times 60}{Ct} \qquad (4)$$

where I is the quantity of injectate (mg), C is mean concentration (mg/l), and t is time in seconds.

Several dyes have been used, notably Evans blue, Cardiogreen, and methylene blue.

Using thermodilution a catheter with a lumen opening via a side hole in the right atrium and with a thermister at the tip, placed in the pulmonary artery, is employed. A bolus of cooled dextrose solution at either 5°C or at room temperature (22°C) is injected rapidly into the right atrium, and a time/temperature curve is recorded via the thermister in the pulmonary artery. Several determinations are usually made and are averaged.

The technique is now largely automated and a computer does the calculations. The volume and temperature of the injectate are critical and the speed of delivery of the bolus is also important. While the method is generally simple and reliable it is important that operators are familiar with the technique and this necessitates that one or more technologists or cardiologists gain experience with using the method on a regular basis. Results have been shown to correlate closely with both dye dilution and Fick methods, though in low cardiac output states the Fick method is considered to be more reliable.

While methods exist for estimating the size of left to right shunts (for example, Qp:Qs) using indicator dilution, the assessment of systemic cardiac output and pulmonary flow is not valid in the presence of shunting.

Common sources of errors

- Slow injection of cooled dextrose

- Operator "selection" of computer results. When the results are "scattered" the operator may elect to reject those that appear to be wide of the anticipated value and to average only those that are closer to that which is expected (it is worthy of note that some degree of "scatter" is frequent with this method)

Calculation of cardiac output and pulmonary blood flow by the Fick method is the routine for use in patients with septal defects and associated shunts. The method depends on the fact that oxygen uptake by the lungs is equal to oxygen consumption in the tissues. Blood flow is calculated by measurement of the oxygen content of venous blood and of arterial blood (in ml/l) and hence estimating the difference between the two, which represents the tissue oxygen utilisation. In general the difference (pulmonary VA O_2 diff. or systemic AV O_2 diff.) tends to be in the order of 20–50 ml/l, depending on conditions and with considerable variability between individuals. If oxygen consumption (V_{O_2}) is known (in an adult usually around 200–250 ml/min) then blood flow is calculated by the simple equation:

$$Q = \frac{V_{O_2}}{VA\ O_2\ diff.} \qquad (5)$$

where Q = blood flow in l/min.

Thus, in the above example, if the content difference is 50 ml/l and oxygen consumption is 250 ml/min then blood flow is 5 l/min.

The same equation allows calculation of either pulmonary blood flow or systemic cardiac output—by substituting pulmonary VA O_2 diff. or systemic AV O_2 diff.

Thus Qp (pulmonary flow) is calculated by the equation:

$$Q_p = \frac{V_{O_2}}{Pulmonary\ VA\ O_2\ diff.} \qquad (6)$$

Similarly systemic flow may be estimated employing the difference in oxygen content between the aorta and a "mixed venous" sample (systemic AV O_2 diff.)

$$Q_s = \frac{V_{O_2}}{Systemic\ AV\ O_2\ diff.} \qquad (7)$$

In practice absolute values for pulmonary and systemic flow are less useful than indexed values (corrected for body surface area). Therefore most paediatric cardiologists will take into account surface area; the simplest way of doing this is to employ a figure for oxygen consumption that has been related to body surface area —for example, ml/min/m². Thus for an adult with a body surface area of 2 m² and a V_{O_2} of 240 ml/min the oxygen consumption may be expressed as being 120 ml/min/m². Flow calculations then produce a result in "litres/min/m²". This correction (for body surface area) is particularly important for estimation of pulmonary and systemic vascular resistance, where the use of indexed flows (pulmonary flow index and systemic cardiac index) produces meaningful resistance calculations without the need for any further "correction".

The critical parts of these equations are the calculation of the oxygen content of the various samples and estimation of oxygen consumption. Oxygen content is calculated by estimating the oxygen carrying capacity of the patient's blood, as haemoglobin bound oxygen. This is the volume of oxygen that could be carried on haemoglobin at 100% saturation. This is calculated by: Hb (g/l) × 1.36.

Usually this is in the order of 200 ml/l, though it varies with Hb. The content of each sample is then computed by multiplying by the saturation. Thus if Hb is 140 g/l and saturation in a sample is 70% the oxygen carrying capacity will be $140 \times 1.36 = 190$ ml/l and content will be $190 \times 70\% = 133$ ml/l.

Providing that the patient is breathing air or an oxygen enriched mixture of 30% or less the amount of dissolved oxygen in plasma is sufficiently small as to be unimportant. Each sample needs to have its oxygen content calculated as above. The pulmonary VA oxygen difference and the systemic AV oxygen difference are thus easily estimated. As in the calculation for Qp:Qs ratio the mixed venous saturation is estimated either using SVC alone or by employing a sample from within the right heart (proximal to any left to right shunt), or by a formula using both the SVC and the IVC saturation. The last of these is our preferred method.

The largest source of error is in the assessment of oxygen consumption. Traditionally this has been measured using a hood and gas pump that extracts all exhaled air and passes it through a mixing system before measuring the oxygen content. The difference between inhaled oxygen content and exhaled oxygen content, coupled with the flow maintained by the pump, allows estimation of oxygen consumption.[4] The method involves several assumptions. Firstly, it assumes that the pump caters for all exhaled air and that none is "lost". Secondly it assumes effective mixing before the oxygen measurement. Thirdly, it assumes (at least with some equipment) that the volume of exhaled air is the same as that of inhaled air, which is only true if carbon dioxide production is identical with oxygen uptake (in some labs a respiratory quotient—respiratory exchange ratio (RER)—of 0.8 is assumed).[5] It also requires very accurate measurement of flow through the pump. Additionally it requires very precise measurement of the oxygen level in exhaled air, which has in the past required the use of large and cumbersome equipment (a mass spectrometer). Patients being catheterised under anaesthesia may require a closed circuit method, which is also laborious and time consuming to perform. In either case it is essential that the medical and technical personnel involved be very familiar with the equipment and the methodology, and that they perform such measurements on a regular basis.[6]

Until recently no commercially available system had been produced that allowed simple and reliable measurements to be made routinely by technologists or physicians without substantial and regular experience of the apparatus and its potential problems. For this reason regular measurement of oxygen consumption has been largely restricted to centres in which there are physicians and/or technical personnel with a major interest in oxygen consumption measurements, and usually an ongoing research programme or project that involves them.

There are now several commercially available methods of measuring oxygen consumption, which employ relatively compact and reasonably simple equipment that eliminates, to some degree, many of the problems detailed above.[7][8]

In the majority of institutions, even when such equipment is available, oxygen consumption is not measured routinely; when measurements are required it is often difficult or impossible to obtain satisfactory measurements—for example, because those staff who are familiar with the apparatus are unavailable, and the personnel involved with the procedure are unfamiliar with the equipment and lack confidence/competence in obtaining the necessary data.

The availability of nomograms for oxygen consumption obtained from children of varying age and sex and at different heart rates has allowed the use of "assumed oxygen consumption" based on such data.[9] Several regression equations and tables of "assumed oxygen consumption" are available and produce normal values, ranging from around 180 ml/min/m^2 in young children (aged 2–3 years) down to around 100 ml/min/m^2 in adult women.[4] Males have higher oxygen consumption (by 10–20%) than females and tachycardia above 150 beats/min is associated with a 10% increase compared with heart rates of 120 or lower. Young children (aged 2–5 years) have oxygen consumption values between around 150 and 200 ml/min/m^2. Older children (for example, adolescents) tend to have values between 120 and 180 ml/min/m^2. The sex difference is less pronounced in the younger age groups and is largest in adults. Infants younger than 3 months may have somewhat lower oxygen consumption values (130 ml/min/m^2) than older infants (170 ml/min/m^2), while children of 1–2 years have values close to 200 ml/min/m^2.

Unfortunately those studies in which direct comparisons have been made between assumed and measured oxygen consumption have shown poor correlation and wide discrepancies in individual cases.[4]

Despite the deficiencies implicit in the use of assumed oxygen consumption this method is employed very widely and is probably adequate for most purposes. A useful practice is to do duplicate calculations—assuming alternative oxygen consumption values—at the upper and lower levels of the likely range for a child of the particular age and sex. Thus, for a 5 year old boy one might use assumed oxygen consumption values of 140 ml/min/m^2 and 200 ml/min/m^2. The calculated flow using these two figures should give values at the extremes of the likely range, and the actual figure is most likely somewhere in between.

Common sources of errors

- Assumed O_2 consumption is notoriously unreliable

- Unfamiliarity with O_2 consumption measurement technique—leads to unpredictable/unreliable results

- Failure to calculate dissolved O_2 when using enriched gas (for example, 100% O_2)

Pulmonary resistance

Calculation of pulmonary resistance and assessment of pulmonary vascular reactivity remains a fundamentally important issue in many patients. The calculation becomes extremely simple once the pulmonary blood flow index has been estimated as indicated above. Resistance is the pressure drop across the pulmonary (or systemic) circulation per unit of flow in a specified time period. As flow is usually measured in l/min/m^2 this is the unit of measurement usually employed. The pressure drop is the difference between mean arterial and mean venous pressure. In the case of pulmonary resistance the equation is therefore:

$$R_p = \frac{PAm - LAm}{Q_p} \qquad (8)$$

where Rp is pulmonary resistance, PAm is mean pulmonary artery pressure, LAm is mean left atrium (or pulmonary vein) pressure, and Qp is the pulmonary blood flow index.

If the left atrium and/or pulmonary veins have not been entered a pulmonary capillary wedge pressure may be used. Alternatively an assumed pressure of around 8 mm may be employed.

The resistance units in this calculation are in "mm Hg/l/min"—referred to usually as Wood units. An alternative is to measure resistance in metric units in "dyne.sec.cm^{-5}". The conversion is achieved by multiplying resistance in Wood units by 80 to achieve the metric units in dyne.sec.cm^{-5}.

It should be appreciated that if the figure for pulmonary blood flow is indexed to body surface area the resistance is also indexed. Values of resistance (in Wood units) are frequently expressed with the simple abbreviation of "u" (units). When indexed to body surface area the appropriate abbreviation is "u.m^2". Unfortunately in much of the published literature this has been misrepresented as "u/m^2", which is misleading as it implies that the calculated resistance in units has been divided by the body surface area to index it. If absolute values for flow (rather than indexed values) are used to calculate resistance it will become clear that smaller patients have much higher levels of resistance (because of the lower flows with smaller surface area). Obviously the use of indexed flows eliminates this disparity. If the value of resistance obtained by using absolute flows is divided by body surface area, however (as the abbreviation "u/m^2" would imply) the disparity is exaggerated. For example, a child with a body surface area of 0.5 m^2 has a pulmonary blood flow (Qp) of 2 l/min and a pulmonary artery mean pressure of 20 mm Hg with a left atrium mean of 8 mm Hg. His absolute resistance is therefore (20 − 8)/2 or 6 u. If this is "corrected" for surface area by dividing by 0.5 the result will be 12 u/m^2. However, if the flow is corrected for surface area it becomes 4 l/min/m^2. The calculation will then produce the correct figure for indexed resistance: (20 − 8)/4 = 3 u.m^2. The same result will be achieved by taking the absolute figure for resistance (6 u) and multiplying (rather than dividing) it by body surface area (6 × 0.5 = 3).

Common sources of errors

- Correction for body surface area by *dividing* by BSA in m^2

- Unstable haemodynamics due to hypoventilation or acidosis, leading to pulmonary vasoconstriction and high pulmonary vascular resistance (check pH and pCO$_2$)

Pulmonary vascular reactivity

The assessment of pulmonary vascular reactivity is sometimes important if the initial value (with the patient breathing air) is greatly elevated, raising concerns about the presence of significant pulmonary vascular disease. The significance of raised levels of pulmonary vascular resistance depends on the patient's age. In the early months of life high resistance is often related to pulmonary vasoconstriction/ increased vasomotor tone (with increased medial smooth muscle in the walls of the pulmonary arterioles). It does not necessarily imply significant obliterative pulmonary vascular disease until later in infancy/childhood. Values of pulmonary resistance above 6 u.m^2 would be a cause for concern on this score in a child above 1 year of age (estimates greater than 10 u.m^2 would be especially sinister). In interpreting such measurements it should be recognised that hypoventilation or acidosis can produce quite intense pulmonary vasoconstriction and may be associated with artificially (misleadingly) elevated resistance. To exclude this as a potential source of error, blood gas measurements need to be carried out at the time of the pressure and saturation measurements, to ensure that pH and pCO$_2$ are within the normal range.

In cases in which a high pulmonary vascular resistance is demonstrated, it is customary to allow the patient to breath an oxygen enriched mixture (80% or 100% oxygen) for 10 minutes and then to repeat the pressure and saturation measurements in order to get a calculation of flow and resistance under these conditions. This is a very important and useful manoeuvre but does introduce a very important potential source of error. With the increased concentration of inspired oxygen the partial pressure of oxygen in pulmonary alveoli and in pulmonary capillary and pulmonary venous blood will rise to supernormal levels. This will result in quite significant amounts of oxygen being transported dissolved in plasma, in addition to that which is bound to haemoglobin. If the calculations do not take this into account the oxygen content difference between pulmonary vein and pulmonary artery blood will be underestimated. The estimated pulmonary blood flow will then be overestimated and pulmonary resistance will appear to be lower than is really the case. To calculate dissolved oxygen is extremely simple. The pO_2 of pulmonary venous blood is measured (in mm Hg) and this value multiplied by 0.03 to provide a volume of dissolved oxygen (in ml/l). Thus if the pulmonary vein pO_2 is 500 mm Hg there will be 15 ml/l of dissolved oxygen ($500 \times 0.03 = 15$). The amount of dissolved oxygen in pulmonary arterial blood should also be estimated by the same method (though in practice it is seldom more than 3 ml/l). Thus there may be as much as 12 ml/l oxygen content difference in the form of dissolved oxygen. In patients with high pulmonary flow this may account for more than 50% of the total oxygen content difference between pulmonary venous and pulmonary arterial blood. Consequently, failure to include dissolved oxygen in the calculations can lead to major errors in the data for pulmonary flow and resistance.

One of the misconceptions concerning the measurements made in 100% oxygen, which is quite widely held, is that patients with significantly labile pulmonary vascular beds (in whom resistance will drop with increased inspired oxygen) will always show a fall in pulmonary artery pressure under these conditions. Thus the assumption may be made that the absence of any fall in pressure demonstrates a lack of lability and implies the presence of advanced pulmonary vascular disease. However, some patients may achieve a substantial increase in pulmonary blood flow, associated with a large drop in resistance, with little change in pulmonary artery pressure. Thus careful assessment of pulmonary blood flow index and resistance (including the calculation of dissolved oxygen) is an essential part of the study in patients being evaluated with 100% oxygen because of pulmonary hypertension.

As an alternative to the use of 100% oxygen (or in addition), other vasodilators may be employed to test vasoreactivity. The most useful of these is probably inhaled nitric oxide —usually given in concentrations between 20 and 80 parts per million (ppm). This is a useful adjunct to (but not a substitute for) use of 100% oxygen. However it should be born in mind that while there is broad agreement about the level of pulmonary vascular resistance which is likely to be "reversible" as demonstrated with the vasodilation and fall in resistance achieved with 100% oxygen (usually a fall to 6 u.m² or less), it is not yet clear whether patients who show a similar fall with nitric oxide (but not with 100% oxygen) will prove to have similarly "reversible" pulmonary vascular damage. Thus, in a patient whose resting resistance is calculated at 10 u.m², in whom 100% oxygen produces a fall to around 8 u.m², and nitric oxide produces a further fall to 6 u.m², it is by no means certain that the outcome after surgery would be the same as might be anticipated if 100% oxygen had produced a fall to 6 u.m².

Common sources of errors

- Hypoventilation/acidosis producing pulmonary vasoconstriction

- Failure to calculate dissolved O_2 when using enriched gas (for example, 100% O_2)

- Assumption that no fall in pulmonary artery pressure means no fall in resistance

---

It may appear from the above brief analysis that the assessment of pulmonary hypertension and pulmonary vascular reactivity is time consuming, complex, and fraught with assumptions that are of doubtful validity. In practice useful assessments can be made rapidly and quite simply. The calculations need to be worked through carefully (usually after the case has been completed), but a rapid estimation can often be made at the time of the procedure, which may produce a useful insight into the severity of the problem.

In a patient in stable haemodynamic state with systemic venous saturations in the normal range (60–75%) it is reasonable to assume that the systemic cardiac index will be in the general range of 3–4 l/min/m². As Qp:Qs can be estimated very simply while the patient is under basal conditions (for example, breathing air) a simple "guesstimate" of pulmonary blood flow index is easily made. If Qp:Qs is 2.5 then Qp must be in the general range of 7–10 l/min/m² ($3 \times 2.5 = 7.5$, $4 \times 2.5 = 10$). If the pulmonary artery mean pressure is 35 mm Hg and left atrium is 10 mm Hg then the pressure drop (transpulmonary gradient) is 25 mm Hg. Resistance in this case is likely to fall between 2.5 and 4 u.m². This calculation is simple, quick, and informative—although it does not eliminate the need to do the complete calculations.

A fairly simple "cross check" can be made by doing a quick mental calculation of pulmonary veno-arterial oxygen content difference and using an assumed oxygen consumption of 150–200 ml/min/m².

This depends on having a value for Hb and for the saturation difference between the pulmonary artery and pulmonary vein. Thus if the pulmonary artery saturation is 90% (in the presence of a left to right shunt) and the left atrium is 99%, with a Hb of 120 g/l the following calculation may be made:
Hb $\times$ 1.36 = 120×1.36 = approximately 160;
Sat PV − Sat PA = 99 − 90 = 9;
$160 \times 9\%$ = approximately 15 ml/l (oxygen content difference).
Pulmonary blood flow index is then likely to be in the general range of 10–13 l/min/m² (150/15 = 10; 200/15 = 13).

If the transpulmonary gradient is 25 mm, as in the earlier example, then the pulmonary vascular resistance is 2–2.5 u.m² (25/10 = 2.5; 25/13 ~ 2).

A similar piece of mental arithmetic will allow estimation of systemic cardiac index as well as systemic vascular resistance.

Similar calculations may be performed with the patient in 100% oxygen, but here the dissolved oxygen needs to be taken into account. A fairly simple way to do this is to assume the "worst case scenario"—which would have a difference in dissolved oxygen between pulmonary vein and pulmonary artery of around 12 ml/l (it would very seldom be any greater than this).

Using the same values for saturation and Hb, as well as the same assumed oxygen consumption as in the earlier example, the equation is now:

Hb × 1.36 = 120 × 1.36 = approximately 160;
Sat PV − Sat PA = 99 − 90 = 9;
160 × 9% = approximately 15 ml/l; dissolved oxygen difference = 12 ml/l (worst case scenario).
Total oxygen content difference = 15 + 12 = 27 ml/l

This now produces a very different result in the blood flow calculation.

Pulmonary blood flow index is now likely to be in the general range of 5.5–7.5 l/min/m^2 (150/27 = 5.5; 200/27 = 7.4).

If the transpulmonary gradient is 25 mm then pulmonary vascular resistance is now 3–4.5 u.m^2 (25/5.5 = 4.5; 25/7.5 = 3.3).

In reality if the dissolved oxygen content difference is lower than the "worst case scenario" the flow will be higher than this (nearer to the value arrived at when the dissolved oxygen is not included in the calculation).

Perhaps surprisingly, considering all the assumptions and approximations contained in these "rough calculations", the results correlate generally very well with the more laborious calculations performed after the case is complete and with the calculations produced by the computer software which is often employed for automating these estimations. Moreover where major discrepancies arise it is often desirable to go back and carefully check the data and the way in which the calculations have been done. Sometimes the "rough result" is the more correct one and errors have been made in the more detailed calculation.

In any case the ability to perform these quick "mental" calculations in the catheter laboratory is an entertaining exercise and demonstrates an understanding of the data.

Valve (orifice) area

Calculation of valve area is based on the hydraulic formula usually referred to as the "Gorlin formula" and published almost 50 years ago.[10]

The calculation depends on obtaining estimates for valve flow in ml/sec during the time that the valve is open.

This is conventionally estimated by measuring the duration (in seconds) of systolic ejection or of diastolic filling, from the pressure wave forms, and multiplying by heart rate—to assess the period of flow through the valve per minute (expressed in secs/min), which is in turn divided into the cardiac output (in ml/min) to obtain flow per second across the valve for which an area calculation is required (in ml/sec).

The mean ventricular pressure during flow through the valve (systole for arterial valves, diastole for atrioventricular (AV) valves) and the mean pressure proximal or distal to the valve are required, in order to estimate the mean transvalvar gradient. These mean pressure measurements need to relate specifically to the period when the valve is open (during systolic ejection for an arterial valve or during diastolic filling for an AV valve). This conventionally requires planimetry and is potentially time consuming and cumbersome.

The formula includes constants, one of which is an "orifice constant coefficient" (0.8 for mitral valve; 1.0 for aortic, pulmonary, and tricuspid valves).

The final formula is:

$$\text{Valve area(cm}^2) = \frac{\text{Flow (ml/sec)}}{\text{Oc} \times 44.3\sqrt{\text{mn Gradient}}} \quad (9)$$

where Oc is orifice constant coefficient (0.8 for mitral valve, 1.0 for other valves); 44.3 is a constant derived from $\sqrt{2g}$ (where g is gravity acceleration = 980 cm/s/s); and mn Gradient is the mean transvalvar gradient (mm Hg), being the difference in mean pressure on each side of the valve during systolic ejection (arterial valve) or diastolic filling (AV valve).

Simplified versions of this formula have been advocated and include the Bache formula for aortic valve area (using peak to peak gradient)[11] and the Hakki formula[12]:

$$\text{Valve area} = \frac{\text{CO}}{\sqrt{\text{mn Gradient}}} \quad (10)$$

In practice these formulae all depend on a number of assumptions and approximations. They permit estimations of valve orifice that are, in our opinion, of limited clinical use. We do not rely on such data for clinical decision making, preferring to use other parameters.

1. **Miller HC, Brown DJ, Miller GA.** Comparison of formulae used to estimate oxygen saturation of mixed venous blood from caval samples. *Br Heart J* 1974;**36**:446–51.
• *Methods of calculating mixed venous oxygen saturation are described.*

2. **Freed MD, Keane JF.** Cardiac output measured by thermodilution in infants and children. *J Pediatr* 1978;**92**:39–42.
• *This provides an important reference on the use of thermodilution to measure cardiac output in children.*

3. **Wood EH.** Diagnostic applications of indicator-dilution technics in congenital heart disease. *Circ Res* 1962;**10**:531.
• *Application of indicator dilution techniques in congenital heart disease is provided.*

4. **Lundell BPW, Casas ML, Wallgren CG.** Oxygen consumption in infants and children during heart catheterization. *Pediatr Cardiol* 1996;**17**:207–13.
• *A useful comparison of measured and assumed oxygen consumption in infants, children, and adolescents during catheter procedures.*

5. **Lindahl SG.** Oxygen consumption and carbon dioxide elimination in infants and children during anaesthesia and surgery. *Br J Anaesth* 1989;**62**:70–6.

- *This describes oxygen consumption measurement using a mass spectrometer.*

6. Kappagoda CT, Greenwood P, Macartney FJ, *et al.* Oxygen consumption in children with congenital diseases of the heart. *Clin Sci* 1973;**45**:107–14.

7. Phang PT, Rich T, Ronco J. A validation and comparison study of two metabolic monitors. *J Parenteral Enteral Nutr* 1990;**14**:259–61.
- *A comparison is provided between Deltatrac and SensorMedics 2900 metabolic monitors.*

8. Tissot S, Delafosse B, Bertrand O, *et al.* Clinical validation of the Deltatrac monitoring system in mechanically ventilated patients. *Intensive Care Med* 1995;**21**:149–53.
- *A comparison of Vo_2, Vco_2, and RQ measurements between Deltatrac, mass spectrometer and Douglas Bag techniques in ventilated patients is provided.*

9. LaFarge CG, Miettinen OS. The estimation of oxygen consumption. *Cardiovasc Res* 1970;**4**:23–30.
- *This provides the basis for the "assumed oxygen consumption" values used in many laboratories around the world.*

10. Gorlin R, Gorlin G. Hydraulic formula for calculation of area of stenotic mitral valve, other cardiac valves and central circulatory shunts. *Am Heart J* 1951;**41**:1–29.
- *The famous (or infamous?) Gorlin formula for valve area.*

11. Bache RJ, Jorgensen CR, Wang Y. Simplified estimation of aortic valve area. *Br Heart J* 1972;**34**:408–11.
- *An easier way to calculate valve area.*

12. Hakki AH. A simplified valve formula for the calculation of stenotic cardiac valve areas. *Circulation* 1981;**63**:1050–5.
- *Another option for calculation of valve formula.*

20 Heart disease and pregnancy

Samuel C Siu, Jack M Colman

Pregnancy in most women with heart disease has a favourable maternal and fetal outcome. With the exception of patients with Eisenmenger syndrome, pulmonary vascular obstructive disease, and Marfan syndrome with aortopathy, maternal death during pregnancy in women with heart disease is rare.[1-4] However, pregnant women with heart disease do remain at risk for other complications including heart failure, arrhythmia, and stroke. Women with congenital heart disease now comprise the majority of pregnant women with heart disease seen at referral centres. The next largest group includes women with rheumatic heart disease. Peripartum cardiomyopathy, though infrequent, will be discussed in view of its unique relation to pregnancy. Two groups of conditions not discussed further are coronary artery disease, infrequently encountered, and isolated mitral valve prolapse, which generally has an excellent outcome.

Cardiovascular physiology and pregnancy

Hormonally mediated increases in blood volume, red cell mass, and heart rate result in a major increase in cardiac output during pregnancy; cardiac output peaks during the second trimester, and remains constant until term. Gestational hormones, circulating prostaglandins, and the low resistance vascular bed in the placenta result in concomitant decreases in peripheral vascular resistance and blood pressure. During labour and delivery, pain and uterine contractions result in additional increases in cardiac output and blood pressure. Immediately following delivery, relief of caval compression and autotransfusion from the emptied and contracted uterus produce a further increase in cardiac output. Most haemodynamic changes of pregnancy resolve by two weeks postpartum.[5]

Outcomes associated with specific cardiac lesions

Congenital heart lesions
Left to right shunts
The effect of increase in cardiac output on the volume loaded right ventricle in *atrial septal defect* (ASD), or the left ventricle in *ventricular septal defect* (VSD) and *patent ductus arteriosus*, is counterbalanced by the decrease in peripheral vascular resistance. Consequently, the increase in volume overload is attenuated. In the absence of pulmonary hypertension, pregnancy, labour and delivery are well tolerated.[2 4] However arrhythmias, ventricular dysfunction, and progression of pulmonary hypertension may occur, especially when the shunt is large or when there is pre-existing elevation of pulmonary artery pressure. Infrequently, particularly in ASDs, paradoxical embolisation may be encountered if systemic vasodilatation and/or elevation of pulmonary resistance promote transient right to left shunting.

Left ventricular outflow tract obstruction
When *aortic stenosis* complicates pregnancy it is usually because of congenital bicuspid aortic valve which may also be associated with aortic coarctation and/or ascending aortopathy. Other causes of left ventricular outflow tract obstruction at, below, and above the valve have similar haemodynamic consequences. Women with symptomatic aortic stenosis should delay pregnancy until after surgical correction.[6] However the absence of symptoms antepartum is not sufficient assurance that pregnancy will be well tolerated. In a pregnant woman with severe aortic stenosis, the limited ability to augment cardiac output may result in abnormal elevation of left ventricular systolic and filling pressures which in turn precipitate or exacerbate heart failure or ischaemia. In addition the non-compliant, hypertrophied ventricle is sensitive to falls in preload. The consequent exaggerated drop in cardiac output may lead to hypotension. In a compilation of many small retrospective series, 65 patients were followed through 106 pregnancies with a maternal mortality of 11% and a perinatal mortality of 4%.[7] Most of the complications were reported in the earlier studies. In 25 pregnancies managed more recently, there was no maternal mortality but deterioration of maternal functional status occurred in 5 (20%).[7] Intrapartum palliation by balloon valvuloplasty may be helpful in selected cases.

In the absence of prosthetic dysfunction or residual aortic stenosis, patients with bioprosthetic aortic valves usually tolerate pregnancy well. Though it had been stated that pregnancy might accelerate the rate of degeneration of bioprosthetic or homograft valves, recent studies have shown that this is not the case.[8] A study of 14 pregnancies in women who underwent pulmonary autograft aortic valve replacement (Ross procedure) reported favourable maternal and fetal outcomes except in one woman who developed postpartum left ventricular dysfunction.[9] Pregnancy in a woman with a mechanical valve prosthesis carries increased risk of valve thrombosis as a result of the hypercoagulable state. The magnitude of this increased risk (3–14%) is greater if subcutaneous unfractionated heparin rather than warfarin is used as the anticoagulant agent and may be a result of inadequate dosing, monitoring or reduced efficacy with subcutaneous unfractionated heparin.[6 10]

138

Coarctation of the aorta

Maternal mortality with uncorrected coarctation has been reported as 3% in an early series, and is higher in the presence of associated cardiac defects, aortopathy, or longstanding hypertension; aortic rupture accounted for eight of the 14 reported deaths and occurred in the third trimester as well as in the postpartum period.[11] More recently, a preliminary report described encouraging maternal and fetal outcome in 87 pregnancies, with no maternal deaths and one early neonatal death.[12] The management of hypertension in uncorrected coarctation is particularly problematic in pregnancy because satisfactory control of upper body hypertension may lead to excessive hypotension below the coarctation site, compromising the fetus. Intrauterine growth restriction and premature labour and delivery are more common. Following coarctation repair, the risk of dissection and rupture is likely reduced but not eliminated.

Pulmonary stenosis

Mild pulmonic stenosis, or pulmonic stenosis that has been alleviated by valvuloplasty or surgery, is well tolerated during pregnancy and fetal outcome is favourable. Though a woman with severe pulmonic stenosis may be asymptomatic, the increased haemodynamic load of pregnancy may precipitate right heart failure or atrial arrhythmias; such a patient should be considered for correction before pregnancy. Even during pregnancy, balloon valvuloplasty may be feasible if symptoms of pulmonary stenosis progress.

Cyanotic heart disease: unrepaired and repaired

In uncorrected or palliated pregnant patients with cyanotic congenital heart disease such as tetralogy of Fallot, single ventricle, etc, the usual pregnancy associated fall in systemic vascular resistance and rise in cardiac output exacerbate right to left shunting leading to increased maternal hypoxaemia and cyanosis. A recent report examining the outcomes of 96 pregnancies in 44 women with a variety of cyanotic congenital heart defects reported a high rate of maternal cardiac events (32%, including one death), prematurity (37%), and a low live birth rate (43%).[13] The lowest live birth rate (12%) was observed in those mothers with an arterial oxygen saturation of $\leq$ 85%.

Tetralogy of Fallot is the most common form of cyanotic congenital heart disease. Pregnancy risk is low in women who have had successful correction of tetralogy.[2 4] However, residua and sequelae such as residual shunt, right ventricular outflow tract obstruction, arrhythmias, pulmonary regurgitation, right ventricular systolic dysfunction, pulmonary hypertension (caused by the effects of a previous palliative shunt), or left ventricular dysfunction (caused by previous volume overload) increase the likelihood of pregnancy complications and require independent consideration.

Atrial repair (Mustard or Senning procedure) was developed for the surgical correction of complete transposition of the great arteries. The anatomic right ventricle supports the systemic circulation. Late adult complications following atrial repair include sinus node dysfunction, atrial arrhythmias, and dysfunction of the systemic ventricle. In 43 pregnancies in 31 women described in recent reports, there was one late maternal death.[14] There was a 14% incidence of maternal heart failure, arrhythmias, or cardiac deterioration. Few recipients of the current repair of choice for complete transposition—the arterial switch procedure—have yet reached reproductive age.

The Fontan operation eliminates cyanosis and volume overload of the functioning systemic ventricle but patients have a limited ability to increase cardiac output. In a recent review of 33 pregnancies in 21 women who were doing well after the Fontan operation, there were 15 (45%) term pregnancies with no maternal mortality although two women had cardiac complications and the incidence of first trimester miscarriage was high (39%).[15] Since the 10 year survival rate following the Fontan operation is only 60–80%, it is important that information regarding long term maternal prognosis be discussed during preconception counselling.

Marfan syndrome

Life threatening aortic complications of Marfan syndrome are caused by medial aortopathy resulting in dilatation, dissection, and valvar regurgitation. Risk is increased in pregnancy because of haemodynamic stress and perhaps hormonal effects. Although older case reports suggested a very high mortality risk in the range of 30%, more recent data suggested an overall maternal mortality of 1% and fetal mortality of 22%. A prospective study of 45 pregnancies in 21 patients reported no increase in obstetrical complications or significant change in aortic root size in the patients with normal aortic roots. Importantly, in the eight patients with a dilated aortic root (> 40 mm) or prior aortic root surgery, three of their nine pregnancies were complicated by either aortic dissection (two) or rapid aortic dilatation (one).[16] Thus, patients with aortic root involvement should receive preconception counselling emphasising their risk, and in early pregnancy should be offered termination. In contrast, women with little cardiovascular involvement and with normal aortic root diameter may tolerate pregnancy well, though there remains a possibility of dissection even without prior evidence of aortopathy. Serial echocardiography should be used to identify progressive aortic root dilatation and prophylactic β blockers should be administered.

Congenitally corrected transposition of the great arteries

Many adult patients will have had surgical interventions, primarily VSD closure and relief of pulmonic stenosis, sometimes requiring a valved conduit from the left ventricle to the pulmonary artery. Potential problems in pregnancy include dysfunction of the systemic right ventricle and/or increased systemic atrioventricular valve regurgitation with heart failure, atrial arrhythmias, and atrioventricular block. In two recent reports on 41 patients, there were 105 pregnancies with 73% live births and no maternal mortality, although seven patients developed either heart failure, endocarditis, stroke, or myocardial infarction.[17][18]

Eisenmenger syndrome and pulmonary vascular obstructive disease
Maternal mortality in Eisenmenger syndrome is approximately 30% in each pregnancy.[19] The preponderance of complications occurs at term and during the first postpartum week. Preconception counselling should stress the extreme pregnancy associated risks. Termination of pregnancy should always be offered to such patients, as should sterilisation. The vasodilation associated with pregnancy will increase the degree of right to left shunting in patients with Eisenmenger syndrome, resulting in worsening of maternal cyanosis with adverse effect on fetal outcome. Spontaneous abortion is common, intrauterine growth restriction is seen in 30% of pregnancies, and preterm labour is frequent. The high perinatal mortality rate (28%) is caused mainly by prematurity.

A recent review of outcome of 125 pregnancies in patients with Eisenmenger syndrome, primary pulmonary hypertension, and secondary pulmonary hypertension reported poor outcomes in all three groups.[20] The maternal mortality observed in the Eisenmenger, primary, and secondary pulmonary hypertension groups was 36%, 30%, and 56%, respectively. The overall neonatal mortality was 13%.

Rheumatic heart disease
Mitral stenosis is the most common rheumatic valvar lesion encountered during pregnancy. The hypervolaemia and tachycardia associated with pregnancy exacerbate the impact of mitral valve obstruction. The resultant elevation in left atrial pressure increases the likelihood of atrial fibrillation. Thus, even patients with mild to moderate mitral stenosis, who are asymptomatic before pregnancy, may develop atrial fibrillation and heart failure during the ante- and peripartum periods. Atrial fibrillation is a frequent precipitant of heart failure in pregnant patients with mitral stenosis, primarily caused by uncontrolled ventricular rate, and equivalent tachycardia of any cause may produce the same detrimental effect. Earlier studies examining a pregnant population comprised predominantly of women with rheumatic mitral disease showed that mortality rate increased with worsening antenatal maternal functional class.[3] A more recent study found no mortality but described substantial morbidity from heart failure and arrhythmia.[4]

Pregnant women whose dominant lesion is rheumatic aortic stenosis have a similar outcome to those with congenital aortic stenosis. Severe aortic or mitral regurgitation is generally well tolerated during pregnancy although deterioration in maternal functional class has been observed.

Maternal cardiac status and risk of cardiac complications during pregnancy
Low risk
- Small left to right shunts
- Repaired lesions without residual cardiac dysfunction
- Isolated mitral valve prolapse without significant regurgitation
- Bicuspid aortic valve without stenosis
- Mild to moderate pulmonic stenosis
- Valvar regurgitation with normal ventricular systolic function

Intermediate risk
- Unrepaired or palliated cyanotic congenital heart disease
- Large left to right shunt
- Uncorrected coarctation of the aorta
- Mitral or aortic stenosis
- Mechanical prosthetic valves
- Severe pulmonic stenosis
- Moderate to severe systemic ventricular dysfunction
- History of peripartum cardiomyopathy with no residual ventricular dysfunction

High risk
- New York Heart Association (NYHA) class III or IV symptoms
- Severe pulmonary hypertension
- Marfan syndrome with aortic root or major valvar involvement
- Severe aortic stenosis
- History of peripartum cardiomyopathy with residual ventricular dysfunction

Peripartum cardiomyopathy
Peripartum cardiomyopathy is a form of idiopathic dilated cardiomyopathy diagnosed by otherwise unexplained left ventricular systolic dysfunction, confirmed echocardiographically, presenting during the last antepartum month or in the first five postpartum months.[21] It usually manifests as heart failure, although arrhythmias and embolic events also occur. Many affected women will show improvement in functional status and ventricular function postpartum, but others may have persistent or progressive dysfunction. The relapse rate during subsequent pregnancies is substantial in women with evidence of persisting cardiac enlargement or left ventricular dysfunction. It remains unclear whether pregnancy is safe in those with recovery of systolic function. Dobutamine stress echocardiography may have a role in evaluating contractile reserve in women with recovered systolic function who are contemplating further pregnancies, but there are, as yet, insufficient data to confirm the validity of this approach.

Management

Risk stratification and counselling
Risk stratification and counselling of women with heart disease is best accomplished before conception. The data required for risk stratifi-

cation can be acquired readily from a thorough cardiovascular history and examination, 12 lead ECG, and transthoracic echocardiogram. In patients with cyanosis, arterial oxygen saturation should be assessed by percutaneous oximetry. In counselling, the following six areas should be considered: the underlying cardiac lesion, maternal functional status, the possibility of further palliative or corrective surgery, additional associated risk factors, maternal life expectancy and ability to care for a child, and the risk of congenital heart disease in offspring.

Defining the *underlying cardiac lesion* is an important part of stratifying risk and determining management. The nature of residua and sequelae should be clarified, especially ventricular function, pulmonary pressure, severity of obstructive lesions, persistence of shunts, and presence of hypoxaemia. Almost all patients can be stratified into low, intermediate, or high risk groups. *Maternal functional status* is widely used as a predictor of outcome, and most often defined by New York Heart Association (NYHA) functional class. In a study of 482 pregnancies in women with congenital heart disease, cardiovascular morbidity was less (8% *v* 30%) and live birth rate higher (80% *v* 68%) in mothers with NYHA functional class I compared to the others.[1] We recently examined 276 pregnancies in 221 women and showed that poor functional status (NYHA > II) or cyanosis, myocardial dysfunction, left heart obstruction, prior arrhythmia, and prior cardiac events were independent predictors of maternal cardiac complications.[4] Poor maternal functional class or cyanosis was also predictive of adverse neonatal events.

Further palliative or corrective surgery. Both maternal and fetal outcomes are improved by surgery to correct cyanosis, which should be undertaken before conception when possible. Similarly, patients with symptomatic obstructive lesions should undergo intervention before pregnancy. A systematic overview of cardiovascular surgical outcomes during pregnancy reported a maternal and fetal mortality of 6% and 30%, respectively.[22] Valve replacement requires weighing the need for ongoing anticoagulation with a mechanical valve against the likelihood of early reoperation if a tissue valve is used. For aortic stenosis, an attractive alternative is the pulmonary autograft.

Additional associated risk factors that may complicate pregnancy include a history of arrhythmia or heart failure, prosthetic valves and conduits, anticoagulant treatment, and the use of teratogenic drugs such as warfarin or angiotensin converting enzyme inhibitors.

Maternal life expectancy and ability to care for her child. A patient with limited physical capacity or with a condition that may result in premature maternal death should be advised of her potential inability to look after her child. Women whose condition imparts a high likelihood of fetal complications, such as those with cyanosis or on anticoagulants, must be apprised of these added risks.

The *risk of recurrence of congenital heart disease in offspring* should be addressed in the context of a 0.4–0.6% risk in the general population.

The risk with a first degree relative affected increases about 10-fold. Left heart obstructive lesions have a higher recurrence rate. Certain conditions such as Marfan syndrome and the 22q11 deletion syndromes are autosomal dominant, conferring a 50% risk of recurrence in an offspring. Patients with congenital heart disease who reach reproductive age should be offered genetic counselling so that they are fully informed of the mode of inheritance and recurrence risk as well as the prenatal diagnosis options available to them. Preventive strategies to decrease the incidence of congenital defects such as preconception use of multivitamins containing folic acid can be discussed at the time of such counselling.[23]

Antepartum management
Pregnant women with heart disease may be at particular risk for one or more of congestive heart failure, arrhythmias, thrombosis, emboli, and adverse effects of anticoagulants.

When ventricular dysfunction is a concern, activity limitation is helpful and in severely affected women with NYHA class III or IV symptoms, hospital admission by mid second trimester may be advisable. Pregnancy induced hypertension, hyperthyroidism, infection, and anaemia should be identified early and treated vigorously. For patients with important mitral stenosis, the use of β blockers or digoxin for control of heart rate should be considered. We also offer empiric treatment with β blockers to patients with coarctation and to Marfan patients.

Arrhythmias
Arrhythmias in the form of premature atrial or ventricular beats are common in normal pregnancy, although sustained tachyarrhythmias have also been reported. In those with pre-existing arrhythmias, pregnancy may exacerbate their frequency or haemodynamic severity. Pharmacological treatment is usually reserved for patients with severe symptoms or when sustained episodes are poorly tolerated in the presence of ventricular hypertrophy, ventricular dysfunction, or valvar obstruction. Sustained tachyarrhythmias such as atrial flutter or atrial fibrillation should be treated promptly, avoiding teratogenic antiarrhythmic drugs. Digoxin and β blockers are antiarrhythmic drugs of choice in view of their known safety profiles.[24] Quinidine, adenosine, sotalol, and lidocaine are also "safe" but published data on their use during pregnancy is more limited. Amiodarone is more problematic and standard texts classify it as contraindicated in pregnancy; however, there are case reports describing successful use with careful follow up including assessment of neonatal thyroid function. Electrical cardioversion is safe in pregnancy. A recent report of 44 pregnancies in women with implantable cardioverter-defibrillators reported favourable maternal and fetal outcomes.[25]

Anticoagulation
When a pregnant woman with mechanical heart valve requires anticoagulation, heparin

and warfarin are used but controversy continues as to which is better at different stages of pregnancy. Oral anticoagulation with warfarin is better accepted by patients, and is effective. However, warfarin embryopathy may be produced during organogenesis, and fetal intracranial bleeding can occur throughout pregnancy. A recent study of 58 pregnancies reported that a daily warfarin dose of ≤ 5 mg was associated with no cases of embryopathy.[10] Fetal intracranial haemorrhage during vaginal delivery is a risk with warfarin unless it has been stopped at least two weeks before labour. Adjusted dose subcutaneous heparin has no teratogenic effects, as the drug does not cross the placenta, but may cause maternal thrombocytopenia and osteoporosis. Claims of inadequate effectiveness of heparin in patients with mechanical heart valves have been countered by arguments that inadequate doses were used. Recent practice guidelines have favoured use of warfarin and low dose aspirin either during the entire pregnancy or substituted by heparin only during the peak teratogenic period (sixth to 12th week of gestation).[6] Low molecular weight heparin is easier to administer and has been suggested as an alternative to adjusted dose unfractionated heparin.[26] Clinical trials examining the optimal anticoagulation strategy are needed.

Eisenmenger syndrome

If a woman with Eisenmenger syndrome does not accept counselling to terminate, or presents late in pregnancy, meticulous antepartum management is necessary including early hospitalisation, supplemental oxygen, and possibly empiric anticoagulation. There have been several case reports describing reduction of pulmonary pressure with the use of nitric oxide in pregnant patients. However, despite haemodynamic improvement, the maternal mortality in this small experience remained high.

Multidisciplinary approach and high risk pregnancy units

Women with heart disease who are at intermediate or high risk for complications should be managed in a high risk pregnancy unit by a multidisciplinary team from obstetrics, cardiology, anaesthesia, and paediatrics. When dealing with a complex problem the team should meet early in the pregnancy. At this time the nature of the cardiac lesion, anticipated effects of pregnancy, and potential problems are explored. Since it is often not possible for every member of the team to be at the patient's bedside at a moment of crisis, it is helpful to develop and distribute widely a written management plan for foreseeable contingencies. Women with heart disease in the "low risk" group can be managed in a community hospital setting. However, if there is doubt about the mother's status or the risk, consultation at a regional referral centre should be arranged.

Labour and delivery

Vaginal delivery is recommended with very few exceptions. The only cardiac indications for caesarean section are aortic dissection, Marfan

Management of pregnancy complicated by maternal heart disease

All patients
- Define the lesion, the residua, and the sequelae
- Assess functional status
- Determine predictors of risk
- Eliminate teratogens
- Arrange genetic counselling when relevant
- Consider consultation with a regional centre
- Assess need for endocarditis prophylaxis during labour and delivery

Intermediate and high risk patients
- Arrange management at a regional centre for high risk pregnancy
- Consider antepartum interventions to reduce pregnancy risk
- Engage a multidisciplinary team, as appropriate
- Consider a multidisciplinary case conference
- Develop and disseminate a management plan
- Anticipate vaginal delivery in almost all cases, unless there are obstetrical contraindications
- Consider early epidural anesthesia
- Modify labour and delivery to reduce cardiac work
- Plan postpartum monitoring, sometimes in a coronary or intensive care unit setting

syndrome with dilated aortic root, and failure to switch from warfarin to heparin at least two weeks before labour. Preterm induction is rarely indicated, but once fetal lung maturity is assured a planned induction and delivery in high risk situations will ensure availability of appropriate staff and equipment. Although there is no consensus on the use of invasive haemodynamic monitoring during labour and delivery, we commonly utilise intra-arterial monitoring (with or without concurrent pulmonary artery catheterisation) in cases where there are concerns about the interpretation and deleterious effects of a sudden drop in systemic blood pressure (such as in patients with severe aortic stenosis, pulmonary hypertension, or more than moderate systemic ventricular systolic dysfunction). Placement of an indwelling pulmonary artery catheter should be considered only when the information sought is not available otherwise and warrants the risk of the procedure, which may be significant especially in the setting of pulmonary hypertension.

Heparin anticoagulation is discontinued at least 12 hours before induction, or reversed with protamine if spontaneous labour develops, and can usually be resumed 6–12 hours postpartum.

Endocarditis prophylaxis is initiated at onset of active labour when indicated. The American Heart Association recommendations state that delivery by caesarean section and vaginal delivery in the absence of infection do not require

142

endocarditis prophylaxis except, perhaps, in patients at high risk. However, many centres with extensive experience in caring for pregnant women with heart disease utilise endocarditis prophylaxis routinely, as an uncomplicated delivery cannot always be anticipated.

Epidural anaesthesia with adequate volume preloading is the technique of choice. Epidural fentanyl is particularly advantageous in cyanotic patients with shunt lesions as it does not lower peripheral vascular resistance. In the presence of a shunt, air and particulate filters should be placed in all intravenous lines.

Labour is conducted in the left lateral decubitus position to attenuate haemodynamic fluctuations associated with contractions in the supine position. Forceps or vacuum extraction will shorten the latter part of the second stage of labour and reduce need for maternal expulsive efforts. As haemodynamics do not return to baseline for many days after delivery, those patients at intermediate or high risk may require monitoring for a minimum of 72 hours postpartum. Patients with Eisenmenger syndrome require longer close postpartum observation, since mortality risk persists for up to seven days.

1. **Whittemore R, Hobbins J, Engle M.** Pregnancy and its outcome in women with and without surgical treatment of congenital heart disease. *Am J Cardiol* 1982;**50**:641–51.
• *The first large study examining pregnancy outcomes in women with congenital heart disease. The relation between maternal functional class and cardiac risk during pregnancy was demonstrated in this study.*

2. **Shime J, Mocarski E, Hastings D,** et al. Congenital heart disease in pregnancy: short- and long-term implications. *Am J Obstet Gynecol* 1987;**156**:313–22.
• *This study, together with reference 1, provided much of the early risk stratification data on pregnancy outcomes in women with congenital heart disease.*

3. **McFaul P, Dornan J, Lamki H,** et al. Pregnancy complicated by maternal heart disease. A review of 519 women. *Br J Obstet Gynaecol* 1988;**95**:861–7.
• *Examining a patient population with predominantly rheumatic heart disease, this study observed a relation between maternal functional class and mortality risk during pregnancy.*

4. **Siu SC, Sermer M, Harrison DA,** et al. Risk and predictors for pregnancy-related complications in women with heart disease. *Circulation* 1997;**96**:2789–94.
• *This retrospective study assessed maternal and neonatal outcomes in a contemporary cohort of pregnant women with heart disease and developed a risk index which can be used to estimate the risk of cardiac complications during pregnancy.*

5. **Hunter S, Robson SC.** Adaptation of the maternal heart in pregnancy. *Br Heart J* 1992;**68**:540–3.

6. **Bonow RO, Carabello B, de Leon AC, Jr,** et al. Guidelines for the management of patients with valvular heart disease: executive summary. A report of the American College of Cardiology/American Heart Association task force on practice guidelines (committee on management of patients with valvular heart disease). *Circulation* 1998;**98**:1949–84.
• *Recently published recommendations on the risk stratification and treatment of pregnant women with valvar heart lesions.*

7. **Lao T, Sermer M, MaGee L,** et al. Congenital aortic stenosis and pregnancy–a reappraisal. *Am J Obstet Gynecol* 1993;**169**:540–5.

8. **North RA, Sadler L, Stewart AW,** et al. Long-term survival and valve-related complications in young women with cardiac valve replacements. *Circulation* 1999;**99**:2669–76.

9. **Dore A, Somerville J.** Pregnancy in patients with pulmonary autograft valve replacement. *Eur Heart J* 1997;**18**:1659–62.

10. **Vitale N, De Feo M, De Santo LS,** et al. Dose-dependent fetal complications of warfarin in pregnant women with mechanical heart valves. *J Am Coll Cardiol* 1999;**33**:1637–41.

11. **Deal K, Wooley CF.** Coarctation of the aorta and pregnancy. *Ann Intern Med* 1973;**78**:706–10.

12. **Connolly H, Ammash N, Warnes C.** Pregnancy in women with coarctation of the aorta [abstract]. *J Am Coll Cardiol* 1996;**27**:43A.

13. **Presbitero P, Somerville J, Stone S,** et al. Pregnancy in cyanotic congenital heart disease. Outcome of mother and fetus. *Circulation* 1994;**89**:2673–6.
• *The largest case series to date examining the pregnancy outcomes of cyanotic women without pulmonary hypertension.*

14. **Genoni M, Jenni R, Hoerstrup SP,** et al. Pregnancy after atrial repair for transposition of the great arteries. *Heart* 1999;**81**:276–7.

15. **Canobbio M, Mair D, van der Velde M,** et al. Pregnancy outcomes after the Fontan repair. *J Am Coll Cardiol* 1996;**28**:763–7.

16. **Rossiter J, Repke J, Morales A,** et al. A prospective longitudinal evaluation of pregnancy in the Marfan syndrome. *Am J Obstet Gynecol* 1995;**173**:1599–606.

17. **Connolly HM, Grogan M, Warnes CA.** Pregnancy among women with congenitally corrected transposition of great arteries. *J Am Coll Cardiol* 1999;**33**:1692–5.

18. **Therrien J, Barnes I, Somerville J.** Outcome of pregnancy in patients with congenitally corrected transposition of the great arteries. *Am J Cardiol* 1999;**84**:820–4.

19. **Gleicher N, Midwall J, Hochberger D,** et al. Eisenmenger's syndrome and pregnancy. *Obstet Gynecol Surv* 1979;**34**:721–41.

20. **Weiss B, Zemp L, Seifert B,** et al. Outcome of pulmonary vascular disease in pregnancy: a systematic overview from 1978 through 1996. *J Am Coll Cardiol* 1998;**31**:1650–7.
• *A comprehensive overview of pregnancy outcomes in women with pulmonary hypertension.*

21. **Pearson GD, Veille JC, Rahimtoola S,** et al. Peripartum cardiomyopathy: National Heart, Lung, and Blood Institute and Office of Rare Diseases (National Institutes of Health) workshop recommendations and review. *JAMA* 2000;**283**:1183–8.
• *A comprehensive overview on the current state of the art knowledge in this area.*

22. **Weiss BM, von Segesser LK, Alon E,** et al. Outcome of cardiovascular surgery and pregnancy: a systematic review of the period 1984-1996. *Am J Obstet Gynecol* 1998;**179**:1643–53.

23. **Czeizel A.** Reduction of urinary tract and cardiovascular defects by periconceptional multivitamin supplementation. *Am J Med Genet* 1996;**62**:179–83.

24. **Chow T, Galvin J, McGovern B.** Antiarrhythmic drug therapy in pregnancy and lactation. *Am J Cardiol* 1998;**82**:58I–62I.
• *A comprehensive overview of the use of antiarrhythmic agents during pregnancy.*

25. **Natale A, Davidson T, Geiger M,** et al. Implantable cardioverter-defibrillators and pregnancy: a safe combination? *Circulation* 1997;**96**:2808–12.

26. **Ginsberg JS, Hirsh J.** Use of antithrombotic agents during pregnancy. *Chest* 1998;**114**:524S–30S.
• *Practice guidelines that incorporate the conflicting opinions and data regarding the choice of anticoagulation regimen during pregnancy.*

website extra

Additional references appear on the Heart website

www.heartjnl.com

21 Dizziness and syncope in adolescence

Karen A McLeod

Classification of syncope in adolescence

- Neurally mediated syncopes
  - reflex syncopes
  - postural orthostatic tachycardia syndrome (POTS)
  - pure autonomic failure
  - multiple system atrophy

- Cardiovascular causes
  - arrhythmic
  - structural
  - vascular

- Noncardiovascular
  - epileptic
  - psychogenic

"The only difference between syncope and sudden death is that in syncope you wake up"—*G L Engels*[1]

Syncope is a common problem in adolescence, with up to one in five experiencing an episode of syncope before adulthood.[2] Whereas the vast majority of syncope is benign, a minority is caused by something potentially more serious or even life threatening. For this reason and also because syncope has such a death-like quality, it often generates extreme anxiety and is often extensively, inappropriately, and unfruitfully investigated.

Classification

There are many causes of syncope and therefore it can be helpful to categorise them. One way of categorising syncope is to divide the causes into three main groups.[2] Neurally mediated syncopes occur when there is a disturbance in the autonomic nervous system's control of heart rate and blood pressure. Generally they can be considered as benign. Cardiovascular causes of syncope are rare in adolescence, but it is important to be aware of them, as they are potential causes of sudden death. Non-cardiovascular syncopes can broadly be divided into the epilepsies and the psychogenic causes. In the latter the child actually fakes the syncope. It is beyond the scope of this article to discuss all the causes of syncope and the aim will be to concentrate on the most common form of syncope, the neurally mediated syncopes.

Neurally mediated syncopes

Although neurally mediated syncope can occur at any age in childhood, the peak age groups are in toddlers and in adolescents. Neurally mediated syncopes are a heterogeneous group of autonomic disorders, which result in orthostatic intolerance. Grubb suggests dividing them into four main groups: the reflex syncopes, postural orthostatic tachycardia syndrome, pure autonomic failure. and multiple system atrophy.[3]

Neurocardiogenic syncope is a form of reflex syncope and also the most common type of syncope in adolescence. A typical history is of syncope that occurs when the child is upright, either sitting or standing. Characteristically the child will experience a prodrome such as dizziness, nausea and pallor, before loss of tone and consciousness. It is important to remember that following loss of consciousness there may be a period of retrograde amnesia and, despite a prodrome, the child might claim "I went straight down without warning". Depending on the duration and severity of cerebral hypoxia secondary to hypotension or profound bradycardia, or both, the child may have an anoxic seizure and may be incontinent. An anoxic seizure is often mistaken for an epileptic seizure but in reality is quite different. During an anoxic seizure the electroencephalogram (EEG) is flat and rather than tonic-clonic movements, there tends to be stiffening, opisthotonos, and fine twitching.[4] On recovery the child will often complain of feeling tired and "washed out" for some time afterwards.

The mechanism of neurocardiogenic syncope is not entirely understood. It has been proposed that in response to being in the upright position, there is peripheral pooling of blood.[2] This results in reduced venous return and an empty heart. The empty heart contracts overvigorously, stimulating so called "C fibres". The brain interprets this as *hyper*tension, resulting in sympathetic withdrawal. There is initially pallor, sweating, often with hyperventilation and tachycardia, followed by relative bradycardia, hypotension, and loss of consciousness.

A type of reflex syncope that has only been recognised relatively recently is cerebral vasoconstrictive syncope.[5] In this condition syncope occurs as a result of cerebral vasoconstriction in the absence of hypotension and bradycardia. The diagnosis is made by showing that cerebral vasoconstriction occurs during symptoms. This can be done by measuring cerebral blood flow with techniques such as transcranial Doppler or near infrared cerebral spectrophotometry.[3 5] Cerebral vasoconstrictive syncope is probably uncommon in adolescence, but probably also underdiagnosed. As blood pressure and heart rate are not significantly altered during symptoms, it can be mistaken for psychogenic pseudosyncope. This mistake can usually be avoided by recording an EEG or measuring cerebral blood flow during tilt testing in individuals who have symptoms despite normal blood pressure and heart rate.

Diagnosis of syncope—history, history, history!

- Eye witness?

- Onset and frequency?

- Circumstances: relation to exercise? posture? precipitating factor?

- Prodrome: dizziness? nausea? pallor? aura?

- Altered consciousness: complete loss? partial impairment? duration?

- Abnormal movements: tonic-clonic? anoxic? fine repetitive?

- Incontinence, injury?

- Recovery: tired? "washed out"? post-ictal? rapid return to normal?

- Family history: fits? faints? sudden death in young person?

Syncope "warning bells"

- Syncope in response to loud noise, fright or extreme emotional stress

- Syncope during exercise

- Syncope while supine

- Syncope associated with tonic clonic or abnormal movements

- Family history of sudden death in young person < 30 years old

- Syncope with an "odd" history

Postural orthostatic tachycardia syndrome (POTS) probably is a heterogeneous group of conditions.[3] Although not common in adolescence, it is almost certainly underdiagnosed. POTS is defined as an excessive tachycardia, either a rise of > 30 beats per minute (bpm) or an increase to > 120 bpm, in response to being upright.[6] In some, the heart rate may be persistently greater than 160 bpm. Symptoms include fatigue, dizziness, and exercise intolerance.[7] POTS is probably a mild form of chronic autonomic failure, such that there is failure of the peripheral vasculature to vasoconstrict adequately in response to upright posture. This results in a compensatory tachycardia. There is a danger of misdiagnosing POTS as inappropriate sinus tachycardia. Radiofrequency modification of the sinus node will usually make symptoms worse.

Pure autonomic failure and multiple system atrophy are very rare in adolescence and are accompanied by other signs of autonomic failure, including loss of sweating, thermoregulatory problems, and bladder and bowel dysfunction.

Diagnosis of syncope

History, history, history!

The key to the diagnosis of syncope is to take a careful and detailed history. If a good history is taken, the physician will obtain a very good idea which of the three categories the syncope is likely to fall into. It is important be on the alert for any "warning bells" from the history that would point towards a potentially more serious or life threatening cause of syncope. Neurally mediated syncope can occur before or following exercise, but syncope that occurs during exercise raises the possibility of a cardiac structural or arrhythmic cause of syncope. Syncope that occurs secondary to a loud noise, fright or extreme emotional stress raises the possibility of the long QT syndrome. Syncope that occurs when supine is of concern as this would be very unusual for neurally mediated syncope. A family history of sudden death in a young person raises the possibility of a hereditary cardiovascular cause such as long QT syndrome or hypertrophic cardiomyopathy. Tonic-clonic or fine repetitive movements suggest a possible epileptic cause. One caveat is that in some susceptible individuals, an anoxic seizure can result in a secondary epileptic seizure, leading to an incorrect diagnosis of primary epilepsy.[8] A careful history should help prevent this mistake.

Investigation of recurrent syncope

Investigations for syncope in adolescents will almost always be normal. The most important investigation is a 12 lead ECG, primarily to exclude a long QT interval. Pre-excitation, heart block or ventricular hypertrophy can also be diagnosed from an ECG. If symptoms are related to exercise, an exercise test should be performed in the hope of inducing symptoms. In reality, they rarely occur during the test. Holter monitoring is usually unhelpful, as symptoms almost never occur in the 24–48 hour period while the monitor is worn. This also tends to be true for cardiac event monitoring. Unless the child has other cardiac signs or symptoms, or any of the warning bells from the history, an echo will almost certainly be normal. Although an EEG is often performed on children with syncope to "exclude epilepsy", this is rarely helpful for even in children with epilepsy the EEG will usually be normal between attacks. Intracerebral causes of syncope are very rare in childhood and would usually be associated with other neurological signs or symptoms; thus magnetic resonance imaging (MRI) or computed tomographic (CT) scan is usually an expensive waste of time.

It is our practise to perform a 12 lead ECG in all adolescents referred with recurrent syncope. If there are any of the "warning bells" from the history or if there are any other cardiac or neurological signs or symptoms, appropriate cardiac or neurological investigations are undertaken. If there is a good history for neurally mediated syncope and the ECG is normal, usually no further investigation is required. For those who have very severe or frequent attacks, who are in need of reassurance or where the history is not entirely clear, tilt testing is probably the most productive investigation.[9] Unfortunately there is no standardised protocol for tilt testing in either children or adults, and protocols vary in terms of duration of tilt, degree of tilt, and whether or not drugs, including isoprenaline or glyceryl trinitrate, are given.[10] The specificity or sensitivity of any given protocol will therefore vary. Our own protocol at The Royal Hospital for Sick Children in Glasgow is very simple and tolerated by most children, as it does not involve any intravenous cannulae or drugs. We rest the child supine for 15 minutes. The child is then tilted to 60° head-up for a maximum of 45 minutes. During this time the blood pressure is continuously but non-invasively monitored using the Finapres system, and a three lead ECG continuously recorded. We always warn the children (and those supervising) that the test is likely to be one of the most boring things they have ever done! Using this protocol, approximately 50% of children with a good history for neurally mediated syncope will have a positive tilt test. The use of drugs increases the sensitivity of the test but reduces its specificity and makes the test more unpleasant for the child. Whatever tilt test protocol is chosen it seems important to have a period of supine rest before tilting, to tilt to between 60–80° to reduce false positive and negative responses, and to tilt for at least 40 minutes of drug-free period.

The most common positive tilt test response is a combination of hypotension and bradycardia before syncope. Hypotension with no significant change in heart rate is the next most common positive response. The least common positive response is asystole before syncope.

In children with suspected psychogenic pseudosyncope it is important to include EEG monitoring or measurement of cerebral blood flow during tilt in order not to miss the diagnosis of cerebral vasoconstrictive syncope. In situations where it is claimed that syncope is occurring several times a day every day, admission to hospital for observation with continuous ambulatory ECG and EEG monitoring is usually the best approach. With this history the ECG, EEG, and measured blood pressure will almost always be normal during the "syncopes" and a diagnosis of psychogenic pseudosyncope can be confirmed.

In situations where the distinction between neurally mediated syncope and potentially serious arrhythmia remains unclear—for example, in a child with a borderline QT interval or slightly worrying history—our approach is now to implant a Reveal monitor (Medtronic Inc, USA). The monitors are extremely easy and quick to implant. Most adolescents find them considerably more acceptable than the non-invasive monitors in that they are less conspicuous and do not restrict activities. The manufacturer recommends that the monitors be implanted in the left parasternal region to reduce artefact from muscle activity. We have found that a pocket made medial to the left

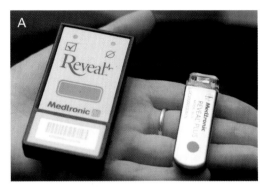

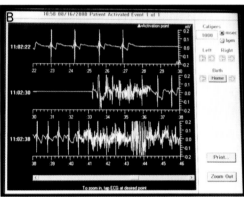

Figure 21.1. The Reveal Plus monitor (A) is easy to implant and tends to be more acceptable to adolescents than the more traditional non-invasive cardiac event monitors. The Reveal Plus can be activated using an external activator or programmed to recognise and record significant bradycardias, tachycardias or pauses. The quality of ECG recording is usually very good (B). Although there may be some artefact from muscle activity, it is rarely sufficient to affect ECG interpretation.

axilla is better cosmetically, and although there can be some artefact on the ECG from muscle activity, we have not found this to be enough to impair ECG interpretation (fig 21.1). The new Reveal Plus monitors have automatic functions and can be programmed to recognise and record significant pauses, bradycardias, and tachycardias even if the patient does not activate the monitor with the external activator. This is a distinct advantage in the adolescent population where there are the inevitable excuses of forgetting the activator or forgetting to use it to record an event.

Management of neurally mediated syncope

The mainstay of treatment is reassurance, specifically that the episodes are not caused by epilepsy or a cardiac problem.[11] Advice should be given to drink plenty (with the exception of caffeine containing drinks as they tend to dehydrate) such that the urine always looks clear. Many families now restrict the amount of salt in the diet because of concerns about future hypertension. We advise an increase in dietary salt to what might be termed a "normal" salt diet. Advice on posture when prodromal symptoms are experienced can be helpful. Manoeuvres such as crossing the legs and folding the arms especially when standing help to maintain blood pressure. Often with the

146

Management of neurally mediated syncope

- Reassurance
- Fluid, posture, salt
- Drugs: fludrocortisone, β blocker, others
- Biofeedback techniques
- Pacemaker

above simple measures of reassurance, fluid, posture and salt, symptoms will improve significantly.

The likelihood of further syncopal attacks depends on the number of episodes of syncope before presentation.[12] For those who present with frequent syncope or continue to have syncope despite the above simple measures, drug treatment should be considered. There are many pharmacological agents available, which no doubt testifies to our lack of understanding of the mechanisms of neurally mediated syncope and probably also reflects a likely placebo effect of drugs. No drug has been adequately evaluated by randomised clinical trials, but fludrocortisone and β blockers are the most favoured first line drugs, with relatively few side effects.[13] My own preference is for fludrocortisone at a dosage of 100 μg daily in the first instance. This seems to be effective in most adolescents in reducing frequency and severity of syncope. Occasionally the drug is not tolerated because of problems of fluid retention and weight gain. If symptoms continue despite fludrocortisone, then the addition of a β blocker can be helpful. Serotonin reuptake inhibitors such as fluoxetine hydrochloride and vasoconstrictors such as midodrine are currently under clinical review. Initial studies suggest they might prove beneficial for some forms of neurally mediated syncope, but the use and safety of the drugs in children has not been established. It would be wise, therefore, to reserve them for those who continue to have symptoms despite first line treatments. Serotonin reuptake inhibitors are thought to act by inhibiting sympathetic neural outflow and reducing susceptibility to certain neurally mediated events.[14] Midodrine is an α_1 agonist which causes peripheral vasoconstriction but with minimal cardiac and neurological effects.[15]

An alternative or adjunct to drugs is biofeedback therapy. Techniques include tilt training and active tension.[16] The latter is best undertaken with the help and supervision of a clinical psychologist.

Cardiac pacing

The use of cardiac pacing for neurocardiogenic syncope remains controversial. The rationale is that pacing should eliminate any contribution of bradycardia to the hypotension that results in syncope. There is little direct evidence, however, that significant bradycardia commonly occurs in spontaneous neurocardiogenic syncope even if it is demonstrated during tilt testing. Pacing would not be expected to affect to any great degree hypotension caused by vasodilation .

An excellent review examining the role of pacing in the treatment of neurocardiogenic syncope is provided by Sheldon.[17] In his summary of clinical studies evaluating the role of permanent pacing for neurocardiogenic syncope, all studies showed a benefit from pacing but only one study successfully addressed the issue of placebo.

The recently published North American vasovagal pacemaker study tested whether dual chamber pacing would reduce frequency of neurocardiogenic syncope.[18] Patients were randomised to pacing or to medical treatment. Pacing did reduce recurrence of syncope by 91% compared with medical treatment, but the important issue of placebo was not addressed.

The only completed study to date that has successfully addressed the problem of placebo was a three way, double blind, randomised, crossover study of dual chamber pacing in 12 children.[19] The children had frequent, severe neurocardiogenic syncopes and a demonstrated asystole of > 4 seconds during a typical attack. The pacemakers were programmed to no pacing, ventricular pacing with hysteresis, and dual chamber pacing with the rate drop algorithm. Each treatment arm lasted four months. Both ventricular pacing and dual chamber pacing with rate drop algorithm were equally effective in preventing syncope, but dual chamber pacing with the rate drop algorithm was more effective in preventing pre-syncope.[20]

It would appear that pacing can be a very effective treatment for children who have severe neurocardiogenic syncope and who have a demonstrated asystole during a typical episode. The question remains as to whether pacing would be effective for the majority of children who have neurocardiogenic syncope but who do not demonstrate prolonged asystole during an event. The vasovagal pacemaker study II might help to answer this question. This study will evaluate adult patients who have had six or more syncopal episodes and who have a positive tilt test with or without bradycardia. All patients will receive a pacemaker and will be randomised to either pacing with the rate drop algorithm, pacing with an escape rate of 45 bpm, or to no pacing. It is expected that the study will be completed by the year 2002.

As cardiac pacing is a significant commitment in a young person it should be reserved for those who have severe, frequent attacks and in whom drug treatment has failed or is declined. Although ventricular pacing with hysteresis should suffice for the younger child, for adolescents who are likely to be more aware of and distressed by symptoms of presyncope, a dual chamber pacemaker with the rate drop algorithm is recommended. Until the question is answered as to whether patients with neurocardiogenic syncope but without demonstrable asystole will benefit from pacing, it seems sen-

Syncope in adolescence: key points

- Common

- Usually benign

- Most common cause is neurally mediated syncope

- Diagnosis primarily from history

- 12 lead ECG is most important investigation

- Investigations usually normal

- Mainstay of treatment for neurally mediated syncope is reassurance

- BEWARE OF "WARNING BELLS" FROM HISTORY

sible to reserve pacing for children who have a recorded asystole or profound bradycardia during a typical attack. It is now our practise to implant a Reveal Plus monitor in any young person with frequent neurally mediated syncope in whom we are considering a pacemaker. The Reveal allows us to determine accurately both the frequency of events and whether asystole or profound bradycardia occurs during a spontaneous syncope. It has been our experience that implantation of the Reveal can have an astonishingly curative effect. Perhaps it works as a placebo or perhaps the awareness of the monitor and activator works as a form of biofeedback. Certainly we been impressed enough to wonder whether the manufacturer should recommend it as a treatment for neurocardiogenic syncope!

1. **Engel GL.** Psychological stress, vasodepressor syncope and sudden death. *Ann Intern Med* 1978;**89**:403–12.

2. **Ross B, Grubb B.** Syncope in the child and adolescent. In: Grubb B, Oshlansky B, eds. *Syncope: mechanisms and management*, New York: Futura, 1998:305–16.
• *This book is well worth reading for anyone interested in syncope. It includes a well written chapter that summarises the mechanisms and management of syncope in the paediatric and adolescent population.*

3. **Grubb BP, Karas B.** Clinical disorders of the autonomic nervous system associated with orthostatic intolerance: an overview of classification, clinical evaluation, and management. *PACE* 1999;**22**:789–810.
• *A helpful overview of the classification, evaluation, and management of neurally mediated syncope and related disorders. It includes discussion on postural orthostatic tachycardia (POTS) and cerebral vasoconstrictive syncope.*

4. **Stephenson J, McLeod K.** Reflex anoxic seizures. In: David TJ, ed. *Recent advances in paediatrics*. Edinburgh: Churchill Livingstone, 2000:1–19.
• *This chapter provides a detailed overview of the pathophysiology, diagnosis, and management of reflex anoxic syncope in childhood.*

5. **Grubb B.** Cerebral syncope: new insights into an emerging entity. *J Pediatr* 2000;**136**:431–2.

6. **Grubb BP.** Pathophysiology and differential diagnosis of neurocardiogenic syncope. *Am J Cardiol* 1999;**84**:3Q–9Q.
• *It is increasingly recognised that neurally mediated syncope is a heterogeneous group of disorders. This excellent overview provides a new classification of the disorders together with a discussion of the pathophysiology and diagnosis.*

7. **Karas B, Grubb BP, Boehm K,** *et al.* The postural orthostatic tachycardia syndrome: a potentially treatable cause of chronic fatigue, exercise intolerance, and cognitive impairment in adolescents. *Pacing Clin Electrophysiol* 2000;**23**:344–51.

8. **Stephenson JBP.** Nonepileptic seizures, anoxic-epileptic seizures and epileptic-anoxic seizures. In: Wallace S, ed. *Epilepsy in children*. London: Chapman and Hall, 1996:5–26.

9. **Sutton R, Bloomfield D.** Indications, methodology, and classification of tilt table testing. *Am J Cardiol* 1999;**84**:10Q–19Q.

10. **Kenny RA, O'Shea D, Parry SW.** The Newcastle protocols for head-up tilt table testing in the diagnosis of vasovagal syncope and related disorders. *Heart* 2000;**83**:564–9.
• *Wide variation in tilt test protocols affects sensitivity, specificity, and reproducibility. The authors suggest a practical and standardised approach to tilt testing, based on their considerable experience.*

11. **Bloomfield DM, Sheldon R, Grubb BP,** *et al.* Putting it together: a new treatment algorithm for vasovagal syncope and related disorders. *Am J Cardiol* 1999;**84**:33Q–39Q.
• *A comprehensive algorithm is given to help guide the diagnosis and subsequent management of patients with neurally mediated syncope.*

12. **Grimm W, Degenhardt M, Hoffman J,** *et al.* Syncope recurrence can be better predicted by history than by head-up tilt testing in untreated patients with suspected neurocardiogenic syncope. *Eur Heart J* 1997;**18**:1465–9.

13. **Benditt D, Fahy G, Lurie K,** *et al.* Pharmacotherapy of neurocardiogenic syncope. *Circulation* 1999;**100**:1242–8.
• *This paper gives an excellent overview of the use of drugs in the management of neurally mediated syncope. It includes discussion of relatively new agents such as serotonin reuptake inhibitors and midodrine.*

14. **Di Girolamo E, Di Iorio C, Sabatini P,** *et al.* Effects of paroxetine hydrochloride, a selective serotonin reuptake inhibitor, on refractory vasovagal syncope: a randomized double-blind, placebo-controlled study. *J Am Coll Cardiol* 1999;**33**:1227–30.

15. **Ward C, Gray J, Gilroy J,** *et al.* Midodrine: a role in the management of neurocardiogenic syncope. *Heart* 1998;**79**:45–9.

16. **Reybrouck T, Heidbuchel H, Van de Werf F,** *et al.* Tilt training: a treatment for malignant and recurrent neurocardiogenic syncope. *Pacing Clin Electrophysiol* 2000;**23**:493–8.

17. **Sheldon R.** Role of pacing in the treatment of vasovagal syncope. *Am J Cardiol* 1999;**84**:26Q–32Q.
• *An excellent and comprehensive review of clinical studies evaluating the efficacy of pacing for vasovagal syncope.*

18. **Connolly SJ, Sheldon RS, Roberts RS,** *et al.* The North American vasovagal pacemaker study: a randomized trial of permanent cardiac pacing for the prevention of vasovagal syncope. *J Am Coll Cardiol* 1999;**33**:16–20.
• *The paper publishes the findings of the North American vasovagal pacemaker study. Patients were randomised to pacing with the rate drop algorithm or to medical treatment. Pacing reduced recurrence of syncope by 91% compared with medical treatment but the issue of placebo was not addressed.*

19. **McLeod K, Wilson N, Hewitt J,** *et al.* Double-blind trial of cardiac pacing for severe childhood neurally mediated syncope with reflex anoxic seizures. *Heart* 1999;**82**:721–6.
• *This study was a three way, double blind, randomised, crossover study of dual chamber pacing in 12 children with frequent, severe neurocardiogenic syncope and demonstrated asystole (median age 2.9 years). The pacemakers were programmed to no pacing, ventricular pacing with hysteresis, and dual chamber pacing with the rate drop algorithm for four month periods. Ventricular pacing and dual chamber pacing were equally effective in preventing syncope but dual chamber pacing was more effective in preventing presyncope.*

20. **Gammage MD.** Rate-drop response programming. *PACE* 1997;**20**:841–3.

147

SECTION VII: IMAGING TECHNIQUES

22 Cardiovascular magnetic resonance

Dudley Pennell

Cardiovascular magnetic resonance (CMR) is a new field in cardiology. CMR has enormous potential because of its major attributes of high image quality and resolution combined with non-ionising radiation and versatility. With recent major technological advances there has been a quantum leap in acquisition speed and image quality that makes its use in ischaemic heart disease robust and clinically valuable. This review will focus on the current clinical indications for CMR, starting with those that are well established, and moving on to the developing indications that are expected to reach clinical maturity soon; finally, the less advanced uses of CMR will be briefly summarised.

> ## Fundamentals of cardiovascular magnetic resonance

What is magnetic resonance?

Magnetic resonance (MR) is a fundamental property of some elements which contain an uneven number of nucleons (protons plus neutrons in the nucleus), and was first described in 1946. These atoms have a property known as net spin, and they absorb radio waves at a resonant frequency which is linearly related to the ambient magnetic field. Nearly all CMR is currently performed at the resonant frequency of hydrogen (63 MHz at 1.5 Tesla) because it is abundant and yields high signal. However, other nuclei can also be interrogated: phosphorus-31, carbon-13, sodium-23, potassium-39, and fluorine-19. These nuclei give lower signal and usually are only examined using MR spectroscopy, a technique which shows the spectrum of the radio signal. Important results in cardiology have been shown using P-31 MR spectroscopy.[1]

For clinical MR, a process of image acquisition occurs which has some parallel with echocardiography. Energy is transmitted into the heart (radio waves), and after a delay an echo (radio waves) is received. In the intervening period, the hydrogen nucleus becomes excited, and subsequently relaxes. The rate of relaxation is defined by two parameters known as T1 and T2, and these can be manipulated to give varying contrast allowing tissue characterisation. Many other parameters also affect the signal, such as temperature and oxygen concentration and flow, and these therefore can also be measured using MR. Transmission and reception of the radio waves is achieved using special aerials known as coils. Conversion of the raw data into images requires fast computers and Fourier transformation.

What is cardiovascular magnetic resonance?

There are essentially three types of imaging sequence which are used in the cardiovascular system:

- *spin echo imaging*—the blood is black and good quality anatomical imaging can be obtained;
- *gradient echo imaging*—the blood is white and high quality cine imaging can be obtained, which is used to identify regional myocardial function and abnormal flow patterns;
- *velocity mapping*—a variant of gradient echo imaging that in its usual form behaves like two dimensional Doppler, but unlike Doppler it can measure flow directly and can be extended into seven dimensional flow imaging for complex flow dynamics problems.[2]

CMR therefore consists of applications of these sequences and their variants, which allows determination of cardiac physiology, anatomy, metabolism, tissue characterisation, and vascular angiography

What is different about CMR compared with normal MR?

A CMR scanner is a large superconducting magnet with its associated radio wave and computer systems. For dedicated CMR, the environment typically also incorporates medical gases, full invasive and non-invasive physiological monitoring telemetry, stress infusion pumps for adenosine and dobutamine, a power injector for contrast studies, and full resuscitation equipment and drugs. Experience has shown that acutely ill and anaesthetised patients can be safely managed within the magnet in experienced centres. State of the art CMR systems are differentiating from standard MR systems in much the same way as echocardiography systems have become specialised compared with general ultrasound systems used for obstetrics and gynaecology, for example. Modern CMR scanners incorporate ultrafast technology which allows real time imaging (up to 50 frames per second ungated), and ultrafast applications for coronary artery disease. Currently most scans are still gated to the ECG, and in some cases also to the respiratory cycle using advanced MR diaphragm monitoring techniques called navigators.

Safety of CMR

CMR is safe, and this marks it out from *x* ray based techniques. MR contrast agents are not nephrotoxic and are much safer than the *x* ray agents. It is safe to scan all prosthetic heart valves, and patients with sternal wires, joint replacements, and retained epicardial pacing leads. There is abundant evidence that stents are safe to scan any time after insertion.[3] Pacemakers are problematic, although recent experience at 0.5 Tesla is encouraging, but this should only be considered in centres of specialist experience. Other implantable devices including defibrillators and cerebrovascular aneurysm clips are currently a contraindication to CMR. Claustrophobia occurs in about 4% of patients but this frequently responds to low dose diazepam, to leave a hard core of refusing patients of approximately 1%.[4]

Current established clinical indications

AORTA

As a large conduit, the aorta is easily investigated by CMR for its entire length in the thorax. Three point plane definition techniques are useful for imaging in the long axis of the aorta as it curves out of the coronal and sagittal planes. Typically, points are taken in the ascending and descending limbs and the arch to achieve this. The hockey stick view so obtained is ideal for showing the extent of dissections and the location of coarctation. Closer interrogation of specific regions can also be made with the orthogonal planes. CMR has been shown in *randomised* trials to be more accurate than transoesophageal echocardiography (TOE) and computed tomography in acute dissection,[5] although rapid access to echocardiography is simpler to organise in most hospitals. CMR is preferred for chronic follow up of these patients, in order to exclude aneurysm formation at the margins of the operation site, and other complications. In coarctation, the location of stenosis frequently makes Doppler problematic, and CMR is ideal in answering clinical issues, as well as being cost effective (fig 22.1).[6] CMR can also demonstrate the net flow in collaterals as an index of stenosis severity.

CONGENITAL HEART DISEASE

Echocardiography is excellent in defining congenital disease in the young, but with growth into adulthood and after corrective surgery, CMR plays a larger role and is often complementary to TOE. Studies show that TOE is better at defining fine structure such as valve morphology, whereas CMR is better at showing flow, conduits, and great vessel anatomy.[7] In centres with expertise in both techniques, invasive catheterisation has greatly reduced in frequency, being required mainly for pressure measurements.

ANGIOGRAPHY

For angiography of all vessels (arterial and venous) other than the coronary tree, CMR is rapidly becoming the clinical test of choice (fig 22.2). MR angiography is fast, simple, and safe, requiring only a peripheral intravenous injection of paramagnetic gadolinium contrast agent without catheterisation, and 4–20 seconds of three dimensional acquisition, according to scanner capability. The data can be displayed in a three dimensional rotating cine, and on the latest scanners, such cines can also be time resolved (four dimensional angiography). This has proved useful for the pulmonary arteries. Major application has been shown for the aorta, renal, and leg arteries,[8] but the technique is not limited to these areas. Recently thrombus imaging with CMR has been shown

to be very sensitive in the venous system,[9] and comparisons with established techniques for detection of deep vein thrombosis and pulmonary embolism are under way.

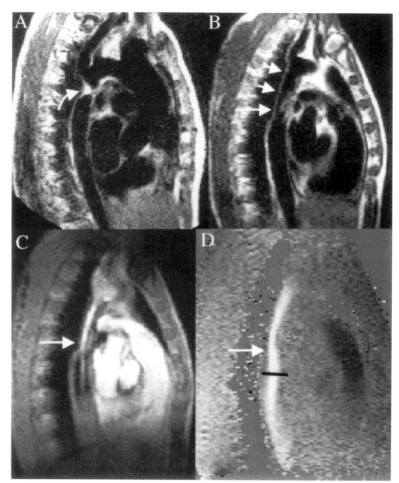

Figure 22.1. CMR in a patient with coarctation. (A) The preoperative spin echo image in an oblique sagittal plane shows the entire thoracic length of the aorta, and the coarctation (curved arrow) just distal to an enlarged left subclavian artery. (B) Appearance of the same region with spin echo imaging some years after repair of the coarctation site with a Dacron graft (short arrows). There is narrowing of the distal end of the graft and this is clearly seen in C with the systolic frame of the gradient echo cine showing bright signal within the graft from increased velocities and flow enhancement. Immediately distal to the graft narrowing (straight arrow) a bright jet is seen exiting into the normal descending aorta surrounded by dark areas which are caused by signal loss from turbulence. The velocity map D, from exactly the same plane as C, shows intense white colouration and a peak velocity measured at 3 m/s (36 mm Hg pressure gradient).

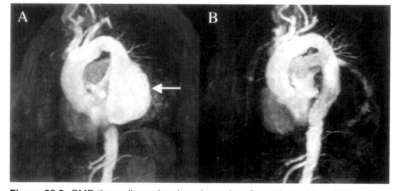

Figure 22.2. CMR three dimensional angiography of a patient with a descending aortic aneurysm (arrow) before (A), and after (B) insertion of a covered stent. The technique involves a peripheral injection of gadolinium contrast agent and data acquisition for eight seconds. Each of the images shown is one from a three dimensional data set which can be rotated to appreciate fully the anatomy, and plan the length and size of stent for this procedure. Reproduced from Stables et al, Circulation 2000;101:1888–9, with permission of the publisher.

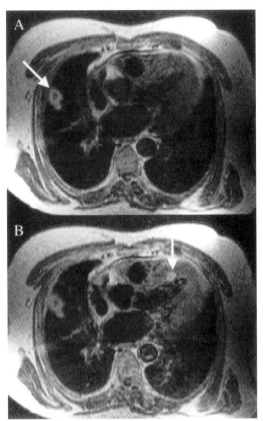

Figure 22.3. CMR before (A) and after (B) gadolinium enhancement in a patient with an abnormal chest *x* ray, and symptomatic ventricular premature beats. After gadolinium a clear enhancing lesion is seen in the subendocardium of the apical septum (vertical arrow). This was a metastatic chondrosarcoma from a chest primary (angled arrow).

MASSES AND TUMOURS
CMR is ideal for defining the size, extent, and relations of masses to surrounding tissues because of the high quality of the three dimensional imaging.[10] There are two other techniques which make CMR useful for assessment of cardiac masses, namely tissue characterisation and the presence of enhancement with gadolinium contrast. T1 and T2 weighted images vary between masses according to their biochemical composition, and this can be used to distinguish between them. For example, pericardial cysts have very characteristic high signal on T2 imaging. In addition, the fat content of tumours can be selectively imaged with the technique of fat suppression. Gadolinium enhancement reflects tumour vascularity and therefore positive enhancement occurs in malignancy (fig 22.3). Some capsular enhancement is expected in benign tumours as well, however, and vascular benign tumours such as myxoma also enhance. Overall, however, these additional characterisation features are very useful clinically for guidance for diagnosis and surgery.

ASSESSMENT OF CARDIAC VOLUMES, MASS, AND FUNCTION
There is abundant evidence linking ventricular function, volumes, and mass with prognosis in coronary artery disease and other cardiac disease. However, current techniques are not ideal. Radionuclide techniques suffer from a radiation burden which is best avoided if possible, and echocardiography is limited by technical issues such as image quality and acoustic windows which hinder quantification. These techniques have now been shown to be less accurate and reproducible than CMR,[11] which has become a new gold standard. The interstudy reproducibility of CMR is now recognised by pharmaceutical companies which are switching to CMR for phase 2 and 3 drug development studies in order to reduce the sample size of their studies (fig 22.4),[11] which saves time on recruitment and reduces costs significantly. Comparisons of established techniques and CMR show that mean values in populations vary between techniques by reasonably small amounts, but that individual variation can be very substantial.[12] This means that the techniques are not interchangeable for *individuals*. If clinical decisions are based on numerical thresholds therefore, CMR is the preferred technique. The acquisition of these parameters by CMR is fast on the most modern scanners and can be achieved in a few minutes. Analysis still remains an area requiring improvement, however, and many centres still perform this manually, but new software with highly automated analysis is now coming on to the market.

FLOW AND SHUNTS
CMR has particular application for the measurement of flow in the cardiovascular system. The normal images obtained reflect the magnitude of the radio signals received, but for each pixel in the image, the relative signal phase can also be measured. The phase can be encoded to relate linearly with velocity, and hence produce two dimensional velocity maps exactly corresponding with the anatomy from the normal images. Because the area of a vessel can easily be measured, and the mean velocity within the vessel calculated, absolute measurements of instantaneous flow can be derived. When run in cine mode throughout the cardiac cycle, flow curves are generated, where the area

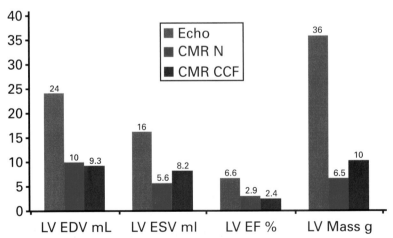

Figure 22.4. Comparison of the standard deviation of inter-study reproducibility between echocardiography and CMR. This standard deviation is central to determining sample size for drug trials. Sample size rises with the square of the ratio in standard deviations between the techniques. For all remodelling parameters of function and mass, the variability of two dimensional echocardiography is greater. The comparative figures come from different patient groups—echocardiography data from Otterstad et al, Eur Heart J 1997;18:507–13, and CMR data from Bellenger et al.[11] N, normals; CCF, congestive cardiac failure; LV, left ventricle; EDV, end diastolic volume; ESV, end systolic volume; EF, ejection fraction.

Key points

- CMR is a rapidly growing new speciality in cardiovascular medicine

- CMR uses radio waves to generate images and is very safe

- CMR is versatile and can assess anatomy, function, flow, and several tissue characteristics

- The latest generation of CMR scanners allow real time scanning

- Applications of CMR in coronary artery disease are increasingly useful clinically

- The high reproducibility of CMR functional measurements has found significant research application in research into mechanisms of disease, and new drugs

low water content, although in acute inflammation it can enhance with gadolinium and appear bright. The thickness of the pericardium needs to be distinguished from any pericardial effusion. Pericardial effusion is commonly black on spin echo images, but bright on gradient echo cines, and this is a useful means of differentiation. Pericardial calcification is not well seen by CMR, as calcium appears black, and therefore may simply appear as a localised area of pericardial thickening. CT is the best technique for showing calcium. Diastolic flow abnormalities can be demonstrated using velocity mapping, which can aid in diagnosis.

Cardiomyopathy

The contributions of CMR to the assessment of cardiomyopathy are in order of importance: arrhythmogenic right ventricular cardiomyopathy (ARVC), thalassaemia, hypertrophic cardiomyopathy, and sarcoidosis.

under the curve represents true flow in the vessel through the cardiac cycle. This is very valuable in the non-invasive measurement of the pulmonary to systemic flow ratio (Qp:Qs) in cardiac shunting (fig 22.5), and in a number of other clinical scenarios.

VALVAR HEART DISEASE

Echocardiography is ideal for investigating most valvar disease, but CMR has some particular uses. In valvar regurgitation, echo identifies the lesion, but it is not straightforward to ascertain the severity of the regurgitant flow. With CMR, the regurgitant flow can be measured directly using reverse flow measurement in diastole with an imaging plane placed just downstream of the aortic and pulmonary valve.[13] Extension to assessment of mitral regurgitation involves the subtraction of aortic flow from true left ventricular stroke volume measured using the multislice technique. The technique is especially useful when surgery is being considered and clinical and echo results are not concordant, or there is doubt. For valvar stenosis, Doppler is more reliable for assessment and CMR is required less often, but again is helpful when conventional assessment has failed, such as in aortic stenosis with a distorted valve when a catheter cannot be passed across the valve. Experience suggests that CMR is a useful alternative to echocardiography for both stenosis and regurgitation, when flow across the valve is very eccentrically orientated.

PERICARDIUM

The thickness of the pericardium is a good guide to the presence of constriction. This can be readily measured using CMR, although the thickness is slightly greater than expected from pathological studies, and this results from an effect known as chemical shift, caused by fat overlying the thin fibrous pericardial tissue. The normal CMR thickness of pericardium is therefore quoted as less than 4 mm. The pericardium appears black on CMR because of its

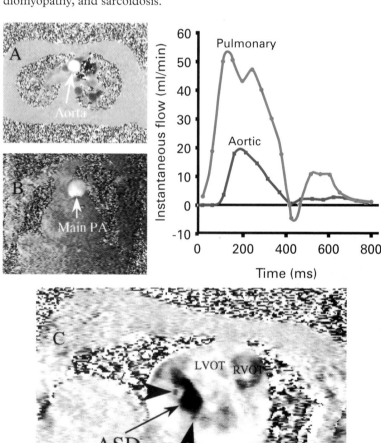

Figure 22.5. CMR of a patient with an atrial septal defect (ASD) in which conflicting echocardiographic and catheterisation results as to the size of the shunt had been obtained. (A) Velocity map (single frame) in a transverse plane for measurement of flow in the aorta; (B) velocity map (single frame) in a coronal plane for measurement of flow in the main pulmonary trunk (main PA); and graph of systemic and pulmonary flow plotted against time. The flow is calculated from the area under each curve, and the Qp:Qs ratio was 4:1 indicating a very substantial shunt. (C) Phase velocity map of the ASD viewed from the right atrium in an oblique transaxial plane (RVOT, right ventricular outflow tract; LVOT, left ventricular outflow tract). The large ASD is seen as black pixels due to transseptal flow into the right atrium, and has a maximum diameter of 3.5 cm and an area of 5.6 cm². The arrow heads indicate adjacent fenestrations. Reproduced from Taylor et al, J Cardiovasc Magn Reson 1999;1:43–7, with permission of the publisher.

ARVC is a complex disorder which typically affects young men causing ventricular tachycardia of right ventricular origin, and sudden death. It is familial and gene abnormalities resulting in ARVC have been discovered. The disease presents with abnormalities of the right ventricle (15% also have left ventricular involvement) and these are best delineated by CMR, as they can be subtle and localised (fig 22.6).[14] The late stages with a large poorly functioning right ventricle and widespread fat infiltration are easy to identify, but in the early stages abnormalities typically include discrete areas of fat infiltration, regional hypokinesia, localised myocardial thinning, and abnormal trabeculations. Considerable experience is required to differentiate these findings from normal variants, and in particular the normal patterns of epicardial fat distribution associated with the right coronary and left anterior descending coronary arteries must be understood. It is important to not overdiagnose the condition because of the significant effects on the patient's insurance status and the psychological wellbeing of the rest of the family. CMR is the technique of choice for the assessment of ARVC, but cases are best assessed in experienced CMR centres seeing several potential early cases per week.

The assessment of myocardial iron overload has been problematic in clinical practice, but recently a T2* CMR technique has been established which allows reproducible quantifi-

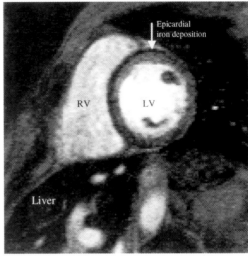

Figure 22.7. Example of iron deposition in a patient with thalassaemia. The dark epicardial rim of iron is arrowed. Note that liver deposition is very heavy, and the liver is therefore black. The signal loss occurs because of disturbances in the relaxation parameters of the tissues brought about by the iron causing alterations in the local magnetic field. There is very poor correlation between iron deposition in the liver and the heart, which prevents adequate management of the cardiac complications of myocardial iron overload (arrhythmia, heart failure, and death) from liver biopsy results. RV, right ventricle; LV, left ventricle. Reproduced from Rajappan et al, Eur J Heart Failure 2000;2:241-52, with permission of the publisher.

cation of the iron concentration (fig 22.7).[15] Results show that iron loading in the myocardium is not correlated with other tissues such as the blood and liver, and must be examined separately. T2* values below 20 ms indicate incipient heart failure, which is frequently precipitous, and requires urgent intensive chelation treatment. This technique is likely to reduce considerably the premature mortality from heart failure in thalassaemia which is the most common cause of death in these patients. The technique can also be used in other iron overload conditions such as haemochromatosis and sickle cell anaemia.

In hypertrophic cardiomyopathy, the diagnosis can usually be made by echocardiography, but there are circumstances when CMR is very useful. If the condition is suspected but not confirmed by echocardiography, CMR is ideal as a second line investigation. CMR also shows the distribution of hypertrophy very well, and is superior for quantification of myocardial mass. CMR appears to be more sensitive than echocardiography for the diagnosis of apical hypertrophic cardiomyopathy and can be considered early in the diagnostic work up of these patients. Finally, CMR is valuable for the assessment of septal ablation techniques in locating the size and extent of infarction and assessing rest and stress outflow tract gradients.

The final area where CMR has utility is in cardiac sarcoidosis. This is a rare condition but one which is important as arrhythmias or ventricular dysfunction may be arrested with steroids. The myocardium appears speckled with CMR spin echo techniques, but enhancement occurs with gadolinium, and this makes infiltration or focal fibrosis more obvious. Little work has been published in this area, but in

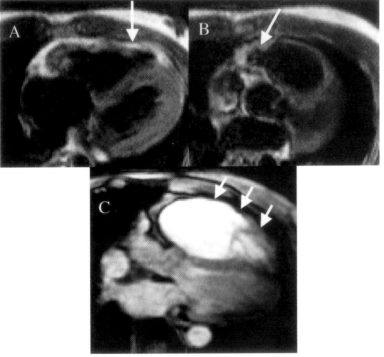

Figure 22.6. CMR features of arrhythmogenic right ventricular cardiomyopathy (ARVC). (A) A mid-ventricular transaxial plane in a patient with early disease who presented with non-sustained ventricular tachycardias of left bundle branch block morphology. The vertical arrow indicates an area of high signal in the right ventricular wall which represents fatty replacement of the myocardium. (B) In the same patient, the angled arrow shows a slightly higher transaxial plane with a bulge in the medial portion of the right ventricular outflow tract. (C) In a different patient, end stage disease is shown in the transaxial plane, with a very large right ventricle pushing the left ventricle posteriorly, and a thinned right ventricular free wall (short arrows). In general, ARVC is best diagnosed in its early stages when regional wall motion abnormalities in the right ventricle are present. In the patient in A and B, the region of fatty infiltration showed dyskinesia during systole, greatly increasing confidence in the diagnosis.

experienced centres, abnormal myocardial enhancement has been shown in a significant proportion of patients with known pulmonary disease.

CORONARY ANOMALIES

Coronary anomalies occur in approximately 1% of the population and are usually clinically silent. There are many anatomical variations which have been recorded and their definition requires not only the origin of the vessel, but also the proximal course. The importance of this condition lies in the occurrence of sudden death in patients who have a coronary artery passing between the great vessels (aorta and pulmonary artery). This may occur because of compression or kinking during exercise. Coronary (x ray) angiography commonly identifies the anomalous origin of the coronary artery, but is poor at defining the proximal course and the relation to the great vessels. Coronary CMR is now a robust technique for showing the origin and course of the proximal coronaries, and also the three dimensional relations of the great vessels. Several studies have shown that CMR is superior to x ray angiography for this purpose. More recently, coronary CMR has been applied to patients with congenital heart disease in whom the incidence of coronary anomaly is up to 30%, and defining the course by x ray angiography is even more complex because of altered positions of the great vessels and ventricles.[16] CMR was shown to be superior to x ray angiography in defining the anomalies, and this is important for operative planning—for example, with vessels that cross in front of the right ventricular outflow tract.

Indications close to clinical reality

DETECTION OF MYOCARDIAL INFARCTION

Recently the technique of late enhancement with gadolinium contrast agent has been described, in which imaging of the heart is performed 15 minutes after an intravenous injection of gadolinium (fig 22.8). The gadolinium concentrates in the necrotic (acute infarction) or scar tissue (chronic infarction) because of an increased partition coefficient, and the infarcted area becomes bright.[17] There is very close correlation of the volume of signal enhancement and infarct size in animal experiments of acute infarction. The technique has high resolution, and can define the transmural extent of necrosis and scar for the first time in vivo. Although the technique has been recently developed, it has obvious applications in defining whether infarction has actually occurred in borderline cases; it also has the major advantage of not being subject to a time window of positivity like cardiac enzymes and pyrophosphate imaging. In addition, a different technique known as *early enhancement* (at 1–2 minutes after gadolinium injection) can be used to define the extent of microvascular obstruction in acute infarctions, which again is now possible for the first time clinically. Microvascular obstruction has already been shown to predict

remodelling and adverse cardiac events after infarction. It is likely these techniques will rapidly find their way into clinical practice in centres with CMR available.

ASSESSMENT OF MYOCARDIAL VIABILITY

The technique of late enhancement has clinical application to the assessment of viability which is under intense current scrutiny. In a recent study, the simple morphological measure of the percentage transmural replacement of normal myocardium by scar has been shown to be a powerful predictor of post-revascularisation contraction recovery. Segments with less than 50% transmural replacement improved function, while those with higher grades of transmural replacement failed to improve.[18] There are many clinical advantages of this technique—it is morphologically based, making analysis straightforward, and there is no radiation burden. It is anticipated that the late enhancement technique will make substantial clinical impact in the management of infarction and its sequelae.

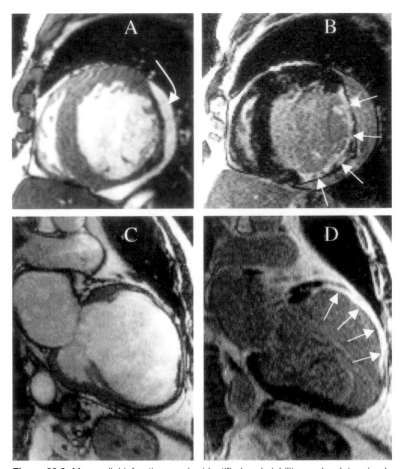

Figure 22.8. Myocardial infarction can be identified and viability can be determined using the late enhancement pattern after intravenous gadolinium. This figure shows two different patients, with the top row showing a lateral infarction, and the bottom row showing an anterior infarction. The left column (A and C) shows single frames from gradient echo cines, and the right column (B and D) shows the gadolinium enhanced images. The bright areas in B and D are infarcted tissue which is brightly enhanced (straight arrows). The infarct in the short axis plane (B) extends from the inferior wall to the anterolateral wall, and is mainly non-transmural. In particular, at 4 o'clock a significant rim of viable epicardial tissue is present and wall thickness is preserved. However, wall thinning has occurred elsewhere where the transmural extent of infarction is greater. The infarct in the anterior wall of the vertical long axis plane (D) is transmural, however, and considerably greater thinning and ventricular remodelling has taken place. This technique allows transmural high resolution infarct depiction in-vivo for the first time. The curved arrow shows a pericardial effusion. Reproduced from Rajappan et al, Eur J Heart Failure 2000;2:241–52, with permission of the publisher. Images courtesy of R Kim and R Judd.

DOBUTAMINE STRESS TESTING

Although it was first shown that dobutamine CMR was useful for detection of ischaemia in coronary artery disease a decade ago, it was not until its application in conjunction with modern scanners that the technique has achieved clinical validity. Comparisons with stress echocardiography have shown significantly improved diagnostic parameters with CMR which are related to greatly improved results from those patients in whom echocardiographic image quality was suboptimal or poor.[19] Results from centres with experience approaching 1000 patients have begun to establish this technique, and, where available, it can be considered as a first line approach if acoustic windows are limited.

CMR techniques in development

MYOCARDIAL PERFUSION

There are approximately six million perfusion studies performed worldwide annually, and all currently involve exposure to ionising radiation. A safer technique would be medically welcome, providing it can maintain the same valuable diagnostic and prognostic information and is cost effective. Perfusion CMR may be a contender for this role (fig 22.9). The CMR technique is fast and simple with a baseline first pass perfusion study and a repeat study during adenosine stress. Gadolinium is used as the contrast agent with a peripheral intravenous injection. Areas of reduced perfusion show as dark areas in the myocardium surrounded by normal enhancing areas. One of the advantages of perfusion CMR is high resolution, which allows the visualisation of subendocardial perfusion defects in vivo for the first time. Quantitative analysis tools have been developed which examine the slope of signal increase during the first pass and the myocardial perfusion reserve index. Analysis on a pixel by pixel basis has allowed the generation of parametric perfusion maps and bullseyes, which are very similar to scintigraphy and aid immediate clinical recognition.[20] Other advantages of perfusion CMR include the speed of the examination (one hour compared with typically 2–6 hours for a nuclear examination), and the easy combination with other techniques such as late enhancement (which depict areas of scar, and is available shortly after the perfusion study), as well as regional wall contraction.

ATHEROSCLEROTIC PLAQUE

Further down the road for clinical use is the technique of plaque imaging. CMR can be used to depict plaques and interrogate their lipid constituents as well as the integrity of the fibrous cap, which are factors that determine the propensity to plaque rupture and thrombus formation. T2 imaging has proved so far to be the most helpful, and validation of results against pathology has been achieved in the aorta and carotids. Latest results have also shown plaques in the coronary arteries

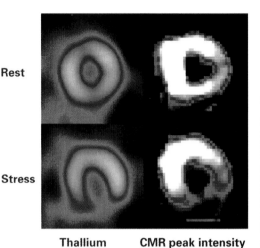

Rest

Stress

Thallium   CMR peak intensity

Figure 22.9. Comparison of thallium (left column) and CMR (right column) perfusion imaging in a patient with right coronary stenosis and inferior reversible ischaemia. The CMR images are parametric maps which are colour coded to appear similar to the thallium scan. Each pixel in the image represents the relative time to peak enhancement and bright colour indicates faster contrast wash-in and therefore better perfusion. The defect in the CMR scan is very similar in size and intensity to the thallium scan.

(fig 22.10).[21] In addition, transoesophageal and intravascular imaging have now become available, and there is currently intense interest in comparison of these techniques with intravascular ultrasound. We will not know for some years the clinical impact of these techniques.

CORONARY IMAGING

Much work has been devoted to the non-invasive assessment of the coronary artery lumen by CMR.[22] There have been tremendous improvements in techniques since the first descriptions in 1993, most notably in the development of "navigators", which allow

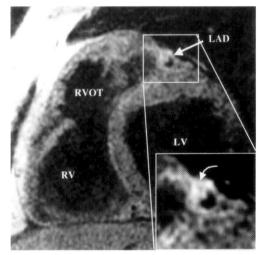

Figure 22.10. Coronary wall imaging in a patient with mild to moderate proximal left anterior descending (LAD) coronary artery stenosis. The enlargement shows eccentric vascular remodelling, as described by Glagov, with minor luminal encroachment. Note the dark area in the plaque (curved arrow). In validation studies, this represents the lipid core. Improvement in this type of imaging may lead to definition of the propensity to plaque rupture in vivo. LV, left ventricle; RV, right ventricle; RVOT, right ventricular outflow tract. Reproduced from Fayad et al, Circulation 2000;102:506–10, with permission of the publisher.

158

Role of CMR in ischaemic heart disease

- Accurate and reproducible ventricular volume and mass measurements in:
    - heart failure
    - hypertension
    - assessment of drug treatment
    - drug research

- Detection of presence and extent of infarction

- Assessment of viability (transmural extent of infarction)

- Assessment of stress induced ischaemia (dobutamine wall motion CMR)

- Under development:
    - myocardial perfusion
    - coronary imaging
    - coronary flow
    - atherosclerosis imaging

patients to breathe freely during the acquisition, with increased resolution and new sequences.[23] Most recently three dimensional breath-hold techniques during contrast agent infusion have shown good results. It is likely that coronary CMR will prove useful in coronary artery disease at some point in the future, but currently its clinical robustness needs improvement, and the issue of preventing coronary motion during the acquisition has to be improved further. However, the success of the technique for coronary anomalies is established and vein graft imaging by CMR is now straightforward. What remains unclear in the longer term is the value of such a technique. With the major advances in depiction of ischaemia using perfusion and dobutamine CMR, there are rational arguments for suggesting that invasive angiography would simply move on to becoming a pre-interventional procedure rather than a diagnostic tool in most cases. The luminogram may not be the holy grail that it was thought to be 10 years ago.

Education in CMR

The rapid development of CMR techniques in cardiology makes the dissemination of the expertise in clinical practice a complex problem. It is likely that major cardiology institutions, with an interest in research, will want to consider the purchase of a dedicated CMR scanner in this decade. Speciality training has, however, barely begun, and there will be a shortage of expertise for some time; however steps in the right direction are happening with the new American College of Cardiology Core Cardiology Training Symposium (COCATS) guidelines for cardiology trainees in the USA recommending training in CMR. Fortunately international bodies such as the Society for Cardiovascular Magnetic Resonance have looked ahead and have published credentialing guidelines to help develop adequate levels of training, whatever the professional background.[24] This is new technology with workings that are not always intuitive, but we have found that newcomers with a good appreciation of cardiac physiology rapidly move through the learning curve.

1. **Neubauer S, Horn M, Cramer M,** *et al.* Myocardial phosphocreatine to ATP ratio is a predictor of mortality in patients with dilated cardiomyopathy. *Circulation* 1997;**96**:2190–6.
- *This is a groundbreaking paper which shows that the phosphocreatine to ATP ratio in the failing heart is a better predictor of adverse outcome than other variables such as ejection fraction and New York Heart Association functional class.*

2. **Kilner PJ, Yang GZ, Wilkes AJ,** *et al.* Asymmetric redirection of flow through the heart. *Nature* 2000;**404**:759–61.

3. **Strohm O, Kivelitz D, Gross W,** *et al.* Safety of implantable coronary stents during H-1 magnetic resonance imaging at 1.0 and 1.5T. *J Cardiovasc Magn Reson* 1999;**1**:239–45.
- *There is much evidence now showing that all stents are safe to image. This paper was one of the first, and used laser techniques to show that no change in temperature occurs in the stent during CMR.*

4. **Francis JM, Pennell DJ.** The treatment of claustrophobia during cardiovascular magnetic resonance; use and effectiveness of mild sedation. *J Cardiovasc Magn Reson* 2000;**2**:139–41.

5. **Nienaber CA, von Kodolitsch Y, Nicolas V,** *et al.* The diagnosis of thoracic aortic dissection by noninvasive imaging procedures. *N Engl J Med* 1993;**328**:1–9.
- *One of the pioneering randomised trials comparing CMR with other imaging techniques for the diagnosis of acute aortic dissection. This showed that CMR was the most accurate technique to make the correct diagnosis.*

6. **Therrien J, Thorne SA, Wright A,** *et al.* Repaired coarctation: a "cost-effective" approach to identify complications in adults. *J Am Coll Cardiol* 2000;**35**:997–1002.

7. **Hirsch R, Kilner PJ, Connelly M,** *et al.* Diagnosis in adolescents and adults with congenital heart disease. Prospective assessment of the individual and combined roles of magnetic resonance imaging and transoesophageal echocardiography. *Circulation* 1994;**90**:2937–51.
- *A seminal paper which showed the complementarity of transoesophageal echocardiography and CMR in the diagnosis of problems in congenital heart disease.*

8. **Owen RS, Carpenter JP, Baum RA,** *et al.* Magnetic resonance imaging of angiographically occult runoff vessels in peripheral arterial occlusive disease. *N Engl J Med* 1992;**326**:1577–81.

9. **Moody AR.** Direct imaging of deep-vein thrombosis with magnetic resonance imaging. *Lancet* 1997;**350**:1073.

10. **Frank H.** Cardiac masses. In: Manning WJ, Pennell DJ, eds. *Cardiovascular magnetic resonance.* Philadelphia: Churchill Livingstone, 2001.

11. **Bellenger NG, Davies LC, Francis JM,** *et al.* Reduction in sample size for studies of remodelling in heart failure by the use of cardiovascular magnetic resonance. *J Cardiovasc Magn Reson* 2000;**2**:271–8.
- *An important paper showing that the improved interstudy reproducibility of CMR compared with echocardiography allows substantial reductions in sample sizes required to prove a hypothesis of change in remodelling parameters, such as ventricular mass and diastolic volume.*

12. **Bellenger NG, Burgess M, Ray SG,** *et al* **on behalf of the CHRISTMAS Steering Committee and Investigators.** Comparison of left ventricular ejection fraction and volumes in heart failure by two-dimensional echocardiography, radionuclide ventriculography and cardiovascular magnetic resonance: are they interchangeable? *Eur Heart J* 2000;**21**:1387–96.
- *This study showed that in comparison with CMR as a gold standard, there is very substantial variation in the results of ejection fraction for individuals between techniques. This implies that management decisions for individuals based on thresholds are best made using CMR, although in groups of sufficient size, the mean values for measurements using all techniques are similar, and then only the sample size determines the ability to detect change between groups.*

13. **Dulce MC, Mostbeck GH, O'Sullivan M,** *et al.* Severity of aortic regurgitation: interstudy reproducibility of measurements with velocity encoded cine MR imaging. *Radiology* 1992;**185**:235–40.

14. **Blake LM, Scheinmann MM, Higgins CB.** MR features of arrhythmogenic right ventricular dysplasia. *AJR* 1994;**162**:809–12.

15. **Anderson LJ, Holden S, Davis B,** *et al.* A novel method of cardiac iron measurement using magnetic resonance T2* imaging in thalassemia: validation and clinical application [abstract]. *Circulation* 2000;**102**(Suppl II):403.

16. **Taylor AM, Thorne SA, Rubens MB,** *et al.* Coronary artery imaging in grown-up congenital heart disease: complementary role of MR and x-ray coronary angiography. *Circulation* 2000;**101**:1670–8.

17. **Kim RJ, Fieno DS, Parrish RB,** *et al.* Relationship of MRI delayed contrast enhancement to irreversible injury, infarct age, and contractile function. *Circulation* 1999;**100**:185–92.

18. **Kim RJ, Wu E, Rafael A,** *et al.* The use of contrast-enhanced magnetic resonance imaging to identify reversible myocardial dysfunction. *N Engl J Med* 2000;**343**:1445–53.
• *Although this group from Chicago has published several validation papers showing the relation between infarct size and gadolinium uptake in animals, this paper extends the concept to viability in humans. In a myocardial segment, viability is preserved and post revascularisation improvement in function occurs, when transmural replacement by scar is less than 50%. This is a simple high resolution technique which clearly shows the importance of residual epicardial muscle in viability.*

19. **Nagel E, Lehmkuhl HB, Bocksch W,** *et al.* Noninvasive diagnosis of ischemia induced wall motion abnormalities with the use of high dose dobutamine stress MRI. Comparison with dobutamine stress echocardiography. *Circulation* 1999;**99**:763–70.
• *A study of 208 consecutive patients undergoing catheterisation who also went on to have dobutamine echocardiography and CMR. CMR significantly outperformed echocardiography because of superior image quality in patients in whom echocardiographic image quality was poor.*

20. **Panting JR, Gatehouse PD, Yang GZ,** *et al.* Echo planar magnetic resonance myocardial perfusion imaging: Parametric map analysis and comparison with thallium SPECT. *J Magn Reson Imaging* 2001;**13**:192–200.

21. **Fayad ZA, Fuster V, Fallon JT,** *et al.* Noninvasive in vivo human coronary artery lumen and wall imaging using black-blood magnetic resonance imaging. *Circulation* 2000;**102**:506–10.
• *First images of coronary wall plaque formation with external remodelling of the arterial wall (as described by Glagov), with only minor luminal encroachment.*

22. **de Feyter PJ, Nieman K, van Ooijen P,** *et al.* Non-invasive coronary artery imaging with electron beam computed tomography and magnetic resonance imaging. *Heart* 2000;**84**:442–8.

23. **Botnar RM, Stuber M, Danias PG,** *et al.* Improved coronary artery definition with T2-weighted, free breathing, three dimensional coronary MRA. *Circulation* 1999;**99**:3139–48.

24. **Pohost GM, Higgins CB, Grist TM,** *et al.* Guidelines for credentialing in CMR (cardiovascular magnetic resonance). Society of Cardiovascular Magnetic Resonance (SCMR) clinical practice committee. *J Cardiovasc Magn Reson* 2000;**2**:233–4.
• *Essential reading for professionals of all backgrounds wishing to train in CMR, to learn of these multidisciplinary guidelines indicating the recommended three month training required in order to satisfy credentialing criteria in this new field.*

23 Transoesophageal Echo-Doppler in cardiology

Peter Hanrath

Transoesophageal echocardiography (TOE) has opened a new sonographic window to the heart and the thoracic aorta. The technical development of this ultrasound based diagnostic tool, as well as its clinical application in a large variety of important cardiovascular diseases, has been cultivated scientifically mainly by European cardiologists within the last 15 years. Miniaturised electronic phased array transducer technology incorporated in a gastroscope-like instrument formed the basis for the breakthrough of TOE in clinical cardiology.[1] The wide clinical application of TOE in the past has without doubt significantly improved our diagnostic possibilities and contributed much to a better understanding of the pathophysiology of many diseases such as aortic dissection or cardiogenic stroke. Both factors influenced significantly the therapeutic management and led to a better outcome of a variety of cardiovascular diseases.

This review will focus on the clinical application of TOE. There is general agreement that a TOE examination is indicated in all patients where conventional transthoracic echocardiography (TTE) fails to provide conclusive diagnostic information (for example, emphysema) or where TTE is impossible (during surgery). Beyond that TOE is generally performed when it is expected to add important information to the data first obtained by TTE, because of the higher image resolution or the potential to acquire images of cardiac or vascular structures that usually are not accessible by the transthoracic approach.

Determining the sources of embolism

Stroke and peripheral embolisation are major causes of morbidity and mortality. Stroke is the third leading cause of death in the USA. Around 80–85% of all strokes are of ischaemic origin, and a fifth of these strokes are caused by cardiogenic embolism. The higher diagnostic sensitivity of TOE in determining sources of embolism is mainly based on the proximity of the oesophagus and the heart, thus allowing unique sonographic views of the atria (especially the left atrial appendage), a better morphological delineation of atrial septal structures and anomalies, and the detection of atherosclerotic lesions within the thoracic aorta.

In a busy referral centre the most frequent indication for TOE examination is the detection of a possible source of embolism. According to their underlying disease patients can be categorised into those with either a high or a low risk of embolic events. In clinical practice TOE plays a major role in the evaluation of patients with high embolic risk, especially in patients with atrial fibrillation, thromboarteriosclerotic changes of the thoracic aorta, infective endocarditis, and prosthetic valve replacement. But the assessment of low risk groups, in particular patients with patent foramen ovale and atrial septum aneurysm, is also possible. In young patients with otherwise unexplained stroke, the delineation of a patent foramen ovale by peripheral contrast injection or the combination of patent foramen ovale with atrial septum aneurysm can be displayed very elegantly by TOE as a potential gate of paradoxical embolisation.[2][3] Several recently published studies have shown a link between these abnormalities and an increased rate of strokes or transient ischaemic attacks. Furthermore, it was shown that patients with major pulmonary embolism and simultaneous patent foramen ovale have in particular a high risk of death and arterial thromboembolic complications compared to those patients with pulmonary embolism and no patent foramen ovale.[4]

About 70% of strokes associated with atrial fibrillation are caused by cardiogenic embolism, most commonly of left atrial origin. TOE is a perfect tool to visualise the left atrium, especially the left atrial appendage, which is the usual site for thrombus formation and which is seldom seen with TTE (fig 23.1).[5] In the past TOE in combination with pulsed wave Doppler has augmented our knowledge and understanding of the thromboembolic risk of patients with atrial fibrillation.[6] A low flow state in the left atrium identified by TOE is characterised by a large left atrium, the presence of left atrial spontaneous echocontrast, and a reduced flow rate within a large left atrial appendage. Low flow conditions are associated with an increased thromboembolic risk and are also associated with a high recurrence rate of atrial fibrillation after initial successful cardioversion. From serial TOE studies we have also learned that, after initial exclusion of thrombotic material within the left atrium, late embolic events after successful cardioversion may occur and are thought to be caused by "atrial stunning". The question of whether early TOE guided cardioversion with preceding short time anticoagulation using heparin and consecutive coumadin is safer and more cost effective than conventional coumadin treatment needs further clarification. The long term effect of early TOE guided cardioversion for the maintenance of sinus rhythm also needs to be studied.[7]

Stroke data banks and textbooks published up to the beginning of the 1990s indicated that in up to 40% of patients with embolic stroke no aetiology was found. Atrial fibrillation and carotid artery disease were considered the two major entities responsible for stroke or peripheral embolisation. Thus "cryptogenic" stroke was a big diagnostic dilemma. In 1990 a new finding in three patients with embolic disease—namely, a protruding plaque in the aortic arch as cause of embolisation, detected by TOE—

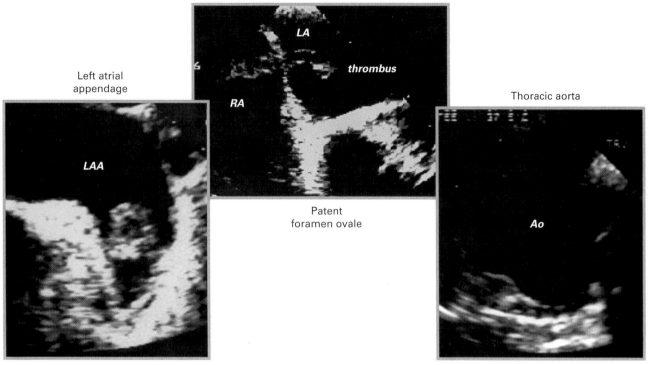

Left atrial
appendage

LA

thrombus

RA

LAA

Thoracic aorta

Ao

Patent
foramen ovale

Figure 23.1. Different sources of embolism detected by transoesophageal echocardiography. Left: clot within the left atrial appendage. Middle: clotting thrombus within the patent foramen ovale. Right: atherothrombotic plaques within the descending thoracic aorta. Ao, aorta; LA, left atrium; LAA, left atrial appendage; RA, right atrium

was reported.[8] Since then atherosclerotic lesions of the thoracic aorta have been recognised as an important cause of stroke and peripheral embolisation (fig 23.2). TOE is now the modality of choice—well ahead of computer tomography or nuclear magnetic resonance tomography—for the diagnosis of these atheromas. The prevalence of these atheromas is about 27% in patients with previous embolic events. The risk of a second embolic event is high—12% have recurrent stroke within one year.

With the more widespread use of TOE it became evident that the prevalence of thoracic atheromas is nearly in the same order of magnitude as other major aetiologies such as atrial fibrillation or carotid artery disease. Plaque thickness and superimposed mobile thrombi are independent risk factors for embolic events. If mobile components are

attached to these atheromas embolic complications may occur in 20–30% of these patients within two years.[9]

Aortic atheromas are an important cause of stroke during open heart surgery. The increasing number of elderly patients with severe atheromatous disease of the aorta has focused clinical interest on the rational management of severe atheroma of the ascending aorta and the associated risk of intraoperative embolisation. Simple palpation of the aorta at surgery underestimates the degree of disease. Intraoperative TOE provides unique information which may alter the conduct of the operation, especially with regard to the site of cross clamping of the aorta. If atheromas are seen in the arch or ascending aorta the intraoperative stroke rate is significantly increased compared to those without atheroma.

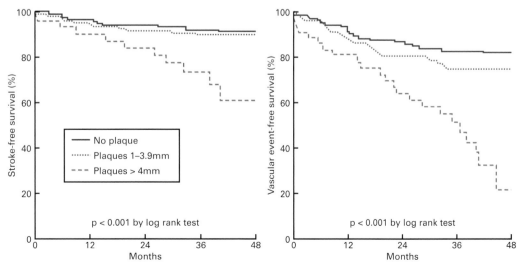

Stroke-free survival (%)

— No plaque
······ Plaques 1–3.9mm
- - - Plaques > 4mm

p < 0.001 by log rank test

Months

Vascular event-free survival (%)

p < 0.001 by log rank test

Months

Figure 23.2. Aortic atheroma. Results of study showing size and event rate of aortic plaques in stroke. From *N Engl J Med* 1996;334:1216–21.

Table 23.1 *Diagnosis proven at surgery, necropsy or by at least two methods (computed tomography/angiography)*[10]

	TOE	CT	Angiography
Sensitivity (%)	99	83	88
Specificity (%)	98	100	94
Positive predictive value (%)	98	100	96
Negative predictive value (%)	99	86	84

CT, computed tomography; TOE, transoesophageal echocardiography.

Aortic dissection

Within the last 15 years TOE has become a valuable modality for the diagnosis and management of diseases of the aorta. This diagnostic tool has also greatly contributed to our present improved understanding of the pathogenesis of diseases of the aorta, especially aortic dissection.

Based on TOE observations intramural haematomas as well as ruptured penetrating arteriosclerotic plaques are suggested to be major precursors of aortic wall dissection.

TOE is the imaging modality of choice for diagnosis and exclusion of thoracic aortic dissection (fig 23.3). In a European multicentre study diagnostic sensitivity (99%) and specificity (98%) in the high 90s have been reported (table 23.1).[10] Compared with aortography, computed tomography, and nuclear magnetic resonance tomography, TOE has the advantage that it can be performed at the bedside.

Combined with colour flow imaging, TOE allows not only the identification of the intimal flap with the true and false lumen, and identification of the entry and re-entry, but also the detection of associated complications such as aortic regurgitation, pericardial effusion, involvement of the coronary arteries, incomplete perforation, and thrombosis in the false lumen. Nowadays in most centres patients with proximal aortic dissection diagnosed by TOE, who are surgical candidates, are taken directly to the operating room, thus saving valuable time. In addition TOE can be used for follow up examinations after surgical or medical treatment to detect late complications such as aneurysm formation at the site of operation, or to provide useful prognostic information in terms of progression of thrombosis in the false lumen.

Infective endocarditis and its complications

Infective endocarditis represents the fourth leading cause of life threatening infections after urosepsis, pneumonia, and intra-abdominal sepsis. There is still a continuous rise in the incidence of infective endocarditis, with a yearly rate of 15–20 000 new cases in the USA despite significant improvement in diagnosis and treatment. This rise is mainly caused by increasing numbers of intravenous drug abusers, patients with artificial valves, and elderly patients.

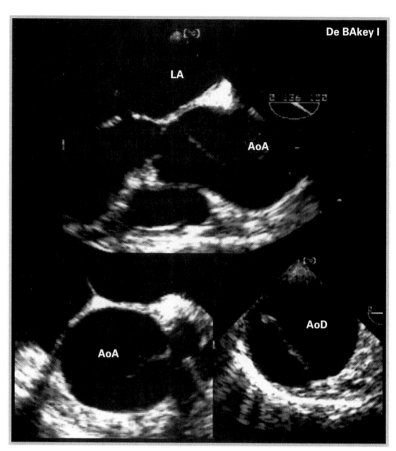

Figure 23.3. Dissection of the thoracic aorta. Upper: dissection of the membrane in the ascending aorta in the long axis view. Lower: ascending (left) and descending (right) aorta showing dissection of the membrane in the short axis view. AoA, ascending aorta; AoD, descending aorta.

By the combination of echocardiographic findings with clinical parameters (history, physical findings, laboratory tests) according to the Duke criteria the diagnostic accuracy to define infective endocarditis has been greatly improved. More then 11 studies in over 2000 patients comparing the von Reyn criteria (excluding echo findings) with the Duke criteria (including echo findings) showed an increased sensitivity and specificity of the Duke criteria, supporting the diagnostic utility of echocardiography—especially TOE—in the clinical setting of infective endocarditis.

TOE has considerably facilitated the process of making a correct diagnosis in the context of suspected endocarditis because TOE has a higher sensitivity (> 90%) compared to TTE (< 70%) for detecting vegetations, especially smaller vegetations < 5 mm.[11]

TOE enhances the visualisation of prosthetic valves, especially the detection of vegetations or valvar and paravalvar insufficiencies, with sensitivities over 80% versus 30% by TTE.[12]

TOE facilitates the detection of left ventricular outflow tract complications (fistula, perforation), especially abscess formation (fig 23.4), with a sensitivity over 80% versus 30% by TTE as proven in several studies (fig 23.5).[13]

Based on these facts—in the setting of suspected infective endocarditis—and according to the American Heart Association guidelines, TOE is the primary diagnostic method of choice, especially in patients with artificial valves, in patients with intermediate or high

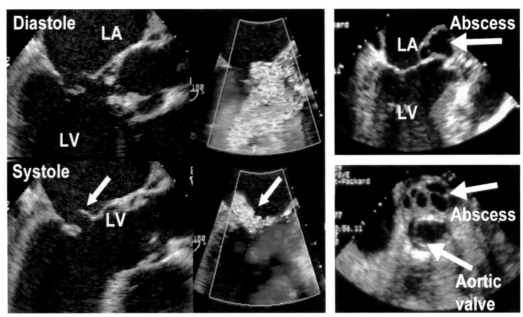

Figure 23.4. Infective endocarditis and abscess detected by transoesophageal echocardiography. Left: mitral valve perforation and aortic regurgitation in infective endocarditis. Right: abscess formation of the aortic valve. LA, left atrium; LV left ventricle.

clinical suspicion of infective endocarditis, and in patients with high risk of infective endocarditis related complications such as *Staphylococcus aureus* bacteraemia.

Evaluation of artificial valves

Prosthetic valve abnormalities, dysfunction or other associated pathologies are being recognised in an increasing number of patients, as the rate of valve replacement surgery grows.

TOE has gained increasing acceptance as a valuable method for assessing prosthetic valve function. The improved signal to noise ratio combined with the high resolution from high frequency transducers and the lack of problems related to acoustic penetration through mechanical valves has made TOE the technique of first choice for the investigation of patients, especially those with mechanical mitral valve replacement.

Additional pathomorphological findings such as thrombi in the left atrium, especially the left atrial appendage, or valvar and paravalvar leakages can be easily detected by TOE and are nearly always missed, especially in mechanical prostheses, by the transthoracic approach because of shadowing. In addition, bioprosthetic degenerations such as thickening or calcification of the leaflets, leaflet tears or prolapse are extremely well visualised by TOE.

Intraoperative application

After introduction of the phased array TOE technology in clinical cardiology this technique was rapidly recognised as a unique imaging modality to view the heart from a surgical perspective. Intraoperative application of TOE allows continuous monitoring of the surgical procedure without disturbing the sterile field, in contrast to epicardial echocardiography.

During myocardial revascularisation procedures TOE allows non-invasive evaluation of global left ventricular function. It can identify regional wall motion abnormalities as possible markers of myocardial hypoperfusion before and immediately after bypass. In the growing area of "off-pump" bypass surgery TOE monitoring is a "must".

In reconstructive mitral valve surgery the information obtained by TOE imaging is of greatest value. The pathomorphology of valvar dysfunction can be clearly defined by TOE, especially in the case of mitral regurgitation, where satisfactory valve repair gives the best short and long term results. Decisions based on TOE made at the time of operation may effect both early and late survival and the need for reoperation or replacement of the valve during the operation.[14]

Intra-aortic balloon pump insertion can be guided by TOE, allowing visualisation of the descending aorta in order to detect severe atheroma and to avoid potential complications.

Intracardiac air can be visualised early and "de-airing" can be continued until TOE no longer detects microbubbles, which may be responsible for most of the neuropsychological syndromes often seen in elderly patients after open heart surgery.[15] In addition, TTE imaging is often unsatisfactory in the early postoperative period for various reasons including the presence of air and tubes in the mediastinum. TOE is the best method for imaging the heart in the postoperative period.

Simple visual assessment of the inotropic state of the left ventricle may be of great clinical value. In patients with hypotension and low cardiac output in the intensive care unit, TOE monitoring of the left ventricle has been shown to be a very practical tool that allows rapid discrimination between depressed myocardial function and hypovolaemia as the underlying cause, or the exclusion of tamponade.[16] Thus immediate availability of the haemodynamic

164

and anatomic information gained from TOE permits rapid adequate therapeutic interventions. With the recent introduction of a miniaturised monoplane TOE probe, which is half the size of a conventional probe, thus allowing nasal insertion, continuous monitoring during the operation and postoperatively seems to be more feasible.

TOE during catheter based interventions

Catheter based interventions for the treatment of congenital lesions in paediatric or adult patients represent an arena in which the use of TOE guidance is beneficial.

The combined use of *x* ray and TOE imaging is in many cases mandatory for the success of a procedure. It provides instantaneous recognition of the morphological and haemodynamic result and its complications. The recent development of commercially available miniaturised biplane or micromultiplane TOE probes opened the door for an increased use of this imaging modality, especially in children and adults. Specific applications include transseptal puncture, catheter positioning during radiofrequency ablation, balloon atrial septostomy, balloon positioning during pulmonary/aortic valvuloplasty or mitral balloon valvuloplasty, balloon dilatation of venous pathways post Mustard or Senning operation, and transcatheter closure of atrial and ventricular septal defects as well as stenting of the thoracic aorta in patients with dissection or aortic coarctation.[17]

In the setting of an atrial septal defect a pre-interventional TOE examination is necessary in order to define the exact morphology and site of the atrial septal defect, as well as its relation to structures in the immediate neighbourhood. Most investigators agree that TOE is superior to fluoroscopy for defining the defect margins and to position the arms of the device. For this reason TOE is routinely used in many centres during these procedures.

Congenital heart disease

Transthoracic two dimensional echocardiography combined with spectral Doppler and colour flow imaging is considered the diagnostic method of choice in the assessment of paediatric patients with congenital heart lesions. In a large series of 240 paediatric patients with congenital heart disease, precordial imaging allowed a correct diagnosis in 93% of all cases, while TOE was necessary in only 7%. However, in 437 adolescent or adult unoperated or postsurgical patients with congenital lesions TTE provided correct morphological and haemodynamic diagnosis in only 57% of cases, TOE being necessary to achieve a diagnosis in the remaining 43%.[18]

The detailed description of systemic and pulmonary venous connections, as well as a precise assessment of pulmonary venous flow

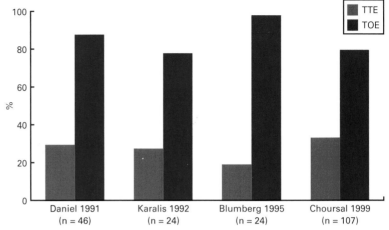

Figure 23.5. Detection rate of abscesses by transoesophageal echocardiography (TOE) versus transthoracic echocardiography (TTE).

patterns and of the structure of the atrial septum in various conditions, constitute one of the strengths of TOE. The distinctive morphology of the right and left atrial appendage provides a reliable guide to determine the atrial anatomy. In addition simple and complex obstructions of the left ventricular outflow tract, including discrete membranous or fibromuscular and long segment tunnel obstruction and their relation to the mitral and aortic valves, are well demonstrated by TOE. The same also holds true for the morphological as well as functional assessment of the subaortic valve apparatus.

Detection of myocardial ischaemia/viability

The diagnostic potential of transthoracic stress echocardiography with its different modalities has become established within the last 15 years for the detection or exclusion of coronary artery disease or to determine viable or non-viable myocardium. However, in 10–15% of patients image quality still remains a diagnostic problem. Based on its unrestricted image quality TOE represents an alternative approach in these cases.

In 1990 transoesophageal atrial pacing combined with simultaneous monoplane two dimensional imaging was introduced.[19] In addition pharmacological stress testing in combination with mono- or multiplane TOE imaging has been reported. Although the reported sensitivities and specificities are somewhat higher compared to transthoracic stress echocardiography, the TOE stress test did not receive wide clinical acceptance and is considered only as a diagnostic method of second choice. This is mainly because of the invasive character of the investigation and the prolonged investigation time, causing inconvenience to the patient.

Apart from the different forms of stress application as an indirect marker of coronary artery disease, TOE in combination with Doppler has been used to verify stenotic lesions as well as to evaluate the coronary flow reserve. In the light of new imaging modalities such as multislice computed tomography and nuclear magnetic resonance tomography, allowing visualisation of all three coronary arteries, and because of the restriction of TOE to the main stem and proximal segments of the left coronary artery, this approach is of less clinical relevance in daily practice.

Three dimensional echocardiography

Although cardiac ultrasound in general has become the most widely used diagnostic imaging method in clinical cardiology during the last three decades, the diagnostic decision making process is based on a mental reconstruction of serial tomographic views into their three dimensional geometry. This is a difficult process, which requires skill and experience.

The most practical approach to three dimensional echocardiography at present is the acquisition of a consecutive series of tomographic views using a multiplane TOE probe together with accurate spatial and temporal information and subsequent off-line reconstruction.[20] Although three dimensional reconstruction after acquisition of the basic data is still rather time consuming, the display of synthetic cross sections in various orientations (any plane echocardiography) is rapidly performed.

Three dimensional reconstruction facilitates the study of structures of complex geometry— the right ventricle, complex congenital heart disease, and aneurysmatic formation of the left ventricle are obvious examples where mental reconstruction is less accurate and most needed. It has already been shown that accurate measurements of cardiac chamber volume and myocardial mass are feasible. Furthermore, calculations of new and complex parameters of regional wall motion throughout the cardiac cycle are possible. The possibility of computer slicing through the beating heart and the display of specific structures and pathological conditions with their three dimensional relation may greatly facilitate the diagnosis. The surgeon can now have a "preview" of what will be found during surgery, which will be of great help in mitral valve reconstruction, aneurysmectomy, myectomy, and congenital defect repair, for example. A logical step forward is the imaging of dynamic three dimensional reconstruction with colour flow imaging and myocardial perfusion. In these days of robotic surgery of the mitral valve, TOE with three dimensional reconstruction are essential for such surgical intervention.

Summary

The success rate of TOE is impressive. In just more than one decade this diagnostic technique has become an integrated part of paediatric and adult cardiology, as well as cardiac surgery and anaesthesiology, with a wide range of indications. With modern transducer and computer technology further improvements

Main cardiovascular applications of transoesophageal echocardiography (TOE)

- Determining sources of embolism
- Aortic dissection
- Complication of infective endocarditis
- Prosthetic valve dysfunction
- Intraoperative monitoring/catheter based interventions

will be achieved in image quality, acquisition, and processing. Modern software packages or new matrix array transducer technology will very soon enable on-line reconstructive or real time three dimensional echocardiography, even of the oesophagus.

The combination of morphological and haemodynamic data of high diagnostic quality, and the possibility to use this diagnostic method at the bedside in the intensive care unit or in the operating theatre, guarantee that this diagnostic tool can survive successfully alongside other modern cardiac image modalities such as nuclear magnetic resonance tomography.

1. **Schlüter M, Langenstein BA, Presta J,** *et al.* Transoesophageal cross-sectional echocardiography with phased array transducer system techniques and initial clinical results. *Br Heart J* 1982;**48**:67–72.
- *Landmark paper describing the technology and first clinical results with miniaturised phased array transducer technology incorporated in an endoscope.*

2. **Hausmann D, Mügge A, Becht J,** *et al.* Diagnosis of patent foramen ovale by transoesophageal echocardiography and association with cerebral and peripheral embolic events. *Am J Cardiol* 1991;**70**:66–72.

3. **Zenker G, Ertel R, Krämer G,** *et al.* Transoesophageal two-dimensional echocardiography in young patients with cerebral ischemic events. *Stroke* 1988;**19**:345–8.

4. **Konstantinides S, Geibel A, Kasper W,** *et al.* Patent foramen ovale is an important predictor of adverse outcome in patients with major pulmonary embolism. *Circulation* 1998;**97**:1946–51.

5. **Aschenberg W, Schluter M, Kremer P,** *et al.* Transoesophageal two-dimensional echocardiography for the detection of left atrial appendage thrombus. *J Am Coll Cardiol* 1986;**7**:163–6.

6. **Manning WJ, Leeman DE, Gotch PJ,** *et al.* Pulsed Doppler evaluations of atrial mechanical function after electrical cardioversion of atrial fibrillation. *J Am Coll Cardiol* 1989;**13**:617–23.
- *Study describing atrial stunning in atrial fibrillation.*

7. **Klein AL, Grimm RA, Murray RD,** *et al.* Use of transoesophageal echocardiography to guide cardioversion in patients with atrial fibrillation. *N Engl J Med* 2001;**344**:1411–20.

8. **Tunick PA, Kronzon J.** Protruding atherosclerotic plaque in the aortic arch of patients with systemic embolization: a new finding seen by transoesophageal echocardiography. *Am Heart J* 1990;**120**:658–60.
- *Landmark article describing the detection of atherosclerotic plaques in the aorta.*

9. **Tunick PA, Kronzon J.** Atheromas of the thoracic aorta: clinical and therapeutic update. *J Am Coll Cardiol* 2000;**35**:545–54.
- *A classic review article describing the published literature on clinical and therapeutic aspects of atheromas of the aorta.*

10. **Erbel R, Rennollet H, Engerding R,** *et al.* Echocardiography in diagnosis of aortic dissection. *Lancet* 1989;i:457–61.
- *Keynote article describing the potential of TOE in aortic dissection in comparison to computed tomography and angiography within a large European multicentre trial.*

11. **Mügge A, Daniel W, Frank W,** *et al.* Echocardiography in infective endocarditis: reassessment of prognostic implications of vegetation size determined by the transthoracic and transoesophageal approach. *J Am Coll Cardiol* 1989;**14**:631–8.

• *Large study showing the diagnostic potential of TOE in the setting of acute endocarditis.*

12. Daniel WG, Mügge A, Groth J, *et al.* Comparison of transthoracic and transoesophageal echocardiography for detection of abnormalities and prosthetic and bioprosthetic valves in the mitral and aortic position. *Am J Cardiol* 1993;**71**:210–15.

13. Daniel W, Mügge A, Martin RP, *et al.* Improvement in the diagnosis of abscesses associated with endocarditis by transoesophageal echocardiography. *N Engl J Med* 1991;**324**:795–800.
• *Keynote article describing the unique diagnostic potential of TOE in the detection of abscess formation. Comparison with intraoperative and postmortem findings.*

14. Sheikh KH, Bengston JR, Rankin JS, *et al.* Intraoperative transoesophageal Doppler color flow imaging used to guide patient selection and operative treatment of ischemic initial regurgitation. *Circulation* 1991;**84**:594–604.
• *Study demonstrating the potential of colour Doppler imaging during operation in patients with mitral insufficiency.*

15. Topol EJ, Humphry LS, Boston AR, *et al.* Value of intraoperative left ventricular microbubbles detected by transoesophageal two-dimensional echocardiography in predicting neurologic outcome after cardiac operations. *Am J Cardiol* 1985;**56**:773–5.

16. Reichert SCA, Visser CA, Koolen JJ, *et al.* Transoesophageal echocardiography in hypotensive patients after cardiac operations. Comparison with hemodynamic parameters. *J Thoracic Cardiovasc Surg* 1992;**104**:321–6.

17. Cheitlin MD, Alpert JS, Armstrong WF, *et al.* ACC/AHA guidelines for the clinical application of echocardiography. A report of the American College of Cardiology/American Heart Association task force on practice guidelines (committee on clinical application of echocardiography). *Circulation* 1997;**95**:1686–744.

18. Sutherland GR, Stumper OF. Transoesophageal echocardiography in congenital heart disease. *Acta Paediatr* 1995;**410**(suppl):15–22.
• *Large study describing the advantage of TOE versus TTE in congenital lesions.*

19. Lambertz H, Kreis A, Trumper H, *et al.* Simultaneous transoesophageal atrial pacing and transoesophageal two-dimensional echocardiography: a new method of stress echocardiography. *J Am Coll Cardiol* 1990;**16**:1143–53.

20. Roelandt JRTC. Three-dimensional echocardiography: new views from old windows [editorial]. *Br Heart J* 1995;**74**:4–6.
• *Review of use of TOE for three dimensional reconstruction.*

SECTION VIII: GENERAL CARDIOLOGY

24 Cardiac tumours: diagnosis and management

Leonard M Shapiro

Until the 1950s, cardiac tumours were merely a curiosity. Diagnosis was academic and outlook poor. With the advent of cardiopulmonary bypass, however, surgical management became possible, particularly of intracavity tumours. More recently, the development of echocardiography, computed tomography, and magnetic resonance imaging has contributed greatly to the process of preoperative diagnosis.

Epidemiology and nomenclature

Primary cardiac tumours are rare, with a necropsy incidence of 0.05%.[1] Secondary deposits are seen more frequently, in 1% of postmortem examinations, but usually in the setting of widely disseminated malignancy.[2] The relative incidence of presentation is shown in table 24.1, and demonstrates that atrial myxoma is by far the most common primary cardiac tumour in adults, and rhabdomyosarcoma is the most common in children. A quarter of all cardiac tumours are malignant, the majority of which are angiosarcomas or rhabdomyosarcomas.

General clinical features
Cardiac tumours are diverse in clinical presentation, and atrial myxomas in particular may cause systemic symptoms mimicking collagen vascular disease, malignancy or infective endocarditis. There are several clinical features, however, that are seen commonly with many cardiac tumours:

- *Embolisation*—This occurs frequently. Either the tumour itself, or adherent thrombus may dislodge and migrate; hence the age old aphorism that all retrieved emboli should be examined histologically.

Table 24.1 *Approximate incidence of benign tumours of the heart in adults and children*

	Incidence (%)	
	Adults	Children
Myxoma	45	15
Lipoma	20	–
Papillary fibroelastoma	15	–
Angioma	5	5
Fibroma	3	15
Haemangioma	5	5
Rhabdomyoma	1	45
Teratoma	< 1	15

Reproduced from data provided in Allard MF, *et al*. Primary cardiac tumours. In: Goldhauber S, Braunwald E, eds. *Atlas of heart diseases*. Philadelphia: Current Medicine, 1995:15.1–15.22.

Epidemiology and presentation

- Primary cardiac tumours are rare

- The most common primary cardiac tumour is the atrial myxoma

- A quarter of primary cardiac tumours are malignant, the vast majority being sarcomas

- Embolisation, obstruction, and arrhythmogenesis are the chief modes of presentation

- Surgically retrieved emboli should be examined histologically

- Sudden death is not uncommon

Multiple small emboli may mimic vasculitis or endocarditis, while larger fragments may lead to cerebrovascular events. Right sided tumours naturally embolise to the lungs producing pleuritic symptoms and possibly right heart failure.

- *Obstruction*—Atrial tumours, once they are large enough, may result in obstruction of atrioventricular valvar flow, and, in particular, may mimic valvar stenosis. Symptoms are often markedly paradoxical and may relate to body positions. Ventricular tumours, though in general less frequent, may obstruct outflow tracts leading to chest pain, breathlessness or syncope.

- *Arrhythmias*—Intramyocardial and intracavity tumours may both affect cardiac rhythm, either through direct infiltration of the conduction tissue, or through irritation of the myocardium itself. Atrioventricular block and ventricular tachycardia are not infrequently seen, and the initial presentation may be with sudden death. The presence of serious ventricular arrhythmias should always lead to a search for structural heart disease and very infrequently a tumour may be found.

Myxoma

Atrial myxoma is the most common cardiac tumour, comprising 50% of tumours. Occurring more commonly in women, myxomas are usually diagnosed between the ages of 50 and 70 years, 90% are left atrial, and 90% are solitary. Sometimes myxomas are familial, in which case they are seen in younger patients. Facial freckling and endocrine adenomas are frequent. The tumours are much more frequently multiple whereas the sporadic cases are almost all single and atrial. Under these circumstances, screening of first degree relatives should be undertaken. Multiple acronyms have been proposed for such syndromes. These include LAMB (lentigines, atrial myxoma, mucocutaneous myxoma, and blue naevi) and NAME (naevi, atrial myxoma, myxoid neurofi-

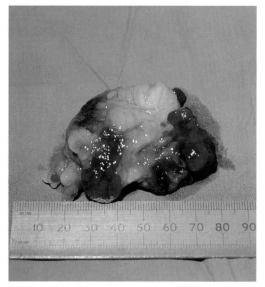

Figure 24.1. Macroscopic specimen of an atrial myxoma. Note the irregular, heterogenous, and polypoid nature of the tumour.

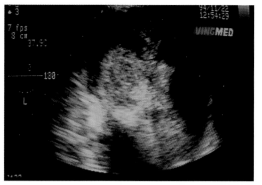

Figure 24.3. Transoesophageal echocardiogram (180° therefore left-to-right inversion) showing a left atrial myxoma, again obstructing the mitral valve orifice but also spreading across the fossa ovalis into the right atrium.

bromata, and ephelides). Recent nomenclature, however, suggests that they should be brought together under a broader category of Carney complex, named after the physician who first described the familial nature of this disorder.[3] A recent study of four relatives with the Carney complex suggests that the disease is caused by a gene deletion at the 17q2 locus.

The cell of origin of the myxoma is not known. Macroscopically they appear irregular, shiny and coloured (fig 24.1). Occasionally they are calcified. Their pedunculated nature means that the tumour may be very mobile and may obstruct a valve orifice (fig 24.2). The majority of myxomas are attached to the left atrial septum around the fossa ovalis, often with a component protruding through the atrial septum to the right side (fig 24.3).

Clinical features

Clinical manifestations are legion, both cardiac and systemic. Symptoms include breathlessness, fever, weight loss, syncope, haemoptysis, and sudden death. Emboli both of tumour fragments and thrombus from the tumour surface may present in a dramatic fashion. Multiple systemic emboli may imitate vasculitis and infective endocarditis. The features may mimic

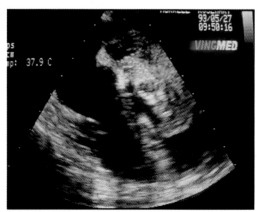

Figure 24.2. Transoesophageal echocardiogram showing a left atrial myxoma prolapsing across and obstructing the mitral valve.

systemic infection with cachexia, fever, arthralgias, and raised inflammatory markers. Very occasionally patients with transient ischaemic attacks or stroke are found to have an isolated myxoma only diagnosed by echocardiography. Right sided tumours embolising to the lungs result in pulmonary hypertension. Physical signs are also very variable and include clubbing, rash, and other features of infection and inflammation. Murmurs are frequently present, as is evidence of pulmonary hypertension, right sided cardiac failure, and pulmonary embolisation. Anaemia, raised acute phase reactants, and erythrocyte sedimentation rate are frequently present. Less frequently, the characteristic "tumour plop" may be detected. This is heard as a loud but rather dull sound as the tumour prolapses into the left ventricle, and may be confused with a third heart sound. Occasionally patients undergoing routine echocardiography for other indications are found to have a myxoma; despite the lack of clinical symptoms and signs they should have a surgical resection.

Diagnosis

Diagnosis depends on a high index of suspicion and can almost always be made by echocardiography. Both transthoracic and transoesophageal imaging should demonstrate a tumour and its relation to the atrial septum. If the exact origin cannot be seen, often an echo of increased amplitude may be visualised or the traction on the atrial septum may be noted as the tumour prolapses through the mitral valve. Differentiation of myxoma from valvar vegetation and, more importantly, from atrial thrombus is important. Usually the echocardiographic appearance of a myxoma is quite distinctive. In addition to the characteristic location and pedicle, myxomas are heterogenous and may have small lucencies. Thrombus is usually homogenous in appearance (though occasionally a liquefied centre may give rise to reduced echo amplitude), and usually arises from the left atrial appendage. Diagnostic confusion may exist when the myxoma arises from the left atrial appendage, as it does in 5% of cases. In this situation, the clinical setting of the illness and corroborating features should help to distinguish myxoma from thrombus. Occasionally, however, the two may be impossible to

Myxoma

- 90% are left atrial

- 90% are solitary

- Associated facial freckling should raise the possibility of the Carney complex, in which case family members should be screened

- The clinical features may mimic infective endocarditis, vasculitis or other inflammatory disorders

- Differentiation from intra-atrial thrombus is important

- Surgical resection is advisable as soon as possible after diagnosis, as the risk of embolisation is high.

- Recurrence is possible, and therefore long term echocardiographic follow up is recommended

distinguish on the basis of clinical and imaging criteria and a surgical approach may be required in the absence of a clear diagnosis. Alternatively, if the mass is small it has been recommended that a period of oral anticoagulation may help in differential diagnosis. Right atrial myxomas are relatively rare, but may cause diagnostic confusion as they may be mistaken for embolised or in situ thrombus. In these cases, it is important to look carefully to see if the mass is growing through the foramen ovale. Where diagnostic confusion persists after echocardiography, magnetic resonance imaging may prove helpful.[4]

Management

The method of choice for treating atrial myxomas is early surgical resection on cardiopulmonary bypass. These tumours are histologically benign but patients may die from obstruction, distal embolisation or rhythm disorders. Dislodgement of tumour fragments can be a significant risk during operative resection,

and to reduce this possibility manipulation of the heart is reduced to a minimum. Atrial myxomas may occasionally recur, either due to a second tumour origin, failure to demonstrate a pre-existing tumour focus or incomplete excision. Surgical survival following resection is excellent, but long term follow up is usually recommended, with echocardiography, to exclude development of a new tumour. However, the rate of reoccurrence is now so low most patients could be safely discharged.

Other benign primary cardiac tumours

Papillary fibroelastoma

These small tumours of the valve apparatus are often incidental postmortem findings. With the developments in echocardiographic imaging, they may be visualised during life, when they may be mistaken for valvar vegetations (fig 24.4). Until recently these tumours were considered to be benign and insignificant, but recent postmortem studies have demonstrated a high incidence of embolisation to cerebral and coronary arteries, and surgical resection is now considered more appropriate.[5] The "sea anemone" appearance, with a short attaching pedicle, is typical. Microscopically, each frond is formed of a central fibroelastic core, an overlying myxomatous layer, and an endothelial covering. Their pathological origin, however, remains elusive.

Rhabdomyoma

This intramyocardial tumour is the most frequent cardiac neoplasm of childhood, and is almost always multiple and ventricular. They may be seen by echocardiography as a pedunculated mass which may obstruct ventricular inflow or outflow. The majority of children with cardiac rhabdomyomas also have tuberous sclerosis.[6] Spontaneous tumour resolution is common, and treatment is therefore usually conservative. Life threatening complications are unusual, but occasionally surgical resection is necessary.[7]

Lipoma

These encapsulated tumours are usually subepicardial and asymptomatic. Rarely they may become large and cause arrhythmias, including atrioventricular block. Occasionally they may extend into the left atrial cavity but tend to avoid the fossa ovalis. If diagnostic confusion exists, magnetic resonance imaging is characteristic.[8] Lipomatous hypertrophy of the interatrial septum is a separate, non-neoplastic condition, usually found in obese patients, in which the atrial septum is heavily infiltrated with adiposity. This is seen by ultrasound as a very thickened atrial septum (2–3 cm) with low echo density. If atrial tachyarrhythmias are problematic, weight loss may be beneficial.

Fibroma

Cardiac fibromas are low grade connective tissue tumours which are usually intraventricular and occur principally in childhood. Firm, grey-

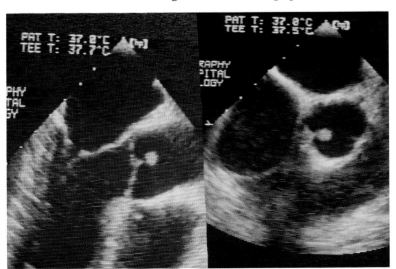

Figure 24.4. Transoesophageal images of an aortic papillary fibroelastoma in (left) longitudinal long axis and (right) short axis transverse views.

Other benign primary cardiac tumours

- Papillary fibroelastomas have a high incidence of embolisation—consideration should be given to surgical resection

- Rhabdomyoma is the most common cardiac neoplasm of childhood, often seen in association with tuberous sclerosis

- Lipomas are usually asymptomatic

- Lipomatous hypertrophy of the interatrial septum should not be mistaken for intracardiac tumour

---

Malignant primary cardiac tumours

- The majority of malignant primary cardiac tumours are sarcomas, usually angiosarcomas or rhabdomyosarcomas

- Most primary cardiac tumours are right atrial in location

- The incidence of primary intracardiac lymphomas is increasing—they are seen as part of the acquired immunodeficiency syndrome

- Treatment is rarely curative

---

white masses, they range from 1–10 cm in diameter. The echocardiographic appearance is of discrete, often obstructive masses. Grossly they appear sharply demarcated, with multiple foci of calcification which may aid diagnosis as they are often well seen by fluoroscopy. Located chiefly in the interventricular septum, these tumours interfere with the conduction system. Ventricular arrhythmic symptoms are common and sudden death is not rare. Surgical excision is sometimes possible, but transplantation has also been advocated.

Angioma

These tumours are extremely rare, and occur principally in the interventricular septum. They are visualised as subendocardial nodules, usually 2–4 cm in diameter. Coronary angiography may reveal a characteristic "tumour blush". Microscopically, they are classified as capillary, cavernous, intramuscular or haemangioendotheliomatous, though this does not seem to influence prognosis. Total surgical excision is not usually feasible because of the highly vascular nature of the tumour. Ventricular tachycardia and cardiac tamponade may intervene.

Malignant primary cardiac tumours

Approximately a quarter of all cardiac tumours exhibit some features of malignancy or behave in a malignant way; 95% of these are sarcomas,[9] the other 5% being lymphomas. Sarcomas are common between the third and fifth decades of life and most frequently affect the right atrium. They display a wide variety of morphologies owing to their mesenchymal origin. The clinical course is usually rapidly progressive, with death occurring as a result of widespread local infiltration, intracavity obstruction or metastases.

Angiosarcomas

These tumours occur more commonly in men, and almost exclusively in the right atrium. Clinical features include congestive cardiac failure, pericardial effusion, and pleuritic chest pain. Occasionally non-specific signs of disseminated malignancy, such as fever, weight loss and lassitude appear before signs of cardiac involvement. Echocardiography usually shows a broad based right atrial mass near the inferior vena cava. Epicardial, endocardial or intracavity extension is common and local spread of the tumour to pleura or mediastinum is often found. Pulmonary metastases are frequent and survival after diagnosis rarely exceeds six months.[10] Adjuvant chemotherapy seems to have little to offer at present.

Rhabdomyosarcomas

These tumours, the second most common primary sarcomas of the heart, are also more common in males, but may involve any cardiac chamber. Non-specific symptoms of malignancy are the rule, though pleuro-pericardial symptoms and distal embolisation may occur. Arrhythmias and obstructive symptoms may develop and raise the suspicion of a primary cardiac lesion. In contrast to angiosarcoma, diffuse pericardial involvement is not a feature and the tumour only rarely infiltrates beyond the parietal pericardium. Response to chemotherapy has been reported, and tumour bulk may be followed sequentially with magnetic resonance imaging,[11] but survival remains poor.

Others

Fibrosarcomas, histiocytomas, and lymphomas constitute the remainder of primary malignant cardiac tumours. Fibrosarcomas are malignant mesenchymal tumours which are primarily fibroblastic in origin, and occur with equal frequency on left and right sides of the heart. Firm, grey-white and nodular, they are often multiple and may invade the cardiac chambers and the pericardium. Survival is poor. Malignant fibrous histiocytomas are differentiated from fibrosarcomas by the typical whorled pattern of spindle cells on histology, but clinically behave in much the same way as fibrosarcomas.

Primary lymphomas must, by definition, involve only the heart and/or pericardium. They are rare, though in the last 20 years the incidence has been rising as they are seen as part of the acquired immunodeficiency syndrome[12] and in transplant recipients on immunosuppressive regimes. Lymphomas may go unrecognised as the chief presentation is with intractable heart failure. Treatment involves surgical resection and radiotherapy, but again with limited success.

Secondary cardiac tumours
• Secondary cardiac tumours are usually epicardial and asymptomatic
• Metastasis is rarely limited solely to the heart
• Pericardial effusion is common
• Melanoma, leukaemia, and lymphoma are most commonly associated with metastasis to the heart

Secondary cardiac tumours

Secondary cardiac tumours may be epicardial, myocardial or endocardial, but the vast majority are epicardial. With an incidence of up to 1% at necropsy, metastatic deposits to the heart are more than 20 times more common than are primary tumours.[2 13] Metastasis is rarely limited solely to the heart. The development of tachycardia, arrhythmias, cardiomegaly or heart failure in a patient with carcinoma should raise the suspicion of cardiac metastases. Rarely, cardiac involvement may be the first clinical feature of malignancy, and when this is the case, the presentation is usually with a large pericardial effusion or incipient cardiac tamponade. Metastases to the heart are, however, clinically silent in 90% of cases.

Local infiltration
Carcinoma of the lung or breast may spread by local infiltration to the pericardium, leading usually to pericardial effusion. Alternatively, carcinoma of the lung may invade the pulmonary veins and grow into the left atrium, occasionally causing symptoms as a result of mitral valve obstruction. Similarly, renal cell carcinoma has a tendency to invade the inferior vena cava, and may embolise to the right atrium, or may even grow as far as the heart.

Metastasis
For reasons which are not clear, melanoma has a particular predilection for metastasising to the heart. Half of all cases of disseminated melanoma will have cardiac deposits at necropsy,[14] and these tend to affect all four chambers of the heart. Leukaemias commonly invade the heart. Leukaemic infiltration between myocardial cells and sometimes larger deposits may be found. Pericardial effusion is sometimes a feature, in which case the fluid is usually haemorrhagic. Lymphomas similarly metastasise to the heart with regularity, forming discrete intramyocardial masses which are usually clinically silent.

173

1. **Reynen K.** Frequency of primary tumors of the heart. *Am J Cardiol* 1996;**77**:107.
• *This study incorporated the results of 22 large necropsy series, in order to provide reliable data on the frequency of the various primary cardiac tumours.*

2. **Lam KY, Dickens P, Chan AC.** Tumors of the heart. A 20-year experience with a review of 12,485 consecutive autopsies. *Arch Pathol Lab Med* 1993;**117**:1027–31.
• *This study analysed data from over 12 000 necropsies to provide accurate data on the incidence of primary and secondary cardiac tumours.*

3. **Carney JA, Hruska LS, Beauchamp GD,** *et al.* Dominant inheritance of the complex of myxomas, spotty pigmentation, and endocrine overactivity. *Mayo Clin Proc* 1986;**61**:165–72.
• *An original description of the Carney complex, comprising in the index family cardiac myxomas, cutaneous myxomas, lentigines, Cushing's syndrome, and acromegaly.*

4. **Hoffmann U, Globits S, Frank H.** Cardiac and paracardiac masses. Current opinion on diagnostic evaluation by magnetic resonance imaging. *Eur Heart J* 1998;**19**:553–63.

5. **Loire R, Donsbeck AV, Nighoghossian N,** *et al.* Papillary fibroelastoma of the heart. A review of 20 cases. *Arch Anat Cytol Pathol* 1999;**47**:19–25.

6. **Webb DW, Thomas RD, Osborne JP.** Cardiac rhabdomyomas and their association with tuberous sclerosis. *Arch Dis Child* 1993;**68**:367–70.

7. **Black MD, Kadletz M, Smallhorn JF,** *et al.* Cardiac rhabdomyomas and obstructive left heart disease: histologically but not functionally benign. *Ann Thorac Surg* 1998;**65**:1388–90.

8. **Rokey R, Mulvagh SL, Cheirif J,** *et al.* Lipomatous encasement and compression of the heart: antemortem diagnosis by cardiac nuclear magnetic resonance imaging and catheterization. *Am Heart J* 1989;**117**:952–3.

9. **Roberts WC.** Primary and secondary neoplasms of the heart. *Am J Cardiol* 1997;**80**:671–82.
• *An excellent and authoritative overview of the incidence, behaviour, and management of primary and secondary cardiac tumours.*

10. **Herrmann MA, Shankerman RA, Edwards WD,** *et al.* Primary cardiac angiosarcoma: a clinicopathologic study of six cases. *J Thorac Cardiovasc Surg* 1992;**103**:655–64.

11. **Szucs RA, Rehr RB, Yanovich S,** *et al.* Magnetic resonance imaging of cardiac rhabdomyosarcoma. Quantifying the response to chemotherapy. *Cancer* 1991;**67**:2066–70.

12. **Holladay AO, Siegel RJ, Schwartz DA.** Cardiac malignant lymphoma in acquired immune deficiency syndrome. *Cancer* 1992;**70**:2203–7.

13. **Abraham KP, Reddy V, Gattuso P.** Neoplasms metastatic to the heart: review of 3314 consecutive autopsies. *Am J Cardiovasc Pathol* 1990;**3**:195–8.

14. **Gibbs P, Cebon JS, Calafiore P,** *et al.* Cardiac metastases from malignant melanoma. *Cancer* 1999;**85**:78–84.

25 Endothelial function and nitric oxide: clinical relevance

Patrick Vallance, Norman Chan

The vascular endothelium is a monolayer of cells between the vessel lumen and the vascular smooth muscle cells. Far from being inert, it is metabolically active and produces a variety of vasoactive mediators. Among these mediators, endothelial derived nitric oxide is essential in the maintenance of vascular homeostasis, and defects in the L-arginine: nitric oxide pathway have been implicated in a variety of cardiovascular diseases.

Historic perspectives

From EDRF to nitric oxide

In 1980, Furchgott and Zawadzki showed that the presence of vascular endothelial cells is essential for acetylcholine to induce relaxation of isolated rabbit aorta.[1] If the vascular endothelium was removed, the blood vessel failed to relax in response to acetylcholine but still responded to glyceryl trinitrate. This endothelium dependent relaxation of vascular smooth muscle to acetylcholine is mediated by an endogenous mediator initially named endothelium derived relaxing factor (EDRF),[1]

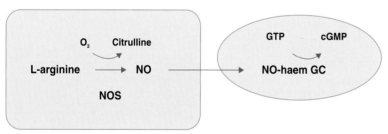

Figure 25.1. The L-arginine: nitric oxide pathway. NO, nitric oxide; NOS, nitric oxide synthase; GC, guanylate cyclase; cGMP, cyclic guanosine-3',5-monophosphate; GTP, guanosine triphosphate

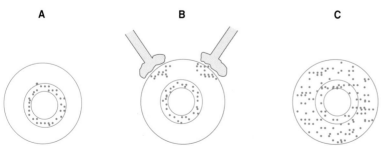

Figure 25.2. (A) In most, if not all, vessels nitric oxide is synthesised within the endothelium. (B) In certain vessels (for example, cerebral vessels) nitric oxide is also synthesised by nerves in the adventitia (nitrogenic nerves). (C) After exposure to endotoxin or cytokines, iNOS is expressed throughout the vessel wall and produces large amounts of nitric oxide.

which was subsequently identified as nitric oxide.[2][3]

L-arginine: nitric oxide pathway

Endothelium derived nitric oxide is synthesised from the amino acid L-arginine by the endothelial isoform of nitric oxide synthase, yielding L-citrulline as a byproduct.[4] Nitric oxide is labile with a short half life (< 4 seconds in biological solutions). It is rapidly oxidised to nitrite and then nitrate by oxygenated haemoglobin before being excreted into the urine.[4] Several co-factors are required for nitric oxide biosynthesis. These include nicotinamide adenine dinucleotide phosphate (NADPH), flavin mononucleotide, flavin adenine dinucleotide, tetrahydrobiopterin (BH_4), and calmodulin. Once synthesised, the nitric oxide diffuses across the endothelial cell membrane and enters the vascular smooth muscle cells where it activates guanylate cyclase, leading to an increase in intracellular cyclic guanosine-3',5-monophosphate (cGMP) concentrations[4] (fig 25.1). As a second messenger, cGMP mediates many of the biological effects of nitric oxide including the control of vascular tone and platelet function. In addition, nitric oxide has other molecular targets which include haem or other iron centred proteins, DNA, and thiols. These additional reactions may mediate changes in functions of certain key enzymes or ion channels. Nitric oxide also interacts with enzymes of the respiratory chain including complex I and II, and aconitase, and through these effects alters tissue mitochondrial respiration. Interaction of nitric oxide with superoxide anion can attenuate physiological responses mediated by nitric oxide and produce irreversible inhibitory effects on mitochondrial function as a result of the formation of peroxynitrite ($ONOO^-$), a powerful oxidant species.

Nitric oxide synthase isoforms

Three isoforms of nitric oxide synthase (NOS) have been identified: the endothelial isoform (eNOS), neuronal isoform (nNOS), and macrophage or inducible isoform (iNOS). All three NOS isoforms play distinct roles in the regulation of vascular tone (fig 25.2). The genes encoding eNOS, nNOS, and iNOS are located on chromosome 7, 12, and 17, respectively.[5] Whereas eNOS and nNOS are normal constituents of healthy cells, iNOS is not usually expressed in vascular cells and its expression is seen mainly in conditions of infection or inflammation.

Biological effects of nitric oxide

Nitric oxide and the vasculature

Endothelium derived nitric oxide is a potent vasodilator in the vasculature, and the balance between nitric oxide and various endothelium derived vasoconstrictors and the sympathetic nervous system maintains blood vessel tone. In addition, nitric oxide suppresses platelet aggregation, leucocyte migration, and cellular

The L-arginine: nitric oxide pathway

- Nitric oxide is synthesised from L-arginine to yield citrulline

- Co-factors required for nitric synthesis:
  - nicotinamide adenine dinucleotide phosphate (NADPH)
  - flavin mononucleotide
  - flavin adenine dinucleotide
  - tetrahydrobiopterin (BH_4)
  - calmodulin

- Enzymes responsible for nitric oxide synthesis:
  - endothelial nitric oxide synthase (expressed in normal cells) (eNOS)
  - neuronal nitric oxide synthase (expressed in normal cells) (nNOS)
  - inducible nitric oxide synthase (expressed during infection/ inflammation) (iNOS)

- Nitric oxide activates guanylate cyclase in vascular smooth muscle cells to synthesise cyclic guanosine-3',5-monophosphate (cGMP) which causes many of its biological effects

adhesion to the endothelium, and attenuates vascular smooth muscle cell proliferation and migration. Furthermore, nitric oxide can inhibit activation and expression of certain adhesion molecules, and influence production of superoxide anion. Loss of endothelium derived nitric oxide would be expected to promote a vascular phenotype more prone to atherogenesis, a concept supported by studies in experimental animals.[6]

Nitric oxide release from the vascular endothelium

There is a continuous basal synthesis of nitric oxide from the vascular endothelium to maintain resting vascular tone. A number of chemical and physical stimuli may activate eNOS and lead to increased nitric oxide production.

Basal nitric oxide release

The synthesis of nitric oxide in vascular endothelial cells in culture or intact vascular tissue can be inhibited by N^G monomethyl-L-arginine (L-NMMA), an analogue of L-arginine in which one of the guanidino nitrogen atoms is methylated. This inhibitory effect of L-NMMA is readily reversed by L-arginine.[7] L-NMMA and similar substrate based inhibitors have been used to examine the role of nitric oxide in various vascular beds in vitro and in both human and animal models.

In rings of rabbit aorta, L-NMMA causes significant endothelium dependent contraction. Intravenous infusion of L-NMMA into experimental animals induces a dose related increase in blood pressure which is reversed by intravenous administration of L-arginine, and in the human forearm vasculature infusion of L-NMMA into the brachial artery causes substantial dose dependent vasoconstriction. Thus continuous generation of nitric oxide is crucial in maintaining peripheral vasodilatation in humans[7] (fig 25.3). This basal nitric oxide mediated dilatation has been seen in every other arterial bed studied including cerebral, pulmonary, renal, and coronary vasculature. In contrast, in the venous system inhibitors of NOS do not lead to an increase in basal tone in a variety of venous preparations from animals or humans,[8] suggesting that basal nitric oxide production does not have a major role in the maintenance of the resting tone in most veins. In conduit vessels, there is some basal nitric oxide mediated dilatation but it appears to be less than that seen in resistance vessels.

Agonist stimulated nitric oxide release

Many chemical substances such as acetylcholine, bradykinin, serotonin, and substance P are able to induce endothelium dependent vasodilatation. In rings of rabbit aorta, endothelium dependent relaxation induced by acetylcholine, calcium ionophore (A23187) or substance P is inhibited by L-NMMA. This provides in vitro evidence that vasorelaxation induced by endothelium dependent agonists is nitric oxide mediated. L-NMMA also attenuates the hypotensive effect of acetylcholine in vivo in animals. However, the blockade is far from complete and there is now growing evidence for additional mechanisms underlying endothelium dependent responses to acetylcholine, particularly in resistance vessels. Similarly in humans, L-NMMA inhibits agonist stimulated relaxation in resistance,[7] conduit, and venous vessels in vivo. However, the degree of inhibition to agonist dependent dilatation varies between vascular beds, and mechanisms (for example, prostaglandins and endothelium derived hyperpolarising factors) other than that mediated by nitric oxide appear to be involved.

Physical forces and nitric oxide release

Haemodynamic shear stress exerted by the viscous drag of flowing blood is an important physiological stimulus in the regulation of nitric oxide release from the endothelium. The mechanisms of shear stress induced nitric oxide release is complex, involving

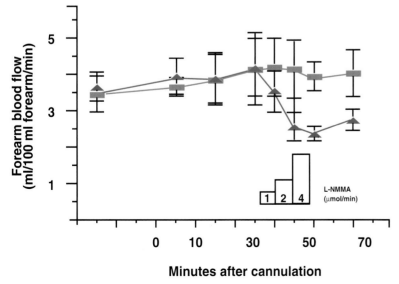

Figure 25.3. Inhibition of endogenous nitric oxide by L-NMMA produces a dose dependent reduction in forearm blood flow.

(1) extremely rapid initiation via ion channel activation, and (2) subsequent events related to signalling pathway activation such as phosphorylation of eNOS protein and increased expression of eNOS mRNA and protein. These complex events allow rapid and short lasting as well as slow onset and sustained vasodilatation in response to changes in shear stress.

Ultra-quick: ion channels

Numerous in vitro studies have provided strong evidence that ion channels—including certain calcium, potassium, and chloride ion channels—open seconds after exposure to haemodynamic shear. Application of shear stress to bovine aortic endothelial cells by fluid perfusion led to an immediate large increase in intracellular free calcium within one minute followed by a rapid decline. Notably, the increase in intracellular calcium occurs only in response to pulsatile flow and not to steady flow. The detection of potassium selective current with whole cell patch clamp recordings of arterial endothelial cells suggests activation of a distinct potassium channel in response to shear stress. Recently, a flow activated, chloride selective membrane current in vascular endothelial cells, distinct from the potassium current, was demonstrated. The balance between anionic and cationic current determines the net membrane potential and the subsequent change in calcium that alters eNOS activation and nitric oxide output.

Quick: phosphorylation

Mechanical activation of eNOS as induced by shear stress occurs also via phosphorylation and the effect is independent of intracellular calcium concentrations. It has been shown that in response to shear stress, the serine/threonine protein kinase B (Akt) directly phosphorylates and activates eNOS with a maximal increase up to sixfold after one hour of exposure to shear stress. The stimulation of Akt phosphorylation by shear stress appears to be mediated by phosphoinositide 3-OH kinase.

Slow: increased transcription

Shear stress also stimulates eNOS gene transcription to maintain long term nitric oxide production. Application of shear stress for three hours resulted in an induction of eNOS mRNA in a dose dependent manner in both bovine and human aortic endothelial cells.

These in vitro experimental data demonstrate the complexity of short medium and long term regulation of nitric oxide release in response to shear stress.

Loss of nitric oxide and predisposition to atherogenesis

A reduction in nitric oxide activity (manifested as impaired endothelial dependent vasodilatation) occurs very early in experimental and human hypercholesterolaemia, even before any structural changes in the vascular wall. In some cases, the impaired endothelial dependent vasodilatation appears to be reversed with L-arginine.[9] The action that nitric oxide normally has as an antiatherogenic factor is supported by studies of long term NOS inhibition. Aortic rings from rabbits fed with cholesterol rich diet showed impaired endothelial dependent vasorelaxation to acetylcholine. Furthermore, blockade of nitric oxide with nitro-L-arginine methylester (L-NAME) causes structural changes with development of greater lesion surface area in the aorta of hypercholesterolaemic rabbits.

Endothelial dysfunction in established cardiovascular disease

Atherosclerosis

Impaired endothelium dependent vasorelaxation to acetylcholine occurs in experimental models of atherosclerosis. In these studies, relaxation to endothelium independent nitric oxide donors such as glyceryl trinitrate and sodium nitroprusside was unaffected, indicating selective impairment of the L-arginine–nitric oxide pathway rather than a generalised reduced vascular smooth muscle cell response to nitric oxide. Similar findings were also confirmed in human coronary and peripheral circulation in vivo.[10] In patients with early coronary artery disease, abnormal responses to acetylcholine were found even in angiographically normal segments of coronary artery. Similarly, in patients with established coronary artery disease, endothelial dysfunction in the peripheral vessels as assessed by flow mediated dilatation is impaired. This impairment correlates with the extent of the coronary artery disease.

Chronic heart failure

Chronic heart failure (CHF) is characterised by a reduced vasodilator response to exercise and increased vasoconstriction; this is primarily a result of an imbalance between endothelium derived vasodilator and constrictor substances. There is general agreement that in CHF synthesis of endothelin-1, a potent vasoconstrictor, is greatly increased and this may contribute to the characteristic haemodynamic abnormalities. However, it remains unclear whether nitric oxide synthesis is decreased in CHF. The fact that endothelium dependent vasodilator response to acetylcholine, methacholine, and serotonin[11] is attenuated in peripheral resistance vessels suggests a reduction in agonist stimulated nitric oxide release. In contrast, response to L-NMMA appears to be either unchanged or even paradoxically exaggerated in CHF. This could be partially explained by an increased basal nitric oxide synthesis in the face of increased vasoconstrictor generation. Interestingly, endothelium independent vasodilator response to nitric oxide donors may also be attenuated,[11] suggesting that vascular smooth muscle sensitivity to nitric oxide might be reduced, with the degree of attenuation correlating with the severity of CHF. It is possible that the underlying mechanism relates to increased vascular generation of superoxide anion (O_2^-) that inactivates nitric oxide.

Treatment of CHF with angiotensin converting enzyme (ACE) inhibitors has been shown to improve endothelium dependent vasodilatation induced by cholinergic stimuli. Furthermore, in a randomised, placebo controlled study of patients with moderate to severe CHF, spironolactone increased vasodilator response to acetylcholine with an associated increase in vasoconstriction to L-NMMA, suggesting enhanced basal nitric oxide mediated dilatation following spironolactone treatment. Whether these beneficial effects on endothelial nitric oxide contribute to the favourable outcome remains to be determined.

Endothelial dysfunction and risk factors for coronary heart disease

Hyperlipidaemia

Experimentally induced hyperlipidaemia by either a fatty meal or intralipid infusion impairs flow mediated dilatation (FMD). In patients with hypercholesterolemia, endothelium dependent vasodilatation in both coronary and peripheral vessels is impaired before the development of clinical atherosclerosis.[9][12] Restoration of normal or near normal endothelium dependent vasodilatation in the forearm resistance vessels of hypercholesterolaemic subjects can be achieved after six months of lipid lowering treatment. Interestingly, reduced vasodilatation in response to acetylcholine has also been seen in patients with raised triglyceride but normal low density lipoprotein (LDL) cholesterol concentrations. In patients with familial combined hyperlipidaemia, lipid lowering treatment improved forearm blood flow in response to serotonin. Finally, raised Lp(a) lipoprotein appears to enhance acetylcholine and cold pressor coronary *constrictor* responses in patients with normal coronary arteries on angiography and impairs basal nitric oxide production in forearm resistance vessels. Thus, there is compelling evidence to indicate that endothelial function is impaired by hyperlipidaemia. However, recently the reversibility of this defect in coronary arteries has been called into question.

Hypertension

Substantial evidence from animal and human studies indicates that acetylcholine induced relaxation is impaired in patients with hypertension. However, no difference was found in endothelium dependent vasodilator response to acetylcholine or carbachol between patients with essential hypertension and matched normotensive controls in at least one study. This may be because of differences in methodology and in population subgroups in this heterogeneous condition. There is, however, evidence that basal nitric oxide synthesis is reduced in essential hypertension and that vasoconstrictor response to L-NMMA is reduced in untreated hypertension, although again this has not been a universal finding.[13] Current data would be most consistent with hypertension causing a decrease in nitric oxide mediated dilatation

rather than the loss of nitric oxide causing essential hypertension. This notion is supported by the observation that impaired endothelium dependent vasodilatation in essential hypertension can be restored with antihypertensive treatment,[13] and that endothelium dependent vasodilatation is impaired following acute elevation of blood pressure in normotensive subjects.

Diabetes mellitus

There is considerable controversy regarding the extent of endothelial dysfunction that occurs in type 1 diabetes mellitus, as endothelial function studies in both animal and human models of type 1 diabetes have produced conflicting results.[14] For example, agonist stimulated, endothelium dependent vasodilatation has been found to be either impaired or unchanged. Endothelial function may be modulated by several factors associated with diabetes such as the degree of acute hyperglycaemia, chronicity of hyperglycaemia (disease duration), accumulation of advanced glycosylated end products, insulin concentrations, and diabetic complications such as autonomic neuropathy and microalbuminuria. Variation in these factors between studies may in part explain the conflicting results. At present, there is no clear consensus about the level at which the disease might alter nitric oxide signalling. Most data would be consistent with a reduced responsiveness to nitric oxide in type 1 diabetes, and large scale definitive studies in the future would be required to show whether this is the case.

Vascular studies in type 2 diabetes have generally shown an impaired muscarinic, agonist stimulated, endothelium dependent response as well as an impaired endothelium independent response, although the impaired endothelium independent response was not confirmed by other investigators. Interestingly, it has recently been shown that even normoglycaemic subjects who are prone to develop type 2 diabetes and insulin resistance syndrome, such as those characterised by previous gestational diabetes and low birth weight, exhibit impaired FMD. This has led to the suggestion that endothelial dysfunction may precede the development of type 2 diabetes.

Hyperhomocysteinaemia

Raised plasma homocysteine is thought to be an independent risk factor for coronary heart disease, and this may be mediated by endothelial dysfunction. Acute methionine induced hyperhomocysteinaemia impairs endothelium dependent FMD in healthy subjects which can be reversed by folic acid supplementation. Impaired FMD has also been found in chronic hyperhomocysteinaemia and homocysteinuric children. The concentration of plasma homocysteine associated with endothelial dysfunction in these in vivo human studies were several folds higher than the normal range. Recently, it has been shown that even mild physiological increments in plasma homocysteine concentrations were sufficient to impair endothelial function.

Links between risk factors and atherogenesis
In addition to various disease states, endothelium dependent vasodilatation is also impaired in old age,[15] and in young healthy subjects with a family history of premature coronary heart disease and cigarette smoking. The age related endothelial dysfunction may partially explain the increased cardiovascular risk in the elderly. In asymptomatic young smokers, impairment of endothelium dependent vasodilatation is reversible with smoking cessation. It may be that tobacco has a direct toxic effect on the vascular endothelium. Additionally, there is growing evidence of a link between infection/inflammation and risk of coronary heart disease. A recent study showed that acute systemic inflammation induced by vaccination causes impaired endothelium dependent vasodilatation in both resistance and conduit vessels. Thus various effects on the L-arginine: nitric oxide pathway exerted by hypertension, diabetes, hyperlipidaemia, hyperhomocysteinaemia, infection/inflammation, aging, cigarette smoking, and family history of coronary heart disease may form a link between risk factors and predisposition to atherogenesis or acute events.

Alteration of the L-arginine: nitric oxide pathway in diseases: potential mechanisms

---

The involvement of the L-arginine: nitric oxide pathway in disease states is complex and it can be altered in several ways.

Reduced nitric oxide production
Deficiency of NOS co-factor
Several conditions are associated with NOS co-factor deficiency which may contribute to endothelial dysfunction. For instance, insulin resistance is associated with deficiency of the essential co-factor BH_4, resulting in impaired vascular relaxation. Additionally, chronic cigarette smoking contributes to depletion of BH_4 resulting in decreased nitric oxide synthesis, and supplementation of this co-factor restores endothelial function in chronic smokers. In hypercholesterolaemia, impaired endothelium dependent vasodilatation can also be restored with BH_4 supplementation, suggesting that BH_4 deficiency plays an important role in impaired vascular function in these conditions.

Role of endogenous inhibitors of NOS
Overproduction of endogenous inhibitors of NOS in certain disease states may contribute to reduced nitric oxide synthesis (fig 25.4). Asymmetric and symmetric dimethylarginine (ADMA and SDMA) have been identified in human plasma. ADMA has properties similar to L-NMMA. It is synthesised by the human endothelial cells from arginine and is metabolised to citrulline before excretion into the urine (fig 25.4). The enzyme responsible for ADMA metabolism in the human vascular endothelial cells is dimethylarginine dimethylaminohydrolase of which two isoforms

(DDAH I and II) have been identified, sequenced, and cloned.[16] Circulating ADMA is increased in certain disease states. This includes animal models of hypertension, diabetes, hypercholesterolaemia, and atherosclerosis. In humans, raised ADMA concentrations were found in chronic renal failure,[17] childhood hypertension, pre-eclampsia, thrombotic microangiopathy, hypercholesterolaemia, and atherosclerosis. The mechanism whereby various disease states are associated with increased ADMA concentrations remains unclear but may involve alteration in DDAH activity, and this may be an important enzyme in atherogenesis. Accumulation of ADMA would be expected to enhance atherogenesis through loss of nitric oxide.

Reduced nitric oxide bioavailability
Role of oxidative stress
Even with adequate production, nitric oxide may not reach its biological targets (vascular smooth muscle and circulating cells) to exert its effect because of the lack of its bioavailability. For example, in hyperlipidaemia, excess LDL synthesis increases the formation of oxidised LDL. The resultant increase of oxidative stress enhances nitric oxide destruction, thereby reducing its biological effects. In atherosclerotic rabbit aorta, despite a threefold increase in total nitric oxide synthesis compared to normal rabbits, there is notably impaired endothelium dependent vasodilatation. This impaired vascular response can be partially restored following treatment with superoxide dismutase, suggesting that superoxide induced nitric oxide inactivation plays a major role. In humans, hypertriglyceridaemia with or without diabetes may have greater potential than cholesterol to increase superoxide production by leucocytes. Other atherogenic factors such as free fatty acids and low concentrations of high density lipoprotein also increase oxidative stress, contributing to reduced nitric oxide bioavailability. In addition to the associated atherogenic phenotype and oxidative stress, hyperglycaemia per se increases free radical production through increased arachidonic acid metabolism.

In human aortic endothelial cells, although prolonged exposure to high glucose concentration causes increased eNOS expression, it also

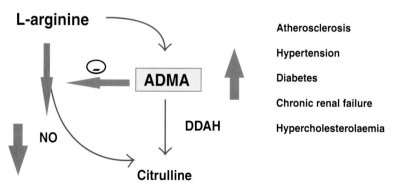

Figure 25.4. Asymmetric dimethylarginine (ADMA) is synthesised from L-arginine by protein methylase I and subsequently metabolised by dimethylarginine dimethylaminohydrolase (DDAH) yielding citrulline. ADMA acts as an endogenous inhibitor of nitric oxide (NO) synthesis and its concentration is increased in certain disease states, possibly as a result of decreased DDAH actions.

leads to a concomitant increase in superoxide anion production (probably from NADH/NADPH oxidase) resulting in nitric oxide inactivation. Oxidative stress may also be a key mechanism for endothelial dysfunction in hyperhomocysteinaemia. Studies in vitro and in animals suggest that elevation of homocysteine enhances lipid peroxidation, which may contribute to impaired endothelium dependent vasodilatation. This potential mechanism is supported by the findings that the antioxidants folic acid and vitamin C rapidly reverse the impaired endothelium dependent vasodilatation without reducing the raised homocysteine concentrations. Similar improvement in endothelial function in type 2 diabetes with antioxidants such as vitamin E have also been observed, suggesting yet again the central role of oxidative stress in endothelial dysfunction under various pathophysiological conditions.

Advanced glycation endproducts
Accumulation of advanced glycation endproducts (AGEs)—the product of non-enzymatic glycation and crosslinking of collagen protein in sustained hyperglycaemia—may lead to quenching (or inactivation) of nitric oxide in diabetes. In experimentally induced diabetic rats, there is in vitro and in vivo evidence that reactive intermediates resulting from glycation quench nitric oxide rapidly. Furthermore, impairment of endothelium dependent vasodilatation in diabetic rats can be partially restored by aminoguanidine, an inhibitor of AGEs formation

Diminished vascular smooth muscle sensitivity

Vascular smooth muscle sensitivity may be decreased even with adequate nitric oxide supply. In human vascular studies, nitrovasodilators or nitric oxide donors (such as glyceryl trinitrate or sodium nitroprusside) have frequently been used as a control for agonist stimulated endothelium dependent vasodilatation. These agents act directly upon vascular smooth muscle and resultant vasodilatation is endothelium independent. There is evidence to suggest that vascular smooth muscle sensitivity to nitric oxide is reduced in diabetes and hyperglycaemia interferes with nitric oxide induced guanylate cyclase activation in vitro. Consistent with this finding, impaired vascular response to nitric oxide donors in vivo have been demonstrated in patients with type 1 diabetes.

Overproduction of nitric oxide in sepsis

Bacterial endotoxin and certain proinflammatory cytokines can lead to profound vasodilatation and decreased vasopressor responsiveness—the main clinical features of septic shock. These cardiovascular effects result from excessive nitric oxide production thought to be caused by induction of iNOS.

Under normal physiological conditions, iNOS is not expressed in the vasculature. Exposure to bacterial lipopolysaccharide or proinflammatory cytokines stimulate iNOS expression. In experimental animals, administration of tumour necrosis factor α (TNFα) in doses similar to those produced endogenously during endotoxaemia rapidly results in a fall in arterial pressure, and longer exposure to TNFα and interleukin-1β (IL-1β) in vitro leads to hyporesponsiveness to vasopressors.

Several animal studies provide evidence for iNOS involvement in the pathogenesis of sepsis. Administration of bacterial lipopolysaccharide to mice causes an increase in nitrite concentration, which is attenuated by a selective iNOS inhibitor. Moreover, selective inhibition of iNOS greatly increases vascular catecholamine reactivity in experimental mice with sepsis but not in control mice. Studies in mice genetically engineered to lack the gene for iNOS also confirm the role of this isoform in septic vasodilatation. In wild type mice, treatment of carotid arteries with lipopolysaccharide leads to impaired constrictor responses which is improved with selective iNOS inhibitors. In contrast, lipopolysaccharide treatment causes no impairment of vasoconstrictor responses in carotid arteries from iNOS deficient mice.

In human sepsis the evidence for iNOS involvement has been less consistent. Some studies have suggested an increased iNOS activity—for example, in urinary leucocytes from patients with urinary tract infection, in alveolar macrophages from patients with acute respiratory distress syndrome following sepsis, and in peripheral blood mononuclear cells and macrophages isolated from putrescent muscle areas in patients with cellulitis. However, other studies have suggested the involvement of eNOS rather than iNOS in human sepsis. In an in vitro study using human umbilical vein endothelial cells cultured with IL-1β and TNFα, the resultant increase in nitric oxide production was shown to originate from eNOS as a result of activation of guanosine triphosphate cyclohydrolase (GTPCH-I), the rate limiting enzyme responsible for the synthesis of BH_4. Similar findings have recently been shown in human veins in vivo. While it is clear that overproduction of nitric oxide contributes to vasodilatation in human sepsis,[18] the molecular mechanisms and isoform of NOS activated are unclear. It is also not known whether inhibition of nitric oxide generation is beneficial. Expression of iNOS in active atherosclerotic plaques has also been detected. It is possible that this iNOS contributes to tissue damage or other features of plaque development or stability.

Therapeutic possibilities

L-arginine
Supplementation of the nitric oxide substrate L-arginine has beneficial effects in certain conditions in laboratory animals and humans. Dietary L-arginine for 10 weeks has been shown to prevent intimal thickening in the

coronary arteries and attenuates platelet reactivity in hypercholesterolaemic rabbits. Furthermore, oral L-arginine administration reduces neointimal formation following balloon catheter induced injury in both hypercholesterolaemic and normocholesterolaemic rabbit models. In humans, dietary L-arginine supplementation reduces the increased platelet reactivity in hypercholesterolaemic subjects. Additionally, intravenous L-arginine infusion reduces peripheral vascular resistance and decreases both systolic and diastolic blood pressure, at least in some studies, improves endothelium dependent coronary vasodilatation in response to intracoronary acetylcholine in hypercholesterolaemic subjects,[9] and improves blood flow in critical lower limb ischaemia.

The arginine paradox

The beneficial effects of exogenous L-arginine to the vasculature in various disease states with increased plasma nitrate and cGMP concentrations during L-arginine administration suggest provision of excess L-arginine supply can stimulate NOS activity. However, it is perplexing that extracellular arginine administration should drive nitric oxide production since the intracellular arginine concentrations are always available in great excess of the needs of NOS, a phenomenon known as the "arginine paradox". This was first demonstrated in hypercholesterolaemic rabbits[19] and has also been observed in patients with pulmonary hypertension. Several explanations have been proposed to account for this paradox. Firstly, it is possible that the endogenous inhibitor of NOS, ADMA, might antagonise the normal intracellular concentrations of L-arginine, and additional arginine supplementation is required to overcome a functional defect of NOS substrate. Secondly, since eNOS is preferentially localised to specific intracellular sites known as caveolae, local concentration of L-arginine in this microenvironment may differ considerably from that within the endothelial cell. It remains unclear how specific localisation of eNOS by caveolae might affect local substrate availability, but the mechanism may involve the co-localisation of eNOS with certain arginine transporters (for example, cationic amino acid transporter-1). The formation of such a caveolar complex seems to facilitate arginine delivery to eNOS.

It is also important to recognise that the vasodilatory effects of L-arginine are not all mediated directly by nitric oxide. L-arginine may inhibit peripheral sympathetic tone leading to vasodilatation via its metabolite, agmatine, which stimulates central α_2 adrenoceptors. Additionally, arginine also stimulates the release of several other hormones such as glucagon, prolactin, and growth hormone which may account for its vasodilatory action. Furthermore, many of the vascular and other actions of L-arginine are shared by its stereoisomer, D-arginine, which is not a substrate for NOS. The complex mechanisms whereby L-arginine appears to improve cardiovascular function in some conditions merits further investigation.

Nitrovasodilators/nitric oxide donors

Nitrovasodilators such as amyl nitrite, glyceryl trinitrate, sodium nitroprusside, and molsidomine are all pro-drugs and exert their pharmacological effects after metabolism to nitric oxide. Hence they are termed "nitric oxide donor". Based on their venodilatory properties, nitrovasodilators have conventionally been used for the treatment of cardiac failure and angina. Nitrosoglutathione, a compound in the class of nitrosothiols, has been studied extensively in humans. It has profound antiplatelet effects and more balanced arterial and venous vasodilatory effects than organic nitrates. Nitrosoglutathione inhibits platelet activation in the coronary artery following angioplasty and in coronary bypass grafts. Hence, nitrosothiols are potential pharmacological agents in the treatment of nitric oxide deficient conditions, and it is possible that novel nitric oxide donors could be developed that differ greatly from existing drugs.

Inhalation of nitric oxide

Administration of nitric oxide as inhalation treatment has been shown to improve several conditions affecting the pulmonary vasculature, including persistent pulmonary hypertension of the newborn, pulmonary hypertension secondary to chronic hypoxia, and adult respiratory distress syndrome (ARDS). In ARDS, selective delivery of nitric oxide to the pulmonary vasculature reduces the pulmonary arterial pressure and increases arterial oxygenation by improving the matching of ventilation with perfusion. As the nitric oxide is rapidly inactivated by haemoglobin, inhalation of nitric oxide gas does not cause systemic vasodilatation. However, whether this form of nitric oxide treatment will improve survival in patients with ARDS remains to be determined by randomised controlled clinical trials. It does have potential adverse effects such as pulmonary oedema and methaemoglobinaemia. There are as yet no clear guidelines regarding the effective dose of inhaled nitric oxide for the above pulmonary conditions.

Antioxidants

Since oxidative stress has been strongly implicated in endothelial dysfunction, numerous studies have examined the role of antioxidants in vascular function and in the prevention of cardiovascular disease. Intrabrachial administration of ascorbic acid (vitamin C) improves endothelium dependent vasodilatation in patients with type 2 diabetes, smokers, patients with hypercholesterolaemia, and patients with heart failure. Similarly, oral administration of ascorbic acid in patients with coronary heart disease also improves flow mediated vasodilatation. This beneficial effect has been shown to occur rapidly after two hours and can be sustained for 30 days. Furthermore, intravenous infusion of ascorbic acid improved endothelium dependent vasodilatation in epicardial arteries in hypertensive patients without

Summary

- Endothelium derived nitric oxide has important antiatherogenic properties:
  - enhancement of vasodilatation
  - inhibition of platelet aggregation
  - inhibition of leucocyte migration
  - inhibition of smooth muscle proliferation and migration
  - inhibition of adhesion molecule activation and expression
  - anti-oxidant

- Three distinct nitric oxide synthase isoforms exist which all have a role in vascular control under different conditions

- Reduced nitric oxide synthesis or defective nitric oxide activities predispose to atherosclerosis

- Different disease processes and risk factors affects the L-arginine–nitric oxide pathway via different mechanisms:
  - decreased synthesis
  - decreased co-factor availability
  - decreased enzyme expression/activity
  - increased endogenous nitric oxide synthase inhibitors
  - decreased nitric oxide bioavailability
  - decreased vascular smooth muscle sensitivity to nitric oxide

- Understanding these mechanisms in diseases may help therapeutic strategies in prevention of atherosclerosis

coronary heart disease. In patients with coronary heart disease, intracoronary co-infusion of vitamin C with L-arginine causes greatly increased vasodilatation. Despite these observations, not all experiments have shown beneficial effects and further studies are required. In addition, agents such as vitamin C can produce pro-oxidant effects in some circumstances.

Gene transfer

The direct transfer of NOS isoform genes to the vessel wall alters vasomotor function and may have a role in the treatment of cardiovascular diseases.[20] This approach has been shown to be effective in a variety of animal models of vascular disease. Vascular gene therapy of eNOS delivered to specific tissues enhances nitric oxide production at the site of interest. In 1995, NOS gene transfer was first reported when eNOS cDNA, in a complex with the haemagglutinating virus of Japan, was delivered to rat carotid arteries intraluminally following balloon injury. This resulted in a pronounced reduction in neointima formation at 14 days. Shortly after, similar results were confirmed by other research groups in iliac and coronary arteries and vein grafts. Gene therapy has also been extended from local to systemic delivery. Delivery of a single injection of naked eNOS cDNA into the systemic circulation through the tail vein of spontaneously hypertensive rats resulted in increased production and excretion of cGMP and nitrite/nitrate, and was associated with a significant reduction in systolic blood pressure lasting up to 12 weeks.

NOS inhibitors

Inhibition of iNOS has been shown to improve nitric oxide mediated haemodynamic changes in experimental models of septic shock.[18]

Intravenous administration of the arginine analogue L-NMMA reverses the decrease in peripheral vascular resistance and fall in arterial blood pressure in endotoxaemic dogs. The same effects with L-NMMA have also been confirmed in humans in a randomised, double blind, placebo controlled trial.[18] A potential pitfall in this therapeutic strategy is that none of the currently available NOS inhibitors are specific for the excess nitric oxide causing pathophysiology, and may therefore lead to potential hazardous effects, by also inhibiting "physiological" nitric oxide. Indeed, both pulmonary hypertension and reduced cardiac output have been reported following NOS inhibition. Future drug development in this area should focus on NOS isoform specificity as well as the degree of inhibition required in order to produce an optimal pharmacological effect.

Conclusions

Nitric oxide is a major player in cardiovascular physiology and pharmacology. Its release from endothelium exerts a tonic hypotensive, antiplatelet, antiatherogenic influence in the arterial tree. Several common cardiovascular disease states or risk factors impair nitric oxide synthesis, increase nitric oxide destruction or affect the ability of cells to respond to this mediator. The net effect is to enhance vascular tone and reactivity and predispose to atherosclerosis. Clinicians already use drugs that either mimic nitric oxide (nitric oxide donors) or enhance its endogenous production (for example, by lowering blood pressure or serum cholesterol). In contrast, overproduction of nitric oxide is an important mechanism of inflammatory vasodilatation. Over the next few years a new generation of drugs will emerge that specifically modify nitric oxide production or mimic its action. Indeed, the first such drug is sildenafil which blocks the phosphodiesterase that degrades cGMP and thereby acts as an amplifier of nitric oxide signalling (fig 25.1). Diagnostic tests based on early assessment of endothelial function may also become part of cardiovascular risk stratification or assessment of novel therapeutics.

This work is supported by the British Heart Foundation.

1. **Furchgott RF, Zawadski JV.** The obligatory role of endothelial cells in the relaxation of arterial smooth muscle by acetylcholine. *Nature* 1980;**288**:373–6.
- *The original paper describing the importance of endothelium in acetylcholine induced vasorelaxation. Furchgott was the recipient of the 1998 Nobel prize in medicine.*

2. **Palmer RMJ, Ferrige AG, Moncada S.** Nitric oxide release accounts for the biological activity of endothelial-derived relaxing factor. *Nature* 1987;**327**:524–6.
- *Novel finding that endothelial derived relaxing factor is nitric oxide.*

3. **Ignarro LJ, Buga GM, Wood KS,** *et al.* Endothelium-derived relaxing factor produced and released from artery and vein is nitric oxide. *Proc Natl Acad Sci USA* 1987;**84** 9265–9.
- *Novel finding that endothelial derived relaxing factor is nitric oxide. Published in the same year as reference 2.*

4. **Moncada S, Higgs EA.** The L-arginine-nitric oxide pathway. *N Engl J Med* 1993;**329**:2002–12.
- *Review article describing in detail the biochemical nitric oxide pathway.*

182

5. **Xu W, Charles IG, Moncada S,** *et al.* Mapping of the genes encoding human inducible and endothelial nitric oxide synthase (NOS2 and NOS3) to the pericentric region of chromosome 17 and to chromosome 7, respectively. *Genomics* 1994;**21**:419–22.
• *Identification of chromosomes encoding nitric oxide synthase isoforms.*

6. **Cayatte AJ, Palacino JJ, Horten K,** *et al.* Chronic inhibition of nitric oxide production accelerates neointima formation and impairs endothelial function in hypercholesterolemic rabbits. *Arterioscler Thromb* 1994;**14**:753–9.
• *The original animal study which demonstrated the antiatherogenic role of endogenous nitric oxide.*

7. **Vallance P, Collier J, Moncada S.** Effects of endothelium-derived nitric oxide on peripheral arterial tone in man. *Lancet* 1989;ii:997–1000.
• *First experimental evidence showing the key role of nitric oxide in maintaining the resting arterial tone in humans.*

8. **Vallance P, Collier J, Moncada S.** Nitric oxide synthesised from L-arginine mediates endothelium-dependent dilatation in human veins in vivo. *Cardiovasc Res* 1989;**23**:1053–7.
• *Experiment demonstrating the dilatatory property of nitric oxide is not only confined to the arteries.*

9. **Drexler H, Zeiher AM, Meinzer K,** *et al.* Correction of endothelial dysfunction in coronary microcirculation of hypercholesterolemic patients by L-arginine. *Lancet* 1991;**338**:1450–6.
• *Early experiment in humans showing that endothelial dysfunction is reversible with L-arginine supplementation. This paper provides important insight to potential therapeutic strategies targeting the nitric oxide pathway.*

10. **Ludmer P, Selwyn A, Shook TL,** *et al.* Paradoxical vasoconstriction induced by acetylcholine in atherosclerotic coronary arteries. *N Engl J Med* 1986;**315**:1046–51.
• *Angiographic evidence that atherosclerotic coronary arteries constrict in response to the conventional vasodilator, acetylcholine.*

11. **Maguire SM, Nugent AG, McGurk C,** *et al.* Abnormal vascular responses in human chronic cardiac failure is both endothelium dependent and endothelium independent. *Heart* 1998; **80**:141–5.
• *Evidence of impaired endothelium dependent and independent vasodilatation as assessed by venous occlusion plethysmography in non-ACE inhibitor treated chronic heart failure.*

12. **Chowienczyk PJ, Watts GF, Cockcroft JR,** *et al.* Impairment of endothelium-dependent vasodilatation of forearm resistance vessels in hypercholesterolaemia. *Lancet* 1992;**340**:1430–2.
• *This paper provides early evidence that raised cholesterol impairs endothelial function.*

13. **Calver A, Collier J, Moncada S,** *et al.* Effect of local intra-arterial NG-monomethyl-L-arginine in patients with hypertension: the nitric oxide dilator mechanism appears abnormal. *J Hypertens* 1992;**10**:1025–31.
• *Vascular study using plethysmography demonstrating impaired vasoconstrictor response to L-NMMA in forearm resistance vessels of hypertensives.*

14. **Chan NN, Vallance P, Colhoun HM.** Nitric oxide and vascular responses in type 1 diabetes. *Diabetologia* 2000;**43**:137–47.
• *A recent review of the conflicting evidence regarding nitric oxide release and response in type 1 diabetes. Potential mechanisms of defective L-arginine: nitric oxide pathway in diabetes are also discussed.*

15. **Celermajer DS, Sorensen KE, Spiegelhalter DJ,** *et al.* Aging is associated with endothelial dysfunction in healthy men years before the age-related decline in women. *J Am Coll Cardiol* 1994;**24**:471–6.
• *This study showed that endothelial function as assessed by flow-mediated dilatation declines with aging, particularly in males.*

16. **Leiper JM, Santa Maria J, Chubb A,** *et al.* Identification of two human dimethylarginine dimethylaminohydrolases with distinct tissue distributions and homology with microbial arginine deaminases. *Biochem J* 1999;**343**:209–14.
• *Novel discovery of dimethylarginine dimethylaminohydrolases, enzymes responsible for metabolism of the endogenous nitric oxide synthase inhibitor, asymmetrical dimethylarginine (ADMA).*

17. **Vallance P, Leone A, Calver A,** *et al.* Accumulation of an endogenous inhibitor of nitric oxide synthesis in chronic renal failure. *Lancet* 1992;**339**:572–5.
• *Identification of ADMA as an endogenous inhibitor of nitric oxide synthase.*

18. **Petros A, Bennett D, Vallance P.** Effects of nitric oxide synthase inhibitors on hypotension in patients with septic shock. *Lancet* 1991;**338**:1557–8.
• *Evidence of cardiovascular effects of NOS inhibition in treatment in human septic shock.*

19. **Girerd Xj, Hirsch AT, Cooke JP,** *et al.* L-Arginine augments endothelium-dependent vasodilatation in cholesterol-fed rabbits. *Circ Res* 1995;**67**:1301–8.
• *Early animal evidence that arginine supplementation improves nitric oxide production in hypercholesterolaemic rabbits.*

20. **Kibbe M, Billiar T, Tzeng E.** Nitric oxide synthase gene transfer to the vessel wall. *Curr Opin Nephrol Hypertens* 1999;**8**:75–81.
• *Excellent review of the potential role of nitric oxide gene transfer in the treatment of cardiovascular disorders.*

website
extra

Additional references appear on the Heart website

www.heartjnl.com

26 Diabetic heart disease: clinical considerations

Adam D Timmis

Diabetes is one of the most common metabolic disorders, and with our aging, sedentary and increasingly obese population, the number of affected individuals will continue to rise. This will have major implications for cardiological practice since much of the excess morbidity and mortality among diabetic patients is attributable to accelerated atherogenesis. Young diabetics are at particular risk and, by the age of 50 years, 33% of those requiring insulin have died from coronary heart disease. Indeed, 75% of all deaths in patients with diabetes are from this cause. Generally speaking, the management of diabetic patients with heart disease is underpinned by the same evidence base as applies to non-diabetic patients, and it is noteworthy that 15–20% of the patients in most of the landmark clinical trials have been diabetic. Recently, however, trials such as the UKPDS, HOPE, and DIGAMI studies (see below) have identified novel strategies for reducing cardiovascular risk in diabetes. These trials have already had a major impact on cardiological practice, emphasising the prime importance of blood pressure control and converting enzyme inhibition for reducing cardiovascular risk in diabetes, and also the value of insulin treatment for reducing mortality in diabetic myocardial infarction. Additional trials, already in progress, are expected to refine further the cardiovascular management of patients with diabetes in order to provide an effective challenge for a problem that shows no signs of going away.

Diabetes and cardiovascular risk

Three large epidemiological studies have shaped current understanding of the natural history of diabetic heart disease. The Framingham study showed that diabetes increased the relative risk of coronary heart disease by 66% in men and 203% in women followed up for 20 years, after controlling for the effects of age, smoking, blood pressure, and cholesterol.[1] The Whitehall study of male civil servants extended these observations by showing that subclinical glucose intolerance, in addition to frank diabetes, also increased coronary risk.[2] The MRFIT trial, with its very large population of middle aged men, was able to provide more detailed information about the interaction between diabetes and other risk factors in determining coronary risk.[3] This trial confirmed the heightened risk attributable to diabetes, and also the independent effects of serum cholesterol, blood pressure, and smoking in men with and without diabetes. MRFIT showed that in men with diabetes, 12 year cardiovascular mortality was much higher at every level of these major risk factors considered singly and in combination, and that with progressively more unfavourable risk factor status the mortality rate rose much more steeply than in men without diabetes (fig 26.1).

Angina and revascularisation in diabetes

Angina may affect up to 40% of adults with diabetes, although its precise prevalence is hard to deduce from the literature. Symptoms are commonly atypical, perhaps because of abnormalities in the perception of angina caused by autonomic neuropathy, and the physician should retain a low threshold for non-invasive investigation. A positive stress test associated with atypical symptoms in the diabetic patient indicates a high probability of underlying coronary disease and the need for specific antianginal treatment, often with additional angiographic assessment. The disease is typically diffuse, affecting both proximal and distal coronary segments (angiographic observations not always borne out by pathological studies), and this has the potential to intensify ischaemia.

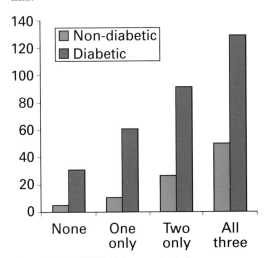

Figure 26.1. MRFIT trial: age adjusted cardiovascular disease death rates (per 10 000 person years) by presence of number of risk factors in men with and without diabetes. Reproduced from Stamler et al[3] with permission of American Diabetes Association.

> **Revascularisation in diabetes**
>
> - Diffuse and distal disease makes revascularisation technically more demanding
>
> - Reduced survival after coronary artery bypass graft (CABG) and percutaneous transluminal coronary angioplasty (PTCA)
>
> - Increased restenosis rates after PTCA
>
> - BARI data indicate that for most diabetics CABG is preferable to PTCA
>
> - Recent EPISTENT data point to an important role for stenting and IIb/IIIa receptor blockers in diabetic patients undergoing PTCA

There is no evidence of reduced responsiveness to medical treatment in patients with diabetes, which should be with nitrates and β blockers in the first instance with the addition of calcium channel blockers or potassium channel openers in more resistant cases. However, diffuse disease makes revascularisation by angioplasty or bypass surgery more difficult and more hazardous. Indeed, diabetes has long been recognised as one of the major independent predictors of long term mortality after surgery. The results of angioplasty also tend to be less good in diabetic compared with non-diabetic patients. Again, diffuse disease makes for technically more difficult angioplasty procedures and, in addition, restenosis rates are consistently higher. In the recent BARI trial of angioplasty versus bypass surgery, subgroup analysis showed that patients with diabetes randomised to angioplasty had a significantly worse five year survival than those randomised to bypass surgery. The investigators concluded that for most diabetics requiring revascularisation coronary bypass surgery was preferable to angioplasty.[4] Nevertheless, BARI antedated the stenting era and recently a predefined subgroup analysis from the EPISTENT trial showed that angioplasty and stenting combined with infusion of abciximab (a glycoprotein IIb/IIIa receptor inhibitor) improves the long term outcome in diabetic patients substantially, with a six month incidence of ischaemic end points comparable to that achieved in non-diabetic patients.[5] The data suggest, therefore, that stenting and IIb/IIIa receptor blockade may have an important role in diabetic angioplasty.

Acute myocardial infarction in diabetes

Framingham data have shown that the risk of acute myocardial infarction is 50% greater in diabetic men and 150% greater in diabetic women than in non-diabetic individuals.[1] Indeed, acute myocardial infarction accounts for 30% of all diabetic deaths. This propensity to myocardial infarction presumably reflects the increased prevalence of coronary artery disease in diabetes, with associated hypertension predisposing to plaque rupture. Moreover, thrombotic responses to plaque rupture are likely to be exaggerated in diabetes because of haematological abnormalities, particularly increased platelet activation.

It has long been recognised that diabetics are prone to "silent" myocardial infarction and this presumably reflects impaired perception of ischaemic cardiac pain caused by autonomic neuropathy. Thus, in diabetes, acute myocardial infarction is silent or presents with atypical symptoms in 32–42% of cases compared with 6–15% of non-diabetic infarcts. This is disadvantageous because it has the potential to delay access to emergency facilities early after coronary events, increasing the risk of out-of-hospital sudden death and morbid complications of myocardial infarction, particularly cardiogenic shock. Abnormalities of circadian and seasonal rhythms of acute myocardial infarction, with attenuation of the morning and winter peaks, may also reflect autonomic dysfunction because these rhythms are largely driven by parallel changes in sympathovagal activity. The consequences of this to the patient with diabetes are unclear.

All the major complications of myocardial infarction occur more commonly in diabetes, particularly heart failure which affects nearly 50% of diabetics compared with under 30% of non-diabetics (fig 26.2). This difference is not accounted for by infarct size but may reflect the more severe and diffuse disease in diabetes that limits coronary reserve and intensifies ischaemia in non-infarcted segments by a watershed effect.[6] Diabetes specific myocardial disease may also have a role. Thus, contractile dysfunction remote from the infarct zone is commonly reported in diabetic myocardial infarction.[6] Since heart failure is one of the major determinants of outcome, it is little surprise that both hospital and long term mortality rates are increased in patients with diabetes. In our own coronary care unit, the 30 day and 12 month mortality rates (95% confidence intervals) for patients with diabetes are 19.2% (15.3% to 23.1%) and 26.6% (22.2% to 31.1%), compared with 12.7% (10.6% to 14.8%) and 19.1% (16.6% to 21.6%) for patients without diabetes.

Patients with acute myocardial infarction who have diabetes, or an admission blood glucose concentration ≤ 11.0 mmol/l, should receive insulin and glucose infusion for at least 24 hours based on the findings of the DIGAMI investigators who showed that this significantly improves survival.[7] Subcutaneous insulin treatment continued for at least three months in this study, a regimen that many units find too unwieldy to apply in practice, largely because of the unwillingness of many patients with mild diabetes to self inject. Certainly treatment during the acute phase of infarction is likely to be particularly beneficial, not only for improving left ventricular function, but also for reducing infarct size and lethal complications, since the shift to anaerobic glucose metabolism that occurs in the myocardium during acute ischaemia is an insulin

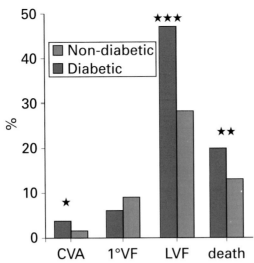

Figure 26.2. Complications of acute myocardial infarction in diabetic and non-diabetic patients (n = 1929). CVA, cerebrovascular accident; 1° VF, primary ventricular fibrillation; LVF, left ventricular failure. *p < 0.05; **p < 0.01; ***p < 0.001. Unpublished data from the Newham General Hospital coronary care unit database.

dependent adjustment that may be deficient in diabetes because of absolute or relative lack of insulin.[8]

In other respects the treatment of myocardial infarction in patients with diabetes should be the same as in those without—responses to thrombolytic treatment and the benefits of secondary prevention being similar in the two groups. The TAMI investigators, for example, reported that patency rates of the infarct related artery 90 minutes after thrombolytic treatment were almost identical in patients with and without diabetes.[6] Similarly, diabetes does not appear to affect the benefits of aspirin, or β blockers and statins which provide protection against recurrent infarction and death comparable to that seen in patients without diabetes. Angiotensin converting enzyme (ACE) inhibitors, in particular, have a special role and should be given to all diabetic patients with acute myocardial infarction, not only because of the heightened risk of left ventricular failure, for which these drugs are of proven benefit, but also because of the protection they afford against microvascular complications.

Sudden death in diabetes

Patients with diabetes are at increased risk of sudden death, and this is not always attributable to complications of plaque events. There is considerable evidence that autonomic neuropathy plays an important pathophysiological role, through prolongation of QT interval and selective reductions in vagal function (increasing sympathetic activity), both of which may increase susceptibility to lethal arrhythmias.[9][10] In addition, altered perception of ischaemic cardiac pain may deprive diabetic patients of the signal to stop exercising, allowing ischaemia to intensify to the point that arrhythmias are triggered.[11] Alterations in pain perception may also prevent the diabetic patient from seeking medical attention in the event of acute

coronary syndromes or lead to inappropriate triage decisions in the emergency room, such that access to defibrillators is denied and specific treatment delayed. This emphasises the importance of retaining low diagnostic thresholds for coronary heart disease in the diabetic patient presenting with atypical symptoms. It also emphasises the importance of strict glycaemic control in diabetes, although whether this indeed protects against neuropathy is unclear.

Heart failure in diabetes

Over 20 years ago, the Framingham investigators reported that the annual incidence of heart failure in diabetic men and women was substantially greater across all age groups than in non-diabetic individuals, even after controlling for underlying coronary and rheumatic heart disease. They concluded that diabetes itself might predispose to heart failure independently of concurrent coronary or rheumatic heart disease. At about the same time postmortem reports appeared on diabetics with heart failure describing normal coronary arteries and heart valves. Histology, however, may reveal a range of abnormalities including myocyte hypertrophy, interstitial fibrosis, increased periodic acid-Schiff (PAS) positive material, and intramyocardial microangiopathy. These are largely indistinguishable from changes found in hypertensive left ventricular disease and emphasise the importance of effective antihypertensive treatment as reported in UKPDS (see below). In further studies, analysis of systolic time intervals provided evidence of both systolic and diastolic left ventricular dysfunction in diabetic individuals in whom there was no clinical evidence of coronary artery disease. Taken together these epidemiological, pathological, and haemodynamic data provide the evidence base for diabetes specific myocardial disease, commonly called "diabetic cardiomyopathy". The pathogenesis is unclear, although possible mechanisms include the synergistic impact of hypertension plus chronic derangement of myocardial metabolism, with increased free fatty acid oxidation and decreased glucose utilisation.[12]

While the existence and clinical importance of diabetic cardiomyopathy is fairly well established, it must be emphasised that coronary heart disease is considerably more important as a cause of heart failure in the patient with diabetes. Certainly some of the epidemiological data summarised above may have been distorted by coexisting but asymptomatic coronary heart disease, and the pathological data do not rule out the possibility of cardiomyopathy as a coincidental diagnosis or as a response to hypertension. In practical terms, however, the distinction is largely unimportant, except insofar as it affects revascularisation decisions, since treatment strategies are unaffected and are the same as for non-diabetic patients with heart failure. Thus, control of provocative factors, particularly arrhythmias and hypertension,

Evidence for diabetic cardiomyopathy

- Pathological evidence
  - in 1972, postmortem findings in diabetics with congestive cardiac failure (CCF) include: myocyte atrophy, interstitial fibrosis, increased PAS positive material, and intramyocardial microangiopathy
  - depletion of myocardial catecholamines

- Epidemiological evidence
  - increased risk of CCF in diabetes, not all explained by coronary heart disease
  - diabetics with coronary artery disease more likely to be hospitalised with CCF than non-diabetics (SOLVD)

- Haemodynamic evidence
  - non-invasive evidence of systolic and diastolic dysfunction

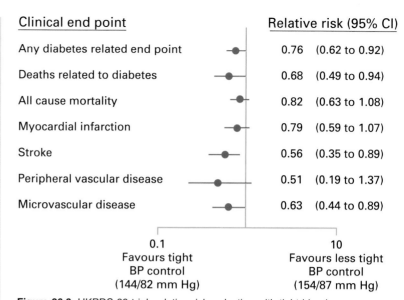

Figure 26.3. UKPDS 38 trial: relative risk reduction with tight blood pressure control.[13]

remains essential and conventional treatment should be applied for correcting fluid retention, increasing exercise capacity, and improving prognosis. Diuretics may adversely influence metabolic control in diabetes but are mandatory for treatment of peripheral oedema and pulmonary congestion. The efficacy of ACE inhibition is undiminished in diabetes, judging by subgroup analyses of the SOLVD prevention and treatment trials, but the heightened risk of renal artery stenosis demands caution when initiating treatment. β Blockers are also recommended, although this is based on generalisation from randomised trials rather than specific data for patients with diabetes.

Risk factor modification for protecting against coronary heart disease in diabetes

Based on their data, the MRFIT investigators recommended "vigorous sustained intervention in people with diabetes to control blood pressure, lower serum cholesterol, and abolish cigarette smoking". These recommendations remain central to the cardiovascular management of diabetes, and their value for primary and secondary prevention has been confirmed in randomised trials. Disappointingly, however, there is not yet clear evidence that the recommendation for more vigorous risk factor modification in diabetes leads to extra protection against coronary heart disease beyond that achieved in non-diabetic individuals, although important protection against microvascular complications (retinopathy, renal disease) does occur. Nevertheless, as our practice evolves from single to multifactorial risk assessment, in which an individual's absolute coronary risk can be readily assessed from simple colour coded charts, the clinical impact of risk factor modification can be expected to increase, particularly with the recent availability of charts for use in men and women with diabetes.

Blood pressure

Hypertension commonly occurs in type 2 diabetes, and contributes importantly to the heightened risk of cardiovascular, renal, and retinal disease. By the age of 50 years more than 40% of patients with type 2 diabetes are hypertensive, the proportion rising to 60% by the age of 75 years. Subgroup analyses of large trials have suggested that the benefits of treating hypertension apply equally to diabetic and non-diabetic patients, a suggestion emphatically confirmed in the hypertensive cohort of UKPDS.[13] Comparison of patients allocated either to tight blood pressure control (< 150/85 mm Hg) using captopril or atenolol, or to less tight control showed that tight control for 8.4 years was associated with significant reduction in the risk of death related to diabetes, and with reductions in all microvascular endpoints. Predictably, reductions in the risk of heart failure and stroke also occurred, but the 21% reduction in the risk of myocardial infarction was not significant (fig 26.3). The HOT study also reported reductions in myocardial infarction in patients treated to a target diastolic blood pressure of ≤ 80 mm Hg compared to targets of ≤ 85 or ≤ 90 mm Hg, but again the changes were not significant. Based largely on these recent trial data, a target blood pressure of < 130 mm Hg systolic and < 80 mm Hg diastolic is now recommended for diabetic patients. Lower targets might be appropriate for diabetic patients with microalbuminuria, in whom considerable data support the use of ACE inhibitors for protecting against deterioration of renal function, a beneficial effect that occurs independently of blood pressure reduction. However, UKPDS reported that captopril or atenolol were similarly effective in reducing the incidence of diabetic complications, and concluded that for most patients blood pressure reduction itself is more important than the agent used.[14]

Lipid modification with fibrates and statins

Hypertriglyceridaemia with reductions in high density lipoprotein (HDL) cholesterol are the typical abnormalities detected on routine laboratory testing in type 2 diabetes. This provides a logic for fibrate treatment in addition to exercise and weight reduction. The Helsinki study suggested a trend towards reduced coronary events in diabetic patients treated with gemfibrozil for five years, but data from other fibrate studies have generally been inconclusive. This contrasts with subgroup analyses of the major statin trials which have shown convincingly that hypercholesterolaemic diabetic patients gain similar relative benefit as non-diabetic patients in the secondary prevention of coronary artery disease, and greater absolute benefit because of their higher event rate. Thus, vigorous treatment of all diabetics with known atherosclerotic disease to achieve a total cholesterol of < 5.0 mmol/l (low density lipoprotein (LDL) cholesterol < 3.0 mmol/l) is recommended, together with correction of hypertriglyceridaemia using additional fibrate treatment, as necessary, In diabetic patients without overt atherosclerotic disease, an absolute risk ⩾ 30% of developing coronary heart disease over the next 10 years, as deduced from colour coded risk prediction charts, is sufficiently high to justify drug treatment.

Smoking

Observational data suggest that the risk of myocardial infarction is reduced by up to 50% within one year of quitting smoking, with favourable effects on mortality maintained for up to 10 years. Since the cardiac risk attributable to smoking is magnified considerably in diabetes, as indeed is the risk attributable to all other risk factors, the benefits of quitting are likely to be as great, if not greater, in diabetic then non-diabetic patients.

Glycaemic control for protecting against coronary heart disease in diabetes

---

Strict glycaemic control has long been recommended in diabetes, based on epidemiological surveys that have reported more favourable clinical outcomes for groups with lower plasma glucose and glycosylated haemoglobin concentrations. However, whether these more favourable outcomes reflected less severe underlying disease rather than the benefits of glycaemic control remained unresolved until publication of UKPDS in which 3867 newly diagnosed patients with type 2 diabetes were randomly assigned to an intensive (sulfonylurea or insulin) or conventional treatment policy.[15] After follow up for 10 years, glycosylated haemoglobin concentrations in the two groups were 7.0% and 7.9%, respectively, a difference of only 11%. Nevertheless, this trial confirmed the close relation between glycaemia and the risk of microvascular and macrovascular complications, including coronary heart disease, and also dispelled concerns about the potential adverse cardiovascular effects of sulfonylureas. Importantly, in the group randomised to intense glycaemic control, significant protection against microvascular complications occurred although macrovascular complications were not similarly affected, the 16% reduction in the risk of myocardial infarction being of only borderline significance. In short, therefore, UKPDS has confirmed the importance of strict glycaemic control (glycosylated haemoglobin 7% or lower) for protection against microvascular complications of diabetes. It is tempting to speculate that more substantial protection against macrovascular end points might have occurred had there been greater differences in glycaemic control (as reflected by glycosylated haemoglobin) between the intensive and conventional treatment groups.

Other strategies for protecting against coronary heart disease in diabetes

---

Antiplatelet treatment

An overview of randomised trials has shown that the benefits of antiplatelet treatment for secondary prevention of coronary heart disease are similar for groups with and without diabetes. Thus patients with diabetic coronary heart disease should all receive a daily aspirin. Though not strictly evidence based, aspirin is now recommended for diabetic adults without clinical manifestations of atheromatous disease (primary prevention) since platelet dysfunction is common and the prevalence of subclinical disease high. Evidence for non-aspirin platelet inhibitors in diabetic subgroups is often unavailable, but it is reasonable to assume that the potential benefits of glycoprotein IIb/IIIa receptor antagonists in non-ST elevation coronary syndromes apply equally to patients with diabetes. At present the proven benefit of these drugs is largely restricted to the catheter laboratory where they have a vital role in high risk angioplasty, particularly as an adjunct to coronary stenting,[5] reducing the rate of adverse events in patients with diabetes to a level comparable to that of patients without diabetes (see above).

ACE inhibition

ACE inhibition protects against the development of atherosclerotic plaque in experimental animals fed lipid rich diets. Potential for similar benefit in humans was reported by the TREND investigators who showed that treatment with quinapril improved coronary endothelial function in patients with coronary disease.[16] This potential has now been confirmed by the HOPE study in which significant reductions in the risk of the combined primary outcome (death, myocardial infarction, and stroke) occurred in high risk patients randomised to treatment with ramipril.[17] Among these high risk patients were 3577 with diabetes who had a previous cardiac event or at least one other cardiovascular risk factor, but not heart failure or proteinuria. Within this diabetic subgroup, randomisation to ramipril reduced the risk of the combined primary outcome by 25%, with an additional reduction in the risk of overt nephropathy.[18] These important findings are

188

Trial acronyms

BARI: Bypass Angioplasty Revascularization Investigation

DIGAMI: Diabetes Mellitus, Insulin Glucose Infusion in Acute Myocardial Infarction

EPISTENT: Evaluation of Platelet IIb/IIIa Inhibitor for Stenting Trial

HOPE: Heart Outcomes Prevention Evaluation

HOT: Hypertension Optimal Treatment

MRFIT: Multiple Risk Factor Intervention Trial

SOLVD: Studies Of Left Ventricular Dysfunction

TAMI: Thrombolysis and Angioplasty in Myocardial Infarction

TREND: Trial on Reversing ENdothelial Dysfunction

UKPDS: United Kingdom Prospective Diabetes Study

now having a major impact on the management of diabetes, providing indications for ACE inhibition with ramipril in any diabetic patient with multiple risk factors, established vascular disease, or microalbuminuria.

Screening for coronary heart disease in diabetes

The prevalence of subclinical coronary artery disease in the general population is high, but is almost certainly higher in the diabetic population because of accelerated atherosclerosis. Thus, people with diabetes have a long term rate of myocardial infarction and cardiovascular death comparable to that of non-diabetic patients with a documented history of myocardial infarction. Subclinical disease is commonly non-obstructive because of outward remodelling of the coronary artery. However, obstructive disease may also be clinically silent, particularly in diabetes when autonomic neuropathy may interfere with the perception of cardiac pain such that symptoms take longer to develop after the onset of myocardial ischaemia (prolonged anginal perceptual threshold) or do not occur at all (silent ischaemia).

The relatively high prevalence of subclinical coronary artery disease associated with diabetes has led to debate about the value of screening programmes using non-invasive tests. As a universal principal, this can scarcely be justified, the sensitivity of stress testing (electrocardiographic or perfusion imaging) for detecting subclinical disease being low with only a 5–10% incidence of obstructive lesions (> 50% luminal narrowing at angiography) among asymptomatic diabetic cohorts. Moreover, the mere demonstration of obstructive coronary disease does not usually affect ongoing management with strict glycaemic control and risk factor modification. Certainly, there is no evidence to support angioplasty in asymptomatic cases, while the potential prognostic benefits of surgery in the minority with three vessel or left

main disease needs to be balanced against the heightened procedural risk and less favourable longer term outcome in patients with diabetes. Nevertheless, in certain subgroups, screening for coronary artery disease is recommended because it can lead to treatment strategies that favourably affect prognosis. These include diabetic patients needing renal transplantation or major non-cardiac vascular surgery in whom coronary revascularisation may reduce the procedural risk.

1. **Kannel WB, McGee DL.** Diabetes and cardiovascular risk factors: the Framingham study. *Circulation* 1979;**59**:8–13.
   • *Subset analysis from the father of all epidemiological studies.*

2. **Fuller JH, Shipley MJ, Rose G,** *et al.* Mortality from coronary heart disease and stroke in relation to degree of glycaemia: the Whitehall study. *BMJ* 1983;**287**:867–70.
   • *The classic Whitehall study which for the first time related the risk of stroke, as well as coronary heart disease, to the degree of ischaemia.*

3. **Stamler J, Vaccaro O, Neaton J,** *et al.* Diabetes, other risk factors, and 12-yr cardiovascular mortality for men screened in the multiple risk factor intervention trial. *Diabetes Care* 1993;**16**:434–44.
   • *The massive MRFIT study confirmed the independent risk attributable to diabetes over and above the effect of smoking, lipids and blood pressure.*

4. **The Bypass Angioplasty Revascularization Investigation (BARI) Investigators.** Comparison of coronary bypass surgery with angioplasty in patients with multivessel disease. *N Engl J Med* 1996;**335**:217–25.
   • *The randomised trial that called into question the use of angioplasty for revascularising diabetic patients with coronary artery disease.*

5. **Marso SP, Lincoff AM, Ellis SG,** *et al.* Optimizing the percutaneous interventional outcomes for patients with diabetes mellitus: results of the EPISTENT (Evaluation of platelet IIb/IIIa inhibitor for stenting trial) diabetic substudy. *Circulation* 1999;**100**:2477–84.
   • *This study produced a sigh of relief from interventionists by showing that stenting plus abciximab in diabetics produces results similar to those achieved in non-diabetic patients, justifying percutaneous revascularisation in this high risk group.*

6. **Granger CB, Califf RM, Young S,** *et al,* **and The Thrombolysis and Angioplasty in Myocardial Infarction (TAMI) Study Group.** Outcome of patients with diabetes mellitus and acute myocardial infarction treated with thrombolytic agents. *J Am Coll Cardiol* 1993;**21**:920–5.
   • *An influential study confirming the equal benefits of thrombolytic treatment for achieving coronary patency in diabetic and non-diabetic patients with acute myocardial infarction.*

7. **Malmberg K, Ryden L, Efendic S,** *et al* **for the Diabetes Mellitus, Insulin Glucose Infusion in Acute Myocardial Infarction (DIGAMI) Study Group.** Randomized trial of insulin-glucose infusion followed by subcutaneous insulin treatment in diabetic patients with acute myocardial infarction: effects on mortality at 1 year. *J Am Coll Cardiol* 1995;**26**:57–65.
   • *One of those studies that had a major impact on clinical practice. Since its publication glucose and insulin infusion has become recommended practice for all diabetic patients with acute myocardial infarction.*

8. **McGuire DK, Granger CB.** Diabetes and ischemic heart disease. *Am Heart J* 1999;**138**:S336–75.
   • *State of the art review of diabetic coronary heart disease.*

9. **Ewing D, Boland O, Neilson J,** *et al.* Autonomic neuropathy, QT interval lengthening, and unexpected deaths in male diabetic patients. *Diabetologia* 1991;**34**:182–5.
   • *One of several classic papers from Ewing highlighting the important interaction between autonomic neuropathy and clinical manifestations of coronary heart disease in diabetes.*

10. **Marchant B, Umachandran V, Stevenson R,** *et al.* Silent myocardial ischaemia: the role of subclinical neuropathy in patients with and without diabetes. *J Am Coll Cardiol* 1993;**22**:1433–7.
    • *Debate about the relation between diabetes and silent ischaemia was resolved by this study which showed that silent ischaemia was largely confined to neuropathic subsets.*

11. **Ranjadayalan K, Umachandran V, Ambepityia G,** *et al.* Prolonged anginal perceptual threshold in diabetes: effects on exercise capacity and myocardial ischemia. *J Am Coll Cardiol* 1990;**16**:1120–4.
    • *This study showed how impaired perception of ischaemic cardiac pain in patients with diabetes deprives them of the signal to stop exercising as ischaemia intensifies.*

12. **Solang L, Malmberg K, Ryden L.** Diabetes mellitus and congestive heart failure: further knowledge needed. *Eur Heart J* 1998;**20**:789–95.
- *An authoritative review of heart failure as it affects patients with diabetes.*

13. **United Kingdom Prospective Diabetes Study (UKPDS) Group.** Tight blood pressure control and risk of macrovascular and microvascular complications in type 2 diabetes (UKPDS 38). *BMJ* 1998;**317**:703–13.
- *A new milestone in diabetic research confirming the protective effects of tight blood pressure control.*

14. **United Kingdom Prospective Diabetes Study (UKPDS) Group.** Efficacy of atenolol and captopril in reducing risk of macrovascular and microvascular complications in type 2 diabetes (UKPDS 39). *BMJ* 1998;**317**:713–20.
- *This study raised a few eyebrows when it reported that ACE inhibitors offered no apparent advantage over β blockers for protecting against microvascular complications in hypertensive diabetics.*

15. **United Kingdom Prospective Diabetes Study (UKPDS) Group.** Intensive blood-glucose control with sulphonylureas or insulin compared with conventional treatment and risk of complications in patients with type 2 diabetes (UKPDS 33). *Lancet* 1998;**352**:837–53.
- *Another landmark publication from the UKPDS investigators confirming unequivocally the benefits of strict glycaemic control for protecting against microvascular complications of diabetes.*

16. **Mancini GB, Henry GC, Macaya C,** *et al.* Angiotensin-converting enzyme inhibition with quinapril improves endothelial vasomotor dysfunction in patients with coronary artery disease. The TREND (trial on reversing endothelial dysfunction) study. *Circulation* 1996;**94**:258–65.
- *The first study in humans to show that ACE inhibition improves endothelial function in diseased coronary arteries.*

17. **Yusuf S, Sleight P, Pogue J,** *et al,* **for The Heart Outcomes Prevention Evaluation (HOPE) Study Investigators.** Effects of an angiotensin-converting-enzyme inhibitor, ramipril, on cardiovascular events in high-risk patients. *N Engl J Med* 2000;**342**:145–53.
- *A landmark study confirming the benefits of ACE inhibition for protecting against ischaemic events in high risk patients.*

18. **Heart Outcomes Prevention Evaluation (HOPE) Study Investigators.** Effects of ramipril on cardiovascular and microvascular outcomes in people with diabetes mellitus: result of HOPE study and MICRO-HOPE substudy. *Lancet* 2000;**355**:253–9.
- *A crucial substudy of HOPE showing the benefits of ACE inhibition in diabetic patients for protecting against microvascular and macrovascular end points.*

27 Pulmonary arterial hypertension: new ideas and perspectives

Nazzareno Galiè, Adam Torbicki

The classic way to describe a disease is to begin with nomenclature, definitions, and classifications. A fortunate coincidence gives us the opportunity today to start from the very early stages of pathophysiologic processes, a gene mutation. In fact, in a recently published paper[1] the gene involved in familial primary pulmonary hypertension (PPH) has been described and the finding has been confirmed by a second independent group.[2]

Genetics

Familial PPH has an incidence of at least 6% among all cases of PPH; it is an autosomal dominant disorder with reduced penetrance and genetic anticipation, and has been mapped to a locus designated *PPH1* on chromosome 2q33. The mutations interest the gene BMPR2, encoding a transforming growth factor β (TGF-β) type II receptor (BMPR-II) that is located in the cell membrane.[3] TGF-β is representative of a large family of small polypeptides that have many different effects on growth and development. In fact, depending on the cell type, the TGF-β pathway influences many different processes such as growth, mobility, angiogenesis, immunosuppression, and apoptosis. Interestingly, mutations in the BMPR-II gene have also been found in more than 20% of human colorectal cancers. A link between PPH and tumorigenesis has been suspected in the past,[4] based on exuberant proliferative vascular changes of pulmonary arteries and on monoclonal endothelial cell proliferation of plexiform lesions.[5] BMPR2 germline mutations have been detected in 55% of cases of familial PPH and also in 26% of sporadic cases of PPH, raising the possibility that familial cases are more frequent than expected.[6] Until now 46 different mutations of BMPR2 have been identified in PPH patients, and most of them produce a loss of function for the BMPR-II receptor.[7] Thus, haploinsufficiency seems to be the molecular mechanism that initiates PPH. On the other hand, the high frequency of "true" sporadic PPH cases and reduced penetrance of familial PPH suggests that additional triggers are required for the development of the disease. Such mechanisms could be a second somatic mutation within an unstable BMPR-II pathway[8] or any stimulus able to disrupt pulmonary vascular cell growth control. It is obvious that the identification of the gene responsible for familial PPH and for some

Genetics of primary pulmonary hypertension

- A family history is detectable in at least 6% of cases of primary pulmonary hypertension (PPH)

- Familial PPH is an autosomal dominant disorder with reduced penetrance and genetic anticipation

- Mutations of type II bone morphogenetic protein receptor gene (BMPR2) have been detected in 56% of families with PPH and 26% of sporadic cases of PPH

- Mutations are likely to produce a loss of function in the transforming growth factor β (TGF-β) pathway that is involved in cell proliferation and apoptosis

- Reduced penetrance suggests that additional triggers besides genetic mutations are required for the development of the disease

cases of sporadic PPH represents a milestone in our understanding of this severe condition, and it will provide new insights into research strategies in pulmonary hypertension.

Pathology and classification

Even if in the future genetic analysis can help us to identify patients at the very early stages of the disease,[9] currently when a PPH patients become symptomatic the characteristic obstructive changes of the pulmonary vascular bed are fully expressed. The lesions are characterised by cellular proliferation that involves the intima, media, and adventitia of the small pulmonary arteries and arterioles.[10] Plexiform lesions that are considered as a proliferation of endothelial cells, smooth muscle cells, and myofibroblasts with formation of microvessels, are often present. Thrombosis in situ, typically involving the small arteries or veins, can coexist with any of the previous findings. This picture has been defined as proliferative pulmonary vascular disease and is characteristic not only of PPH but is present in other conditions with precapillary pulmonary hypertension—for example, collagen vascular disease, congenital systemic to pulmonary shunts, portal hypertension, and HIV infection.

The identical pathologic features represent a strong rationale for categorising all the above conditions in a single group of diseases defined according to the new World Health Organization classification as pulmonary arterial hypertension (PAH) (table 27.1).[11] In addition, all these patients share a similar clinical picture and are treated medically in the same way. These aspects underscore the philosophy of the new WHO classification that is intended to group diseases with similar pathologic, pathophysiologic, clinical, and therapeutic features.

Table 27.1   World Health Organization new diagnostic classification[11]

1. Pulmonary arterial hypertension
  1.1 Primary pulmonary hypertension
    (a) Sporadic
    (b) Familial
  1.2 Related to:
    (a) Collagen vascular disease
    (b) Congenital systemic to pulmonary shunts
    (c) Portal hypertension
    (d) HIV infection
    (e) Drugs/toxins
      (1) Anorexigens
      (2) Other
    (f) Persistent pulmonary hypertension of the newborn
    (g) Other

2. Pulmonary venous hypertension
  2.1 Left sided atrial or ventricular heart disease
  2.2 Left sided valvar heart disease
  2.3 Extrinsic compression of central pulmonary veins
    (a) Fibrosing mediastinitis
    (b) Adenopathy/tumours
  2.4 Pulmonary veno-occlusive disease
  2.5 Other

3. Pulmonary hypertension associated with disorders of the respiratory system and/or hypoxemia
  3.1 Chronic obstructive pulmonary disease
  3.2 Interstitial lung disease
  3.3 Sleep disordered breathing
  3.4 Alveolar hypoventilation disorders
  3.5 Chronic exposure to high altitude
  3.6 Neonatal lung disease
  3.7 Alveolar-capillary dysplasia
  3.8 Other

4. Pulmonary hypertension caused by chronic thrombotic and/or embolic disease
  4.1 Thromboembolic obstruction of proximal pulmonary arteries
  4.2 Obstruction of distal pulmonary arteries
    (a) Pulmonary embolism (thrombus, tumour, ova and/or parasites, foreign material)
    (b) In situ thrombosis
    (c) Sickle cell disease

5. Pulmonary hypertension caused by disorders directly affecting the pulmonary vasculature
  5.1 Inflammatory
    (a) Schistosomiasis
    (b) Sarcoidosis
    (c) Other
  5.2 Pulmonary capillary haemangiomatosis

The second category—pulmonary venous hypertension—identifies all the conditions characterised haemodynamically by postcapillary pulmonary hypertension that are usually caused by left heart diseases. The third category includes cases in which pulmonary hypertension is associated with disorders of the respiratory system and/or hypoxaemia. The fourth category—pulmonary hypertension caused by chronic thrombotic and/or embolic disease—lists the states characterised by mechanical obstruction situated in the main, lobar, and segmental pulmonary arteries. Interestingly, patients with chronic thromboembolic pulmonary hypertension (CTEPH) seem to develop in the unobstructed arteries and arterioles, submitted to high flow-high pressure stress, pathological changes similar to those considered specific for PAH. Those changes are probably responsible for progressive haemodynamic deterioration, despite the absence of recurrent embolic episodes. The final category—pulmonary hypertension caused by disorders directly affecting the pulmonary vasculature—comprises inflammatory diseases such as sarcoidosis, schistosomiasis, and a rare condition called pulmonary capillary haemangiomatosis.

The new WHO classification will help the diagnostic process as well as the definition of categories to be included in treatment trials. Interestingly the term "secondary" pulmonary hypertension, widely used in the past, is no longer recommended as pathophysiologic links between the underlying conditions remain unproven beyond epidemiological clustering of some diseases with pulmonary hypertension. Recent genetic advances give insights and new impetus to research into why patients with similar associated conditions may or may not develop pulmonary hypertension.

Diagnosis and assessment

Relatively early detection of pulmonary hypertension would be possible in the era of Doppler echocardiography if only appropriate diagnostic work up was not so commonly delayed, especially in "healthy" young individuals stubbornly complaining of unexplained mild functional impairment. New classification and uniform treatment for patients with PAH, together with availability of non-invasive imaging tests, greatly simplified the diagnostic procedures required for therapeutic decision making. Venous and hypoxic pulmonary hypertension are readily diagnosed within the framework of routine clinical tests such as chest radiography, echocardiography, and pulmonary function tests. A perfusion lung scan is essential for identifying patients with chronic thromboembolic disease who should follow different diagnostic pathways towards assessing the indications for surgical intervention. In PAH patients right heart catheterisation is still considered mandatory for initial prognostic evaluation and assessment of pulmonary vasoreactivity.

Of the various drugs available, inhaled iloprost and inhaled nitric oxide are increasingly used for this purpose in referral centres. Nitric oxide is particularly interesting because it does not affect systemic circulation and hardly modifies cardiac output, despite significant pulmonary vasodilatation observed in some responders. Therefore, calculation of the true effect on vascular tone is more reliable. However, with emerging potent oral and inhaled drugs, combining vasodilatory and antiproliferative properties, the issue of invasive testing for pulmonary vasoreactivity in selecting treatment may lose its importance. "True" responders, represented by patients in whom the acute fall of both pulmonary artery pressure and pulmonary vascular resistance is in the range of 30–50%, will likely be identified by real time Doppler echocardiography performed during inhalation of nitric oxide or iloprost. There is a tendency to avoid treatment with calcium channel blockers in patients with severe pulmonary hypertension, because of concern that the potentially detrimental side effects of this class of drugs will outweigh their benefits in less responsive patients.

In the prostanoids era the main challenge is now to assess the results of long term treatment. This is especially important for intravenous epoprostenol in order to steer between, on the one hand, unnecessary dose escalation leading to side effects, faster tachyphylaxis, and excessive costs, and on the other, ineffective doses of the active substance. Repeated catheterisation is clearly a poor option, while the six minute walk test has a growing importance, especially in the light of recent data indicating the prognostic implications of this test in patients with PPH.[12] While standard echocardiography virtually failed as a non-invasive test for long term monitoring of effects of treatment in severe pulmonary hypertension,[13] new ideas based on Doppler assessment of indices of pulsatile right heart haemodynamics offer some promise.[14] There is no alternative to Doppler echocardiography when screening high risk populations. Importantly, recent WHO recommendations allow the diagnosis of mild pulmonary hypertension based on systolic pulmonary pressure exceeding 40 mm Hg, which corresponds to a tricuspid regurgitant velocity on Doppler echocardiography of 3.0–3.5 m/s.[11] However, anecdotal reports on false positive Doppler diagnosis of pulmonary hypertension as well as the risk of missing early stages of the condition, apparent only during exercise, must be taken into account.[15] On the other hand, stress Doppler echocardiography seems to be able to identify genetically predisposed subjects with normal rest haemodynamics and an abnormal rise in systolic pulmonary artery pressure on exercise.[9] However, evaluation of the level and changes in mean pulmonary pressure is virtually impossible using the Doppler method.

Therapeutic strategy

Medical treatment

The treatment of PPH until a few years ago was only symptomatic and based on the experiences of few specialised centres. In fact, the evidence of the favourable effect of oral anticoagulation and calcium channel blockers came from studies experiencing methodological problems. In any case, anticoagulation may not be enough to revert or even stabilise vascular changes, and calcium channel blockers are effective in only a small proportion of PPH patients that respond to acute pharmacological challenges (15–25% according to response definition).[16]

The 1990s can be considered as the prostacyclin era, even if the first experiences with this compound started a decade earlier. Two randomised studies showed that continuous intravenous infusion of epoprostenol, a stable preparation, improved functional capacity, haemodynamics, and survival of New York Heart Association (NYHA) functional class III/IV PPH patients when compared to "conventional" treatment.[17 18] Epoprostenol treatment can be considered "unconventional" because its very short half life (3–5 minutes) means it has to be administered intravenously, which requires "tunnelled" central venous catheters and portable pumps for the continuous administration of the drug. However, significant clinical and functional improvement

---

Diagnosis and assessment

- Non-invasive early detection of pulmonary hypertension is possible by traditional Doppler echocardiography at rest or on exercise

- Venous and hypoxic pulmonary hypertension are diagnosed with routine clinical tests such as chest radiography, echocardiography, and pulmonary function tests

- Segmental defects on perfusion lung scan suggest chronic thromboembolic pulmonary hypertension and require a different diagnostic pathway addressing the feasibility of surgical thromboendarterectomy

- Right heart catheterisation is still considered mandatory for initial prognostic evaluation and assessment of pulmonary vasoreactivity in patients with PAH

- Nitric oxide is the substance of choice to test for acute vasoreactivity

- The current tendency is to define acute responders as patients in whom the acute fall of both pulmonary artery pressure and resistance is in the range of 30–50%

- Six minute walk test is useful in the assessment of functional impairment and prognosis, and in the evaluation of long term therapeutic response

- The usefulness of Doppler parameters of pulsatile right heart haemodynamics as indices of prognosis and treatment effect is under scrutiny

---

may be expected, also in patients not responding to pulmonary vasodilatation during acute tests and previously considered to have irreversible vascular changes.

Initially, epoprostenol treatment was viewed as providing a bridge to transplantation in advanced cases of PPH, but recent experience has established this approach as a possible alternative to transplantation. In fact, the improvement in some patients is so great that they no longer fulfil the criteria for being put on a waiting list for transplantation. A reasonable approach may therefore be to consider patients in NYHA functional class III/IV for initiation of epoprostenol treatment and concurrent listing for transplantation, and then maintain on the waiting list only those patients who do not improve substantially or who deteriorate after an initial improvement. By limiting the number of waitlisted patients in this way, it may be possible to reduce the waiting time for lung transplantation.

The favourable effects of epoprostenol have been shown not only in PPH patients but also in almost all the conditions in the PAH category according to the WHO classification (table 1).[11] Nevertheless, epoprostenol treatment requires that patients and relatives are given adequate training for the appropriate management of the delivery system, in order to minimise severe side effects such as sepsis and pump malfunctions, which may be life threatening. Moreover, the development of tolerance to the drug means that the doses must be increased over time in order to maintain efficacy, thus increasing both side effects and costs. Alternative ways of administering prostacyclin are under active investigation in order to improve the risk–benefit profile and cost effectiveness of treatment. Currently, three stable prostacyclin compounds—uniprost, iloprost, and beraprost, administered by the subcutaneous, inhaled and oral routes, respectively—are under scrutiny by controlled clinical trials.

Uniprost is infused subcutaneously by small portable pumps similar to those used for administering insulin to diabetic patients; the system requires no more than 15 minutes every three days for management. A randomised, placebo controlled, double blinded study involving 470 patients with NYHA class III/IV PAH has been recently completed and preliminary results have been reported in recent meetings of the European Society of Cardiology and American Heart Association. Favourable and significant effects were observed on functional capacity (as assessed by the six minute walk test), symptoms, and haemodynamics. The most frequent side effect was pain and redness at the infusion site, which limited the dose increase in a proportion of cases and prevented use of the drug in about 8% of patients.

Iloprost is a stable analogue of prostacyclin available for intravenous, oral, and inhalation use. Several open, uncontrolled studies have reported favourable effects of inhaled iloprost on functional capacity and haemodynamics of patients with PAH.[19 20] Administration of iloprost requires a special inhalation device in order to produce particles of a certain diameter and to limit ambient spillover of the drug. A major limitation of this administration method is the short duration of effect, requiring up to 12 inhalations a day to achieve consistent clinical efficacy in some patients. A randomised, placebo controlled, double blind study is currently underway in Europe in patients with PAH. The results should be available in 2001 and they will indicate definitively the extent of the long term effects of this new treatment.

Beraprost sodium is the first chemically stable and orally active prostaglandin I_2 analogue available for clinical studies. Preliminary, uncontrolled experiences mainly in Japan have shown that long term treatment with this compound is able to determine favourable clinical haemodynamic and prognostic effects in patients with PPH.[21] Currently, two randomised, placebo controlled, double blind studies in PAH patients are in progress in the USA and Europe.

Recently, endothelin-1 (ET-1) receptor antagonists, a class of drug available for oral administration, have undergone evaluation in PAH patients. The rationale for using these drugs is linked to the raised concentrations of ET-1, a potent vasoconstrictor and mitogenic substance, both in plasma[22] as well as in lung tissue[23] of PAH patients. A pilot, randomised, placebo controlled, double blind phase III study on bosentan, an ET-A and ET-B receptor antagonist, administered orally in PAH patients has been recently completed. Preliminary reports show favourable effects on functional capacity and haemodynamics, leading to the initiation of a larger trial currently underway in the USA and Europe.

A phase II open study on the acute haemodynamic effects of intravenous sildenafil, a type V cGMP phosphodiesterase inhibitor, in patients with pulmonary arterial hypertension is in progress in Europe. The drug is available also for oral administration and, if supported by preliminary findings,[24] a long term study could be initiated in the future.

Other substances to be evaluated in phase I, II, and III studies include nitric oxide, L-arginine, and elastase inhibitors. Finally, gene transfection strategies for the treatment of pulmonary hypertension are in preclinical phase of development. Encouraging results have been shown in animal models promoting the expression of both prostacyclin and nitric oxide synthase.

Non-drug treatment

Besides medical treatment and lung transplantation, two additional procedures have been utilised in patients with PAH and CTEPH—balloon atrial septostomy (BAS) and pulmonary artery thromboendarterectomy.

BAS is an invasive procedure that is intended to create an interatrial defect in order to produce a right to left shunt. Experimental and clinical observations suggest that such intervention can reduce right atrial pressure and increase systemic output, improving exercise capacity and survival in PAH patients.[25] Balloon atrial septostomy is performed by the transeptal Brockenbrough technique and stepwise multiple balloon dilatation of increasing size, tailored to produce a maximal systemic oxygen saturation fall of 5–10%. The procedure related failure and death rates are not negligible and therefore BAS should be performed in centres experienced in both interventional cardiology and pulmonary hypertension. Even if BAS may represent a real alternative or a bridge to transplantation for selected patients with severe PAH who are unresponsive to medical treatment, the procedure is still considered investigational.

Pulmonary circulation in patients with CTEPH is affected both by gross central obstructive lesions caused by unresolved organised thrombi, as well as by proliferative changes similar to those found in PAH, involving remaining unobstructed small arteries and arterioles.[26] Pulmonary thromboendarterectomy in deep hypothermia is the treatment of choice. In survivors it offers excellent long term results, with sustained improvement in haemodynamics and exercise tolerance.[27–29] Unfortunately, not all patients are appropriate candidates for this operation. Advanced age and severe functional impairment, as well as severe pulmonary hypertension and high pulmonary vascular resistance, increase the risk of proce-

194

Therapeutic strategies

- Oral anticoagulation is indicated if no contraindication is present, while the use of calcium channel blocking agents is restricted to the minority of patients (15–25%) who are responders to the vasoreactivity test

- Continuous intravenous infusion of prostacyclin is indicated in NYHA class III/IV patients

- Lung transplantation is currently indicated in the case of failure of prostacyclin treatment

- Stable prostacyclin analogues for subcutaneous, inhaled, and oral routes and endothelin-1 receptor antagonists are in the advanced stages of clinical development

- Balloon atrial septostomy is an investigational procedure that can be effective in selected cases unresponsive to other therapeutic options

- Pulmonary artery thromboendarterectomy is indicated in patients with chronic thromboembolic pulmonary hypertension and proximal obstructive lesions

dure related mortality. More importantly, some patients with coexisting distal lesions inaccessible to surgery may in fact fail to improve despite removal of the central lesions.[30] Because chronic distal changes are difficult to either confirm or exclude, even with angiography and angioscopy, the overall mortality related to pulmonary thromboendarterectomy has not decreased below 7% even in the most experienced centres.

In patients with documented isolated distal organised post-thromboembolic obstructions, new prostanoid derivatives are currently tested in the hope of preventing progression or even reversing proliferative changes affecting the patent part of the pulmonary circulation.

A recent paper reports on successful percutaneous balloon dilatation of surgically inaccessible organised thrombotic lesions. This would open new perspectives for patients who are not good candidates for surgical treatment.

In conclusion, with the beginning of the third millennium a wide range of new treatment modalities for pulmonary hypertension are expected in a relatively short time. Our knowledge of the pathophysiology, diagnosis, assessment, and treatment of this condition will probably advance rapidly in the coming years. Compared to the very slow rate of progress previously in this field, we can consider to have entered a totally new era.

1. **PPH International Consortium.** Heterozygous germline mutations in BMPR2, encoding a TGF-beta receptor, cause familial primary pulmonary hypertension. *Nat Genet* 2000;**26**:81–4.
- *First paper reporting that familial primary pulmonary hypertension is caused by mutations of BMPR2 gene.*

2. **Deng Z, Morse JH, Slager SL,** et al. Familial primary pulmonary hypertension (gene PPH1) is caused by mutations in the bone morphogenetic protein receptor-II gene. *Am J Hum Genet* 2000;**67**:737–44.

3. **Zhou S, Kinzler KW, Vogelstein B.** Going mad with Smads. *N Engl J Med* 1999;**341**:1144–6.

4. **Voelkel NF, Cool C, Lee SD,** et al. Primary pulmonary hypertension between inflammation and cancer. *Chest* 1998;**114**:225S–30S.

5. **Lee SD, Shroyer KR, Markham NE,** et al. Monoclonal endothelial cell proliferation is present in primary but not secondary pulmonary hypertension. *J Clin Invest* 1998;**101**:927–34.
- *The finding of a frequent monoclonal endothelial cell proliferation in PPH suggests that a somatic genetic alteration similar to that present in neoplastic processes may be responsible for the pathogenesis of PPH.*

6. **Thomson JR, Machado RD, Pauciulo MW,** et al. Sporadic primary pulmonary hypertension is associated with germline mutations of the gene encoding BMPR-II, a receptor member of the TGF-beta family. *J Med Genet* 2000;**37**:741–5.
- *First article reporting that 26% of sporadic cases of PPH are caused by mutations of BMPR2 gene.*

7. **Machado RD, Pauciulo MW, Thomson JR,** et al. BMPR2 haploinsufficiency as the inherited molecular mechanism for primary pulmonary hypertension. *Am J Hum Genet* 2001;**68**:92–102.
- *Comprehensive spectrum of all BMPR2 mutations and analysis of their functional impact. The considerable heterogeneity of BMPR2 mutations that cause PPH strongly suggests that additional factors, genetic and/or environmental, may be required for the development of the clinical phenotype.*

8. **Thomson JR, Trembath RC.** Primary pulmonary hypertension: the pressure rises for a gene. *J Clin Pathol* 2000;**53**:899–903.

9. **Grunig E, Janssen B, Mereles D,** et al. Abnormal pulmonary artery pressure response in asymptomatic carriers of primary pulmonary hypertension gene. *Circulation* 2000;**102**:1145–50.
- *Detection of abnormal elevation of systolic pulmonary artery pressure in asymptomatic carriers of PPH gene by stress Doppler echocardiography.*

10. **Pietra GG, Edwards WD, Kay JM,** et al. Histopathology of primary pulmonary hypertension. A qualitative and quantitative study of pulmonary blood vessels from 58 patients in the National Heart, Lung, and Blood Institute, primary pulmonary hypertension registry. *Circulation* 1989;**80**:1198–206.
- *Systematic "historical" description of the pathologic changes of proliferative pulmonary vascular disease.*

11. **Rich S.** Primary pulmonary hypertension: executive summary from the world symposium—primary pulmonary hypertension 1998. World Health Organization http://www.who.int/ncd/cvd/pph.html.
- *A landmark document presenting results of a consensus on new classification of pulmonary hypertension reached during the WHO endorsed meeting of world experts in the field of pulmonary circulation held in Evian, France in 1998.*

12. **Miyamoto S, Nagaya N, Satoh T,** et al. Clinical correlates and prognostic significance of six-minute walk test in patients with primary pulmonary hypertension. Comparison with cardiopulmonary exercise testing. *Am J Respir Crit Care Med* 2000;**161**:487–92.
- *Prospective analysis of prognostic significance of six minute walk test showing that patients with primary pulmonary hypertension walking < 332 m had a significantly lower survival rate at a mean follow up of 21 months than those walking further.*

13. **Hinderliter AL, Willis PW, Barst RJ,** et al. Effects of long-term infusion of prostacyclin (epoprostenol) on echocardiographic measures of right ventricular structure and function in primary pulmonary hypertension. Primary pulmonary hypertension study group. *Circulation* 1997;**95**:1479–86.
- *First multicentre study trying to assess in 75 patients whether echocardiography might be helpful in monitoring effects of long term prostacyclin treatment.*

14. **Naeije R, Torbicki A.** More on the noninvasive diagnosis of pulmonary hypertension: Doppler echocardiography revisited. *Eur Respir J* 1995;**8**:1445–9.
- *Comprehensive review of the current role and future perspectives of Doppler echocardiography in the diagnosis and assessment of patients with pulmonary arterial hypertension.*

15. **Vachiery JL, Brimioulle S, Crasset V,** et al. False-positive diagnosis of pulmonary hypertension by Doppler echocardiography. *Eur Respir J* 1998;**12**:1476–8.
- *A well documented case report indicating the possibility of overestimation of pulmonary arterial systolic pressure with tricuspid regurgitant jet method, leading to false diagnosis of pulmonary hypertension.*

16. **Galie N, Ussia G, Passarelli P,** et al. Role of pharmacologic tests in the treatment of primary pulmonary hypertension. *Am J Cardiol* 1995;**75**:55A–62A.
- *Review of the technical aspects and theoretical concepts of vasoreactivity tests in pulmonary arterial hypertension.*

17. **Rubin LJ, Mendoza J, Hood M,** *et al.* Treatment of primary pulmonary hypertension with continuous intravenous prostacyclin (epoprostenol). Results of a randomized trial. *Ann Intern Med* 1990;**112**:485–91.

18. **Barst RJ, Rubin LJ, Long WA,** *et al.* A comparison of continuous intravenous epoprostenol (prostacyclin) with conventional therapy for primary pulmonary hypertension. The primary pulmonary hypertension study group. *N Engl J Med* 1996;**334**:296–302.
   • *Randomised study on the effect of continuous intravenous infusion of prostacyclin in 80 patients with NYHA class III/IV PPH. Active treatment improved functional capacity, haemodynamics, and survival.*

19. **Olschewski H, Ghofrani HA, Schmehl T,** *et al.* Inhaled iloprost to treat severe pulmonary hypertension. An uncontrolled trial. German PPH study group. *Ann Intern Med* 2000;**132**:435–43.

20. **Hoeper MM, Schwarze M, Ehlerding S,** *et al.* Long-term treatment of primary pulmonary hypertension with aerosolized iloprost, a prostacyclin analogue. *N Engl J Med* 2000;**342**:1866–70.
   • *Unblinded study on the effect of 12 months treatment of inhaled prostacyclin analogue iloprost in 22 PPH patients. Improvements in functional capacity and haemodynamics were shown.*

21. **Nagaya N, Uematsu M, Okano Y,** *et al.* Effect of orally active prostacyclin analogue on survival of outpatients with primary pulmonary hypertension. *J Am Coll Cardiol* 1999;**34**:1188–92.
   • *Retrospective study on the effects of orally active prostacyclin analogue beraprost in 24 PPH patients compared to 34 conventionally treated controls. Improvements in haemodynamics and survival were shown.*

22. **Stewart DJ, Levy RD, Cernacek P,** *et al.* Increased plasma endothelin-1 in pulmonary hypertension: marker or mediator of disease? *Ann Intern Med* 1991;**114**:464–9.

23. **Lutz J, Gorenflo M, Habighorst M,** *et al.* Endothelin-1- and endothelin-receptors in lung biopsies of patients with pulmonary hypertension due to congenital heart disease. *Clin Chem Lab Med* 1999;**37**:423–8.

24. **Abrams D, Schulze-Neick I, Magee AG.** Sildenafil as a selective pulmonary vasodilator in childhood primary pulmonary hypertension. *Heart* 2000;**84**:e4.(electronic only)

25. **Sandoval J, Gaspar J, Pulido T,** *et al.* Graded balloon dilation atrial septostomy in severe primary pulmonary hypertension. A therapeutic alternative for patients nonresponsive to vasodilator treatment. *J Am Coll Cardiol* 1998;**32**:297–304.
   • *Effect of graded balloon dilation atrial septostomy in 15 patients with NYHA class III/IV PPH. Improvements in functional capacity, haemodynamics, and survival were shown.*

26. **Moser KM, Bloor CM.** Pulmonary vascular lesions occurring in patients with chronic major vessel thromboembolic pulmonary hypertension. *Chest* 1993;**103**:685–92.
   • *Report suggesting that changes in the patent arteries of patients with chronic thromboembolic pulmonary hypertension are of the same character as those found in PPH.*

27. **Archibald CJ, Auger WR, Fedullo PF,** *et al.* Long-term outcome after pulmonary thromboendarterectomy. *Am J Respir Crit Care Med* 1999;**160**:523–8.
   • *Experience on long term effect of thromboendarterectomy in 420 patients operated on in a single centre. A consistent improvement in functional capacity and quality of life was shown in survivors.*

28. **Moser KM, Daily PO, Peterson K,** *et al.* Thromboendarterectomy for chronic, major-vessel thromboembolic pulmonary hypertension. Immediate and long-term results in 42 patients. *Ann Intern Med* 1987;**107**:560–5.

29. **Kramm T, Mayer E, Dahm M,** *et al.* Long-term results after thromboendarterectomy for chronic pulmonary embolism. *Eur J Cardiothorac Surg* 1999;**15**:579–83.
   • *European single centre experience indicating excellent long term (mean 60 months) effect of pulmonary thromboendarterectomy in 22 survivors of this intervention.*

30. **Moser KM, Fedullo PF, Finkbeiner WE,** *et al.* Do patients with primary pulmonary hypertension develop extensive central thrombi? *Circulation* 1995;**91**:741–5.
   • *A first report indicating the difficulties in differentiating between embolic and local pulmonary arterial thrombi, the latter being a consequence and not the cause of pulmonary hypertension.*

31. **Feinstein JA, Goldhaber SZ, Lock JE,** *et al.* Balloon pulmonary angioplasty for treatment of chronic thromboembolic pulmonary hypertension. *Circulation* 2001;**103**:10–13.

195

28 Diseases of the thoracic aorta

Raimund Erbel

New imaging techniques such as computed tomography (CT), magnetic resonance imaging (MRI), transoesophageal echocardiography (TOE), and intravascular ultrasound (IVUS) have improved the detection of diseases of the aorta. These techniques not only provide a better visualisation of the aorta but also a better understanding of the pathogenesis of aortic diseases, which have led to new strategies for decision making and patient management.

Arteriosclerosis of the aorta

Arteriosclerosis of the aortic wall begins with the development fatty streaks, with intermediate lesions being found in children and young adults. In necropsy studies up to 15% of the latter group have been found to have advanced lesions such as atheroma and fibroatheroma. Early intracellular and extracellular calcification develops in intermediate lesions and atheroma. Complicated lesions are characterised by plaque erosion or rupture forming plaque ulcers, mural thrombus formation, and intramural haemorrhage/haematoma.

The development of arteriosclerosis of the aorta is related to traditional risk factors—hypertension, hypercholesterolaemia, and smoking.[1] In addition, fibrinogenaemia and homocysteinaemia are related to the development of aortic sclerosis. Not surprisingly, aortic arteriosclerosis is a marker of coronary artery disease. High sensitivity and positive predictive accuracy have been found for presence of significant coronary artery stenosis in patients in whom TOE could demonstrate atheroma of the aortic wall. A grading from I to V (table 28.1) has been developed which is related to the risk of embolisation and the development of strokes.

A significant relation between plaque morphology and the risk of stroke has been found. The risk is high in patients with signs of lipid pools, calcification, and plaque thickness of more than 4 mm, but plaque ulceration by itself was not found to increase embolic risk. Thus, the detection of plaques at risk (vulnerable plaques) seems to be important.[1] The prevalence of atheromas in the aortic arch was 20–30% in stroke patients and 9–13% in control subjects. Thus, the presence of arteriosclerosis of the aorta in stroke patients is as high as the prevalence of atrial fibrillation (18–30%) and carotid artery disease. If the plaque thickness exceeds 4 mm the risk increases, with an odds ratio as high as 13.8, whereas plaque thickness in the range of 1–3.9 mm has an odds ratio of only 3.9, when plaque formation below 1 mm is regarded as normal with an odds ratio of 1.[1]

Calcification of the aortic wall usually combined with aortic elongation or kinking is visualised by chest x ray and can be regarded as a sign of arteriosclerosis of the aorta. This should be taken as a sign (1) of high risk of ischaemic strokes in women and men, and (2) of coronary disease in men. This relation was detected in a large follow up study after adjustment for race, cigarette smoking, alcohol consumption, body mass index, serum cholesterol concentration, hypertension, diabetes, and family history of myocardial infarction.[2]

Transoesophageal or intraoperative epicardial echocardiography is the method of choice for visualising aortic arteriosclerosis of the aorta, but in the future MRI using transoesophageal probes to improve the resolution may become an alternative method.

Free floating structures within the aorta are best visualised by TOE and represent initial flaps or thrombus formation. In these patients there is an increased risk of embolic events during left heart catheterisation and intra-aortic balloon pumping. During bypass surgery cross clamping of the aorta is often necessary. The injury to the aortic wall increases the risk of stroke in patients with arteriosclerosis of the aorta. The risk reaches 14% in patients with atheromas, which are found by palpitation or epicardial intraoperative ultrasound. Undetected atheromas may be the reason for the particularly high risk in patients who are older than 70 years, as the degree of arteriosclerosis is related to age.[1] In the case of severe arteriosclerosis of the aorta, arterial graft surgery using the arteria mammaria interna or arteria gastroepiploica is an alternative to venous aortocoronary bypass grafting. Surgery, usually atherectomy, has yielded very disappointing results.

If grade IV arteriosclerosis of the aorta is present, anticoagulation is the method of choice for preventing subsequent embolic events. In the future aortic stent implantation may provide an alternative strategy for free floating structures in the arterial wall.

Aortic aneurysm

For the aorta normal values which are related to body surface area and age have been reported. The mean (SD) normal value for the aortic annulus in men is 2.6 (0.3) cm and in women is 2.3 (0.2) cm, and for the proximal ascending aorta 2.9 (0.3) cm and 2.6 (0.3) cm, respectively. The upper normal limit for the

Table 28.1 Grading of aortic diseases

	Aortic atheroma	Aortic trauma
Grade I	Minimal intimal thickening	Intimal haemorrhage
Grade II	Extensive intimal thickening	Intimal haemorrhage with laceration
Grade III	Sessile atheroma	Medial laceration
Grade IV	Protruding atheroma	Complete laceration
Grade V	Mobile atheroma	False aneurysm formation

ascending aorta is 2.1 cm/m². A value beyond 4 cm is regarded as an aneurysm, a lower value as ectasia. The normal value for the descending aorta is 1.6 cm/m², and aneurysm is present when a value of 3 cm is exceeded. Wall thickness should be below 4 mm.

The aortic diameter gradually increases over time. The normal expansion rate over 10 years is between 1–2 mm and is greater for patients with an aorta that is larger than normal.

All diseases which result in a weakening of the aortic wall can lead to an aortic dilatation. Aneurysms of the aorta can be subdivided into localised and diffuse, true and false aneurysm (pseudoaneurysm). In the latter, the aortic wall is penetrated completely and the wall of the aneurysm formed by surrounding tissue. As long as the aortic wall is intact, the aneurysm represents a true aneurysm. Aortic aneurysms typically present in the ascending aorta, the area of the origin of the ductus arteriosus Botalli, and the aortic isthmus just distal to the subclavian artery.

Aortic dissection

Aortic dissection is defined as a disruption of the aortic wall, forming an intimal flap and therefore separating a true from a false lumen. Aortic dissection is differentiated into type A and B according to the Stanford classification. In type A the ascending and descending aorta are involved, while in type B only the descending aorta is involved. Further subdivision was previously initiated by DeBakey using three types: type I—involvement of the total aorta (same as type A); type II—involvement of the ascending aorta only; and type III—involvement of the descending aorta (same as type B). Using newer imaging techniques, aortic dissection can be further subdivided into five classes taking into account the aetiology of the aortic disease[3] (see box below).

> **New classification of aortic dissection (according to Svensson and colleagues[3])**
> **Class 1** Classic aortic dissection with true and false lumen with or without communication of the two lumina
> **Class 2** Intramural haemorrhage or haematoma
> **Class 3** Subtle or discrete aortic dissection with bulging of the aortic wall
> **Class 4** Ulceration of aortic plaque following plaque rupture
> **Class 5** Iatrogenic or traumatic aortic dissection

Pathological spectrum of aortic dissection

Class 1 aortic dissection is characterised by an intimal flap and may be present as a communicating or non-communicating dissection depending on whether or not a tear between the

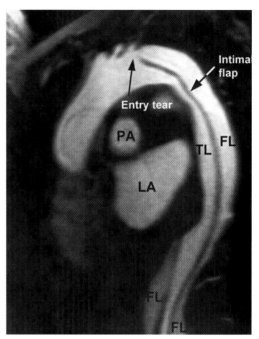

Figure 28.1. Aortic dissection type B, class 1 with visualisation of the intimal flap separating the true lumen (TL) from the false lumen (FL) in a magnetic resonance view. The entry tear is just distal to the subclavian artery. LA, left atrium; PA, pulmonary artery.

true and false lumen is present (fig 28.1). The tears can be regarded as an entry or re-entry tear, but flow is quite often multidirectional depending on the pressure difference between the two lumina. Doppler echocardiography has revealed that the pressure gradient between the two lumina is in the range of 10–25 mm Hg, and a high pressure and wall stress is also present in the false lumina. This explains the tendency of the false lumen to enlarge over time, to form aneurysms, dissection, or to even rupture.

The degree of communication can be assessed indirectly by the extent of thrombus formation within the false lumen, which can be graded into four groups ranging from no thrombus formation up to complete obliteration of the false lumen. This grading has become an important feature for image interpretation, as surgery and stent graft implantation is directed at occluding the tear and inducing thrombus formation in the false lumen, thus starting a healing process. Therefore it is necessary not only to describe the presence of communication, but also to localise the tear position for further treatment.

Class 2 dissection is diagnosed when intramural haematoma or haemorrhage (fig 28.2) is present, which has been induced by rupture of the vasa vasorum leading to wall thickening, which in turn may progress to class 1 dissection, rupture, or may heal.[4] Two types are differentiated according to the aetiology—either cystic medial necrosis Erdheim-Gsell or atherosclerosis.[5] Because angiography as a contour method is not able to visualise aortic wall morphology, newer imaging techniques are required for diagnosis.

Class 3 (discrete/subtle) aortic dissection has been well recognised at pathological examination, but could not be diagnosed clinically until recently in patients with persistent chest pain when, despite exclusion of class 1, 2, and 4 dissection, a localised bulging was demonstrated by angiography and confirmed by surgery or pathology.[3]

Class 4 dissection was first detected in the abdominal aorta, but has also been demonstrated in the whole thoracic aorta.[6] Penetration leading to aortic rupture or class 1 dissection may occur. Plaque ulcers (fig 28.3) develop when plaque rupture occurs and the lipid core is washed out, which may lead to cholesterol embolisation. Usually more than one plaque ulcer can be detected.

Class 5 dissection can be the result of traumatic injury of the aorta, which may be iatrogenic, and can also lead to class 1 or 2 dissection or even rupture of the aorta.

Clinical complications of aortic dissection

In all patients the following emergency signs are looked for: pericardial effusion, pleural effusion, periaortic fluid extravasation, and compression of the left atrium. Patients have a mortality of more than 50% when these signs are present, so treatment has to start without delay and any further diagnostic work up.

The detection and grading of the aortic regurgitation is important, as the surgeon has to take into account a resuspension of the aortic valve or implantation of a conduit containing a valve prosthesis, when severe regurgitation is present.

Involvement of coronary arteries in aortic dissection is rare, with signs of myocardial ischaemia being detected in 3–4% of cases. But the intimal flap may occlude the coronary ostium, or the true lumen may collapse during diastole inducing myocardial ischemia. Haemodynamic deterioration can also lead to myocardial ischaemia caused by pre-existing coronary artery disease. If the patient is stable, coronary angiography may be performed, but usually this is not necessary or advisable because of the invasive nature of the procedure, which may cause the patient's condition to deteriorate. If wall motion is normal, it can be assumed that, during this acute stage of the disease, no significant coronary stenosis is present. Thus, the perioperative situation will only rarely be compromised by the development of myocardial ischaemia.

Side branch involvement can include all arteries which are connected to the aorta. As the major aim of aortic surgery is the replacement of the ascending aorta with or without replacement of the aortic valve, in order to prevent rupture into the pericardium and thus cardiac tamponade, the detection of side branch involvement is not a first line prerequisite for surgery. The recently introduced interventional techniques such as aortic fenestration and stent graft implantation have opened up new therapeutic options, so that the development of ischaemia in visceral organs or legs can be avoided either before or after surgery.[3]

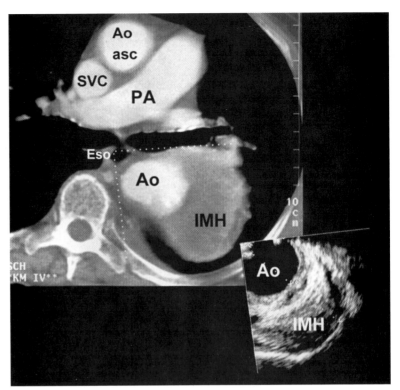

Figure 28.2. Aortic dissection type B, class 2 visualised by spiral CT and TOE. The wall of the aorta (Ao) is thickened by an intramural haematoma/haemorrhage (IMH) which developed and induced acute symptoms. Ao asc, ascending aorta; SVC, superior vena cava; PA, pulmonary artery; TOE sector scan illustrated.

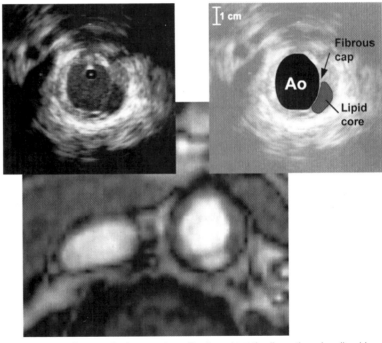

Figure 28.3. Ruptured atheroma type B, class 4 aortic dissection visualised by IVUS (invasively during aortic catheterisation) and by MRI (non-invasively). (Original IVUS images upper left; schematic drawing upper right, MRI lower part). The fibrous cap, lipid pool, aortic lumen, and atheroma are indicated. Ao, aorta.

Imaging of aortic dissection

Many imaging techniques can be used in order to confirm the diagnosis of aortic dissection and describe the extent of dissection, the localisation of tears, the presence of aortic regurgitation, pericardial effusion, emergency signs, and side branch involvement. It is important that the diagnostic strategy is standardised and leads to quick decisions concerning the most appropriate therapeutic options..

Transoesophogeal echocardiography

A recent international multicentred study has shown that TOE is highly accurate in detecting class 1 aortic dissection. All information necessary for decision making is provided by this technique.[7] Sensitivity and specificity are more than 90%. Duplex sonography can be used to detect involvement of abdominal arteries as well as carotid arteries. But the imaging quality in these areas rarely reaches the quality necessary for decision making. Importantly, the negative predictive accuracy of TOE is nearly 100%. Also class 2, 4, and 5 dissections can be diagnosed. Presence of a class 3 dissection should be suspected when a very localised bulging of the aortic wall can be seen in patients with persistent chest pain.[3]

Computed tomography

CT is widely available and commonly used in patients with aortic dissection. The drawback of CT is the inability to diagnose aortic regurgitation and to localise entry tears precisely. The advantage of this technique is that the total extent of the aortic dissection and side branch involvement can be visualised as well as pericardial and pleura effusion. The sensitivity is not as high as for TOE, but the specificity is similar. Also class 2, 4, and 5 dissections can be detected. The visualisation of class 3 dissection is not possible, however.[3]

Magnetic resonance imaging

MRI seems to be the most sensitive method for diagnosing aortic dissection, and has the same specificity as TOE and CT.[9] Until now only a few centres used the technique in acute dissections, owing to the difficulties in handling emergency cases, but in stable patients, particularly chronic dissection during follow up, MRI seems to be the method of choice.[8] Nearly all diagnostic requirements can be fulfilled; tears are detected and side branch involvement even of coronary arteries can be described. Class 3 dissection, however, cannot be detected.[3]

Angiography and intravascular ultrasound

For a long time angiography was the gold standard for imaging patients with aortic dissection. It has now been replaced by the newer imaging methods, as they are non-invasive and avoid the use of radiographic contrast agents. The sensitivity and specificity of angiography is lower than that for the newer imaging techniques. In particular, there are problems in detecting class 2 and 4 dissection with angiography, but it has been helpful in detecting discrete or subtle class 3 dissection and traumatic class 5 dissection. IVUS was introduced in order to overcome the shortcomings of angiography, and to guide interventions, particularly those involving coronary arteries.[10] IVUS has a high resolution for visualising the aortic wall when transducer frequencies of 7.5–10 MHz are used. The total extent of aortic dissection can be analysed. The intimal flap can be visualised, and large entries and re-entries detected. The method seems to be the best technique to visualise side branch involvement and intramural haematoma, as well as plaque ulceration (class 2 and 4) dissection. However, it has not been used so far for visualising class 3 dissections. As it is an invasive method, IVUS is usually undertaken at the same time as angiography. It is currently indicated for guiding aortic fenestration and graft stenting. Newer linear array transducers fixed to a steerable tip allow not only two dimensional imaging but also Doppler, colour Doppler, and even tissue Doppler imaging. The shortcoming of conventional IVUS—no flow visualisation—is now being overcome.

Management of aortic dissection

Medical assessment and stabilisation

When aortic dissection is suspected, treatment to lower blood pressure has to be started, in combination with sedatives as well as analgesics[8]. Blood pressure lowering is the main aim except in patients with haemodynamic deterioration. β Blocking agents are the drugs of choice because they decrease the acceleration of blood pressure and aortic wall stress. Esmolol and metoprolol can be injected to achieve rapid results. Esmolol has a short half life, so that optimal titration can be achieved.[8] Usually it is necessary to combine these drugs with other agents such as sodium nitroprusside or clonidine in order to achieve a constant lower blood pressure. It is important that the blood pressure control is continued during subsequent patient management. This means that the patient's heart rate and blood pressure must be closely monitored. An ECG is regularly performed, in order to detect signs of myocardial ischaemia. In less than 1% of patients with signs of acute myocardial infarction, thrombolytic treatment had been started when aortic dissection was present. The physical examination may detect signs of aortic regurgitation, and a difference in blood pressure between the right and left arm owing to side branch involvement. Painless limb ischaemia is typical for the Leriche syndrome. Visceral ischaemia is followed by severe abdominal pain and involvement of renal arteries, indicated by the development of renal failure. Stroke and paraplegia may be the first manifestations of aortic dissection.

Surgery

The patient should be transferred to the operating theatre as soon as possible. Involvement of the surgeon in the emergency department or imaging department can prove very helpful to shorten time for decision making and to answer the most important questions before surgery.[8] In emergency situations, it may be helpful to move the patient directly to the operating theatre, when the suspicion of type A dissection is present based on transthoracic echocardiography. TOE can be performed just before surgery in the operating theatre. This strategy is recommended when signs of emergency are present and further diagnostic steps may delay surgery.[8]

Surgery is indicated in type A, class 1 dissection because the natural history demonstrates a high mortality, which can be reduced but not completely eliminated. Nowadays the perioperative surgical mortality is still between 20–35%.[11] However, quick decision making made possible by the new imaging techniques has already reduced the preoperative mortality by 50%.[8] The surgical aim is to prevent aortic rupture and tamponade caused by pericardial effusion, and to repair aortic regurgitation and re-establish flow if arteries are blocked. For class 2, 3, and 4 dissection surgery is recommended when pain is persisting and emergency signs are present. Class 5 dissection often heals spontaneously but may require surgery if it progresses and symptoms persist. In blunt chest trauma, however, surgery is indicated when intimal or medial dissections are present, in order to prevent transection of the aortic wall and further fatal events.

Surgery will lead to replacement of the ascending aorta with or without aortic valve prosthesis.[11 12] Nowadays the full aortic root is replaced because, during follow up, aneurysm formation between the aortic valve and the conduit has been observed, when this part of the aorta is left in place. The surgical procedure has improved in recent years by using French glue, which allows attachment of different aortic layers to the aortic prosthesis, eliminating the formation of haematomas, and strengthens the aortic wall.[12] Surgery involves the aortic arch when the tear is found in this area. A reimplantation of the innominate artery or other arteries may be necessary. Some authors have suggested implanting an "elephant trunk", which ends open in the proximal descending aorta and can later be connected to a graft prosthesis.[13] After surgery, the false lumen is open in more than 90% of the patients. Rarely, complete occlusion of the false lumen is found during follow up.

Surgery in aortic dissection type B, class 1 is restricted to patients with signs of aortic expansion, persistence or recurrence of chest pain, and emergency signs. Surgery in acute type B dissection has a mortality of more than 30%.[11] A drawback is the high rate (up to 30%) of paraplegia, which can be observed after this procedure, despite the availability of more sophisticated techniques for spinal cord protection.[8] The same holds true for class 2, 4, and 5 dissections. Thus, the decision is made on a very individual basis.

Fenestration for management of ischaemia

New interventional techniques have been introduced, particularly in order to improve the outcome in patients with aortic dissection and to treat complications. Aortic fenestration is performed in order to create a communication between the true and false lumen, whenever the true lumen is compressed by the false lumen and an intimal flap is occluding the ostium of one of the abdominal or limb arteries.[14] The procedure is indicated when signs of bowel or limb ischaemia are present. Another indication is in the event of renal failure developing. The intimal flap is passed via the true lumen using stiff wires or a Brockenbrough needle. The needle is switched for regular guide wires. Balloons between 10–14 mm are introduced into the false lumen and inflated in order to create a tear in the intimal flap. Usually one puncture is sufficient, in order to improve and relieve the signs of ischaemia. Rarely, multiple punctures are necessary. In stable situations the procedure is performed after surgery, when signs of ischaemia develop. Meanwhile, it has been suggested that the procedure should be undertaken even before surgery, when signs of ischaemia are predominant such as in bowel ischaemia or in the presence of neurological deficits. More than 200 procedures have now been performed worldwide, with evidence of improved safety and low complication rates as experience increases.

Stent implantation

Stent graft implantation was first used to treat true and false aneurysms of the abdominal and later thoracic aorta, and subsequently has been introduced for treatment of patients with aortic dissection type B, class 1, 4, and 5. The aim is to cover the entry tear or aortic ulcer and induce thrombosis of the false lumen in order to stimulate the healing process. The aim is not to push the intimal flap to the aortic wall, but to close the tear or tears. The indication for graft stenting is seen in dissection of the descending aorta of more than 5.5–6 cm, intramural haematoma, or even class 5 dissection. The procedure is in development, but it has already shown encouraging results; only rarely have signs of paraplegia or neurological deficits been observed despite use of long graft stents.[15 16] The average size of the stents being used is between 25–35 mm, according to the size of the true lumen, and the length is between 10–20 cm. While a number of problems still need to be resolved, this new option for treating patients with acute or chronic type B dissection looks set to improve their future prognosis.[8]

Traumatic aortic disease

Blunt chest trauma is mainly related to car accidents, but may be observed as a result of other forms of deceleration trauma, such as sports injuries. It may also occur after aortic cross clamping or after the use of intra-aortic balloon pumping in cardiac surgery. Traumatic injury has also been reported following catheterisation of the aorta. Coarctation angioplasty is regularly followed by intimal disruption but may extend to aortic dissection or rupture. After coronary angioplasty antegrade dissection from the ostium of the coronary arteries to the ascending aorta has been observed.

Following high speed accidents 15–20% of deaths are secondary to aortic injury. Traumatic aortic disease has a high mortality and therefore urgent diagnosis and treatment is necessary.[17] This can be performed in the emergency room with TOE, which is able to show the early stages of the traumatic injury, starting with intimal disruption and transection of the aorta. It is important to determine the distance between the aorta and the oesophagus. If this distance exceeds 1 cm the presence of mediastinal haematoma has to be taken into account. If the mediastinal haematoma is progressive, compression of the left atrium can occur as a sign of an advanced stage of the mediastinal bleeding. Flow transecting the aortic wall can be visualised by colour Doppler echocardiography, forming pseudoaneurysms (false aneurysms) in the chronic stage. Periaortic fluid accumulation can be imaged by TOE. Echolucent areas around the adventitia of the aorta are found and represent a sign of ongoing penetration and pending rupture.

CT can also be used to detect disruption of the aorta in cases of blunt chest trauma. This technique has a high specificity to detect transection of the aorta, but small ruptures may be missed. In addition the injection of contrast material in patients who are severely haemodynamically unstable may be deleterious. Recent analysis suggested using CT if mediastinal widening is detected by chest *x* ray for its better spatial orientation, and TOE when this sign is absent for its better resolution.[17]

Whether or not TOE or CT are used will depend on the emergency teams' expertise, and the availability of expert personnel around the clock. Urgent surgery in patients with blunt chest trauma does improve the prognosis, as interposition of graft prothesis is helpful to stabilise the patient and prevent aortic rupture or lethal bleeding.[16]

Inflammatory aortic diseases

Inflammatory disease of the aorta can lead to a weakening of the aortic walls. Bacterial and fungal aortitis are rare, but focal disruption of the vessel wall can result in aneurysm formation, dissection or rupture.

Autoimmune diseases of the aorta include vasculitis in large and medium size vessels, such as Takayasu aortitis, giant cell arteritis, Behçet's disease, Cogan's disease, rheumatoid disease, and aortitis with retroperitoneal fibrosis (Ormond's disease).

Inflammation related to infectious diseases such as luetic aortitis is followed by a thickening of the aortic wall and can lead to severe chest pain, which can last for several weeks until the condition heals. Aortitis is the principal cardiovascular manifestation of syphilis and is found in both the proximal and distal parts of the aorta.[8]

The diagnosis can be made using high resolution imaging techniques, with demonstration of thickening of the aortic wall, aneurysm formation (pseudoaneurysm), and signs of rupture or dissection. Similarly the healing process can be visualised.[8]

Toxicity related aortic diseases

Experimental studies have shown that the injection of β-aminopropionitril can lead to morphological changes similar to mucoid degeneration of the aortic wall found in Marfan syndrome. Zinc administration has also resulted in aortic diseases, even aortic dissection.

In recent years it became obvious that the presence of aneurysm formation and aortic dissection in drug addicts may be related to the use of cocaine and amphetamines. Thus, involvement of large vessels, in addition to the heart, has to be taken into account in drug addicts.[8]

Inherited aortic diseases

Marfan syndrome

Marfan syndrome is an autosomal dominant connective tissue disease with a prevalence of 1 in 5000 persons. The Gent nosology describes the characteristic clinical features (table 28.2). If four of eight major criteria for the skeletal system are met, the clinical diagnosis is established.[18] As variant forms are not included, the Gent nosology has to be taken as a proposal. A protein called "fibrillin" in the extracellular matrix is a component of microfibrils with or without contact with the elastin fibres, for which more than 100 fibrillin gene mutations have been identified in Marfan patients. The mutations were found in patients with complete and incomplete Marfan syndrome but also in overlapping diseases. A second gene in Marfan syndrome type was found recently. As 7–16% of Marfan patients have normal fibrillin metabolism, other gene mutations also have to be taken into account.[19]

Family studies with specific fibrillin polymorph markers can be used to identify mutation-bearing haplotypes, and are useful in families with several affected individuals (at least four). Such studies may be possible in 6% of cases.

Mutation identification requires a molecular test, which can be performed after the protein analysis or when the family studies have conclusively shown the presence of a fibrillin gene defect. The analysis is very time consuming and costly. Each family has its own specific defects. Point mutations have been detected. It is also possible to perform prenatal diagnosis or offer presymptomatic diagnosis in children of affected subjects.

Mitral valve prolapse and aortic root dilatation are predominant signs of Marfan syndrome. Subsequently mitral and aortic regurgitation may develop. Mitral valve prolapse is found in up to two thirds of all patients using two dimensional echocardiography. Severe regurgitation occurs earlier and more frequently in Marfan syndrome than in other patients without a connective tissue disease. Mitral annulus calcification also develops. Mitral valve reconstruction is attempted which may be difficult because of severe prolapse and

Table 28.2 Gent nosology describing typical clinical and imaging features of patients with Marfan syndrome

Skeletal system
Major criteria (presence of at least 4 of the following manifestations)
- pectus carinatum
- pectus excavatum requiring surgery
- reduced upper to lower segment ratio or arm span to height ratio greater than 1.05
- wrist and thumb signs
- scoliosis of greater than 20° or spondylolisthesis
- reduced extension at the elbows (< 170°)
- medial displacement of the medial malleolus causing pes planus
- protrusio acetabulae of any degree (ascertained on radiographs)

Minor criteria
- pectus excavatum of moderate severity
- joint hypermobility
- highly arched palate with crowding of teeth
- facial appearance (dolichocephaly, malar hypoplasia, enophthalmos, retrognathia, down slanting palpebral fissures)

Ocular system
Major criteria
- Ectopia lentis

Minor criteria
- Abnormally flat cornea (as measured by keratometry)
- Increased axial length of globe (as measured by ultrasound)
- Hypoplastic iris or hypoplastic ciliary muscle causing decreased miosis

Cardiovascular system
Major criteria
- dilatation of the ascending aorta with or without aortic regurgitation and involving at least the sinuses of Valsalva or
- dissection of the ascending aorta

Minor criteria
- mitral valve prolapse with or without mitral valve regurgitation
- dilatation of the main pulmonary artery, in the absence of valvar or peripheral pulmonic stenosis or any other obvious cause, below the age of 40 years
- calcification of the mitral annulus below the age of 40 years or
- dilatation or dissection of the descending thoracic or abdominal aorta below the age of 50 years

Pulmonary system
Major criteria
- none

Minor criteria
- spontaneous pneumothorax or
- apical blebs (ascertained by chest radiography)

Skin and integument
Major criteria
- none

Minor criteria
- striae atrophicae (stretch marks) not associated with major weight changes, pregnancy or repetitive stress, or
- recurrent or incisional herniae

Dura
Major criteria
- lumbosacral dural ectasia by CT or MRI

Minor criteria
- none

Family/genetic history
Major criteria
- having a parent, child or sibling who meets these diagnostic criteria independently
- presence of a mutation in *FBN1* known to cause the Marfan syndrome or
- presence of a haplotype around *FBN1*, inherited by descent, known to be associated with unequivocally diagnosed Marfan syndrome in the family

Minor criteria
- none

When the diameter exceeds the upper normal limit by more than 1.5, annual examinations are necessary.

Aortic dissection is rare during childhood but poses a threat during adulthood. Most occur in the ascending aorta but the descending aorta may also be involved. Typical and atypical clinical features have been observed. Therefore, a high suspicion of aortic dissection in Marfan syndrome has to be present, including detailed patient information.

Aortic surgery is recommended when the diameter has reached or exceeded 5 cm independent of symptoms. Composite grafts are used to repair the ascending aorta. Resuspension of the aortic valve and ring is commonly used in order to avoid long term anticoagulation. Even replacement of the total aorta has successfully been performed in Marfan syndrome.

Ehlers-Danlos syndrome

The prevalence of Ehlers-Danlos syndrome is similar to that of Marfan syndrome and has typical clinical features. In the autosomal dominant type IV a structural defect in the pro α 1(III) chain of collagen type III was found, explaining the development of aortic aneurysm and aortic dissection. In Ehlers-Danlos syndrome abnormal collagen type III could be demonstrated in fibroblast cultures, and polymorphic markers were found. No phenotype/genotype correlations have yet been identified. The mutations do not predict the aortic disease type, course, and severity. Even a normal collagen III metabolism has been shown in typical individuals.[20]

Annuloaortic ectasia

In annuloaortic ectasia isolated diseases of the ascending aorta with or without aortic regurgitation are found, and aortic rupture and dissection may occur. More than one third of patients have an autosomal dominant transmission. First mutations of the gene COL 3 A1 have been found, but clear evidence of gene involvement has not yet been found in the majority of patients. Only two of the genes involved in annuloaortic ectasia have been identified. Both are very large and there is no evidence of a clustering of mutations within specific regions of the gene. However, since antibodies are available against collagen III and fibrillin-1, structural or metabolical abnormal proteins can be looked for in cell cultures.

Conclusions

The development of new imaging techniques has led to further insight into the pathogenesis of aortic diseases and opened the field for the development of new interventional techniques. Early stabilisation of patients should be followed by an extensive analysis (staging) of the patient's arteriosclerosis, including the aorta and the coronary, carotid, and peripheral arteries. This is important in order to stratify the patient's further management, because the

chordae tendinea rupture. Therefore, residual regurgitation and prosthesis leakages are not rare.

Aortic root dilatation is detected by echocardiography. Standard measurements are performed and aortic size related to nomograms.

prognosis is poor with a mortality rate of 50–70% within 3–5 years. Coronary and peripheral artery revascularisation by interventional techniques or surgery have to be improved in order to increase organ perfusion and/or induce thrombus formation in the false lumen. The treatment of patients with aortic diseases should be carried out by specialists, including cardiologists, interventional radiologists, and vascular/cardiovascular surgeons, who should work as a team and be involved in all steps of decision making.

I thank Dr Jörg Barkhausen and Prof. Dr Debatin (department of radiology) for the excellent magnetic resonance images, as well as Dr Holger Eggebrecht (department of cardiology) for his great help in preparing the figures, and Mrs Celesnik and Mrs Stephanie Gerstberger for their secretarial assistance.

1. **Tunick PA, Kronzon I.** Atheromas of the thoracic aorta: clinical and therapeutic update. *J Am Coll Cardiol* 2000;**35**:545–54.
   • *Excellent review of aortic sclerosis describing the prevalence of the disease, correlation to carotid artery disease, atrial fibrillation, and coronary artery disease. The importance of aortic plaque morphology in regard to the embolic risk is described as well as the different imaging techniques and therapeutic consequences.*

2. **Iribarren C, Sidney S, Sternfeld B,** *et al.* Calcification of the aortic arch. Risk factors and association with coronary heart disease, stroke, and peripheral vascular disease. *JAMA* 2000;**283**:2810–15.

3. **Svensson LG, Labib SB, Eisenhauer AC,** *et al.* Intimal tear without haematoma. *Circulation* 1999;**99**:1331–6.
   • *First description of the clinical features of discrete/subtle aortic dissection using angiography and confirmation by surgery and pathology. A new five stage classification system of aortic dissection is proposed which has been taken over by the Task Force of the European Society of Cardiology.*

4. **Maraj R, Rerkpattanapipat P, Jacobs LE,** *et al.* Meta-analysis of 143 reported cases of aortic intramural haematoma. *Am J Cardiol* 2000;**86**:664–8.

5. **Mohr-Kahaly S, Erbel R, Puth M,** *et al.* Aortic intramural haematoma visualized by transesophageal echocardiography. Follow-up and prognostic implication. *J Am Coll Cardiol* 1994;**23**:658–64.
   • *First large scale prospective study for the diagnosis of intramural haemorrhage/haematoma with the differentiation of two subtypes according to the aetiology of the disease—cystic medial necrosis and aortic sclerosis. Important clinical features and prognostic implication are presented and confirmed by recent meta-analysis (reference 4).*

6. **Stanson AV, Kamier FJ, Chollier LG.** Penetrating atherosclerotic ulcer of the thoracic aorta: natural history and clinicopathology correlation. *Ann Vasc Surg* 1986;**1**:15–23.
   • *Description of the clinical, radiographic and pathological anatomical features of aortic plaque rupture which has been taken over as class 4 dissection by Svensson et al and the Task Force of the European Society of Cardiology.*

7. **Erbel R, Engberding R, Daniel W,** *et al.* Echocardiography in diagnosis of aortic dissection. *Lancet* 1989;ii:457–61.
   • *First European multicentre prospective study for assessment of the sensitivity and specificity of TOE in comparison to CT and angiography in 164 patients with suspected aortic dissection.*

8. **Erbel R, Alfonso F, Boileau C,** *et al.* Diagnosis and management of aortic dissection. Recommendations of the task force on aortic dissection. European Society of Cardiology. *Eur Heart J* (in press).

9. **Nienaber CA, von Kodolitsch Y, Nicolas V,** *et al.* The diagnosis of thoracic aortic dissection by noninvasive procedures. *N Engl J Med* 1993;**328**:1–9.

10. **Weintraub AR, Erbel R, Görge G,** *et al.* Intravascular ultrasound imaging in acute aortic dissection. *J Am Coll Cardiol* 1994;**24**:495–503.

11. **Hagan PG, Nienaber CA, Isselbacher EM,** *et al.* The international registry of acute aortic dissection (IRAD). New insights into an old disease. *JAMA* 2000;**283**:897–903.
   • *Multicentre registry of patients with aortic dissection in the USA and Europe demonstrating the high mortality and morbidity of the disease despite progress and imaging and surgical techniques.*

12. **Bachet J, Gogou F, Laurien C.** Four-year clinical experience with gelatin-resorcine-formol biological glue in acute aortic dissection. *J Thorac Cardiovasc Surg* 1982;**83**:212–7.

13. **Borst HG, Walterbusch G, Schaps D.** Extensive aortic replacement using "elephant trunk" prosthesis. *Thorac Cardiovasc Surg* 1983;**31**:7–14.

14. **Williams DM, Lee DY, Hamilton BH,** *et al.* The dissected aorta: percutaneous treatment of ischaemic complications—principles and results. *J Vasc Intervent Radiol* 1997;**8**:605–65.

15. **Dake MD, Miller DC, Semba CP,** *et al.* Transluminal placement of endovascular stent-grafts for the treatment of descending thoracic aortic aneurysms. *N Engl J Med* 1994;**331**:1729–34.

16. **Nienaber CA, Fattori R, Lund G,** *et al.* Nonsurgical reconstruction of thoracic aortic dissection by stent-graft placement. *N Engl J Med* 1999;**340**:1539–45.

17. **Vignon P, Boncoeur MP, Francois B,** *et al.* Diagnosis of blunt traumatic cardiovascular injuries: a noninvasive approach. Multiplane transesophageal echocardiography versus helical computed tomography. *Crit Care Med* (in press)
   • *A randomised study in blunt chest trauma with assessment of the diagnostic value of TOE in comparison to CT. The results directly influence clinical daily practice.*

18. **de Paepe A, Devereux R, Dietz HC,** *et al.* Revised diagnostic criteria for the Marfan syndrome. *Am J Med Genet* 1996;**62**:417–26.
   • *Gent nosology listing the typical clinical and imaging features of Marfan syndrome. These signs can be used in order to describe the typical forms of the syndrome, but it has to be taken into account that forms also exist which do not fit perfectly well into this scheme but may show a family dominance and even characteristic gene mutations.*

19. **Boileau C, Jondeau G, Babron MC,** *et al.* Familial Marfan-like aortic dilatation and skeletal anomalies are not linked to the fibrillin genes. *Am J Hum Genet* 1993;**53**:46–57.

20. **Beighton P, de Paepe A, Steinmann B,** *et al.* Ehlers-Danlos syndromes: revised nosology, Villefranche, 1997. *J Vasc Surg* 1997;**25**:506–11.

29 Management of pericardial effusion

Jordi Soler-Soler, Jaume Sagristà-Sauleda,
Gaietà Permanyer-Miralda

Pericardial effusion is a common finding in everyday practice. Sometimes, its cause is obviously related to an underlying general or cardiac disease, or to a syndrome of inflammatory or infectious acute pericarditis. On other occasions, pericardial effusion is an unexpected finding that requires specific evaluation. In these cases, the main issues are aetiology, the clinical course, and the possibility of evolution to haemodynamic embarrassment. This is especially relevant in cases of large pericardial effusions, in which echocardiographic recordings not infrequently show findings suggestive of subclinical haemodynamic derangement, mainly right atrial or right ventricular wall collapse. These uncertainties have led to a heterogeneous approach to the management of the syndrome of pericardial effusion by different groups of investigators.

The main goal of this article is to give a comprehensive review of aetiology, haemodynamic findings, and management of pericardial effusion. In addition, some comments on the management of neoplastic pericardial effusion are also provided.

Approach to mild pericardial effusion

In an asymptomatic patient, a pericardial effusion of less than 10 mm on the echocardiogram may be an incidental finding, especially in elderly women, as shown in the Framingham study.[1] In these patients, neither invasive studies nor treatment are required. A follow up echocardiogram is probably warranted to see if the echocardiographic findings are unchanged. Further investigation or treatment of these patients is not necessary if the echo findings are stable.

Aetiologic spectrum and prognosis of moderate and large pericardial effusion

A wide variety of conditions may result in pericardial effusion. All types of acute pericarditis (inflammatory, infectious, immunologic or of physical origin) can be associated with pericardial effusion.[2] In addition, pericardial effusion of varying degrees can be seen in other conditions such as neoplasia (with or without direct pericardial involvement), myxoedema, renal insufficiency, pregnancy, aortic or cardiac rupture, trauma, chylopericardium, or in the setting of chronic salt and water retention of many causes, including chronic heart failure, nephrotic syndrome, and hepatic cirrhosis. Only three major studies[3-5] have addressed one of the most common clinical problems—the aetiology of large pericardial effusion of unknown origin. These three studies (table 29.1) are prospective and were done in general medical centres, but differ in respect to the criteria used to define a pericardial effusion as large, in the number of patients included and, in particular, in the study protocol applied to the patients.

Colombo and colleagues[3] consider effusions greater than 10 mm by M mode echocardiography as large, whereas Corey and associates[4] considered large effusions if they were greater than 5 mm. In the series by Sagristà-Sauleda and colleagues[5] moderate effusions were defined as an echo-free space of anterior plus posterior pericardial spaces of 10–20 mm during diastole, and severe effusions as a sum of echo-free spaces greater than 20 mm.

The series by Colombo and colleagues[3] included 25 male patients, all of whom were submitted to an invasive pericardial procedure. Of these patients, 44% presented with cardiac tamponade. The most frequent causes of pericardial effusion were: neoplastic (36%), idiopathic (32%), and uraemic (20%). The prognosis was strongly determined by the patients' underlying disease, and was particularly poor in patients with neoplastic pericardial effusion, none of whom survived longer than five months after the initial pericardial drainage.

Corey and associates[4] investigated the aetiology of pericardial effusion in 57 patients. The prevalence of cardiac tamponade was not reported. Each patient was assessed by a comprehensive preoperative evaluation followed by subxiphoid pericardiotomy. Microscopic examination of the samples of pericardial fluid and tissue was undertaken; the samples were also cultured for aerobic and anaerobic bacteria, fungi, mycobacteria, mycoplasma, and viruses. Aetiologic diagnosis was made in 53 patients (93%). The most common diagnoses were malignancy (23% of patients), viral infection (14%), radiation induced inflammation (14%), collagen–vascular disease (12%), and uraemia (12%). In only four patients was no diagnosis made. Prognosis was not assessed in this study.

Table 29.1 Moderate-large pericardial effusion trials

	Corey[4]	Colombo[3]	Sagristà[5]
Effusion	> 5 mm	> 10 mm	> 10 mm
n	57	25	322
Tamponade	Not reported	44%	37%
Idiopathic	7%	32%	20%*
Chronic idiopathic effusion	?	?	9%
Neoplastic	23%	36%	13%
Uraemia	12%	20%	6%
Iatrogenic	0%	0%	16%
Post-acute myocardial infarction	0%	8%	8%
Viral	14%	0%	0%
Collagen vascular disease	12%	0%	5%
Tuberculosis	0%	0%	2%
Other	9%	4%	21%

*Acute idiopathic pericarditis; ? no distinction between acute idiopathic pericarditis and idiopathic chronic pericardial effusion.

The study by Sagristà-Sauleda and colleagues[5] included 322 patients, 132 with moderate and 190 with severe pericardial effusion. Cardiac tamponade was present in 37%. The patients were studied following our own protocol for the management of pericardial diseases,[6] in which invasive pericardial procedures were not systematically performed but were only undertaken under precisely defined indications. In this series, the most common diagnosis was acute idiopathic pericarditis which accounted for 20% of patients. The next most prevalent diagnoses were iatrogenic effusion (16%), neoplastic effusion (13%), and chronic idiopathic pericardial effusion (9%). As in the series by Colombo and colleagues,[3] the prognosis was related to the underlying disease, deaths occurring mainly among patients with malignancy.

Other series are limited to patients with clinical[7] or echocardiographic[8] tamponade. Among the 56 patients with tamponade included in the study of Guberman and colleagues,[7] the most common diagnoses were metastatic cancer in 18 patients, idiopathic pericarditis in eight patients, and uraemia in five. Once again, the worst prognosis was in the group of patients with cancer. Finally, in the study by Levine and associates[8] involving 50 patients, the most frequent aetiologies of pericardial effusion were malignancy (58%), idiopathic effusion (14%), and uraemia (14%). The ultimate survival of patients identified in this study did not correlate with initial haemodynamic status, but with the underlying aetiology, with a 17% cumulative probability of survival at one year for the group with malignancy and 91% for the group without malignancy.

Therefore, the main causes of large pericardial effusion in general medical centres are idiopathic pericarditis and malignancy. Remarkably, iatrogenic effusion accounted for 16% and chronic idiopathic pericardial effusion for 9% of patients in the largest series.[5] Nowadays tuberculosis is a rare cause of pericardial effusion in western societies (table 1), although this may not be the case in developing countries with a high prevalence of tuberculosis. In fact, the aetiologic spectrum of pericardial effusion largely depends on the source of the patients, the relative size and activity of the different departments in general hospitals (especially the different number of patients with neoplastic disease who attend each hospital), and, of course, on the frequency distribution of the different aetiologies of pericardial diseases in each geographical area.

Clinical clues to aetiology

When a clinician is faced with a patient who presents with large pericardial effusion, the challenge is to identify its aetiology. In some instances, it can be easily related to an associated condition or iatrogenic procedure, but often the aetiology may be difficult to establish. Agner and Gallis,[9] in a retrospective

> ### Aetiology of moderate and large pericardial effusion
>
> - A wide variety of conditions may result in pericardial effusion. The aetiologic spectrum in different series largely depends on the source of the patients, the characteristics of the centre, and on the frequency distribution of the different aetiologies in each geographic area
>
> - In many cases, pericardial effusion is associated with a previous known condition or underlying cardiac disease, which are finally proven to be the cause of the pericardial effusion
>
> - In patients with no apparent cause of pericardial effusion, the presence of inflammatory signs is predictive of acute (idiopathic) pericarditis; on the other hand, severe effusion with absence of inflammatory signs and absence of tamponade is predictive of chronic idiopathic pericardial effusion. Tamponade without inflammatory signs is suspicious for neoplastic pericardial effusion
>
> - The prognosis of pericardial effusion is related to the underlying disease, being especially poor in patients with malignancy

series of 133 patients, observed that haemodynamic compromise, cardiomegaly, pleural effusion, and large pericardial effusion were more common in patients with tuberculous or malignant disease than in patients with idiopathic pericarditis. In the series of Posner and colleagues,[10] dealing with 31 patients with cancer and pericardial disease, patients with malignant pericardial disease had tamponade more frequently, whereas fever, a pericardial friction rub, and improvement following treatment with non-steroidal anti-inflammatory drugs characterised patients with idiopathic pericarditis. Haemorrhagic pericardial effusion has been associated with neoplasia and a poor survival in some studies,[3] but haemorrhagic effusions can be seen in patients with idiopathic pericarditis. The predictive value of these different clinical findings for assessing the aetiology of pericardial effusion has not been established.

In our recent prospective study of 322 patients with moderate and severe pericardial effusion,[5] we investigated the value of selected clinical data (underlying disease, development of cardiac tamponade, and presence or absence of inflammatory signs) for inclusion of the patients in a likely major aetiologic diagnostic category. In 60% of the patients a known previous condition that could cause pericardial effusion was present. The pericardial effusion was shown to be related to the underlying disease in all but seven of these patients. In the patients with no apparent cause of pericardial effusion at the time of diagnosis (40%) we found that the presence of inflammatory signs (characteristic chest pain, pericardial friction rub, fever or typical electrocardiographic

206

changes) was predictive for acute idiopathic pericarditis (p < 0.001, likelihood ratio 5.4), irrespective of the size of effusion and presence or absence of tamponade. Furthermore, a large effusion with absence of inflammatory signs and absence of tamponade was predictive of chronic idiopathic pericardial effusion (p < 0.001, likelihood ratio 20), and tamponade without inflammatory signs predictive of neoplastic pericardial effusion (p < 0.001, likelihood ratio 2.9). The search for evidence of a previous effusion can be particularly helpful, as it may help to distinguish neoplastic disease from chronic idiopathic pericardial effusion, which sometimes presents with tamponade. Therefore, although the final aetiologic diagnosis should certainly be based on specific clinical data in individual patients, we think that the data afforded by this study (fig 29.1) may be helpful in the initial assessment and in the decision to perform invasive pericardial studies.

Special attention should be given to tuberculous pericarditis. Most patients with acute pericarditis will turn out to have idiopathic pericarditis, but a few cases will be tuberculous in origin. Identification of these cases is important because of the obvious therapeutic implications. The diagnosis can be established through general examination, including the search of tubercle bacilli in sputum or gastric aspirate (which provided the diagnosis in four of our eight cases[5]), or by means of pericardial fluid or pericardial tissue examination (indicated in patients with tamponade or with persistent active illness for more than three weeks).

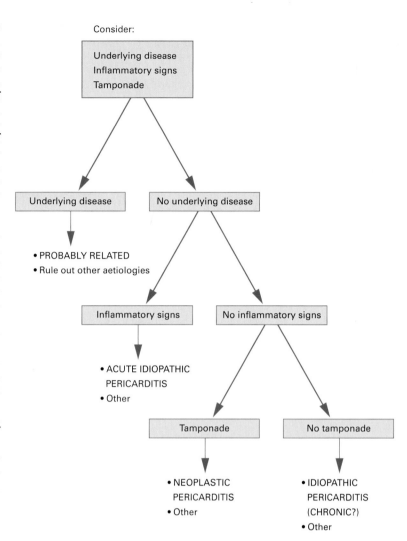

Figure 29.1. Initial approach to aetiologic diagnosis of large pericardial effusion. This flow chart shows the aetiologic likelihood of large pericardial effusion depending on simple clinical data (presence of underlying disease, inflammatory signs, and tamponade). Modified from Sagristà-Sauleda *et al.*[5]

Clinical correlation of echocardiographic and catheterisation findings

Before the advent of echocardiography and cardiac catheterisation, the haemodynamic compromise caused by pericardial effusion could be recognised only through physical findings such as jugular venous distension, hepatomegaly, hypotension, or pulsus paradoxus. These clinical findings defined the condition known as classical clinical tamponade. With the availability of echocardiography it was soon realised[11][12] that some patients with pericardial effusion but without clinical tamponade show findings suggesting raised intrapericardial pressure—namely, collapse of the right sided cardiac chambers. Cardiologists were puzzled about the clinical relevance of these findings, especially regarding the indication of pericardial drainage, since these findings were interpreted as "impending" cardiac tamponade. Studies correlating clinical, echocardiographic, and catheterisation data helped to clarify this problem, although some doubts remain.

In the study by Levine and colleagues,[8] 50 consecutive patients with pericardial effusion and echocardiographic findings suggestive of tamponade (defined as the presence of right heart chamber collapse) underwent combined right sided cardiac catheterisation and percutaneous pericardiocentesis. Right atrial collapse was present in 92%, and right ventricular collapse in 57% of patients, respectively. The initial pericardial pressure was raised in all patients (range 3–27 mm Hg) and was equal to right atrial pressure in 84% of patients. However, many patients had minimal evidence of haemodynamic compromise. For example, systolic blood pressure was higher than 100 mm Hg in 94% of patients, elevation of the jugular venous pressure was found in only 74%, hepatomegaly was present in 28%, and pulsus paradoxus was found in only 36% of patients. In comparison with the series of Guberman and associates,[7] which included patients with classical clinical tamponade, the patients in the series of Levine and colleagues[8] had a significantly lower prevalence of hypotension, abnormal pulsus paradoxus, jugular venous pressure elevation, and hepatomegaly. In fact, in 25 patients (50%) tamponade had not been suspected before the echocardiographic study. Pericardiocentesis was associated with reduction of mean (SD) pericardial pressure in all patients (15 (5) to 1 (5) mm Hg), but frequently did not alleviate dyspnoea or correct tachycardia.

These findings suggest that echocardiography can identify patients with pericardial effusion causing elevation of pericardial pressure before overt haemodynamic embarrassment develops, as the majority of these patients had only mild to moderate clinical tamponade. Subsequent studies have also shown that some patients with moderate or severe pericardial effusion and without any sign of clinical tamponade have chamber collapse at echocardiographic examination. For example, in the study by Mercé and colleagues,[13] which included 110 patients with moderate or severe pericardial effusion, 34% of 72 patients without clinical tamponade showed collapse of one or more cardiac chambers. Specifically, right atrial collapse had a low positive predictive value (50%) for clinical cardiac tamponade. However, these patients consistently show elevation of intrapericardial pressure when they undergo catheterisation study. Patients with asymptomatic large pericardial effusions without echocardiographic collapse show elevation of intrapericardial pressure, which equalises with right atrial pressure and becomes normal after pericardiocentesis. This situation is often found in patients with chronic massive pericardial effusion, as discussed below. Experimental[14–17] and clinical[18 19] studies have shown that cardiac tamponade is not an "all or nothing" phenomenon but a continuum that goes from slight elevation of intrapericardial pressure with subtle haemodynamic changes to severe haemodynamic embarrassment and even death.

Indications for invasive pericardial procedures in the absence of clinical tamponade

The prognosis of pericardial effusion mainly depends on the underlying aetiology, provided that haemodynamic compromise is not life threatening. The optimal management of large pericardial effusion without clinical tamponade is controversial. Some authors[3 4] advise routine pericardial drainage by pericardiocentesis or surgical pericardiotomy, claiming diagnostic and therapeutic benefits. However, these procedures are not innocuous and some fatalities have been reported. Our opinion is that in patients without haemodynamic compromise, routine pericardial drainage would only be justified if it might provide relevant diagnostic information or help to avoid further tamponade. In a study by our group,[20] which included 71 patients with large pericardial effusion without clinical tamponade or suspected purulent pericarditis, we found that pericardial drainage procedures (performed in 26 patients) had a diagnostic yield of only 7%. On the other hand, no patients developed cardiac tamponade or died as a result of pericardial disease, nor did any new diagnosis become apparent in the 45 patients who did not have pericardial drainage initially. Furthermore, moderate or large effusions persisted in only two of 45 patients managed conservatively. In

Indications for pericardiocentesis/surgical drainage

- Pericardiocentesis is indicated in patients with overt clinical tamponade, in patients with suspicion of purulent pericarditis, and in patients with idiopathic chronic large pericardial effusion

- The indications for surgical drainage are tamponade, either unresolved or relapsing after pericardiocentesis, and persistent active illness three weeks after hospital admission

- Pericardial drainage does not seem warranted in the initial management of patients with large pericardial effusion without clinical tamponade because of its low diagnostic yield and its poor influence on the evolution of pericardial effusion. Even the presence of echocardiographic right chamber collapse (suggesting raised intrapericardial pressure) does not warrant by itself pericardial drainage as most of these patients do not evolve to overt tamponade

another study by our group,[12] we found that even patients with echocardiographic collapse rarely require pericardial drainage for therapeutic purposes during initial admission. Accordingly, we think that routine pericardial drainage is not justified in the initial management of patients with large pericardial effusion without clinical tamponade, especially if the aetiology is known. The exceptions would be those patients with suspected purulent or tuberculous pericarditis.

Idiopathic chronic pericardial effusion

When a large pericardial effusion persists for more than three months, the prognosis, even in asymptomatic patients, is less good. Sagristà-Sauleda and colleagues[21] have reported that up to 29% of such patients may develop unexpected, overt cardiac tamponade. In these patients medical treatment, particularly corticosteroids or antituberculous therapy, is not useful. The trigger of tamponade is unknown, but hypovolaemia, paroxysmal tachyarrhythmias, and intercurrent acute pericarditis may precipitate tamponade; accordingly, these events should be vigorously managed.

Role of pericardiocentesis
Pericardiocentesis is the first option in patients with overt tamponade. Elective pericardiocentesis is warranted in asymptomatic patients as well, as a prophylactic measure to prevent unexpected tamponade. In these patients pericardiocentesis may result in the disappearance of chronic pericardial effusion as was the case in eight of 19 patients with effusions present for at least four years.[21] Pericardiocentesis should drain as much pericardial fluid as possible. In

Idiopathic chronic pericardial effusion

- Large (echo-free spaces > 20 mm), chronic (longer than three months) idiopathic pericardial effusion may evolve to unexpected clinical tamponade in spite of a previous prolonged (years) good clinical tolerance

- Anti-inflammatory drugs and corticosteroids are unsuccessful. Pericardiocentesis may allow the resolution of effusion in a third of patients. When large effusion reappears after two pericardiocenteses, wide anterior pericardiectomy has to be considered

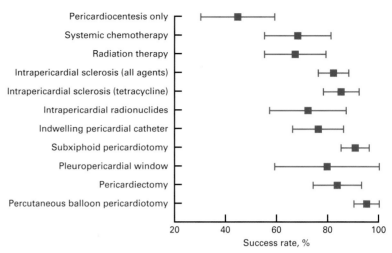

Figure 29.2. Success rates with 95% confidence intervals for different treatment modalities of malignant pericardial effusions to prevent further pericardial complications. Reproduced form Vaitkus et al[28] (Treatment of malignant pericardial effusion. *JAMA* 1994;**272**:59–64). Copyrighted (1994), American Medical Association.

some cases with a relapsing effusion, it has been shown that a second pericardiocentesis is usually followed by complete resolution of the effusion.

Role of pericardiectomy

Surgical drainage with wide anterior pericardiectomy is very effective in the long term.[21 22] At the present time, we recommend this procedure only in patients, with or without symptoms, in which repeat pericardiocentesis is not followed by notable or complete diminution of the effusion.

Management of neoplastic pericardial effusion

Symptoms and signs suggestive of pericardial involvement may be the presenting clinical feature of either primary[23] or secondary[24] malignant cardiac disease, but they are much more frequently present in patients under treatment for advanced malignancy. Life expectancy is short as concomitant metastases are nearly always present elsewhere. In these instances, adequate management of pericardial effusion may contribute to palliation of the symptoms—in a significant number of patients—and possibly to prolonged survival (in an undefined number of cases). Although the main causes of death in patients with malignancy are unrelated to cardiac involvement, in some necropsy series pericardial metastases are commonly found, particularly in lung cancer (35%)[25] and breast cancer (25%)[26]; on the other hand, cardiac symptoms are mainly related to the presence of tamponade, which is present in a significant number of patients, although it has no negative impact on survival if it is correctly managed.

In patients with malignancy and pericardial effusion the first step is to determine whether the effusion is secondary to neoplastic pericardial involvement or if it is an epiphenomenon (non-malignant effusion) related to the management of the cancer (such as previous thoracic irradiation) or effusions of unknown origin. In these two latter situations, an invasive procedure may be warranted in the absence of tamponade as the diagnostic yield of both pericardial fluid and tissue is high for malignancy.[27]

The management of cardiac tamponade in patients with secondary neoplastic pericardial involvement has two targets—relief of symptoms, and prevention of recurrences. Pericardiocentesis alleviates symptoms in most cases. It is a safe, simple, and widely available procedure with few complications if it is done under echocardiographic guidance. Probably it is the procedure of choice in end stage patients, when recurrence of effusion is not a real issue. In patients surviving longer the pericardial fluid may re-accumulate, and isolated pericardiocentesis prevents this in only about 50% of cases.[28] In such patients a more aggressive approach with surgery may be warranted. Patient management has to be individualised (type and stage of neoplasm, general condition, etc)[28 29] as even the best possible treatment for responsive types of tumour (for example, lymphoma) with neoplastic pericardial involvement is associated with survival of only about one year.

Procedures to prevent tamponade

Among the several procedures suggested to prevent tamponade, none has emerged as the treatment of choice (fig 29.2)[28]; adequate controlled trials for the different procedures in the several types of neoplasm are not available. The rate of success (defined as a procedure without mortality, no recurrent cardiac symptoms, and no additional pericardial procedure) of the above mentioned treatment modalities is depicted in fig 29.2. Taking into consideration the poor prognosis of these patients we favour the less invasive procedures, although a surgical approach may occasionally be indicated.

1. **Savage DD, Garrison RJ, Brand F,** *et al.* Prevalence and correlates of posterior extra echocardiographic spaces in a free-living population based sample (The Framingham Study). *Am J Cardiol* 1983;**51**:1207–12.
- *This study showed that the prevalence of echocardiographic-free spaces in 5652 people increased with age, being higher than 15% in those older than 80 years.*

2. **Oakley CM.** Myocarditis, pericarditis, and other pericardial diseases. *Heart* 2000;**84**:449–54.

3. **Colombo A, Olson HG, Egan J,** *et al.* Etiology and prognostic implications of a large pericardial effusion in men. *Clin Cardiol* 1988;**11**:389–94.

4. Corey GR, Campbell PT, Van Trigt P, *et al*. Etiology of large pericardial effusions. *Am J Med* 1993;**95**:209–13.

5. Sagristá-Sauleda J, Mercé J, Permanyer-Miralda G, *et al*. Clinical clues to the causes of large pericardial effusion. *Am J Med* 2000;**109**:95-101.
• *A prospective study of 322 consecutive patients with large pericardial effusions, which provides simple clinical clues (amount of pericardial effusion, presence of inflammatory signs, and presence of tamponade) useful for establishing aetiology.*

6. Soler-Soler J, Permanyer-Miralda G, Sagristà-Sauleda J. Pericardial disease. New insights and old dilemmas. Appendix I. Protocol for the diagnosis and management of pericardial diseases. Dordrecht, the Netherlands: Kluwer Academic Publishers, 1990:217–22.

7. Guberman BA, Fowler NO, Engel PJ, *et al*. Cardiac tamponade in medical patients. *Circulation* 1981;**64**:633–40.

8. Levine MJ, Lorell BH, Divier DJ, *et al*. Implications of echocardiographically assisted diagnosis of pericardial tamponade in contemporary medical patients: detection before hemodynamic embarrassment. *J Am Coll Cardiol* 1991;**17**:59–65.
• *A study showing the correlation between echocardiographic findings, haemodynamic parameters, and clinical signs of tamponade.*

9. Agner RC, Gallis HA. Pericarditis. Differential diagnosis considerations. *Arch Intern Med* 1979;**139**:407–12.

10. Posner MR, Cohen GI, Skarin AT. Pericardial disease in patients with cancer. The differentiation of malignant from radiation-induced pericarditis. *Am J Med* 1981;**7**:407–13.

11. Shiina A, Yaginuma T, Kondo K, *et al*. Echocardiographic evaluation of impending cardiac tamponade. *J Cardiography* 1979;**9**:555–63.

12. Engle PJ, Hon H, Fowler NO, *et al*. Echocardiographic study of right ventricular wall motion in cardiac tamponade. *Am J Cardiol* 1982;**50**:1018–21.

13. Mercé J, Sagristá Sauleda J, Permanyer Miralda G, *et al*. Correlation between clinical and Doppler echocardiographic findings in patients with moderate and large pericardial effusion: implications for the diagnosis of cardiac tamponade. *Am Heart J* 1999;**138**:759–64.
• *A further study showing that echo-Doppler findings suggestive of raised intrapericardial pressure are very common in patients with large pericardial effusions without clinical tamponade.*

14. Leimgruber PP, Klopfenstein HS, Wann LS, *et al*. The hemodynamic derangement associated with right ventricular diastolic collapse in cardiac tamponade: an experimental echocardiographic study. *Circulation* 1983;**68**:612–20.

15. Klopfenstein HS, Cogswell TL, Bernath GA, *et al*. Alterations in intravascular volume affect the relation between right ventricular diastolic collapse and the hemodynamic severity of cardiac tamponade. *J Am Coll Cardiol* 1985;**6**:1057–63.

16. Rifkin RD, Pandian NJ, Funai JT, *et al*. Sensitivity of right atrial collapse and right ventricular diastolic collapse in the diagnosis of graded cardiac tamponade. *Am J Noninvasive Cardiol* 1987;**1**:73–80.

17. Gonzalez MS, Basnight MA, Appleton CP. Experimental pericardial effusion: relation of abnormal respiratory variation in mitral flow velocity to hemodynamics and diastolic right heart collapse. *J Am Coll Cardiol* 1991;**17**:239–48.

18. Singh S, Wann LS, Schuchard GH. Right ventricular and right atrial collapse in patients with cardiac tamponade: a combined echocardiographic and hemodynamic study. *Circulation* 1984;**70**:966–71.

19. Reddy PS, Curtiss EI, Uretsky BF. Spectrum of hemodynamic changes in cardiac tamponade. *Am J Cardiol* 1990;**66**:1487–91.
• *This study provides elegant clinical and haemodynamic observations that show tamponade is a continuum and not an "all or nothing" phenomenon.*

20. Mercé J, Sagristá-Sauleda J, Permanyer-Miralda G, *et al*. Should pericardial drainage be performed routinely in patients who have a large pericardial effusion without tamponade? *Am J Med* 1998;**105**:106–9.
• *In a prospective series of 71 patients with large pericardial effusions without clinical tamponade, pericardial drainage procedures had a very low diagnostic yield and a poor influence on the evolution of effusion.*

21. Sagristà-Sauleda J, Angel J, Permanyer-Miralda G, *et al*. Long-term follow-up of idiopathic chronic pericardial effusion. *N Engl J Med* 1999;**341**:2054–9.
• *This 20 year follow up prospective study provides the haemodynamic pattern, clinical evolution, and prognosis of this unusual form of pericardial disease, and proposes an apparently effective management approach.*

22. Loire R, Goineau P, Fareh S, *et al*. Épanchements péricardiques chroniques d'apparance idiopatique: evolution à long terme de 71 cas. *Arch Mal Coeur* 1996;**89**:835–41.

23. Galve E, Permanyer-Miralda G, Tornos MP, *et al*. Self limited acute pericarditis as initial manifestation of primary cardiac tumor. *Am Heart J* 1992;**123**:1690–2.

24. Soler-Soler J, Permanyer-Miralda G, Sagristà-Sauleda J. A systematic diagnostic approach to primary acute pericardial disease. The Barcelona experience. In: Shabetai R, ed. *Diseases of the pericardium. Cardiology Clinics.* Philadelphia: WB Saunders Company, 1990:609–20.

25. Senkai T, Tomenagu K, Saijo N, *et al*. The incidence of cardiac metastases in primary lung tumors and the management of malignant pericardial effusion. *Jpn J Clin Oncol* 1982;**12**:23–30.

26. Buck M, Ingle JN, Guilani ER, *et al*. Pericardial effusion in women with breast cancer. *Cancer* 1987;**60**:263–71.

27. Permanyer-Miralda G, Sagristà-Sauleda J, Soler-Soler J. Primary acute pericardial disease: a prospective series of 231 consecutive patients. *Am J Cardiol* 1985;**56**:623–30.

28. Vaitkus PT, Herrmann H, LeWinter MM. Treatment of malignant pericardial effusion. *JAMA* 1994;**272**:59–64.
• *An excellent review of different therapeutic options of malignant pericardial disease.*

29. Hancock EW. Neoplastic pericardial disease. *Cardiol Clin* 1990;**8**:673–82.

30 Cardiovascular complications of renal disease

Alan G Jardine, Kevin McLaughlin

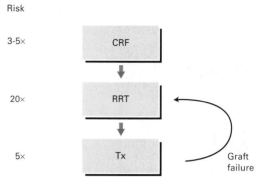

Figure 30.1. Phases of progressive renal disease with estimates of cardiovascular disease risk compared with the general population. CRF, chronic renal failure; RRT, renal replacement therapy; Tx, transplantation.

Advances in the technology and delivery of renal replacement therapy (dialysis and transplantation) have revolutionised the outcome of patients with progressive renal disease. However, the paradox of this success has been to uncover a greatly increased risk of cardiovascular disease (CVD), up to 20 times that of the normal population, a pattern similar to that seen in diabetes following the discovery of insulin. However, the magnitude of the problem is greater in renal disease and there is less agreement on the mechanisms or evidence on which to base interventional strategies.

The importance of CVD in this population is reflected by recent publications[1-3] and a report from a specific task force of the US National Kidney Foundation. The recognition that large scale outcome studies are required has resulted in the initiation of several studies that will report over the next few years. This review is a personal view in which we will cover the background to CVD at different stages in the natural history of progressive renal disease, current treatments, unresolved problems, and ongoing studies

Why patients with renal disease are different from the general population

To appreciate the problems and management of CVD in progressive renal disease it is necessary to consider the key differences between patients with renal disease and other patient groups. The first is the course of renal disease (fig 30.1). Patients with progressive renal disease suffer a period of deteriorating renal function, over months to many years (depending on the underlying disease) and leading ultimately to end stage renal disease (ESRD) in a proportion of patients. Most patients with ESRD (around 100 per million population per annum) currently enter renal replacement therapy programmes involving either peritoneal dialysis or haemodialysis. Thereafter, approximately one third will be considered for renal transplantation and, over a period of years, the majority of these will proceed to have a successful cadaveric or living donor transplant. The current predicted half life for renal allograft survival is around 10 years; those patients whose grafts fail are considered for retransplantation. The importance of the natural history of renal disease is that CVD risk and risk factors vary at different stages (fig 30.1), as does their management and the

opportunities for intervention. A unique feature of CVD in patients with primary renal disease is that retarding or preventing progression of progressive renal disease will reduce cardiac risk.

The second feature of specific importance in progressive renal disease is the role of volume dependent mechanisms involved in hypertension and heart failure. The most extreme example of this is seen in anuric patients on haemodialysis, who accumulate on average 2–3 litres of fluid (a proportion of which will be intravascular) between dialysis sessions. Hypertension in such patients is volume dependent, and high weight gains are also associated with the development of pulmonary oedema in susceptible individuals. Fluid retention increases progressively with deteriorating renal function and thus contributes to the development of heart failure and hypertension.

The third unique feature is the nature of vascular disease in this population, which has led to scepticism about the adoption of treatments and treatment strategies proven in the general population. The characteristic feature of the vessels is calcification—to a large extent the result of hyperparathyroidism in renal disease (fig 30.2)—in peripheral and coronary vessels.[4] The extent to which atherosclerosis in such vessels differs from the general population, and the efficacy of established treatments—such as statins—remains uncertain and unproven.

Finally, the mode of death in advanced renal disease is atypical, classical myocardial infarction being relatively unusual, and sudden death and progressive heart failure being more common. Thus, abnormalities of the myocardium (for example, left ventricular hypertrophy, systolic dysfunction, and ventricular dilatation) that predispose the patient to sudden death, and their determinants, may be of much greater importance than atherosclerotic coronary artery disease in determining the high cardiovascular mortality in this population.

Cardiovascular disease in uraemia: natural history and epidemiology

The scale of the problem of CVD has been demonstrated in publications from the European and US renal disease registries. In

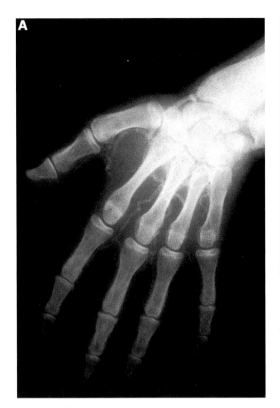

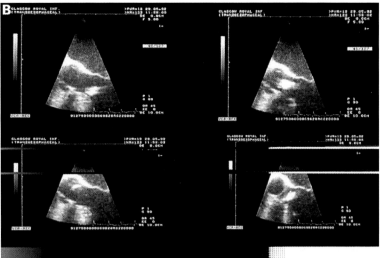

Figure 30.2. Calcified vessels and valves. Atherosclerosis in progressive renal disease has features that suggest conventional interventions may be ineffective. These panels show calcification of digital vessels in a patient with end stage renal failure, and a calcified valvar lesion.

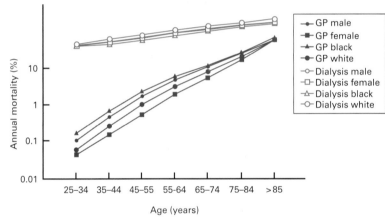

Figure 30.3. Data from the US Renal Disease Service (USRDS) showing CVD mortality rates in patients on renal replacement therapy compared with normal background population. The most dramatic relative increase is seen in the youngest patients on dialysis programmes.[3]

Europe, Raine reported an increase in CVD risk of approximately 20-fold, while a recent study from the US Renal Disease Service provides a more dramatic illustration of the scale of the problem (fig 30.3).[2][3] This report examined patients on dialysis and shows a major increase in all groups, but with the greatest increase in the youngest patients. Thus, a young adult on dialysis has a similar CVD risk to an elderly patient without renal disease. Moreover, risk increases progressively with deteriorating glomerular filtration rate (GFR) and is increased significantly by the time serum creatinine is elevated.[5] Patients with a functioning transplant have a much smaller increase in relative risk of around fivefold, but this group is highly selected and graft failure is associated with a dramatic increase in risk and mortality.

In the general population, a number of risk factors for CVD are well established, based on large scale epidemiological studies, including cigarette smoking, hyperlipidaemia, hyper-

tension, and past or family history of premature CVD. Relating these factors to the development of CVD, and specifically coronary artery disease, in patients with progressive renal disease has proved difficult for a variety of reasons. The first is that it is likely that CVD evolves at different rates during the different stages of renal disease (fig 30.1), and the relative importance of risk factors such as hyperlipidaemia and hypertension differs at each stage. Secondly, some potential risk factors, such as hypertension (using standard definitions) are so common as to have no discriminatory potential. Finally, there are unique CVD risk factors in this population including progression between stages in the natural history and the effect of graft failure (and its determinants—for example, acute rejection, chronic rejection, and graft function at specific time points following transplantation (fig 30.4)[6]). An additional consideration is the increasing age of patients entering renal replacement therapy programmes and the associated increase in pre-existing disease.

These issues have been intensively studied by Kasiske whose longitudinal follow up studies in transplant recipients have greatly increased understanding of CVD risk in, at least, this subset of patients on renal replacement therapy. Although his early studies identified age, diabetes, male sex, and pre-existing vascular disease as the main determinants of outcome, together with a history of acute rejection (a marker for early graft failure), more recent work (using the Framingham equation) confirms the importance of conventional risk factors such as smoking, high cholesterol, and high blood pressure (when absolute lipid and blood pressure readings are used rather than diagnostic labels[7] (table 30.1)).

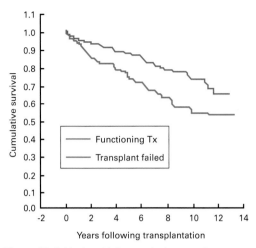

Figure 30.4. Kaplan–Meier survival curves from patients receiving cadaveric transplants at the Western Infirmary, Glasgow. Comparison of patients with continuing graft function and all transplants including graft failures.[6]

Table 30.1 Estimated relative risk of cardiovascular disease event in renal transplants recipients. Impact of individual risk factors.[7]

Risk factor	Increase relative risk
• Age	3% per annum
• Diabetes	2-fold
• Male	2-fold
• Pre-existing IHD, PVD or CVD	5–10-fold
• Smoking	2-fold
• Graft failure	5-fold
• BP (> 160/100 v < 130/80 mm Hg)	1.5-fold
• Total cholesterol (> 7.4 v < 4.2 mmol/l)	2-fold

Other risk factors (unknown relative risk)
• Homocysteine
• Lp (a)
• Parathyroid hormone
• Anaemia
• C-reactive protein
• Acute rejection episodes

BP, blood pressure; CVD, cardiovascular disease; IHD, ischaemic heart disease; PVD, peripheral vascular disease.

Conventional CVD risk factors and patterns of CVD disease

Hypertension

Hypertension is a common presenting feature in all forms of primary renal disease, even in patients with near normal GFR. In the initial phases of progressive renal disease, increased or inappropriately high activity of the renin angiotensin and other vasoconstrictor systems plays a major role. However, with progressive fall in GFR, salt and water retention predominate. Thus, it is possible to control high blood pressure in some dialysis patients by careful attention to fluid balance, either by limiting intake, or effective fluid removal by dialysis and ultrafiltration. Following transplantation, "hypertension" is almost universal; in addition, the influence of longstanding hypertension is a consequence of allograft dysfunction, and of the direct and indirect effects of immunosuppressive agents—specifically the calcineurin inhibitors (cyclosporin A and tacrolimus) and corticosteroid treatment.

Hypertension is associated with increased rate of progression of primary renal disease;

blood pressure reduction (specifically with angiotensin converting enzyme (ACE) inhibitors[8]) retards progression. Whether ACE inhibitors have independent beneficial effects, over and above their effects on blood pressure, remains unresolved. The issue of patient survival and hypertension in progressive renal disease has not been formally addressed in adequately powered studies, although the increasing CVD risk associated with progression to end stage renal failure (ESRF) will be delayed by effective antihypertensive treatment. Target blood pressure levels are also poorly defined. In cohort studies (such as the modification of diet in renal disease (MDRD) study) and in diabetic nephropathy[9] blood pressures below 125–130/75–80 mm Hg are associated with significant benefits. However, whether these targets are achievable in clinical practice remains to be established.

The situation is even more complex in patients receiving dialysis. When fluid balance is tightly regulated,[2 3 10] CVD risk increases with increasing levels of blood pressure, regardless of whether the patient is "hypertensive". However, the opposite has also been reported most recently from the US Renal Disease Service (that is, those with the lowest blood pressure being at highest risk[2 3]). This may be a reflection of pre-existing cardiac disease in patients with low blood pressure, specifically symptomatic heart failure—itself an independent risk factor for poor outcome.[3] However, an alternative explanation is that ventricular hypertrophy places critical importance on diastolic coronary perfusion. Thus, blood pressure control in this group is achieved by judicious fluid balance, with the addition—if necessary—of antihypertensive agents.

Finally, in transplant recipients there is strong evidence linking absolute blood pressure levels with graft failure.[11] Recent studies demonstrate increased CVD risk associated with higher levels of blood pressure and suggest that targets below 130/80 mm Hg are likely to be associated with reduced risk; whether such targets are readily achievable need to be established by interventional trials.

The choice of antihypertensive agent is also unclear. Thiazide diuretics are ineffective in the presence of even modest renal impairment, whereas loop diuretics are effective antihypertensive agents in patients with volume dependent hypertension. ACE inhibitors are proven agents of choice in patients with chronic renal failure, diabetic nephropathy, and glomerulonephritis because of their ability to retard progression and reduce proteinuria. However, they may have catastrophic effects in patients with renovascular disease and their use may be limited by hyperkalaemia in patients with renal impairment. ACE inhibitors should be used with caution and it is worthwhile excluding transplant artery stenosis by Doppler ultrasound before initiating treatment.

Smoking

Until recently there was little evidence linking smoking to CVD in patients with progressive renal disease and a reluctance to restrict the lifestyle of patients (particularly those on haemodialysis) who are already on restrictive fluid and dietary regimens. However, it is now clear that smoking has a similar impact on CVD risk to the general population[7] and may also promote progression of primary renal disease. Although the newer anti-smoking treatments have not been formally assessed in this population, they are likely to be safe and will add to non-pharmacological approaches to smoking cessation.

Lipids and renal disease

Hyperlipidaemia is a feature of progressive renal disease; the pattern and severity of which varies with the stage of renal disease.[2] For example, the nephrotic syndrome may occur in patients with well maintained renal excretory function, and is associated with severe mixed hyperlipidaemia. Patients with non-nephrotic primary renal disease also have raised total cholesterol and low density lipoprotein (LDL) cholesterol, concentrations of which tend to rise with rising serum creatinine and urinary protein excretion. In patients with ESRF the pattern of lipid abnormalities depends on the mode of renal replacement therapy. Haemodialysis may result in low total and LDL cholesterol, while peritoneal dialysis is associated with raised total and LDL cholesterol and triglycerides. Overall the pattern of lipoprotein abnormalities in patients with advanced chronic renal failure or ESRF is a shift towards triglyceride rich and atherogenic (for example, small dense LDL) particles, regardless of concentrations of total or LDL cholesterol. Following transplantation, restoration of renal function, appetite, and the effects of steroids and cyclosporin A contribute to the observed increase in triglycerides, LDL, and total cholesterol, particularly in the early post-transplant period. One problem of the shifting patterns of lipid abnormalities that accompany progressive renal disease is that it is difficult to integrate lipid concentrations in individual patients and their absolute importance on CVD risk over time. As a consequence there have been surprisingly few studies that associate lipids and risk or outcome.

Dietary intervention is of limited use in patients whose diet is already restricted. Fibrates and statins have similar relative efficacy to other patient populations but are associated with an increase risk of side effects. The association of renal failure with fibrates has limited their use and statins are now the agents of choice for patients at any stage of progressive renal disease. The only caveat is that there is a higher incidence of myositis and rhabdomyolisis (albeit small), and a significant interaction with calcineurin inhibitors (that inhibit the microsomal enzyme CyP-3A4) and simvastatin, lovastatin, and atorvastatin (but not fluvastatin or pravastatin), resulting in increased plasma concentrations of these agents. Thus, statins should be initiated at low doses in transplant patients.[2 12]

Table 30.2 Influence of immunosuppressive agents on cardiovascular disease risk factors, including rejection rate, blood pressure, lipids, and post-transplant diabetes. Nearly all immunosuppressive agents impact on risk factors, thus the use of combinations allows maximisation of immunosuppressive effects while minimising side effects

	Rejection	High BP	Lipids	Diabetes mellitus
Steroid	+	++	++	++
Cyclosporin	++	+++	++	+
Tacrolimus	++	+++	++	++
Rapamycin	+++	–	+++	–
MMF	+/++	–	–	–
Azathioprine	+	–	–	–

BP, blood pressure; MMF, mycophenolate mofetil

Diabetes

Diabetic nephropathy is the leading cause of ESRF (accounting for approximately one third of all patients starting renal replacement therapy and about 10% of all transplant recipients). Most patients have type I diabetes as patients with nephropathy caused by type II diabetes rarely survive to require dialysis or transplantation. The 2–3 fold increase in CVD risk (attributable to diabetes) multiplied by the risk associated with ESRF results in an increased CVD risk of around 50-fold in patients with ESRF caused by diabetic nephropathy.

A second issue is that of diabetes following transplantation which affects around 10% of all transplant recipients[13] and is associated with an increase in risk similar to diabetes in the general population, with a lag time of about 8–10 years from the development of disease to onset of complications. Post-transplant diabetes is a complication of immunosuppressive therapy (table 30.2) and is discussed below.

Other risk factors

Much less is known about other risk factors and their influence on treatment. Thus, although patients with progressive renal disease have increased concentrations of homocysteine, acute phase proteins, and lipoprotein Lp(a), and reduced antioxidant concentrations, the associated risks are not known. There has been considerable interest in the role of parathyroid hormone that contributes to extra-articular calcification. However, although vascular calcification is a major problem, the role of parathyroid hormone remains unresolved.

Following transplantation, the use of immunosuppressant drugs alters a number of CVD risk factors. Thus, the immunosuppressant agents themselves become risk factors, and modifying immunosuppressive treatment becomes an aspect of CVD risk factor management. The impact of these effects is offset by benefits on acute rejection rates and graft survival, that also have an impact on patient survival and CVD risk (fig 30.4). However, it is a measure of the increasing importance of CVD in this population that these effects are now considered when prescribing and licensing immunosuppressive agents.

214

Uraemic cardiomyopathy

Echocardiographic abnormalities are more strongly associated with outcome than conventional risk factors. There is a high prevalence of echocardiographic abnormalities in patients starting renal replacement therapy.[2 3 14] Parfrey has characterised uraemic cardiomyopathy into three groups: systolic dysfunction, hypertrophic cardiomyopathy, and dilated cardiomyopathy. On initiation of dialysis they found the prevalence of these abnormalities to be 16%, 41%, and 28%, respectively, with 16% of patients having a normal echocardiogram.[15] Median survival was 38 months in patients with systolic dysfunction, 48 months in concentric hypertrophy, 56 months in left ventricular dilatation, and 66 months in the normal group.[15] The echocardiographic abnormalities may co-exist and overlap for methodological reasons that may limit comparison with other populations; however, each is strongly associated with reduced patient survival. A similar pattern has been reported in patients undergoing renal transplantation (approximately 75% of whom have hypertrophic cardiomyopathy, and over 50% systolic dysfunction or dilated cardiomyopathy) with a similar adverse effect on patient outcome. The characteristic pathophysiological feature of uraemic cardiomyopathy is fibrosis, which is well established by the time patients reach ESRF, raising questions about the reversibility that have not been systematically investigated.

It is recommended that echocardiographic studies be performed on the post-dialysis day with patients close to their "ideal weight" and, by inference, at a normal intravascular volume. This reflects theoretical and observed difficulties in the interpretation of echocardiographic measurements, particularly in patients receiving dialysis treatment. Because of the changes in intravascular volume during haemodialysis (and in the interdialytic period), and the dependence of standard algorithms for the estimation of left ventricular mass index (LVMI) on chamber diameters, calculated LVMI may differ by up to 50 g in the same individual. Echocardiographic measurements of chamber volume will also vary with time in the dialysis cycle, resulting in variable classification of dilated cardiomyopathy, and systolic function. Thus, although echocardiographic abnormalities have prognostic importance in population studies, it is difficult to identify targets for intervention in individuals or an estimate of risk to an individual at a given time point (for example, pre-transplant assessment).

An important development in this area is the use of cardiac magnetic resonance imaging (MRI), which permits the direct estimation of left ventricular mass, independent of chamber diameters.[16] In a comparison with echocardiographic measurements of LVMI we found (fig 30.5) that as left ventricular mass and chamber diameter increase, echocardiographic measurements progressively overestimate mass. The more widespread availability of MRI may result

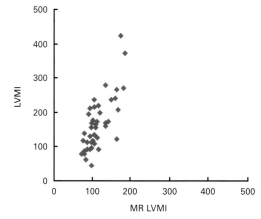

Figure 30.5. Comparison of magnetic resonance (MR) (x axis) and echocardiographic (y axis) estimates of left ventricular mass index (LVMI) in haemodialysis patients. Because of the dependence of echocardiographic estimates of left ventricular mass on chamber diameter, echocardiography progressively overestimates left ventricular mass with increasing mass.

in revision of the definition of uraemic cardiomyopathy and its management.

There are other issues regarding cardiac abnormalities: when do they develop, what happens following transplantation, can they be reversed, and how are they linked to death? There are no longitudinal studies on the natural history of uraemic cardiomyopathy. However, left ventricular hypertrophy is present in patients from the earliest stages of progressive renal disease, in many cases before there is a significant reduction in renal function,[17] a consequence of hypertension, although other contributing factors have not been fully investigated.

Several small studies have examined the change in LVMI following transplantation but without consistent findings, reflecting inconsistencies in methodology, and specifically the reduction in intravascular volume that follows successful transplantation. The reported regression of left ventricular hypertrophy associated with erythropoietin use may also be, at least partly, methodological. The link between echocardiographic findings and mode of death (specifically progressive heart failure and sudden death) is more intuitive. Left ventricular hypertrophy is associated with increased QT dispersion which is increased in patients on all forms of renal replacement therapy. Moreover, QT dispersion is increased by dialysis and may contribute to an increased risk of sudden death in the hours following a haemodialysis treatment.[18]

Coronary artery disease

Prevalence

The cumulative incidence of coronary artery disease, in surviving patients with functioning transplants, is reported to be around 23% in the first 15 years following transplantation. The rates for peripheral and cerebrovascular disease are similar, at 15% over 15 years. However, the cumulative incidence is likely to be much higher in those patients who return to mainte-

> **Cardiac assessment of patients with end stage renal failure**
>
> - Echocardiography: good prognostic indicator but varies during dialysis cycle
>
> - Standard exercise test: little use because of poor exercise capacity and resting ECG abnormalities
>
> - Isotope scanning: useful when combined with dipyridamole or dobutamine stress
>
> - Coronary angiography: required for most patients

nance dialysis after graft failure[6] and in patients starting renal replacement therapy, reflecting the increasing age of patients entering renal replacement therapy programmes with pre-existing disease.

Morphology of atheroma in patients with progressive renal disease

Although the distribution of atherosclerotic lesions appears similar to the general population, the morphology in coronary artery disease is unique[19] with striking medial calcification in addition to intimal hyperplasia. A recent study compared the postmortem morphology of atheromatous lesions in 27 patients with progressive renal disease (average age 69.5 years) and appropriate controls.[20] The major differences in renal patients were that coronary vessels had significantly increased media thickness with atheroma consisting of calcified plaques in contrast to the fibroatheromatous plaques of control patients. However, coronary artery calcification is not exclusive to elderly patients with progressive renal disease, and a recent study of dialysis patients aged 20–30 years had evidence of coronary artery calcification[21] detected by electron beam computed tomography. Coronary calcification was 17.5 times that of the general population and was associated with length of time on dialysis, average serum calcium × phosphate product (a determinant of calcium phosphate deposition), and intake of calcium containing phosphate binders. Moreover, the chemical composition of calcified plaques in dialysis patients is primarily hydroxyl apatite and calcium phosphate, and the calcium × phosphate product has previously been identified as an independent predictor of mortality in this population.[22] The morphology of coronary lesions in patients with progressive renal disease (that is, calcified versus fibroatheromatous plaques) is an important factor when considering the likely re-

sponse to either medical or invasive treatments and the adoption of strategies proven in the general population.

Assessment and diagnosis

Screening for coronary artery disease in patients with progressive renal disease has been performed principally in the assessment of patients for renal transplantation. The incidence of asymptomatic coronary artery disease is perhaps 10 times higher in this group than in the general population. A small study in patients with diabetic ESRF demonstrated benefits of routine angiography (followed by surgery if required) in asymptomatic patients. This has been generally adopted in patients with diabetic nephropathy awaiting transplantation and also, to a variable extent, in patients with other forms of progressive renal disease despite the absence of specific evidence. The American Society of Transplantation recently published guidelines to address this issue (table 30.3). These recommendations are based on a prospective study evaluating five risk factors: history of coronary artery disease; history of heart failure; abnormal resting ECG; diabetes; and age > 50 years. The absence of all five risk factors was associated with a negative predictive value of 0.99 at 46 months, the recommendation being that such individuals do not require screening tests. For patients with multiple risk factors screening is recommended. For symptomatic patients screening should include coronary angiography. However, the investigation of asymptomatic patients with multiple risk factors should initially involve non-invasive investigations.

The choice of non-invasive testing for coronary artery disease is plagued by similar problems to that of interpretation of echocardiography. Few patients with ESRF, have adequate exercise capacity for conventional electrocardiographic exercise tests, and almost invariably have abnormal resting ECGs. Thallium imaging and non-exercise based stress tests involving dobutamine or dipyridamole are preferable. For patients with advanced chronic renal failure or ESRF in our experience, difficulties in interpreting non-invasive tests often lead to coronary angiography being performed. In patients with modest renal impairment or good renal function following transplantation, conventional investigational strategies should be used.

Management

The management of coronary artery disease in patients with early renal failure is the same as for the normal population. In patients with ESRD, the decision of whether or not to inter-

Table 30.3   American Society of Transplantation cardiac screening recommendations

	Risk category		
	Low risk	*High risk*	
Risk history	No history of CAD or CHF	History of CAD or CHF	Symptomatic CAD
Risk factors	Non-diabetic, age < 50 years	Diabetic, age < 50 years; non-diabetic, age > 50 years	Diabetic, age > 50 years
Stress testing?	No	Yes	No, proceed to angiography

CAD, coronary artery disease; CHF, congestive heart failure.

216

vene is usually based on data from the general population. There is no consensus on the management of lesions identified during screening of asymptomatic, potential transplant recipients. In patients with advanced renal failure or ESRF, the success of non-surgical intervention is poor. Primary angioplasty in patients with advanced renal failure is associated with an increased primary failure rate, and a restenosis rate at six months in excess of 40%.[23] Reasons for the high restenosis rate include calcified plaques, more severe artery narrowing, more extensive disease, and a relatively thrombophilic state seen in dialysis patients with increased platelet and fibrin deposition. Although a recent report by Le Feuvre suggests that angioplasty associated with a "stent-like" success (stenosis < 30%) is as achievable in dialysis patients as it is in control patients,[24] overall the chance of similar success in patients with advanced chronic renal failure before dialysis and on various forms of renal replacement therapy is reduced. Many centres consider primary angioplasty inappropriate in this population.

Stenting offers a more effective treatment and may be as successful (technically) in patients with progressive renal disease as it is in the general population. Further studies are needed to assess the efficacy in comparison to coronary artery bypass grafting. For many patients with advanced progressive renal disease coronary artery bypass grafting remains the only viable option. However, there is a significant increase in morbidity and mortality following bypass grafting in patients receiving dialysis and a significant risk of precipitating renal failure in patients with advanced chronic renal failure or poor graft function.[25 26] Thus, these risks must be offset by the potential benefits of successful revascularisation to the patient and in many cases it may be appropriate to opt for stenting as the primary procedure. Whether or not conventional thresholds for intervention are appropriate in patients with ESRF is also uncertain, particularly in view of the difficulties in assessing left ventricular function non-invasively. While most physicians would recommend revascularisation for left main stem lesions and severe triple vessel disease, other strategies including correction of anaemia and regression of left ventricular hypertrophy may have benefits in patients with symptomatic angina and less extensive disease.

The medical management of coronary artery disease in this population is essentially the same as for the general population. However, it is important to reinforce the need to assess factors such as anaemia and its correction by the use of erythropoietin and parenteral iron.

Myocardial infarction

The diagnosis of myocardial infarction in patients with advanced chronic renal failure and ESRF (regardless of the form of renal replacement therapy) is complicated by the high prevalence of ECG abnormalities. More-

---

Intervention for coronary artery disease

- High risk in patients with end stage renal failure

- Angioplasty has unacceptably high failure rate

- Coronary stenting unproven

- Coronary bypass graft surgery remains treatment of choice for most patients

---

over, the ECG may change across a dialysis session[18] reflecting changes in intravascular volume and electrolytes. Serum creatinine kinase concentrations also tend to be slightly higher than normal, even in the absence of myocardial infarction. The management of myocardial infarction is generally the same as for the general population, despite the absence of specific studies in patients with advanced renal disease. Furthermore the outcome of patients with ESRF following myocardial infarction is much worse than patients without renal disease.[27]

Secondary prevention
Similar considerations apply to secondary prevention. Although renal patients have been excluded from large outcome studies of CVD, there is a general consensus that patients with ESRF should not be denied proven secondary prevention measures (for example, statin treatment following myocardial infarction or ACE inhibitors for chronic heart failure).

Valve disease

Another feature of extra-articular calcification in renal disease is accelerated valve calcification and an increased prevalence of aortic valve disease. The decision to intervene is generally based on conventional criteria but, like coronary bypass surgery, preoperative complications are more common and mortality and morbidity substantially increased (fig 30.2).

Ongoing trials

Although long overdue there are now several ongoing trials with cardiovascular end points in patients with primary renal disease. The ALERT (a study of Lescol and renal transplantation) has recruited 2100 stable renal transplant recipients, in northern Europe and Canada, to a five year study with death and major adverse cardiac events as the primary end points. The patients were randomised to 40 mg (increasing to 80 mg) per day of fluvastatin or placebo. The study is based on the 4S (Scandinavian simvastatin survival study) trial, with the assumption that the event rate in this population will be approximately twice that of 4S. Recruitment closed in the autumn of 1997 and the trial should report in 2002. The UK-HARP (heart and renal protection) study is a 2×2 study of aspirin and simvastatin versus placebo in patients with chronic renal failure, patients on dialysis programmes, and renal transplant recipients. After an extensive pilot phase to ensure safety and the logistics of the study design in this population, a full scale study is planned. In dialysis patients the CHORUS (cerivastatin heart outcomes in renal disease: understanding survival) study will examine the effects of cerivastatin (400 µg/day) or placebo in a two year study of 690 dialysis patients. The small size of this study reflects the annual CVD event rate in this population, although the absence of similar interventional studies, and thus information on recruitment profiles and event rates, makes it difficult to provide accurate targets for power calculations. One recent study merits comment. The SPACE study examined the effects of vitamin E supplementation in patients on haemodialysis with a reported benefit in CVD end points.

Conclusions

Accelerated CVD is now the leading cause of death in patients with progressive renal disease. Risk increases progressively from the earliest stages of renal disease, when serum creatinine is close to normal values. Appropriate management is unclear because of the absence of specific studies and the issue of whether or not strategies established in the general population can be applied in a population with atypical CVD. However, we believe that prevention should begin in the earliest phases of progressive renal disease, when serum creatinine rises outwith the normal range with the use of statins and antihypertensive treatment—with the aim of achieving lower targets for blood pressure control that limit the development of left ventricular hypertrophy. In patients with advanced disease strategies should aim to limit, or regress, ventricular abnormalities, rather than simply "control" blood pressure, and should involve antihypertensive agents and meticulous control of fluid balance. Finally, there should be a low threshold for the investigation of patients with advanced renal disease (even in the absence of symptoms).

Overall, the message is clear. Improved understanding and management of CVD in this population will have more immediate benefits that the foreseeable advances in dialysis, transplantation or the treatment of primary renal disease.

1. **London GM, Loscalzo J.** *Cardiovascular disease in end-stage renal failure.* Oxford Clinical Nephrology Series. Oxford: Oxford University Press, 2000.
• *An up-to-date review of all aspects of CVD in renal failure from the leading clinical researchers in this area.*

2. **Baigent C, Burbury K, Wheeler D.** Premature cardiovascular disease in chronic renal failure. *Lancet* 2000;**356**:147–52.
• *A UK perspective dealing with risk factors and epidemiology of CVD.*

3. **Foley RN, Parfrey PS, Sarnak MJ.** Clinical epidemiology of cardiovascular disease in chronic renal disease. *Am J Kidney Dis* 1998(suppl 3):S112–19.

4. **Goodman WG, Goldin J, Kuizon BD,** *et al.* Coronary artery calcification in young adults with end-stage renal disease who are undergoing dialysis. *N Engl J Med* 2000;**342**:1478–83.
• *Atypical coronary artery disease in dialysis patients.*

5. **Schillaci G, Reboldi G, Verdecchia P.** High normal serum creatinine concentration is a predictor of cardiovascular risk in essential hypertension. *Arch Intern Med* 2001;**161**:886–91.

6. **Woo YM, Jardine AG, Clark AF,** *et al.* The influence of early graft function on patient survival following renal transplantation. *Kidney Int* 1999;**55**:692–9.
• *Impact of graft function and failure on patient survival.*

7. **Kasiske BL, Chakkera HA, Roel J.** Explained and unexplained ischaemic heart disease after renal transplantation. *J Am Soc Nephrol* 2000;**11**:1735–43.

8. **Lewis EJ, Hunsicker LG, Bain RP,** *et al.* The effect of angiotensin converting enzyme inhibition on diabetic nephropathy. *N Engl J Med* 1993;**329**:1456–62.

9. **McLaughlin K, Jardine AG.** Clinical management of diabetic nephropathy. *Diabetes, Obesity & Metabolism* 1999;**1**:307–15.

10. **Charra B, Calemard M, Laurent G.** Importance of treatment time and blood pressure control in achieving long-term survival on dialysis. *Am J Nephrol* 1996;**16**:35–44.

11. **Opelz G, Wujciak T, Ritz E.** Association of chronic kidney graft failure with recipient blood pressure. *Kidney Int* 1998;**53**:217–22.

12. **Jardine AG, Holdaas H.** Fluvastatin in combination with cyclosporin in renal transplant recipients: a review of the clinical and safety experience. *J Clin Pharm Ther* 1999;**24**:397–408.

13. **Jindal RM, Hjelmesaeth J.** Impact and management of post-transplant diabetes. *Transplantation* 2000;**70**:SS58–63.

14. **Foley RN, Parfrey PS, Harnett JD,** *et al.* Clinical and echocardiographic disease in patients starting end-stage renal disease therapy. *Kidney Int* 1995;**47**:186–92.

15. **Parfrey PS, Foley RN, Harnett JD,** *et al.* Outcome and risk factors for left ventricular disorders in chronic uraemia. *Nephrol Dial Transplant* 1996;**11**:1277–85.
• *Description of uraemic cardiomyopathy and its impact.*

16. **Stewart GA, Forster J, Cowan M,** *et al.* Echocardiography overestimates left ventricular mass in haemodialysis patients—a comparison with magnetic resonance imaging. *Kidney Int* 1999;**56**:2248–53.

17. **Levin A, Thompson CR, Ethier J,** *et al.* Left ventricular mass index increase in early renal disease: impact of decline in hemoglobin. *Am J Kidney Dis* 1999;**34**:125–34.

18. **Morris STW, Galiatsou E, Stewart GA,** *et al.* QT dispersal before and after dialysis. *J Am Soc Nephrol* 1999;**10**:160–3.

19. **Ibels LS, Alfrey AC, Huffer WE,** *et al.* Arterial calcification and pathology in uremic patients undergoing dialysis. *Am J Med* 1979;**66**:790–6.

20. **Schwarz U, Buzello M, Ritz E,** *et al.* Morphology of coronary atherosclerotic lesions in patients with end-stage renal failure. *Nephrol Dial Transplant* 2000;**15**:218–23.

21. **Goodman WG, Goldin J, Kuizon BD,** *et al.* Coronary-artery calcification in young adults with end-stage renal disease who are undergoing dialysis. *N Engl J Med* 2000;**342**:1478–83.

22. **Block GA, Hulbert-Shearon TE, Levin NW,** *et al.* Association of serum phosphorus and calcium x phosphate product with mortality risk in chronic hemodialysis patients: a national study. *Am J Kidney Dis* 1998;**31**:607–17.

23. **Marso SP, Gimple LW, Philbrick JT,** *et al.* Effectiveness of percutaneous coronary interventions to prevent recurrent coronary events in patients on chronic hemodialysis. *Am J Cardiol* 1998;**82**:378–80.

24. **Le Feuvre C, Dambrin G, Helft G,** *et al.* Clinical outcome following coronary angioplasty in dialysis patients: a case-control study in the era of coronary stenting. *Heart* 2001;**85**:556–60.

25. **Liu JY, Birkmeyer NJO, Sanders JH,** *et al.* Risks of morbidity and mortality in dialysis patients undergoing coronary artery surgery. *Circulation* 2000;**102**:2973–7.
• *Risks of intervention in coronary artery disease.*

26. **Rinehart A, Herzog C, Collins A,** *et al.* A comparison of coronary angioplasty and coronary artery bypass grafting outcomes in chronic dialysis patients. *Am J Kidney Dis* 1995;**25**:281–90.

27. **Herzog CA, Ma JZ, Collins AJ.** Poor long term survival after myocardial infarction among patients on long term dialysis. *N Engl J Med* 1998;**339**:799–805.
• *Poor outcome of patients with ESRF who suffer myocardial infarction.*

217

31 The athlete's heart

David Oakley

Over the last decade the culture of physical exercise has changed. While elite athletes are training to ever more rigorous schedules, our middle aged sedentary population, no doubt seeing the writing on the wall, are hurrying to sign up for the fashionable, local fitness centres. When talking about athletes' hearts, we must distinguish between elite athletes, recreational sports men and women, non-athletes who wish to maintain cardiovascular fitness, and athletic patients with known cardiovascular disease. This article is mainly about athletes with serious sporting ambitions at club or higher level, who train most days for more than one hour. I will make it clear when I am referring to other types of athletes.

A regular training programme causes favourable changes in skeletal muscle performance (the realm of the sports physiologist) and two clear cut cardiovascular effects—namely, enlargement of the heart and a slow pulse rate at rest. These are the components of a characteristic clinical picture known as the "athlete's heart".[1]

Athletes, as a group, tend to be somewhat introspective about their health and will frequently consult doctors complaining of palpitations, dizziness, fatigue, chest pain, and undue dyspnoea. Physical examination may reveal some unusual signs, which will do little to reassure the doctor, already aware of widely publicised high profile cases of sudden death in association with sporting activity. The finding of an apparently abnormal ECG will cause further anxiety. A knowledge of the characteristic features of the athlete's heart is therefore important if the patient is to be advised wisely.[2]

Cardiac enlargement

Regular training causes the heart to enlarge. This is the result of a combination of left ventricular cavity enlargement (dilatation) and increased wall thickness (hypertrophy). The stimuli and processes involved are complex but appear to be akin to the normal growth of the heart in childhood.[3] It is widely held that resistance or isometric training (weight lifting, etc) stimulates hypertrophy with normal cavity dimensions (concentric), whereas aerobic, isotonic training (running, etc) stimulates hypertrophy and cavity dilatation (eccentric).[4] Athletes include both types of training in their schedules, so the distinction is blurred but it is probably a genuine phenomenon, as demonstrated by a recent meta-analysis of the available data.[w1] When the cardiac dimensions are corrected for surface area or lean body mass, it becomes more difficult to demonstrate concentric hypertrophy in resistance athletes. There is a large body of literature concerning the extent of these changes and what might be considered within the normal range for an athlete.[w2] The evidence is inconsistent, but a useful meta-analysis of the available data by Fagard suggests that a wall thickness more than 1.6 cm is very unusual in a healthy athlete, most of whom will be less than 1.3 cm.[5] Oarsmen, cyclists, and Nordic skiers appear to have the largest hearts, but the degrees of hypertrophy observed do not correlate well with the intensity of training or the performance of the athletes. Many Olympic champions have cardiac dimensions within the normal range, whereas a college athlete may exhibit pronounced hypertrophy. This observation implies that the cardiac response to training is not simply induced by the haemodynamic stresses during exercise, which is hardly surprising bearing in mind the much longer periods of rest during which, by the same argument, hypertrophy should regress.

Other influences including hormonal stimuli and genetic susceptibility are thought to play a part. Indeed, there is increasing evidence that the propensity to hypertrophy is partly genetically determined, with physical training acting as the trigger. Studies of identical twins support this thesis.[w3] Also, there is some indication that ACE gene (and probably other) polymorphism affect the hypertrophic response to training. For instance the DD genotype seems to predispose to greater hypertrophy in response to training and the I allele occurs more frequently in elite athletes and high altitude mountaineers.[6]

Whatever the mechanism, it is evident that hypertrophy is a genuine response to training. Athletes who train seasonally exhibit a seasonal variation in left ventricular dimensions[7]. Regression of hypertrophy, even after many years of training, can frequently be observed on de-training.

Cardiac dilatation and hypertrophy may be sufficiently pronounced to resemble a pathological state, but markers of left ventricular function, both systolic and diastolic, are consistently normal.[8 w4] There is no convincing evidence that healthy subjects can train themselves into a pathological state manifest by fibrosis or fibre disarray.[w5]

Most published reports of cardiac enlargement refer to young male athletes but similar, though less notable, changes are reported in children, elderly subjects, and women.[w6-8]

Bradycardia

A resting bradycardia is characteristic of the trained athlete. In exceptional cases this may be less than 40 beats/min (bpm). While denervated hearts beat slower in response to training the bradycardia in athletes is mainly mediated by increased parasympathetic and reduced sympathetic input during the resting state.[9] [w9] This may result in sinus pauses with junctional escape rhythms, first degree heart block and Wenckebach type second degree block especially at night.[10] Resting bradycardia may predispose to increased atrial or ventricular ectopic activity and, in some cases, atrial fibrillation.[1]

As with hypertrophy, there is little evidence to support the view that bradycardia is harmful. The separation of athlete's bradycardia from sick sinus syndrome is somewhat academic if the latter is asymptomatic. One large series of athletes monitored continuously revealed no pauses in excess of 4 seconds.[10] Some subjects do develop symptoms of dizziness or syncope in response to training and require de-training or even permanent pacing. Careful characterisation of this subgroup, however, reveals a previously subclinical sick sinus syndrome rendered symptomatic by the additional stimulus of training.[11]

The effects of increasing age may modify some of the adaptations discussed above. Many athletes maintain their training into middle age and compete in "master" and "veteran" competitions. There is evidence that continued training results in improved diastolic function in the elderly but in one study some left ventricular dysfunction was seen in veteran Japanese cyclists.[12] It was not possible to say whether this was related to training or the development of some other problem such as coronary artery disease. It has also been shown that bradycardias are more pronounced in the older athlete whose maximum heart rate is also less. This may account in part for the drop off in performance with age.[w10]

The patient

Athletes can present with symptoms, or because an "abnormality" has been noted incidentally during screening, etc. Symptoms frequently have a relatively benign explanation—dizziness caused by dehydration or post-exercise hypotension, chest pain due to tracheitis or musculoskeletal pain (particularly in contact sports and heavy weight trainers), palpitations caused by benign premature contractions, and shortness of breath due to chest infection or exercise induced bronchospasm. Nevertheless, thorough investigation is often needed to provide patient and physician with the reassurance they need.

Investigational procedures

PHYSICAL EXAMINATION

A physical examination reveals a normal or slow pulse. Loss of the resting bradycardia may be seen in overtrained subjects. The venous pressure and arterial blood pressure are normal. The left ventricle may be prominent to feel and displaced laterally. Third and fourth sounds are permissible, as is a soft midsystolic flow murmur.[2]

INTERNATIONAL BASKETBALL

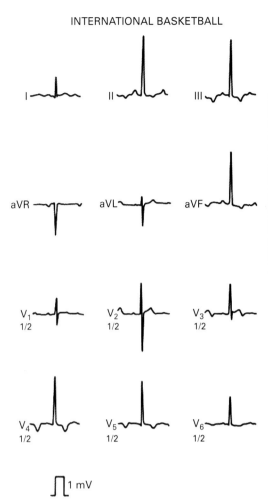

Figure 31.1. Twelve lead ECG of an international basketball player. Note the left ventricular hypertrophy and inferior T wave changes.

ECG

The ECG is usually normal, but left ventricular hypertrophy on voltage criteria is common. Many abnormal ECG patterns have been described. Two of the most common are illustrated here:

- Pronounced left ventricular hypertrophy on voltage with inferolateral T wave changes (fig 31.1)
- Early depolarisation changes with biphasic T waves in the anterior leads (fig 31.2).

The second pattern presents a particularly characteristic biphasic T wave morphology with early repolarisation, convex proximally. These changes reflect non-homogenous repolarisation caused by reduced resting sympathetic drive and resolve rapidly on exercise.[13]

Incomplete RBBB, deep anterolateral T wave inversion, and "left ventricular hypertrophy and strain" pattern are described elsewhere.[14] [15] The latter is rare.

Various slow rhythms as previously mentioned may be present (fig 31.3).

The ECG is a constant source of confusion in athletes with numerous variations on the basic patterns. The changes are related to the extent of training and vary in athletes whose training is seasonal. Even quite gross changes may not indicate cardiovascular disease, though thorough further evaluation will often be needed to prove this point. It seems that

PROFESSIONAL BOXER

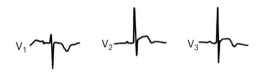

⎍ 1 mV

Figure 31.2. Twelve lead ECG of a European boxing champion. Note the large voltage complexes and bizarre early repolarisation changes in V2–V4.

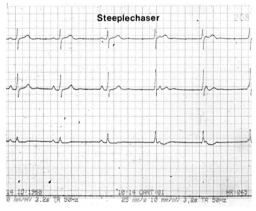

Figure 31.3. Short rhythm strip of a national steeplechaser. Note the bradycardia and junctional escape rhythm.

such changes are more common in athletes of African Caribbean origin.[w11] The unpredictability and variability of the ECG in athletes seriously limits its value in screening for cardiac disease in these subjects.

RADIOGRAPHY
The chest radiograph is usually normal or may show mild cardiac enlargement.

ECHOCARDIOGRAPHY
Cardiac ultrasound will frequently reveal a modest uniform increase in wall thickness seldom to more than 1.6 cm and usually less than 1.3 cm.[w12] Mild left ventricular cavity dilatation is also observed. Trivial regurgitation of mitral and tricuspid valves is reported more fre-

quently than in the sedentary population. Indices of systolic and diastolic function are normal. In some extreme cases, however, a pattern indistinguishable from hypertrophic cardiomyopathy is observed, even though exhaustive further investigations of the subject and immediate family yield no confirmatory evidence. Echocardiographic features of other confounding conditions may be present. Transoesophageal echocardiography has a role in excluding a patent foramen ovale in scuba divers.

24 HOUR ECG
Dynamic ECG monitoring may show some of the bradycardic features mentioned above.[w13] Complete heart block and ventricular tachycardia (sustained or unsustained) are not features of the athlete's heart and should be investigated thoroughly. Premature atrial and ventricular contractions are common,[w14] and more complex forms are seen, especially in the elderly.[w15]

EXERCISE ECG
Stress testing reveals an outstanding exercise capacity with rapid recovery of heart rate in the resting phase. The heart rate response is slower than in untrained people, but the eventual maximum rate is the same. Previously abnormal early repolarisation changes (thought to be related to reduced resting sympathetic tone) and T wave inversion will usually "normalise". It is widely known that patients with coronary disease may develop pseudonormalisation of T wave changes on exercise, but in the context of a fit young athlete this response is reassuring (fig 31.4). The blood pressure response is normal which may be a helpful distinguishing feature from hypertrophic cardiomyopathy.

OTHER INVESTIGATIONS
Radionuclide studies, cardiac catheterisation, and magnetic resonance imaging provide useful insight into the athlete's heart but, in clinical practice, are largely reserved for specific cases where some suspected cardiac pathology requires elucidation. Multiple gated imaging shows that the increment in stroke volume on exercise in athletes is the result of a normal ejection fraction and increased end diastolic volume, rather than any demonstrable enhancement in contractility.

Vigorous exercise can cause elevation in cardiac enzymes including creatine phosphokinase (CPK). Small rises in MB CPK have also been reported.[w16] This can be confusing if an athlete is admitted having collapsed. The rises are modest, however, and the time scale of enzyme release is not typical of myocardial infarction. Troponin T and I are more specific and should be used in cases of doubt.[w17]

Reversibility

Reversibility of these changes in the detrained athlete can occur quite rapidly in athletes whose training is seasonal (fig 31.5) or over

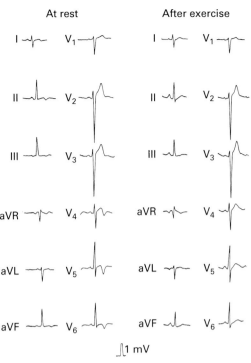

At rest · After exercise

Figure 31.4. Twelve lead ECG before and after exercise of a county squash player. The striking T wave changes in V4–V6 become normal immediately after exercise.

PROFESSIONAL FOOTBALLER

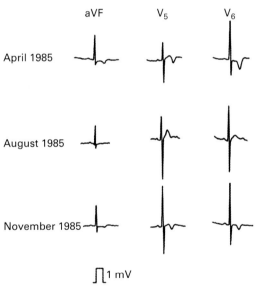

Figure 31.5. Selected leads of a premier league football player while training (April) after a period of detraining (August) and after resumption of training.

longer periods of time. It can be used as a distinguishing feature between athlete's heart and hypertrophic cardiomyopathy. A very long term follow up of competitors in the Tokyo Olympics showed eventual regression of hypertrophy in virtually all subjects.[16] Athletes frequently carry on training into middle and old age, competing in veteran and master events. These subjects are particularly confusing as the features of the athlete's heart are superimposed on other changes associated with aging.

Normal or abnormal?

The obvious concern facing a physician consulted by an athlete is "am I overlooking a potentially fatal cardiac condition?". In the young athlete exhibiting extreme hypertrophy or bradycardia the differential diagnosis will lie between hypertrophic cardiomyopathy and sick sinus syndrome, respectively. No single test can be guaranteed to separate athlete's heart from hypertrophic cardiomyopathy; not surprisingly, bearing in mind the great clinical variability of the latter. Helpful features include the extent and symmetry of hypertrophy on echocardiography, the response to three months detraining, the finding of unexplained hypertrophy in close relatives, the blood pressure and metabolic responses to exercise,[17] and other echocardiographic features such as the left ventricular filling profiles.

Asymptomatic bradycardia is less of a problem, but symptoms may merit a period of detraining monitored with serial 24 hour tapes.

In the older subject, coronary disease is more important and such patients with symptoms will require investigation for this with the usual battery of investigations whose fallibility is only too well known.

Sudden death

The death of a fit young athlete is extremely rare. The frequency is estimated as around 1 in 200 000, with considerable variability depending on different reports.[w18–20] Death rates will, of course be higher in recreational athletes and middle aged joggers, but even in these groups the risk is very small and less than in the sedentary population. When death occurs, however, it is more likely to be in association with exercise than during the resting period.[18 w20]

Death can be non-cardiac—for example, traumatic, hypo- or hyperthermia, dehydration or associated with drug abuse. Sudden death is usually cardiovascular, however, and careful necropsy frequently reveals an underlying cause. In younger subjects hypertrophic cardiomyopathy is the most frequent cause of death, though some authors claim that arrhythmogenic right ventricular dysplasia is even more common.[w21] Other causes include anomalous origins of the coronary arteries,[w22] aortic stenosis, myocarditis (possibly related to exercise during the febrile phase of a viral illness), Marfan syndrome, Wolff-Parkinson-White syndrome, long QT syndromes, mitral valve prolapse, and coronary disease. The estimated number of people who might be at risk from these conditions is summarised in a useful paper by Sharma.[17] In older subjects coronary disease assumes greater importance.

No sport has a monopoly of sudden death, though squash has been singled out as posing special risks, perhaps related to its very vigorous and competitive nature.[w23] There is also now a growing interest in extreme sports (for example, triathlons, 24 hour races, and fell running). The state of complete physical exhaustion encountered by some participants can lead to metabolic changes which adversely affect cardiac performance.[w24]

Screening athletes for cardiovascular disease

The frequent finding of pathology in necropsies of athletes who die suddenly implies that a prior diagnosis of their cardiac condition might have been made on routine screening.[19] Appropriate treatment and advice to avoid extreme exertion could have prevented death. In some countries, such as Italy, screening is mandatory and evidence from this country shows that the programme can be effective.[w25] There are, however, critics of this approach who point out that we are screening for rare abnormalities, for which there is often no curative treatment, with imperfect tests.[20] [w26] Even if a screening programme is embraced, there is no general agreement as to how it should be organised and which tests employed, though some attempts have been made in this area.[w27] The tests we have at our disposal are insensitive and non-specific, and the pre-test probability of cardiac disease is extremely low. This will inevitably lead to missed diagnoses and, more importantly, numerous false positive results. The misdiagnosis of a cardiac problem in a normal athlete is disastrous in someone for whom the state of physical fitness is, by definition, all important. Once the suggestion of cardiac disease has been raised, it is extremely difficult to eradicate it.

While the arguments about the merits of screening continue, it is clear that symptoms or suspicious signs in athletes demand thorough investigation.

Conclusion

Athletes are a challenging group for the cardiologist both in terms of diagnosis and management. The stakes are high. The cardiovascular system is going to be pushed to the limit. The consequences of an erroneous diagnosis are potentially devastating, be it the death of the athlete or a career and way of life in ruins. These patients always merit the most careful evaluation. When still in doubt, the physician is well advised to seek help from others. The author of this paper certainly does!

1. **Huston TP, Puffer JC, MacMillan Rodney W.** The athletic heart syndrome. *N Engl J Med* 1985;**313**:24–32.
- *A good general review of the clinical features of the athlete's heart.*

2. **Crawford MH, O'Rourke RA.** The athlete's heart. *Adv Intern Med* 1979;**24**:311–29.

3. **Schaible TF, Scheuer J.** Cardiac adaptations to chronic exercise. *Prog Cardiovasc Dis* 1985;**27**:297–324.
- *An extensive review of the physiological consequences of prolonged training on the cardiovascular system.*

4. **Morganroth J, Maron BJ, Henry WL,** *et al.* Comparative left ventricular dimensions in trained athletes. *Ann Intern Med* 1975;**85**:521–4.

5. **Fagard RH.** Athlete's heart: a meta-analysis of the echocardiographic experience. *Int J Sports Med* 1996;**17**(suppl 3):S140–4.
- *A useful meta-analysis of the many papers on hypertrophy in response to training.*

6. **Alvarez R, Terrados N, Ortolano R,** *et al.* Genetic variation in the renin-angiotensin system and athletic performance. *Eur J Appl Physiol* 2000;**82**:117–20.

7. **Fagard R, Aubert A, Lysens J,** *et al.* Noninvasive assessment of seasonal variations in cardiac structure and function in cyclists. *Circulation* 1983;**97**:896–901.

8. **Shapiro LM.** Physiological left ventricular hypertrophy. *Br Heart J* 1984;**52**:130–5.
- *One of several good papers showing that hypertrophy in response to training is not pathological.*

9. **Hammond HK, Froelicher VF.** Normal and abnormal heart rate responses to exercise. *Prog Cardiovasc Dis* 1985;**27**:271–96.
- *An extensive review of bradycardia in athletes, and its mechanism.*

10. **Zehender M, Meinertz T, Keul J,** *et al.* ECG variants and cardiac arrhythmias in athletes: clinical relevance and prognostic importance. *Am Heart J* 1990;**119**:1378–91.

11. **Ector H, Verlinden M, Vanden Eynde E,** *et al.* Bradycardia, ventricular pauses, syncope and sports. *Lancet* 1984;ii:591–4.
- *A good paper exploring the significance of symptomatic bradycardias.*

12. **Nishimura T, Yamada Y, Kawai C.** Echocardiographic evaluation of long-term effects of exercise on left ventricular hypertrophy and function in professional bicyclists. *Circulation* 1980;**61**:832–40.

13. **Zeppilli P, Pirrami MM, Sassara M,** *et al.* T wave abnormalities in top ranking athletes: effects of isproterenol, atropine, and exercise. *Am Heart J* 1980;**100**:213–22.

14. **Oakley DG, Oakley CM.** The significance of abnormal electrocardiograms in highly trained athletes. *Am J Cardiol* 1982;**50**:985–9.

15. **Pelliccia A, Maron BJ, Culasso F,** *et al.* Clinical significance of abnormal electrocardiographic patterns in trained athletes. *Circulation* 2000;**102**:278–84.
- *A useful, well referenced paper on the ECG in athletes.*

16. **Murrayama M, Kuroda Y.** Cardiovascular future in athletes. In: Lubich T, Venerando A, eds. *Sports cardiology.* Bologna: Aulo Gaggi, 1980:401–13.
- *An old, but useful study on the reversibility of the athlete's heart.*

17. **Sharma S, Whyte G, Mckenna WJ.** Sudden death from cardiovascular disease in young athletes: fact or fiction. *Br J Sports Med* 1997;**31**:269–76.
- *A helpful review article on sudden death in athletes and the pathological conditions which may be responsible.*

18. **Thompson PD, Funk E, Carleton RA,** *et al.* Incidence of death during jogging in Rhode Island from 1975 through 1980. *JAMA* 1982;**247**:2535–8.

19. **Corrado D, Basso C, Schiavon M,** *et al.* Screening for hypertrophic cardiomyopathy in young athletes. *N Engl J Med* 1998;**339**:364–9.

20. **Maron BJ, Shirani J, Poliac LC,** *et al.* Sudden death in young competitive athletes. Clinical, demographic, and pathological profiles [see comments]. *JAMA* 1996;**276**:199–204.
- *Maron has published extensively on sudden death in athletes, this well referenced paper being an example.*

website extra

Additional references appear on the Heart website

www.heartjnl.com

32 Acute pulmonary embolism 1: pathophysiology, clinical presentation, and diagnosis

Martin Riedel

Thrombotic pulmonary embolism is not an isolated disease of the chest but a complication of venous thrombosis. Deep venous thrombosis (DVT) and pulmonary embolism are therefore parts of the same process, venous thromboembolism. Evidence of leg DVT is found in about 70% of patients who have sustained a pulmonary embolism; in most of the remainder, it is assumed that the whole thrombus has already become detached and embolised. Conversely, pulmonary embolism occurs in up to 50% of patients with proximal DVT of the legs (involving the popliteal and/or more proximal veins), and is less likely when the thrombus is confined to the calf veins. Rarely, the source of emboli are the iliac veins, renal veins, right heart, or upper extremity veins; the clinical circumstances usually point to these unusual sites.

Risk factors, epidemiology, and risk stratification

As pulmonary embolism is preceded by DVT, the factors predisposing to the two conditions are the same and broadly fit Virchow's triad of venous stasis, injury to the vein wall and enhanced coagulability of the blood (table 32.1). The identification of risk factors not only aids clinical diagnosis of venous thromboembolism, but also guides decisions about prophylactic measures and repeat testing in borderline cases.

Table 32.1   Risk factors for venous thromboembolic disease

Venous stasis or injury, secondary hypercoagulable states:
   Immobilisation or other cause of venous stasis—for example, stroke
   Major trauma or surgery within 4 weeks
   Active cancer (treatment within previous 6 months or palliative therapy)
   Prior history of thromboembolism
   Reduced cardiac output (congestive heart failure)
   Obesity, advanced age
   Pregnancy, early puerperium, contraceptive pill with high oestrogen content
   Indwelling catheters and electrodes in great veins and right heart
   Acquired thrombotic disorders—for example, antiphospholipid antibodies, heparin induced thrombocytopenia, thrombocytosis, post-splenectomy
Primary hypercoagulable states (thrombophilia):
   Deficiency of antithrombin III, protein C or S
   Resistance to activated protein C (factor V Leiden)
   Elevated plasminogen activator inhibitor
   Hyperhomocysteinaemia
   High plasma concentration of factor VIII
   Prothrombin gene mutation (G20210A polymorphism)

Primary "thrombophilic" abnormalities are usually discovered after the thromboembolic event. Therefore, the risk of venous thromboembolism is best assessed by recognising the presence of known "clinical" risk factors. However, investigations for thrombophilic disorders at follow up should be considered in those without another apparent explanation. In many patients, multiple risk factors are present, and the risks are cumulative.

The overall incidence and mortality of pulmonary embolism in the population is unknown because the clinical diagnosis is unreliable, many events are asymptomatic, variable methods of prophylaxis are applied, necropsy rates are low, and death certification is inaccurate. Nevertheless, DVT and pulmonary embolism constitute some of the most common cardiovascular diseases in the western world. Many cases go unrecognised and hence untreated, with serious outcomes. The case fatality rate is less than 5% in treated patients who are haemodynamically stable at presentation but approximately 20% in those with persistent hypotension. Most deaths directly attributable to acute pulmonary embolism occur before the diagnosis can be confirmed and effective treatment implemented, which makes prevention in high risk patients imperative.

Although the overall frequency of pulmonary embolism cannot be accurately estimated, it is possible to assess incidence in particular groups at risk (table 32.2). In surgical series the risk of venous thromboembolism rises rapidly with age, length of anaesthesia, and the presence of previous venous thromboembolism or cancer. The incidence is highest in those undergoing emergency surgery following trauma (for hip fractures, for example) and pelvic surgery. Fatal pulmonary embolism occurs in 0.5–0.8% of unprotected patients older than 40 years undergoing major abdominal surgery. About one in 20 patients after total hip replacement will have a pulmonary embolism, nearly half of these being fatal. In obstetrics there is a high incidence of venous thromboembolism, particularly if operative delivery is used. Clinically important pulmonary embolism occurs in at least 3% of patients after coronary bypass surgery. Surgery predisposes patients to pulmonary embolism even as late as one month postoperatively.

In medical patients, venous thromboembolism is frequent in cardiorespiratory disorders (for example, congestive cardiac failure, irreversible airways disease), with leg immobility (caused by stroke and other neurological diseases), and in cancer. The increase in the prevalence of pulmonary embolism with increasing age may be only due to the relation between age and other comorbidities, which are the actual risk factors for venous thromboembolism.

The relative risk of suffering a venous thromboembolism episode is about three times higher in oral contraceptive users compared with non-users. This risk has to be interpreted in light of a low basal risk in the non-user population (about 2 per 10 000 women years)

Table 32.2   Incidence of thromboembolic disease in various risk categories

Risk category	Low risk	Medium risk	High risk
General surgery	Age < 40 years Surgery < 30 minutes No risk factors	Age > 40 years Surgery > 30 minutes No other risk factors	Age > 60 years Surgery > 60 minutes Plus additional risk factors
Orthopaedic surgery, traumatology	Minor trauma	Leg plaster cast	Hip or knee surgery, hip fracture, polytrauma
Medical conditions	Pregnancy	Heart failure, stroke, malignancy	Long immobility
Incidence (%)			
Distal DVT	2	10–40	40–80
Proximal DVT	0.4	6–8	10–15
Symptomatic PE	0.2	1–2	5–10
Fatal PE	0.002	0.1–0.8	1–5

DVT, deep vein thrombosis; PE, pulmonary embolism.

and the fact that fatal pulmonary embolism occurs only in a minority of treated cases. The third generation oral contraceptives carry an excess risk of 1.5–2 for venous thromboembolism as compared with the second generation preparations containing low doses of oestrogens. This may transfer to one extra death per million women per year.

Pathophysiology and clinical presentation

The effects of an embolus depend on the extent to which it obstructs the pulmonary circulation, the duration over which that obstruction accumulates, and the pre-existing state of the patient, which has been defined only imprecisely. Some humoral mediators (for example, serotonin or thromboxane from activated platelets) can probably produce vasospasm in non-embolised segments of the lung. As a result, a degree of pulmonary hypertension may develop disproportionate to the amount of vasculature that is mechanically occluded. In general, a patient who has pre-existing cardiopulmonary disease or who is old, frail or debilitated will be more sensitive to the effects of pulmonary embolism than a patient who was well until the embolic event occurred. Most emboli are multiple. As both the extent and chronicity of obstruction vary so widely, pulmonary embolism can produce widely differing clinical pictures. Disregarding chronic thromboembolic pulmonary hypertension, it is convenient to classify pulmonary embolism into three main types (table 32.3). The first and most common presentation is dyspnoea with or without pleuritic pain and haemoptysis (acute minor pulmonary embolism). The second presentation is haemodynamic instability, which is associated with acute massive pulmonary embolism. The third and least common presentation mimics heart failure or indolent pneumonia, especially in the elderly (subacute massive pulmonary embolism).

Acute minor pulmonary embolism

If an embolus obstructs less than 50% of the pulmonary circulation, it often produces no symptoms. For example, about 40% of patients with DVT who have no symptoms of pulmonary embolism have evidence of the condition on lung scans. If symptoms do develop the most common is dyspnoea, possibly upon minor exertion. Sometimes, the first abnormality the patient notes results from pulmonary infarction, which occurs in obstruction of medium sized pulmonary artery branches. Sharp pleuritic pain develops, and there may be associated haemoptysis. Pulmonary infarction occurs in only about 10% of patients without pre-existing cardiopulmonary disease. If, however, there is already compromise of the oxygenation of the embolised area—either because the airways are abnormal or pulmonary venous outflow is impaired as a result of pre-existing left heart disease—then the incidence of infarction rises to 30%.

If there are any physical signs, they are those of pulmonary infarction. The patient is distressed with rapid and shallow breathing because of the pleuritic pain, but is not cyanosed because the disturbance of gas transfer is only slight. Signs of pulmonary infarction may be found in the lungs: a mixture of consolidation and effusion, possibly with a pleural rub. Fever is common and sometimes differentiation from infective pleurisy is difficult. The fever and pain often produce a sinus tachycardia. Pulmonary artery mean pressure rarely exceeds 25 mm Hg. As minor pulmonary embolism does not compromise the right ventricle, cardiac output is well maintained,

Table 32.3   Clinical forms of pulmonary embolism

Pulmonary embolism	History	Vascular obstruction	Presentation	Typical pressures	
				PAP	RAP
Acute minor	Short, sudden onset	< 50%	Dyspnoea with or without pleuritic pain and haemoptysis	Normal	Normal
Acute massive	Short, sudden onset	> 50%	Right heart strain with or without haemodynamic instability and syncope	45/20	12
Subacute massive	Several weeks	> 50%	Dyspnoea with right heart strain	70/35	8

PAP, pulmonary artery pressure; RAP, mean right atrial pressure.

hypotension does not occur, and the venous pressure and heart sounds are normal. A common misapprehension is that there is often a loud pulmonary component of the second heart sound; this is not the case because the right heart pressures are normal or only slightly elevated.

Acute massive pulmonary embolism

When more than 50% of the pulmonary circulation is suddenly obstructed, the pathophysiology and clinical signs become dominated by the severe derangement of cardiac and pulmonary function. Obstruction of the pulmonary artery and mediator induced vasoconstriction cause a substantial increase in right ventricular afterload and, if the cardiac output is to be maintained, consequent elevation of pulmonary artery systolic pressure and an increase in right ventricular work. If this work cannot be sustained, acute right heart failure occurs. The thin walled right ventricle is designed to work against the normally low pulmonary vascular resistance; it performs poorly against a sudden obstruction. As a result, it dilates, and a moderate rise in the right ventricular and pulmonary artery systolic pressure occurs which rarely exceeds 55 mm Hg because the ventricle, lacking time to develop compensatory hypertrophy, is unable to generate a higher pressure. The right ventricular end diastolic pressure and right atrial pressure rise to about 15–20 mm Hg as the ventricle fails. Right ventricular dilatation leads to tricuspid regurgitation and may compromise the filling of the left ventricle. Cardiac output falls and the patient becomes hypotensive. This may occur so rapidly that syncope is either the presenting feature or easily induced by a relatively minor cardiovascular stress. If the degree of obstruction is sufficient, death occurs almost immediately. The fall in aortic pressure and the rise in right ventricular pressure may cause ischaemia of the right ventricle through a critical reduction of right coronary perfusion. Electromechanical dissociation is the most frequent cause of final cardiac arrest.

Arterial hypoxaemia correlates roughly with the extent of embolism if there is no prior cardiopulmonary disease. Massive pulmonary embolism without hypoxaemia is so rare that if the arterial oxygen tension (Pao_2) is normal an alternative diagnosis should be considered. Hypoxaemia decreases tissue oxygen delivery and can impede circulatory adaptation through its vasodilating effects.

The main causes of hypoxaemia in pulmonary embolism seem to be as follows:

(1) *Ventilation–perfusion mismatch.* Unembolised areas of the lung are relatively overperfused, so that the ventilation in these areas may be insufficient to oxygenate fully the extra blood flow.

(2) *Shunting* occurs through areas of collapse and infarction that are not ventilated but retain some blood flow. This may become more important a few days after the initial episode. In patients with a patent foramen ovale, raised right atrial pressure may open the foramen and cause right-to-left shunt-ing at the atrial level. This should be considered if the degree of hypoxaemia is more profound than would be expected from other clinical features, if it cannot be corrected by oxygen administration and if it is accompanied by hypercapnia.

(3) *Low mixed venous oxygen saturation* caused by the reduced cardiac output causes hypoxaemia because there is insufficient time for the extremely desaturated blood to become fully saturated as it passes through the alveolar capillaries in the over-perfused areas of the lung.

Although pulmonary embolism impairs the elimination of CO_2, hypercapnia is rare because compensatory hyperventilation eliminates CO_2 in all but the most extensive embolism. In cases with a sufficient degree of vascular obstruction to produce hypercapnia, the haemodynamic sequelae of acute right ventricular failure usually prove fatal.

The clinical features of acute massive pulmonary embolism can be explained in terms of these pathophysiological changes (table 32.3). The patient becomes acutely distressed, severely short of breath, and may be syncopal because of the combination of hypoxaemia and low cardiac output. The combination of hypotension, hypoxaemia, and increased cardiac work may cause anginal chest pain. The physical signs are those of reduced cardiac output—that is, pronounced sinus tachycardia, hypotension, and a cool periphery, sometimes with confusion. The patient is obviously dyspnoeic (but not orthopnoeic), cyanosed both centrally and peripherally, and has signs of acute right heart strain: a raised venous pressure, which is often difficult to appreciate because of the respiratory distress; a gallop rhythm at lower sternum; and a widely split second heart sound due to delayed right ventricular ejection, which is difficult to detect because of the accompanying tachycardia. The pulmonary component of the second heart sound is usually not loud because the pulmonary artery pressure is only moderately raised.

Subacute massive pulmonary embolism

This is caused by multiple small or moderately sized emboli that accumulate over several weeks. Because the obstruction occurs slowly, there is time for the right ventricle to adapt and for some hypertrophy to develop; consequently, the right ventricular systolic pressure is higher than in acute pulmonary embolism. The rises in the right ventricular end diastolic and right atrial pressures are of a lesser extent than in acute massive pulmonary embolism since there is time for adaptation to occur and the degree of right ventricular failure is less for a given degree of pulmonary artery obstruction. The main symptoms are increasing dyspnoea and falling exercise tolerance. There is often an associated dry cough. The breathlessness is usually out of proportion to all other findings, and there may be central cyanosis. The blood pressure and pulse rate are usually normal because the cardiac output is well maintained. Commonly, the venous pressure is raised and a third heart sound is audible at the

Table 32.4   Estimation of the (pretest) clinical likelihood of pulmonary embolism

High (> 85% likely)	Otherwise unexplained sudden onset of dyspnoea, tachypnoea, or chest pain and at least 2 of the following:
	    Significant risk factor present (immobility, leg fracture, major surgery)
	    Fainting with new signs of right ventricular overload in ECG
	    Signs of possible leg DVT (unilateral pain, tenderness, erythema, warmth, or swelling)
	    Radiographic signs of infarction, plump hilum, or oligemia

Intermediate (15-85% likely)	Neither high nor low clinical likelihood
Low (< 15% likely)	Absence of sudden onset of dyspnoea and tachypnoea and chest pain Dyspnoea, tachypnoea, or chest pain present but explainable by another condition Risk factors absent Radiographic abnormality explainable by another condition Adequate anticoagulation (INR > 2 or aPTT > 1.5 times control) during the previous week

INR, international normalised ratio; aPTT, activated partial thromboplastin time

lower sternum which may be accentuated by inspiration. The pulmonary component of the second heart sound is sometimes loud. There may also be intermittent symptoms and signs of pulmonary infarction that occurred during the build up of the obstruction. In advanced cases, cardiac output falls and frank right heart failure develops. A further pulmonary embolus may change the picture to that resembling acute massive pulmonary embolism.

Diagnostic procedures

The clinical diagnosis of pulmonary embolism is difficult, particularly when there is coexisting heart or lung disease, and it is notoriously inaccurate when based on clinical signs alone. About two thirds patients who present with suspected DVT or pulmonary embolism do not have these conditions.[1][2] Very rarely, pulmonary embolism presents in such a dramatic fashion that the diagnosis is intuitively obvious and treatment will be started, but the usual presentation is frequently vague and variable in severity, so that further testing is necessary to establish or exclude the diagnosis.[2] Diagnostic evaluation is best carried out by first attempting to identify a provable alternative diagnosis that can explain the patient's symptoms.

Estimating pretest clinical likelihood of venous thromboembolism

Until the 1970s, the diagnosis or exclusion of pulmonary embolism was made on clinical grounds alone. In the UPET (urokinase pulmonary embolism trial) study, several clinical findings, previously considered valuable in the diagnosis of pulmonary embolism, were not present in many patients with the condition, and less than one third of the 2200 patients with suspected pulmonary embolism actually had the disease after objective testing.[1] These results led clinicians to virtually abandon clinical examination and diagnose pulmonary embolism solely based on the results of objective tests. A number of recent studies, however, have suggested that combining the individual components of clinical assessment, risk factors for venous thromboembolism, and simple investigations reliably categorises the likelihood of pulmonary embolism as low, moderate, or high in an individual patient.[3-6]

By adopting a thorough stratification system the clinician can more appropriately select further investigations to prove or exclude pulmonary embolism. Establishing the pretest clinical likelihood of pulmonary embolism is especially helpful in interpreting the scintigraphy. Clinical likelihood of pulmonary embolism is determined after consideration of risk factors (the most common being immobilisation, a history of previous venous thromboembolism, lower limb fractures, and recent surgery), presentation, and basic investigations (ECG and plain chest radiograph). Although the characteristics of these clinical estimates have not been extensively validated, those generally accepted are given in table 32.4.

Nearly all patients with pulmonary embolism will have one or more of the following clinical features—dyspnoea of sudden onset, tachypnoea (> 20 breaths/minute), or chest pain (pleuritic or substernal)[2]; if the clinician remembers these three features, the possibility of pulmonary embolism will rarely be overlooked. When these clinical features are associated with ECG signs of right ventricular strain and/or radiologic signs of plump hilum, pulmonary infarction or oligaemia, the likelihood of pulmonary embolism is high, and it is further strengthened in the presence of risk factors for venous thromboembolism and arterial hypoxaemia with hypocapnia.[4] On the contrary, the absence of all these three clinical features virtually excludes the diagnosis of pulmonary embolism.

Electrocardiography

ECG changes are usually non-specific. In minor pulmonary embolism there is no haemodynamic stress and thus the only finding is sinus tachycardia. In acute or subacute massive pulmonary embolism, evidence of right heart strain may be seen (rightward shift of the QRS axis, transient right bundle branch block, T wave inversion in leads V1-3, P pulmonale), but the classic $S_I Q_{III} T_{III}$ pattern occurs in only a few cases.[2] The main value of ECG is in excluding other potential diagnoses, such as myocardial infarction or pericarditis.

Chest radiography

Chest radiograph findings are also non-specific but may be helpful. A normal film is compatible with all types of acute pulmonary embolism; in fact, a normal film in a patient with severe acute dyspnoea without wheezing is very suspicious of pulmonary embolism. The lung fields may show evidence of pulmonary infarction: peripheral opacities, sometimes wedge shaped or semicircular, arranged along the pleural surface (so called Hampton's hump). Atelectasis, small pleural effusions, and raised diaphragm have low specificity for pulmonary embolism. In massive pulmonary embolism a plump pulmonary artery shadow may be seen when the pulmonary artery pressure is elevated. It may be possible to detect areas of oligaemia in the parts of the lung affected by emboli (Westermark sign), but this is difficult on the type of film usually available in the acute situation. The radiograph is especially valuable in excluding other conditions mimicking pulmonary embolism (pneumothorax, pneumonia, left heart failure, tumour, rib fracture, massive pleural effusion, lobar collapse), but pulmonary embolism may coexist with other cardiopulmonary processes. The radiograph is also necessary for the proper interpretation of the lung scan.

Echocardiography

Transthoracic echocardiography rarely enables direct visualisation of the pulmonary embolus but may reveal thrombus floating in the right atrium or ventricle. With transoesophageal echocardiography, it is possible to visualise massive emboli in the central pulmonary arteries. In the presence of thrombi in right heart chambers, pulmonary angiography is not necessary and, indeed, is contraindicated because of risk of thrombus dislodgement.

In massive pulmonary embolism the right ventricle is dilated and hypokinetic, with abnormal motion of the interventricular septum. The inferior vena cava does not collapse during inspiration. Unfortunately, the finding of right ventricular dysfunction is non-specific and certain conditions commonly confused with pulmonary embolism (such as chronic obstructive pulmonary disease (COPD) exacerbations or cardiomyopathy) are also associated with abnormal right ventricular function. There is some evidence that regional right ventricular dysfunction (akinesia of the mid-free wall with apical sparing) may be more common in acute pulmonary embolism. The Doppler technique allows the pulmonary artery pressure to be estimated and together with contrast echocardiography it is useful in diagnosing patent foramen ovale which may indicate impending paradoxical embolism.

Although direct echocardiographic visualisation of intraluminal thrombi in patients with suspected pulmonary embolism is not frequent, and even when echocardiography provides only indirect signs compatible with haemodynamic consequences of massive pulmonary embolism, it is helpful in excluding or suggesting alternative causes for haemodynamic instability (aortic dissection, ventricular septal rupture, cardiac tamponade, etc). In an unstable hypotensive patient requiring immediate treatment, such information is of great importance. However, because the right ventricle may show no dysfunction even in patients with massive pulmonary embolism, echo-

cardiography should be considered an ancillary rather than a principal diagnostic test for the diagnosis of pulmonary embolism.

Arterial blood gases

The characteristic changes are a reduced Pao_2, and a $Paco_2$ that is normal or reduced because of hyperventilation. The Pao_2 is almost never normal in the patient with massive pulmonary embolism but can be normal in minor pulmonary embolism, mainly due to hyperventilation. In such cases the widening of the alveolo-arterial Po_2 gradient ($AaPo_2$ > 20 mm Hg) may be more sensitive than Pao_2 alone. Both hypoxaemia and a wide $AaPo_2$ may obviously be due to many other causes. Blood gases, therefore, may heighten the suspicion of pulmonary embolism and contribute to the clinical assessment, but they are of insufficient discriminant value to permit proof or exclusion of pulmonary embolism.[2]

Biochemistry

No blood test will diagnose venous thromboembolism. Although endogenous fibrinolysis is indicated by the sensitive assay of cross linked fibrin degradation products (D-dimers), this test has low specificity and is positive not only when there is venous thromboembolism but also in the presence of disseminated intravascular coagulation, malignancy, and after trauma or surgery. Although a negative test may be strong enough evidence that clotting has not occurred and that anticoagulants can be withheld, a positive test cannot confirm venous thromboembolism. The test could reduce the number of investigations in outpatients with suspected pulmonary embolism and a low pretest likelihood for venous thromboembolism, and may be useful as a screening test in an emergency unit when lung scintigraphy or computed tomography (CT) is not immediately available. However, if there is a high clinical suspicion of acute pulmonary embolism, diagnostic tests should proceed in spite of a normal D-dimer. In elderly or inpatients, D-dimer retains a high negative predictive value, but is normal in less than 10% of patients, and, hence, not very useful. Not all D-dimer testing methods have equal and sufficient sensitivity (the latex agglutination test is not reliable in excluding pulmonary embolism), but the rapid assays with a negative predictive value approaching 100% are comparable to the reliable but labour and time consuming ELISA (enzyme linked immunosorbent assay) tests.

Lung scintigraphy

A normal perfusion scan essentially excludes the diagnosis of a clinically relevant recent pulmonary embolism because occlusive pulmonary embolism of all types produces a defect of perfusion. Normal results are almost never associated with recurrent pulmonary embolism, even if anticoagulants are withheld. However, many conditions other than pulmonary embolism, such as tumours, consolidation, left heart failure, bullous lesions, lung fibrosis, and obstructive airways disease, can also produce

227

Table 32.5   Probability (%) of underlying pulmonary embolism according to the criteria of PIOPED study[3]

	Scan probability			
	Normal/very low	"Non-diagnostic"		
		Low	Intermediate	High
Clinical likelihood:				
Low	2	4	16	56
Intermediate	6	16	28	88
High	0	40	66	96

Table 32.6   Probability (%) of underlying pulmonary embolism (PE) according to the criteria of PISA-PED study[8]

	Scan probability	
	PE−	PE+
Clinical likelihood:		
Low	3	55
Intermediate	12	92
High	39	99

perfusion defects. Addition of a ventilation scan increases the specificity of scintigraphy. Pulmonary embolism usually produces a defect of perfusion but not ventilation ("mismatch") while most of the other conditions produce a ventilation defect in the same area as the perfusion defect (matched defects). Pulmonary embolism can also produce matched defects when infarction has occurred, but in this situation the chest radiograph nearly always shows shadowing in the area of scan defect.

The lung scan is an indirect method of diagnosis since it does not detect the embolus itself but only its consequence, the perfusion abnormality. The probability that perfusion defects are caused by pulmonary embolism can be assessed as high, intermediate or low depending on the type of scan abnormality (although there are significant variations in the interpretative patterns and diagnostic accuracy even between experienced readers using standard algorithms).[3 7] If the scan is of a high probability type (basically multiple segmental or larger perfusion defects with a normal ventilation scan) there is a more than 85% chance that the patient has pulmonary embolism. However, the majority of patients with clinically suspected pulmonary embolism do not have high probability scans and instead have ones that suggest either low or intermediate probability (= non-diagnostic scans); in these patients the prevalence of pulmonary embolism is about 25%. Taking the clinical assessment into account improves diagnostic accuracy (when the clinical likelihood of pulmonary embolism and scan interpretation is concordant, the ability to diagnose or exclude pulmonary embolism is optimised (table 32.5)), but the diagnosis can still be made or excluded with accuracy in only about a third of patients. A low probability scan does not rule out pulmonary embolism, but in fact there is up to a 40% probability of pulmonary embolism when clinical likelihood is high.[3]

In theory the addition of ventilation scanning should improve the usefulness of perfusion imaging, but the PIOPED (prospective investigation of pulmonary embolism diagnosis) study showed such benefit to be marginal. Perfusion defects caused by pulmonary embolism are most often wedge shaped. In the PISA-PED (prospective investigation study of acute pulmonary embolism diagnosis) study, when only wedge-shaped defects were classified as suspect for pulmonary embolism, perfusion scintigraphy without the use of ventilation scans, combined with clinical as-

sessment of pulmonary embolism likelihood (table 32.6), made it possible to confirm or exclude the condition in 76% of patients with abnormal scans, with an accuracy of 97%.[4 8] Angiography was then required only in about one fourth of patients with abnormal scans. This suggests that where ventilation imaging is unavailable, perfusion scanning alone is acceptable. The simple PISA-PED criteria are likely to become an attractive alternative to the complex PIOPED criteria.

Although the lung scan is often an imprecise guide it is useful in clinical decision making: a normal scan or a low probability scan with low clinical likelihood of pulmonary embolism means that treatment for suspected pulmonary embolism can be withheld, and a high probability scan with a high clinical likelihood of pulmonary embolism means that treatment is mandatory. Objective tests for DVT and pulmonary angiography or CT must be used to decide on the treatment in patients between these extremes and in whom the clinical likelihood of pulmonary embolism and scan interpretation are discordant.

Planar scintigraphy is the standard technology in most institutions. With SPECT (single photon emission CT) technology, pictures can be reconstructed in any plane and the specificity of scintigraphy substantially improves because of the reduction in the frequency of non-diagnostic scans.[9]

Scanning should be performed within 24 hours of the onset of symptoms of pulmonary embolism, since some scans revert to normal quickly. A follow up scan at the time of discharge is helpful in establishing a new baseline for subsequent episodes of suspected pulmonary embolism. The only clinically important cause of a false positive study is prior pulmonary embolism that has not resolved, leaving a lung scan pattern that remains in the high probability category.

Computed tomography (CT, spiral or electron beam CT)

Contrast enhanced spiral or electron beam CT have emerged as valuable methods for diagnosing pulmonary embolism and, because of its availability, spiral CT is becoming the first choice method at many institutions. The technique is faster, less complex, and less operator dependent than conventional pulmonary angiography, and has about the same frequency of technically insufficient examinations (about 5%). The thorax can be scanned during a single breath hold. There is better interobserver agreement in the interpretation of CT than for

Pulmonary scintigraphy

- Significant variations in scan interpretation exist even between experienced readers using standard algorithms

- Normal perfusion scan excludes clinically important pulmonary embolism and makes further testing unnecessary. It is safe to withhold anticoagulants in patients with suspected pulmonary embolism and normal perfusion scan

- Scan is diagnostic in a minority of cases. Only normal and high probability scans are clear in terms of clinical implications. The utility of scans is optimised when interpreted as representing a low or high probability of pulmonary embolism with concordant clinical likelihood of pulmonary embolism

- Patients with non-diagnostic scans require further imaging rather than management based on clinical features

scintigraphy. Another advantage of CT over scintigraphy is that by imaging the lung parenchyma and great vessels, an alternative diagnosis (for example, pulmonary mass, pneumonia, emphysema, pleural effusion, mediastinal adenopathy) can be made if pulmonary embolism is absent. This advantage of CT also pertains to pulmonary angiography, which images only the arteries. CT can also detect right ventricular dilatation, thus indicating severe, potentially fatal pulmonary embolism.

Criteria for a positive CT scan result include a partial filling defect (defined as intraluminal area of low attenuation surrounded by a contrast medium), a complete filling defect, and the "railway track sign" (masses seen floating in the lumen, allowing the flow of blood between the vessel wall and the embolus). The procedure has over 90% specificity and sensitivity in diagnosing pulmonary embolism in the main, lobar, and segmental pulmonary arteries. When CT is used to evaluate patients with a non-diagnostic lung scan, the sensitivity is lower.[10] [11]

Although recent advances in CT technology enable better visualisation of subsegmental arteries, these small vessels remain difficult to evaluate. The clinical significance of isolated subsegmental emboli is unclear, and it is not current practice to ignore them. They may be of importance in patients with poor cardiopulmonary reserve, and their presence is an indicator for current DVT, which thus potentially heralds more severe emboli. One recent study showed, however, that patients with pulmonary embolism negative spiral CT do well without anticoagulation treatment.[12] This should be especially true when these patients also have a leg venous study that is negative for thrombus.

Other reasons for falsely negative results may be inadequate visualisation of a portion of the lung, difficulty in evaluating non-vertically ori-

ented arteries (particularly of the lingula and the middle lobe), and difficulty in opacifying the arteries in patients with superior vena caval obstruction or intracardiac or intrapulmonary shunts. These sources of falsely negative results are significant and one cannot therefore regard CT as a new "gold standard" to replace angiography. If clinical suspicion for pulmonary embolism is high and the CT is interpreted as negative or inconclusive, further investigation should be performed.

CT may also be falsely positive for pulmonary embolism. Enlarged hilar lymph nodes and volume averaged atelectatic lung or mediastinal fat may be misinterpreted as emboli. Perivascular oedema (such as occurs in congestive heart failure) may appear as an embolus. An insufficient delay from the administration of contrast to the initiation of the scan can lead to filling defects that can be misinterpreted as emboli.

Additional research is required to establish the place of CT in clinical practice. In particular, the sensitivity of CT for small clots should be carefully examined and the utility of testing strategies employing CT must be determined in outcome studies and compared with currently employed algorithms. Because of the small number of non-diagnostic results and a potentially greater out-of-hours availability, spiral CT may replace scintigraphy as the primary test in patients with suspected pulmonary embolism.

After performing lung CT (involving intravenous injection of contrast medium) to diagnose pulmonary embolism, sufficient opacification of the venous system remains to evaluate the veins of the legs, pelvis, and abdomen for DVT, without additional venepuncture or contrast medium. Such an examination is a continuous study, adding approximately five minutes to pulmonary scanning, with the added expense of only one sheet of film. The pelvic and abdominal images screen the iliac veins and vena cava for thrombosis, an important advantage over sonography, particularly when caval filter placement is considered. This potential for performing in a single study both venography and pulmonary CT angiography is promising. If the accuracy of venous imaging after lung scanning is confirmed in large studies, its use should be considered whenever CT pulmonary angiography is indicated.

Magnetic resonance imaging

Magnetic resonance imaging (MRI) offers both morphological and functional information on lung perfusion and right heart function, but its image quality still needs improvement to be comparable with CT. MRI has several attractive advantages, including the avoidance of nephrotoxic iodinated contrast and ionising radiation, and excellent sensitivity and specificity for DVT, together with the potential for performing lung perfusion imaging. This technique may ultimately allow simultaneous and accurate detection of both DVT and pulmonary embolism. Additional data are needed, however. A disadvantage of MRI compared to CT is the long time (15–30

229

Spiral or electron beam CT

- Emerging as a non-invasive testing modality to complement or replace the standard lung scintigraphy

- Can directly visualise intravascular thrombus, but smaller, subsegmental emboli can be overlooked

- Greater sensitivity and specificity for pulmonary embolism than lung scintigraphy. Agreement among readers of CT better than among readers of scintigrams

- CT scans, like angiograms, are either positive or negative for pulmonary embolism in the majority of cases. Only 10% of CT scans are non-diagnostic (compared to 70% non-diagnostic scintigrams)

- Can diagnose alternative causes of dyspnoea

- Currently, because of significant sources of both false negative and false positive examinations, CT cannot yet be regarded as a gold standard alternative to angiography.

minutes) needed to perform the examination, which is not suitable for clinically unstable patients. Improvements in MRI angiographic techniques will inevitably produce better results in the future.

Pulmonary angiography

Catheter pulmonary angiography remains the "gold standard" and the only technique that can diagnose or exclude pulmonary embolism with relative certainty. It should be considered, first, if cardiovascular collapse or hypotension are present and, second, when other investigations are inconclusive. However, angiography has disadvantages of limited availability and a small (< 0.3%) but definite risk of mortality.[7 13] This risk gets higher the more seriously ill the patient is, particularly when there is significant pulmonary hypertension. Relative contraindications include pregnancy, significant bleeding risk, renal insufficiency, and known right heart thrombus. The presence of a left bundle branch block is an indication for a temporary pacemaker during the procedure. The safety of the procedure is enhanced by monitoring (ECG, pulse oximeter, automated blood pressure device), ready oxygen availability, and by reducing the amount of contrast material given at lower pressure.

Injection of low osmolar non-ionic contrast through a pigtail catheter into the main pulmonary artery, with radiographs of the whole chest in two projections taken in rapid succession using an automatic film changer, is sufficient to delineate the emboli in most cases. Where prior scintigraphy is non-diagnostic, angiography can be first confined to the more abnormal side. When the embolus is small, selective injections into subdivisions of the arteries, oblique views and cineangiography, which can separate superimposed vessels as they move apart due to the pulsation of the arteries, improves diagnostic accuracy. The digital subtraction technique makes the examination easier and faster (because of the cinematic review and work station manipulation) and results in comparable image quality and improved interobserver agreement compared with conventional cut-film angiography. An embolus appears as an abrupt vessel cutoff or a convex filling defect often with contrast leaking beyond its edges and the sides of the vessel containing it. The overall perfusion of the affected region is reduced.

The assumption that life threatening pulmonary embolism is not missed by pulmonary angiography seems to hold true. However, although false positives are difficult to prove and probably scarce, false negative examinations can occur despite important intravascular embolus. Non-diagnostic pulmonary angiography can also occur.

Pulmonary angiography can be performed by the femoral, brachial, subclavian or internal jugular approaches. The femoral venous approach is useless in patients who have had an inferior caval interruptive procedure. Disadvantages of the femoral approach relate to the possibility of dislodging iliofemoral or caval thrombus and a high risk of bleeding from a fresh femoral venous puncture site during thrombolytic treatment. This risk can be reduced by leaving the catheter in the vein for mechanical haemostasis during the thrombolysis. The main difficulty with catheterisation from the brachial approach relates to the possibility of catheter induced venous spasm with inability to advance the catheter into the central veins; this may be particularly problematic in patients with excessive circulating catecholamines caused by shock or vasopressor administration. In fully anticoagulated patients the internal jugular and, especially, the subclavian approach are contraindicated.

The changes in the right heart pressures that occur in pulmonary embolism are summarised in table 32.3. It is important to measure the pressures and oxygen saturations before angiography so that the haemodynamic situation, including cardiac output and any intracardiac shunting, can be assessed. This facilitates determination of the patient's underlying cardiopulmonary reserve, identification of any haemodynamic derangements that might require specific treatment to increase the safety of angiography, and more careful selection of the contrast agent and dose to maximise diagnostic information while minimising the risk of hypotension, myocardial depression or a further increase in ventricular filling pressures. Occasionally if the diagnosis of pulmonary embolism before catheterisation is wrong the haemodynamic data may suggest the correct diagnosis and lead to appropriate treatment.

The use of intravenous digital subtraction angiography (DSA) avoids the need for pulmonary artery catheterisation but has been disappointing because opacification of the pulmonary vessels is poor. Although intravenous DSA may be adequate for showing large proximal arterial occlusions, resolution is usually inadequate to identify an embolus in the segmental vessels and beyond. Thus minor pulmonary embolism cannot be excluded on the basis of a normal DSA with peripheral contrast application.[13]

Search for deep venous thrombosis

DVT cannot be reliably diagnosed on the basis of the history and physical examination. Patients with lower extremity DVT often do not exhibit pain, tenderness, erythema, warmth, or swelling. When present, however, these findings merit further evaluation. Impedance plethysmography, compression ultrasonography with venous imaging (colour duplex ultrasound), and MRI are established non-invasive methods for diagnosing DVT. While contrast venography remains the gold standard, it is rarely performed because it is invasive and difficult to carry out in the acutely ill patient. Venography is no longer appropriate as the initial diagnostic test for the evaluation of symptoms that suggest acute DVT; it should be performed whenever non-invasive testing is non-diagnostic or impossible to perform. While plethysmography and ultrasound are reliable for the diagnosis of symptomatic proximal DVT, they are much less reliable for recognising asymptomatic DVT. They are also not able to detect floating thrombus in the vena cava. Plethysmography also has other limitations and is inferior to the latest ultrasound techniques; it is now used in only a few institutions.

Although all the above methods for detecting thrombus in the deep veins do not establish the diagnosis of pulmonary embolism, the confirmation of DVT is of major importance in management decisions. The logic of leg vein imaging is that many patients with pulmonary embolism have residual proximal clot even in the absence of clinical evidence of DVT, itself an indication for treatment even if there is no direct proof of pulmonary embolism. If there is no thrombosis in the proximal leg or pelvic veins the chance of a further significant pulmonary embolism is low; therefore, even if a small pulmonary embolism has occurred already, anticoagulation can be omitted. This approach needs caution if the patient has inadequate cardiorespiratory reserve, is likely to remain immobile, or if there could be an embolic source elsewhere (for example, right atrium or vena cava).[14]

Failure to identify thrombosis of the calf veins rarely has serious sequelae, and the investigation can be repeated if there is persisting clinical concern. In patients with documented isolated calf vein thrombosis, repeated impedance plethysmography or compression ultrasonography can be used to separate the 20% of patients who develop proximal extension (and require treatment) from the remaining 80% of patients who do not and in whom the risks of anticoagulant treatment may outweigh the benefits (for example, in patients at high risk of bleeding).[14]

The integrated diagnostic approach with management options

The diagnosis requires a high level of clinical suspicion, estimation of the pretest clinical likelihood of pulmonary embolism, and the judicious use of objective investigations to confirm or refute the suspicion. Pulmonary angiography is justly regarded as the final arbiter but is not often performed, because of its limited availability, costs, and invasiveness. Therefore, treatment is often based on the clinical probability of pulmonary embolism rather than on a definite diagnosis or a ruling out of the condition. Consequently, some patients receive anticoagulants without proof of pulmonary embolism and other patients are not treated although they may have it. In either situation, the chance for proper disease management may be lost. For these reasons, much effort has been invested to determine how clinicians could reliably use non-invasive tests, alone or in combination, to replace pulmonary angiography as a diagnostic tool.[15 16]

Basic tests

Basic tests include the ECG and plain chest radiograph. These must be performed in all patients both to support clinical suspicion of pulmonary embolism and, in particular, to exclude alternative diagnoses. As ECG and chest radiographic abnormalities in pulmonary embolism may be non-specific, absent, transient, or delayed, they cannot be used to confirm the diagnosis. Normal blood gases do not rule out pulmonary embolism; findings of hypoxaemia or hypocapnia may increase the physician's level of suspicion, but they are not specific for pulmonary embolism. More specific investigations are always required, but choosing which road to follow from the myriad of possibilities of imaging examinations can be confusing.

Various combinations of tests have resulted in several elaborate algorithms which, however, are seldom followed in clinical routine. Algorithms that inevitably result in large numbers of patients being referred for angiography are unhelpful. The availability of and familiarity with certain technology may influence the diagnostic approach. The specific clinical scenario also impacts on the diagnostic procedure that is chosen. There is no single algorithm to be recommended for all situations; rather, the investigations should be chosen according to the haemodynamic state of the patient (suspicion of massive versus minor pulmonary embolism), the onset of symptoms (in versus out of hospital), the presence or absence of other cardiopulmonary diseases, and the availability of specific tests.[15 16]

Haemodynamic instability

In critically ill patients suspected of having a massive pulmonary embolism, particularly those with cardiovascular collapse, echocardiography can be rapidly performed at the bedside to exclude other diseases or, occasionally, to establish the diagnosis by finding clots in the central pulmonary arteries or the right heart. By visualisation of thrombi further investigations are not necessary. When evidence of right heart strain without clots is present on echo, spiral CT or pulmonary angiography should follow, depending on faster availability.

In patients with life threatening instability where emergency treatment is necessary and CT or cardiac catheterisation is unavailable, intravenous DSA may be adequate for showing large proximal arterial occlusions. Image quality can be improved by delivering the contrast to the pulmonary artery via a flow directed, balloon tipped catheter. The floating catheter may also be useful in showing the characteristic haemodynamic changes with massive pulmonary embolism and suggesting an alternative diagnosis.

Haemodynamically stable patients

The principal challenge in stable patients is to develop a logical sequence of investigations that allow early, cost effective diagnosis and are associated with the most favourable markers of outcome. Depending on timely availability of tests and patient presentation, several approaches are possible.

Proof of DVT without definitive diagnosis of pulmonary embolism

This should be the preferred first procedure in patients with clinical suspicion of DVT in addition to the suspicion of pulmonary embolism. If duplex sonography, MRI, or impedance plethysmography confirms thrombosis, treatment can be started without recourse to lung imaging. Because the treatment of DVT and pulmonary embolism is the same in most patients with stable circulation, establishing the diagnosis of DVT, although it does not confirm that pulmonary embolism has occurred, is sufficient reason for full anticoagulation and avoids the need for additional studies. Leg vein imaging can also be performed as the initial investigation for suspected pulmonary embolism in patients with previous pulmonary embolism or chronic cardiopulmonary disease, where the frequency of non-diagnostic scans is high. If the leg study is negative or inconclusive, however, further investigations are imperative.

Lung scintigraphy

In about one third of cases, lung scan either rules out the diagnosis (normal perfusion or low probability scan with low clinical likelihood of pulmonary embolism) or suggests a high enough probability of pulmonary embolism that, in case of concurrent high clinical likelihood of pulmonary embolism, treatment can be undertaken on the basis of its results without further investigations. The frequency of such diagnostic scans is greater in outpatients with no prior cardiopulmonary disease who have a normal chest radiograph, and especially in these patients scintigraphy is the preferred initial examination. By limiting the patients who undergo scintigraphy to those without demonstrable lung disease at chest radiography, one can reduce the number of indeterminate studies and select a group of patients whose scintigrams are likely to show normal or high probability results. However, the presence of cardiopulmonary disease or indeed any critical illness should not deter clinicians from requesting a lung scan, if it is readily available.

In patients with a non-diagnostic scan, or whose clinical likelihood of pulmonary embolism does not correlate with the scan result, further investigation is necessary. Of these patients, about 25% will prove to have pulmonary embolism and require anticoagulants; the other 75% will have another disease as the cause of the lung scan defects. CT is especially useful in these patients owing to its efficacy in imaging alternative pulmonary pathology.

If clinical likelihood is intermediate and the scan non-diagnostic, long term anticoagulation treatment can probably be withheld if repeated examination of leg veins over a week is normal and the patient has no underlying cardiopulmonary disease. If the leg veins are clear it is reasonable to assume that the patient is not in imminent danger of a fatal recurrence. Those with underlying cardiopulmonary disease, where only a medium sized embolus could be fatal, require a more aggressive diagnostic approach.[14]

In outpatients with a non-diagnostic scan, low clinical likelihood of pulmonary embolism, and no prior cardiopulmonary disease, the finding of a normal D-dimer concentration (measured by a test with nearly 100% sensitivity) can be used to reliably exclude venous thromboembolism. A raised D-dimer concentration, however, is a frequent non-specific finding in hospitalised patients and its clinical usefulness in this setting is low.

Spiral CT

Because the results of scintigraphy are inconclusive in most cases, some authors suggest that CT should be the initial imaging modality of choice, especially in patients known to have a high rate of indeterminate scintigrams (for example, all inpatients, patients with radiographic abnormalities, and patients with COPD). If CT is positive for pulmonary embolism, no further examination is necessary. Also, if it is negative down to the subsegmental arteries, it is not necessary to perform another investigation. However, if the CT findings are normal in the presence of a high clinical likelihood of pulmonary embolism, the patient may undergo leg imaging to detect the presence of a DVT. If this test is negative and the clinical likelihood of pulmonary embolism remains high, catheter angiography that focuses on the distal pulmonary vasculature should be performed. It is important to identify small peripheral emboli not detected by CT, because a major embolus may ensue unless anticoagulation is initiated.

Pulmonary angiography

Depending on local capabilities, this may sometimes be the most readily available investigation. It pinpoints the diagnosis in cases of high clinical likelihood of pulmonary embolism despite non-diagnostic findings on lung and leg

Diagnosing pulmonary embolism

- Clinical assessment is the initial step in identifying patients with possible acute pulmonary embolism. However, objective diagnostic tests are necessary to establish or refute the diagnosis

- The presence of risk factors for thromboembolism should always be rigorously scrutinised

- Clinical features of pulmonary embolism are deceivingly non-specific, but pulmonary embolism is highly unlikely in the absence of all of the following: dyspnoea, tachypnoea, and chest pain

- Pulmonary infarction is a relatively rare complication of pulmonary embolism

- Clinical information, ECG, and chest radiography should be used to derive a clinical estimate of prior likelihood of pulmonary embolism before learning the results of imaging studies

imaging. Occasionally, pulmonary angiography is used when the clinical likelihood is low despite the fact that other tests indicate pulmonary embolism. Angiography is also indicated if there are special reasons why the diagnosis must be confirmed beyond doubt (for example, when the risk from anticoagulation is higher than normal or when suspected recurrent emboli have led to frequent admissions to hospital, often in the absence of any firm evidence of venous thromboembolism).

Other combinations of non-invasive tests
Other combinations of non-invasive tests may be useful. For instance, a normal D-dimer and leg imaging can help rule out venous thromboembolism, whereas an echocardiogram showing right ventricular hypokinesis combined with positive leg study is very suspicious of pulmonary embolism.

Finally, if there is no apparent predisposing cause for venous thromboembolism, and particularly if it is recurrent, occurring at a young age (< 50 years) or in an unusual site, or if there is a family history of venous thromboembolism, the patient with pulmonary embolism should be investigated for thrombophilia. If an abnormality is found, consideration should be given to a longer duration of anticoagulation. With limited resources, the testing could be restricted for the activated protein C resistance, because it is the most common cause of thrombophilia; antiphospholipid antibodies, because if present, particularly intensive anticoagulation may be required; and hyperhomocysteinemia, because it can be readily treated with B vitamins. An extensive screening for occult cancer is usually unrewarding and rarely prolongs life in patients with newly diagnosed venous thromboembolism, because in most cases the cancer has already metastasised and the prognosis is ominous. A pragmatic recommendation is to use only simple methods of screening (including abdominal CT and sonography, mammography in women, and the test for prostate specific antigen in men) and to look for cancer in patients with symptoms or signs. An idiopathic thromboembolic event should be regarded as a contraindication to use of an oestrogen containing contraceptive.

1. **Urokinase Pulmonary Embolism Trial Study Group.** Urokinase pulmonary embolism trial: a national cooperative study. *Circulation* 1973;**47**(suppl II):1–108.

2. **Stein PD, Terrin ML, Hales CA**, *et al.* Clinical, laboratory, roentgenographic, and electrocardiographic findings in patients with acute pulmonary embolism and no pre-existing cardiac or pulmonary disease. *Chest* 1991;**100**:598–603.
- *This study compared the clinical characteristics of 117 patients with pulmonary embolism with the characteristics of 248 patients suspected of having pulmonary embolism, but in whom the diagnosis was excluded.*

3. **PIOPED Investigators.** Value of the ventilation/perfusion scan in acute pulmonary embolism. *JAMA* 1990;**263**:2753–9.
- *The importance of clinical likelihood (made without knowledge of the scan results) combined with the V/Q scintigraphy was the crucial aspect of the investigation. A high or low clinical likelihood combined with a matching high or low probability scan made a pulmonary embolism highly likely or unlikely as diagnosed by angiography. Such diagnostic certainty, however, applied to only a minority of patients. Pulmonary embolism was often present in patients with a non-diagnostic scan when associated with a high clinical suspicion of pulmonary embolism.*

4. **Miniati M, Prediletto R, Formichi B**, *et al.* Accuracy of clinical assessment in the diagnosis of pulmonary embolism. *Am J Respir Crit Care Med* 1999;**159**:864–71.
- *An excellent study on 750 patients with suspected pulmonary embolism, aiming at identification of clinical findings that are useful to select patients for further diagnostic testing. Three symptoms (sudden onset of dyspnoea, chest pain, and fainting, singly or in combination), associated with ECG signs of right ventricular overload and/or radiographic signs of oligaemia or infarction, enabled correct clinical classification in 90% of patients; combining this clinical assessment with independent interpretation of lung perfusion scans restricts the need for angiography to a minority of patients with suspected pulmonary embolism.*

5. **Wells PS, Ginsberg JS, Anderson DR**, *et al.* Use of a clinical model for safe management of patients with suspected pulmonary embolism. *Ann Intern Med* 1998;**129**:997–1005.
- *In a prospective study in 1239 patients, a structural clinical model combining the assessment of symptoms and signs, risk factors for venous thromboembolism, and the presence or absence of an alternative diagnosis as likely as pulmonary embolism, was reproducible and predictive of the frequency of objectively established pulmonary embolism.*

6. **Perrier A, Desmarais S, Miron M-J**, *et al.* Non-invasive diagnosis of venous thromboembolism in outpatients. *Lancet* 1999;**353**:190–5.
- *Patients with suspected pulmonary embolism underwent pre-test probability assessment on the basis of risk factors for venous thromboembolism, symptoms and signs, the likelihood of alternative diagnosis, and the results of chest radiography and arterial blood gases, before the performance of objective tests. The pre-test probability assessments were predictive of the frequency of pulmonary embolism. The study also relied on D-dimer to guide management; negative D-dimer excluded pulmonary embolism.*

7. **Worsley DF, Alavi A.** Comprehensive analysis of the results of the PIOPED study. *J Nucl Med* 1995;**36**:2380–7.
- *A clear summary of the much cited PIOPED investigations on 1487 patients.*

8. **Miniati M, Pistolesi M, Marini C**, *et al.* Value of perfusion lung scan in the diagnosis of pulmonary embolism: results of the prospective investigative study of acute pulmonary embolism diagnosis (PISA-PED). *Am J Respir Crit Care Med* 1996;**154**:1387–93.
- *This study on 890 patients demonstrated that clinical assessment combined with perfusion scan evaluation (without the use of ventilation scans) established or excluded pulmonary embolism in the majority of patients. Only wedge shaped perfusion defects were regarded as pulmonary embolism positive.*

9. **Corbus HF, Seitz JP, Larson RK**, *et al.* Diagnostic usefulness of lung SPECT in pulmonary thromboembolism: an outcome study. *Nucl Med Commun* 1997;**18**:897–906.
- *SPECT images of 985 patients with suspected pulmonary embolism provided accurate diagnostic information in 96% of patients and specificity was greatly improved compared to planar imaging.*

10. **Remy-Jardin M, Remy J.** Spiral CT angiography of the pulmonary circulation. *Radiology* 1999;**212**:615–36.

11. Mullins MD, Becker DM, Hagspiel KD, *et al.* The role of spiral volumetric computed tomography in the diagnosis of pulmonary embolism. *Arch Intern Med* 2000;**160**:293–8.
- A critical review of studies comparing CT with pulmonary angiography and/or high probability scan combined with high clinical suspicion for pulmonary embolism.

12. Goodman LR, Lipchik RJ, Kuzo RS, *et al.* Subsequent pulmonary embolism: risk after a negative helical CT pulmonary angiogram—prospective comparison with scintigraphy. *Radiology* 2000;**215**:535–42.
- This prospective outcome study in 198 patients with pulmonary embolism negative spiral CT scans who were not anticoagulated showed subsequent pulmonary embolism in only two patients at three months. This assures us that patients with pulmonary embolism negative CT scans do well without anticoagulation.

13. Greenspan RH. Pulmonary angiography and the diagnosis of pulmonary embolism. *Progr Cardiovasc Dis* 1994;**37**:93–105.

14. Hull RD, Raskob GE, Ginsberg JS, *et al.* A non invasive strategy for the treatment of patients with suspected pulmonary embolism. *Arch Intern Med* 1994;**154**:289–97.
- In the management of patients with non-diagnostic lung scan and without cardiorespiratory disease, serial non-invasive investigation of leg veins offers an effective alternative to angiography.

15. British Thoracic Society, Standards of Care Committee. Suspected acute pulmonary embolism: a practical approach. *Thorax* 1997;**52**(suppl 4):S1–24.
- Comprehensive guidelines with practical algorithms on diagnosis and management.

16. Task Force on Pulmonary Embolism, European Society of Cardiology. Guidelines on diagnosis and management of acute pulmonary embolism. *Eur Heart J* 2000;**21**:1301–36.
- A comprehensive and authoritative "consensus" review with extensive literature references.

234

33 Acute pulmonary embolism 2: treatment

Martin Riedel

Patients with pulmonary embolism are at risk for death, recurrence of embolism or chronic morbidity. Appropriate treatment can reduce the incidence of all. The mortality attributable to pulmonary embolism can be up to 30% in untreated patients, more than 10 times the annual mortality for patients treated with anticoagulant drugs (2.5%). Balanced against the danger of non-treatment are the risks of treatment.

As the primary process leading to pulmonary embolism is deep venous thrombosis (DVT), antithrombotic regimens are the mainstay of treatment. These include drugs that inhibit blood coagulation (heparin, oral anticoagulants, direct thrombin inhibitors), and thrombolytic drugs. Anticoagulation, by preventing clot propagation, allows endogenous fibrinolytic activity to dissolve existing thromboemboli. Anticoagulant treatment is essentially prophylactic, since these agents only interrupt progression of the thrombotic process; unlike thrombolytic agents, they do not actively resolve it. Direct mechanical resolution of the pulmonary vascular obstruction caused by pulmonary embolism can be performed by surgical embolectomy or catheter techniques.

Unfractionated heparin (UFH), low molecular weight heparin (LMWH), direct thrombin inhibitors, and thrombolytic agents in appropriate doses, as well as surgical or catheter embolectomy, are used to treat acute pulmonary embolism. Oral anticoagulants, dextran, physical techniques that counteract venous stasis, inferior vena caval procedures, and lower doses of UFH or LMWH are used for prevention, but these prophylactic regimens are not appropriate for treatment of acute disease.

A general scheme for the treatment of pulmonary embolism is shown in fig 33.1. When there is a suspicion of pulmonary embolism and no strong contraindication to heparin it is wise to start treatment with a bolus of 5000–10000 U while the diagnostic work up is pursued. If subsequent tests rule out the diagnosis then heparin can be stopped. With established diagnosis, the treatment depends on the circulatory state of the patient. With severely impaired circulation—that is, in patients with hypotension or shock—the relief of pulmonary vascular obstruction must be as fast as possible, and in these patients thrombolytic treatment, perhaps combined with mechanical fragmentation of the clot, is indicated. If these measures fail or if thrombolysis is contraindicated, then emergency embolectomy should be undertaken. If thrombolysis is successful, it is followed by heparin and oral anticoagulants. Patients with minor embolism, or even massive embolism but stable circulation, are treated with heparin followed by oral anticoagulants. If recurrent pulmonary embolism occurs during this treatment or if anticoagulation is contraindicated, then venous interruption should be considered.

General supportive measures in acute massive pulmonary embolism

Patients in pain should receive analgesia but opiates should be used with caution in the hypotensive patient. When hypoxaemia is refractory to oxygen supplementation by face mask, intubation and mechanical ventilation may be necessary, but this may cause the haemodynamic situation to deteriorate further by impeding venous return. When the cardiac output is reduced, the dilated right ventricle is hypoxic and already near maximal stimulation from the high concentration of endogenous catecholamines; it is unlikely to respond to inotropic agents, which may do no more than precipitate arrhythmias. When necessary because of a dangerous fall of systemic pressure, the judicious use of noradrenaline (norepinephrine) titrated against a moderate increase in blood pressure might be beneficial in improving right ventricular function and systemic haemodynamics. The right atrial pressure should be maintained at a high level (15 mm Hg) since this filling pressure is necessary for the failing right ventricle to maintain its output; if the right atrial pressure falls for any reason, administration of fluid is helpful. However, fluid loading might be detrimental in case of frank right ventricular distention and high filling pressure, since it may augment ventricular interaction both by increasing pericardial pressure and by shifting the ventricular septum leftwards, thus decreasing left ventricular preload and output. Vasodilators should be avoided at all times; an exception to this rule may in the future be selective pulmonary vasodilatation by inhalation of nitric oxide or prostacyclin.

In the absence of circulatory failure, routine monitoring is sufficient. In patients with shock, at least a central venous line should be inserted to permit repeated measurements of pressure and the administration of drugs. Monitoring with a pulmonary artery catheter is useful in estimating the response to treatment. When thrombolytic treatment is considered, the antecubital route should be preferred and insertion of arterial lines avoided.

Heparin

UFH is the standard treatment after thrombolysis and for all patients who do not have severe circulatory embarrassment. Heparin acts by catalysing the effect of antithrombin III (ATIII), so that this inhibitor efficiently combines with and inactivates a number of serine

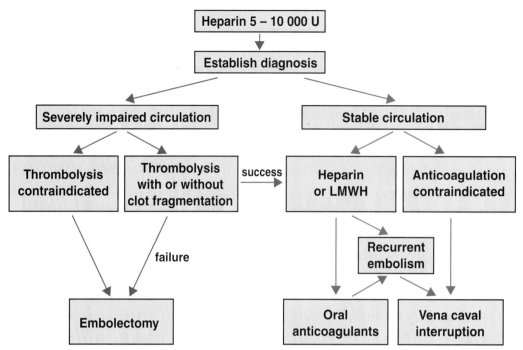

Figure 33.1. A general scheme for the treatment of pulmonary embolism.

proteases, notably thrombin (factor IIa), factor Xa (fXa), and factor IXa. Of these three enzymes, thrombin is the most sensitive to inhibition by heparin-ATIII. In addition, heparin catalyses the inactivation of thrombin by another plasma cofactor, heparin cofactor II, which acts independently of ATIII.[1 2]

Heparin actually constitutes "secondary prevention" of recurrent pulmonary embolism rather than primary treatment. It substantially reduces morbidity and mortality from pulmonary embolism by preventing further fibrin deposition on the thrombus. This stops the formation and growth of thrombi and allows the patient's native fibrinolytic mechanisms to destroy both the emboli that have occurred already and thrombi that are potential further emboli. However, heparin does not directly dissolve thrombus that already exists.

The efficacy of heparin treatment depends on achieving a critical therapeutic concentration of heparin within the first few hours of treatment. Prompt and adequate treatment with UFH, followed by oral anticoagulation for at least three months, results in an 80–90% risk reduction for both recurrent venous thromboembolism and death. UFH also rapidly reduces the mediator induced pulmonary vasoconstriction and bronchoconstriction from thrombin activation and platelet aggregation.

UFH can be given by subcutaneous injection, by continuous infusion or as intermittent boluses four hourly. Haemorrhage is slightly more common with the bolus technique; however, because patients receiving UFH in boluses usually receive greater doses of the drug, it is uncertain whether the difference noted in the rates of bleeding is related to the method of heparin administration or to the difference in the total dose of UFH given. With subcutaneous injection an adequate anticoagulant response is not achieved in the first 24 hours unless a starting dose of at least 17 500 U (or 250 U/kg) every 12 hours is used.[1]

Before initiation of heparin treatment, a screening test for the activated partial thromboplastin time (aPTT), prothrombin time, and platelet count are usually sufficient. The main purpose of the screen is to obtain a pretreatment aPTT from the individual patient as a basis of therapeutic control. The presence of antiphospholipid antibodies can be suspected by a prolongation of the aPTT. It is also important to establish a baseline platelet count should heparin induced thrombocytopenia complicate subsequent treatment. Pretherapeutic screening is particularly desirable in patients with a high risk of bleeding, and those with liver or renal disorders.

Because UFH binds to several plasma, platelet, and endothelial proteins (some of them are acute phase reactants, the concentrations of which are raised in sick patients), its plasma concentrations and anticoagulant response are unpredictable, even with weight based dosing. Therefore, careful control of the level of anticoagulation and dose adjustments for the prevention of complications and for the improvement of therapeutic efficacy are mandatory.

The most commonly used clotting test is the aPTT, which is a global coagulation test (sensitive to the inhibitory effects of heparin on thrombin, fXa, and fIXa). Different reagents and coagulation timers make the aPTT quite variable relative to a given heparin concentration. The current recommendation is to give sufficient UFH to prolong the aPTT to a range that corresponds to a plasma heparin concentration of 0.2–0.4 U/ml by protamine titration. This relation can be established a priori by a simultaneous comparison of aPTT and plasma heparin concentrations in 20–30 patients receiving heparin. Once the therapeutic range for the aPTT is known, monitoring of plasma heparin concentrations is seldom necessary. If the laboratory changes its coagulation timer or uses a different thromboplastin for the aPTT,

Table 33.1   Weight based heparin dosing nomogram

Initial dose	Bolus 80 U/kg, then 18 U/kg/h
aPTT < 35 s (< 1.2 × control)	Bolus 80 U/kg, increase infusion by 4 U/kg/h
aPTT 35–45 s (1.2–1.5 × control)	Bolus 40 U/kg, increase infusion by 2 U/kg/h
aPTT 46–70 s (1.5–2.3 × control)	No change
aPTT 71–90 s (2.3–3 × control)	Decrease infusion rate by 2 U/kg/h
aPTT > 90 s (> 3 × control)	Hold infusion 1 hour, then decrease rate by 3 U/kg/h

aPTT is measured 6 hours after change of dosage, or at least once daily. Data from Raschke *et al.*
Ann Intern Med 1993;**119**:874.

the correlation between aPTT and plasma heparin concentrations should be reestablished.

The aPTT test should be performed 4–6 hours after initiation of the treatment and repeated six hours after any change of dosage, and subsequently at least daily. The aPTT should be maintained at 1.5–2.5 times the patient pretreatment or the laboratory mean control value. Failure to achieve this range is associated with an increased risk of recurrent venous thromboembolism. In contrast, there is only a weak association between supratherapeutic aPTT response and the risk of bleeding. A weight based UFH dosing nomogram is useful in rapidly achieving therapeutic goals while avoiding prolonged periods of excessive anticoagulation (table 33.1). When the bolus method is used, control is difficult because of the wide swings that occur in the plasma heparin concentrations. The best that can be achieved to prevent gross over- or under-anticoagulation is ensuring that there is only a slight prolongation of clotting just before the next dose. If the aPTT is prolonged before UFH is started the possibility of antiphospholipid antibodies should be considered, and in these circumstances the concentration of heparin itself should be assayed. A heparin dose greater than 40 000 U/day should not be administered unless a heparin concentration < 0.2 U/ml is confirmed. True heparin resistance is mainly caused by ATIII deficiency.

The correct duration of heparin treatment for a major pulmonary embolism should be at least a week. Oral anticoagulants are started together with heparin treatment and these should be administered jointly for at least five days; heparin then may be discontinued when the prothrombin time yields an international normalised ratio (INR) above 2.0 on two consecutive days.

Recurrent pulmonary embolism may occur during the first few days of heparin treatment before the clot becomes adherent to the endothelium and does not constitute a therapeutic failure. Many patients who suffer recurrence while receiving heparin will be found to be inadequately anticoagulated as reflected by an aPTT below the therapeutic range. Increasing the dose of heparin should be the initial alteration in treatment in these patients.

Haemorrhagic complications occur in up to 15% of patients on full dose heparin, but are serious in less than 5%. They are most likely if the patient has a potential source of bleeding such as an active peptic ulcer or any of a wide variety of risk factors, the most important of which are a pre-existing bleeding tendency, uraemia, advanced age, recent surgery or trauma, severe hypertension, previous gastrointestinal haemorrhage, and concomitant antiplatelet treatment. Blood transfusion will correct massive blood loss, but protamine in a slow infusion (10–20 minutes) is the specific antidote. One milligram of protamine neutralises about 100 U of UFH, but no more than 50 mg should be given with a single infusion unless a large overdose of heparin is known to have occurred. Heparin treatment is absolutely contraindicated if the patient has had a recent haemorrhagic stroke.

Occasionally, prolonged administration of high dose heparin (over two months at > 15 000 U daily, used mainly in pregnant patients) leads to osteoporosis. The patient receiving long term heparin should be monitored with tests of bone density, and heparin should be discontinued when bone loss is shown to be progressive. No preventive treatment has been proven effective for heparin induced osteopenia, although supplements of calcium and vitamin D are often given. Skin necrosis and hypersensitivity reactions to heparin are rare. Very rarely, continuous heparin infusion over a few days causes aldosterone depression by an unknown mechanism, which may cause clinically important hyperkalaemia in certain patients—for example, those with renal failure or diabetes.

UFH causes transient mild thrombocytopenia in about 10% of patients and severe thrombocytopenia in less than 5%. The milder variety occurs within the first four days of heparin administration and is the result of the direct aggregation effect of UFH on platelets. The platelet count is generally $100–150 × 10^9/l$. The patient is usually asymptomatic and thrombocytopenia resolves spontaneously in spite of continuation of heparin treatment. The severe heparin induced thrombocytopenia occurs five or more days after starting heparin treatment (or sooner with re-exposure to heparin). It is caused by heparin dependent IgG antibodies that activate platelets leading to arterial or venous thrombus formation. It differs from other types of drug induced thrombocytopenia as it gives rise to both arterial or venous thrombosis as well as haemorrhagic complications. The platelet count is below $100 × 10^9/l$ or less than half of the pretreatment value. In established cases, heparin must be stopped, and danaparoid (a heparinoid said to be free of contaminating heparin) or recombinant hirudin (lepirudin) given for temporary anticoagulation. Administering oral anticoagulants in the acute phase of heparin induced thrombocytopenia may actually aggravate the thrombotic tendency, possibly by suppressing protein C synthesis. Adjunctive measures include manoeuvres to salvage ischaemic limbs (thrombectomy or thrombolysis), plasmapheresis, and antiplatelet drugs. Platelet transfusion may worsen the problem and should be avoided. The complications and morbidity related to the heparin induced thrombocytopenia can be prevented if thrombocytopenia is recognised and heparin stopped immediately. It is therefore essential to

> **Heparin in pulmonary embolism**
>
> - The risk of recurrence of thromboembolism is high in patients receiving inadequate initial heparin treatment (aPTT ratio < 1.5)
>
> - The use of a heparin dosing nomogram assures that all patients will achieve the therapeutic range for the aPTT
>
> - Heparin administered by the subcutaneous route cannot be recommended as the initial treatment of pulmonary embolism
>
> - Heparin should be given for at least seven days; oral anticoagulants should overlap with heparin for at least five days. For massive pulmonary embolism, a longer duration of heparin treatment may be considered
>
> - Heparin can be discontinued if the INR > 2.0 for two consecutive days
>
> - Measurement of plasma heparin concentration is useful in patients with baseline elevated aPTT caused by antiphospholipid antibodies and in those requiring large daily doses of heparin (> 40 000 U)

monitor the platelet count in all patients receiving heparin.[1][2]

Low molecular weight heparin

LMWH is progressively replacing standard UFH for treatment of venous thromboembolism. LMWH is obtained by depolymerisation of UFH, yielding molecules of smaller size. Like UFH, LMWH produces its major anticoagulant effect by activating ATIII. A minimum chain length of 18 saccharides is needed for ternary complex formation of heparin, ATIII, and thrombin. Fewer than half of the LMWH molecules of the different commercial preparations contain > 18 saccharide units needed to inhibit thrombin. In contrast, all LMWH chains catalyse the inhibition of fXa. Consequently, LMWHs have ratios of anti-fXa to anti-fIIa that vary between 4:1 and 2:1, depending on their molecular size distribution. Because virtually all molecules of UFH have > 18 saccharide units, UFH has a ratio of anti-fXa to anti-fIIa of 1:1.[1]

Because of reduced binding to plasma proteins, macrophages, platelets, and endothelial cells, the bioavailability of LMWH after subcutaneous injection is better and the half life longer than that of UFH. Therefore, LMWH produces a more predictable anticoagulant response than UFH. The anticoagulant response of a given dose correlates with body weight, so that LMWH may be given in standard doses (anti-fXa U/kg) once or twice daily subcutaneously without laboratory monitoring. Monitoring is usually necessary only in the presence of renal failure or extreme obesity.

Because of its relatively more pronounced anti-fXa effect, LMWH in the therapeutic doses cannot be monitored using the aPTT, which is determined by the antithrombin activity, and anti-fXa assay must be used. For treatment of active venous thromboembolism, the anti-fXa activity should be targeted to the range of 0.4–1.0 U/ml.

The therapeutic index of LMWH (the potential for benefit versus the risk of bleeding) appears to be higher than that of standard UFH. The treatment is cost-effective (despite the higher costs of LMWH) and convenient since it allows early mobilisation and requires less nursing and laboratory supervision. LMWH interacts with platelets and platelet factor 4 less readily and the incidence of heparin induced thrombocytopenia is lower than with standard UFH. The incidence of osteopaenia during long term use also appears to be less than with UFH.

LMWH once or twice daily subcutaneously has been shown to be as effective and safe as standard full dose UFH in the treatment of proximal DVT and acute pulmonary embolism.[3-6] Some unsolved issues remain to be addressed in specific trials before LMWHs can definitively replace UFH in the treatment of all forms of PE. The therapeutic role of LMWH in patients with massive pulmonary embolism who are haemodynamically unstable remains to be determined. Different preparations of LMWH vary with respect to their mean molecular weights, ratios of anti-fXa to anti-fIIa activity, and degree of binding to plasma proteins (table 33.2). Properties associated with one LMWH cannot be extrapolated to a different LMWH. For this reason, the findings of clinical trials apply only to the particular LMWH evaluated and should not be generalised to the LMWH at large.[1][2]

Direct thrombin inhibitors

Clinical evaluation of highly specific, ATIII independent thrombin inhibitors, such as hirudin or hirudin fragments, is just beginning. Hirudin is a progenitor of a family of peptides that directly inhibit thrombin independent of an interaction with ATIII. These peptides, particularly the low molecular weight analogues, more effectively inhibit fibrin deposition in the interstices of a thrombus than does the larger heparin-ATIII complex. They are therefore more effective than heparin in inactivating thrombin bound to fibrin which is a potent stimulus for thrombus growth. Their dose–response curve exhibits linearity over a range greater than that of UFH, and the aPTT test is well suited to monitor their anticoagulant effect. Recombinant hirudin (lepirudin) is available for treatment of heparin induced thrombocytopenia. The half life of lepirudin is relatively short (about 1.3 hours), which is helpful in patients who develop bleeding or who require surgery or invasive procedures. There is no known antidote.

Thrombolytic treatment

Thrombolytic treatment, by actively dissolving the clot, has several potential advantages over anticoagulation in the treatment of patients with pulmonary embolism. By relieving pulmonary artery obstruction, thrombolysis can quickly reduce the load on the right ventricle and reverse right heart failure; consequently, it has the potential to prevent death in the haemodynamically unstable patient who would otherwise not survive the many hours or days required for spontaneous fibrinolysis. Thrombolytic treatment is reserved mainly for patients in whom there is evidence of a severely compromised circulation—for example, hypotension, oliguria or severe hypoxaemia. In patients with pulmonary embolism who also have major proximal DVT, thrombolytic treatment reduces the late morbidity from the thrombosis that often can be considerable. A further potential but unproven advantage of thrombolytic treatment over heparin in such patients is that it may reduce the chance of recurrent embolism by dissolving thrombus before it embolises, and so may reduce the chances of chronic thromboembolic pulmonary hypertension developing at a later date. Although some authorities widen the indication of thrombolysis to patients with pulmonary embolism who have echocardiographic evidence of right ventricular dysfunction, additional information is needed to determine whether right ventricular dysfunction, by itself, is an indication for thrombolysis.

Thrombolytic agents dissolve thrombi by activating plasminogen to plasmin. Plasmin, when in proximity to a thrombus or a haemostatic plug, degrades fibrin to soluble peptides. Circulating plasmin also degrades soluble fibrinogen and, to some extent, factors II, V, and VIII. Moreover, raised concentrations of fibrin and fibrinogen degradation products contribute to the coagulopathy by both inhibiting the conversion of fibrinogen to fibrin and interfering with fibrin polymerisation.

The thrombolytic agents currently in use are streptokinase, urokinase, recombinant tissue plasminogen activator (rt-PA, alteplase), anisoylated plasminogen streptokinase activator complex (APSAC, anistreplase), and reteplase. Streptokinase is a purified bacterial protein; it binds to plasminogen non-covalently to form an activator complex, which converts other plasminogen molecules to plasmin. Streptokinase is antigenic and cannot be readministered for at least six months, as circulating antibodies may both inactivate the drug and produce allergic reactions. Urokinase is isolated from human urine or cultured embryonic renal cells; unlike streptokinase, urokinase is not antigenic and produces a lytic state by directly converting plasminogen to plasmin. rt-PA is produced by recombinant DNA technology; like urokinase, it is non-antigenic and directly converts plasminogen to plasmin, but it is more fibrin specific (that is, it produces less systemic plasminogen activation) than either streptokinase or urokinase. Fibrin specificity is relative, however, and systemic fibrinogenolysis may occur after the administration of rt-PA. Other thrombolytic agents are either not approved or only seldom used for the treatment of pulmonary embolism in most countries. Some new agents (so called second generation thrombolytics), notably mutants of t-PA (tenecteplase, lanoteplase), staphylokinase, and saruplase (prourokinase) are in clinical testing.

With the exception of one small study that is difficult to interpret, none of the trials comparing thrombolytic agents with UFH in pulmonary embolism has been large enough to detect any significant difference in the most important end point—mortality. Consequently, the degree of angiographic or scintigraphic resolution and changes in haemodynamics were used as surrogate measures. Accelerated early resolution of pulmonary embolism as compared with UFH has been proven in all these agents.[7] However, this benefit is short lived and there is no difference after several days. Definite evidence that thrombolytic treatment as opposed to heparin reduces mortality in pulmonary embolism is lacking and it is unlikely to be forthcoming because of the logistic problems involved in mounting such a study. The low mortality at three months (< 10%) of patients treated with UFH and oral anticoagulants has

Table 33.2 Low molecular weight heparins (LMWH)

LMWH	Brand name	Mean molecular weight (daltons)	Ratio of anti-Xa to anti-IIa	Dosage in prophylaxis of VTE (subcutaneously)	Dosage in treatment of VTE (subcutaneously)
Ardeparin	Normiflo	6000	1.9	50 U/kg q12h	130 U/kg q12h
Certoparin	Mono-Embolex	5200		3000 U qd	8000 U q12h
Dalteparin	Fragmin	6000	2.7	2500–5000 U qd	120 U/kg q12h or 200 U/kg qd
Enoxaparin	Lovenox, Clexane	4200	3.8	2000–4000 U qd	100 U/kg q12h
Nadroparin	Fraxiparin	4500	3.6	3100 U qd or 40-60 U/kg qd	< 55 kg: 4000 U q12h 55–80 kg: 6000 U q12h > 80 kg: 8000 U q12h
Reviparin	Clivarin	4000	3.5	1750 U qd	< 60 kg: 4200 U q12h > 60 kg: 6300 U q12h
Tinzaparin	Innohep, Logiparin	6500	1.9	3500 U qd or 50 U/kg qd	175 U/kg qd

VTE, venous thromboembolism; U, international anti-fXa units; qd, every day; q12d, every 12 hours

always precluded the identification of a mortality effect of thrombolytic treatment when a relatively small number of patients were studied. A further factor contributing to the lack of significant reduction of mortality despite impressive early acceleration of thrombus resolution is that patients who survive long enough to be entered into a clinical trial probably make up a group with an improved prognosis, since the most severely affected patients will have died before receiving treatment. Therefore, the numbers of patients required to demonstrate a difference in mortality far exceeds the numbers treated in the centres.

There is only some indirect evidence of better prognosis with thrombolysis. The rate of treatment failure (that is, progression to another form of treatment such as heparin to thrombolysis or thrombolysis to embolectomy) in patients with very severe pulmonary embolism is lower in those treated with thrombolytics than in those who receive UFH. Further indirect evidence comes from a non-randomised study (multicentre registry) of 719 patients without shock, in which 169 patients initially received thrombolytics and 550 were treated with heparin alone. In the group undergoing thrombolysis, mortality at 30 days was significantly lower (4.7% v 11.1%) and recurrent pulmonary embolism significantly less frequent (7.7% v 18.7%) than in the heparin treated group.[8] Therefore, a more rapid resolution of pulmonary embolism seems desirable, because prolonged haemodynamic disturbance can only cause harm, and if further emboli develop their haemodynamic effect will be lessened if previous emboli have been partially removed.

Several trials compared different thrombolytics or different dosages of a given thrombolytic. No clear cut advantage of a given drug or a given dosage has been found. rt-PA produces a faster improvement at 2–4 hours than urokinase, but at 12–24 hours there is no significant difference. All thrombolytics appear to be equally effective and safe when equivalent doses are delivered. It probably matters little which agent is used; it is much more important to ensure that patients receive it quickly.[7]

With experiments showing that rt-PA produces continuing thrombolysis after it is cleared from the circulation, and that thrombolysis is both increased and accelerated, and bleeding reduced when the drug is administered over a short period, interest was awakened in using very high doses over a short interval. The rationale supporting such treatment as opposed to prolonged infusion is that the initially high concentration of the drug overwhelms plasminogen activator inhibitor-1 and renders negligible any attenuating effects of this inhibitor on the drug activity. The higher peak plasma concentration results in a higher concentration of the activator on the surface and inside the thrombi. Further, the bolus is cleared rapidly from the circulation, thus preventing large amounts of degradation products from the lysed emboli interacting with continuously infused plasminogen activator which converts circulating (rather than fibrin bound) plasminogen to plasmin, and in turn, induces the systemic lytic state. However, all studies to date failed to show any significant difference in the early resolution of pulmonary embolism or in bleeding complications. No trial has assessed use of a large bolus dose of streptokinase which, as in the treatment of myocardial infarction, would probably be just as effective and considerably cheaper.[7]

Before initiation of thrombolytic treatment, prothrombin time, aPTT, fibrinogen, and platelets should be measured to make sure that there is no pre-existing coagulation disorder which would complicate thrombolysis. Contraindications include intracranial or intraspinal disease, active internal bleeding, recent major surgery or trauma (within 10 days), and uncontrolled severe hypertension. A blood sample should also be obtained for haemoglobin and for blood typing in case transfusion is required. When streptokinase or APSAC is used, 100 mg hydrocortisone reduces the incidence of side effects. Both agents are not recommended for repeated use or after a recent streptococcal infection.

In contrast to myocardial infarction, thrombolysis in acute massive pulmonary embolism appears effective for up to 10–14 days after the onset of symptoms. Thrombolytics are equally effective when given through a peripheral vein or via a catheter in the pulmonary artery. Generally accepted fixed dosage regimens are given in table 33.3. There is no need to obtain clotting tests during treatment as such tests are of no value in predicting complications or adjusting dosage. After the conclusion of the thrombolytic treatment, measurements of aPTT and fibrinogen are mandatory in order to determine when heparin (without a bolus) should be instituted. If the post-thrombolysis aPTT exceeds twice the upper limit of normal or the fibrinogen concentration is below 1 g/l, these tests should be repeated every four hours until they reach these concentrations, at which point heparin can be started (or resumed) safely. After the patient has been adequately heparinised, oral anticoagulation is initiated; even if the prothrombin time quickly reaches the target range, it should overlap with heparin for at least five days.

The main complication of thrombolytic treatment is bleeding. All thrombolytics are administered in regimens that are designed to activate fibrinolysis systematically throughout the body. None of these agents will distinguish a pathologic thrombus from a beneficial haemostatic plug. Although rt-PA and APSAC are somewhat more fibrin specific than streptokinase and urokinase, all agents have the

Table 33.3 Thrombolytic regimens for massive pulmonary embolism

Streptokinase	250000 to 500000 U as a loading dose over 15 mins, followed by 100 000 U/h for 24 hours
Urokinase	4400 U/kg as a loading dose over 10 min, followed by 4400 U/kg/h for 12 hours
rt-PA	10 mg as a bolus, followed by 90 mg in a continuous infusion over 2 hours
APSAC	30 mg in 5 mins
Reteplase	Two bolus injections of 10 U, 30 mins apart

Before treatment, stop heparin

potential to lyse a fresh platelet–fibrin plug anywhere and cause bleeding at this site. The two major factors which increase bleeding risk are prolonged administration of thrombolytics and the use of procedures which involve vessel puncture.

The reported incidence of haemorrhage has varied greatly. If major haemorrhage is arbitrarily defined as fatal bleeding, intracranial haemorrhage, or bleeding that requires either surgery or transfusion, the average overall incidence of major haemorrhage with pulmonary embolism thrombolysis is about 10%, and is similar among the thrombolytic agents used.

The incidence of cerebral bleeding is about 0.5–1.5 % irrespective of the agent or ancillary treatment used. The elderly, patients with uncontrolled hypertension, and those with recent stroke or craniotomy appear to be at especially high risk for cerebral bleeding. Acute profuse gastrointestinal bleeding is usually the consequence of giving thrombolytics to a patient with unsuspected active peptic ulcer. Late bleeding (2–3 days) may be caused by stress ulceration, particularly in very ill patients; thrombolysis is probably irrelevant but subsequent anticoagulation makes things worse. More common than profuse gastrointestinal bleeding is "coffee ground" vomiting, which is often the result of a combination of thrombolysis and superficial gastric mucosal congestion and erosions, and tends to follow a benign clinical course. Iatrogenic bleeding ranges from trivial to life threatening. Rupture of the heart, liver or spleen during attempted resuscitation may lead to fatal bleeding. Arterial or venous puncture should be avoided if possible. Retroperitoneal bleeding can occur during the femoral vein catheterisation for pulmonary angiography if an artery is inadvertently punctured above the inguinal ligament. Microscopic haematuria is common; macroscopic haematuria is rare and may indicate an unsuspected urinary tract neoplasm.

Bleeding from vascular sites can usually be controlled with manual pressure or compression dressings. Management of severe bleeding from an inaccessible site dictates the reversal of thrombolysis. The basic principles are to stop the administration of the thrombolytic and any concomitant anticoagulation, to inhibit plasmin activity, and to replenish fibrinogen and coagulation factors. There is seldom time for elaborate laboratory tests but a prolonged cutaneous bleeding time is a useful bedside marker of continuing plasmin generation. Plasmin activity is inhibited with intravenous aprotinin, with or without additional tranexamic acid orally. Fibrinogen is replaced with fresh frozen plasma or fibrinogen concentrate, but since both of these contain plasminogen it is prudent to give a plasmin inhibitor first, or at least concurrently. Intracranial bleeding is an emergency, and a neurosurgical consultation must be obtained at the first sign of altered mental status or focal neurologic findings.

The second complication of thrombolytic treatment is an allergic reaction to either streptokinase or APSAC, which are bacterial proteins that regularly induce an antigenic

---

Thrombolysis in pulmonary embolism

- Thrombolysis is indicated in massive pulmonary embolism with right ventricular overload and hypotension

- Thrombolysis is effective up to 10 days after pulmonary embolism

- Laboratory monitoring and dosage adjustments during treatment are not necessary

response in man. Anaphylaxis is very rare (< 0.5%) but flushing, rashes, and fever are relatively common (5–7%). It is unclear whether these are true allergic reactions; they usually respond to hydrocortisone and an antihistamine.

Pulmonary embolectomy

Embolectomy continues to be undertaken in emergency situations when more conservative measures have failed. The only indication for embolectomy is to prevent death. Unfortunately, it is difficult to identify accurately those who will die without embolectomy. Certainly patients in extremis requiring prolonged resuscitation are indicated for embolectomy; there are only very few reports suggesting that such patients may survive with thrombolytic treatment. Patients who deteriorate haemodynamically after the start of thrombolytic treatment, and whose blood pressure remains below 90 mm Hg in spite of vasopressors, would also seem candidates for surgical intervention. Further, there are still patients in whom thrombolytic treatment is contraindicated or too slow in producing benefit. In all these patients, every attempt should be made to confirm the diagnosis of massive pulmonary embolism before surgery, even if it requires partial cardiopulmonary bypass while definitive diagnostic procedures are being performed. Mortality of patients referred for embolectomy with an incorrect diagnosis approaches 100%.

Statistics regarding mortality following embolectomy are difficult to compare. Data are largely derived from retrospective reviews of historical series, often predating the advent of thrombolysis. In some series, considerable numbers of patients have been operated on more than 24 hours after embolism, questioning the need for the procedure. The results depend greatly on the indications used and the haemodynamic impairment of the patients. Mortality will be high in those patients most in need of embolectomy, and low in patients who would survive without it. Until 1985, the overall mortality was 51% for those done without, and 40% for those done with cardiopulmonary bypass. These results have been improved in recent years, mainly due to routine administration of vasopressors before the induction of anaesthesia and to the use of partial (femoro-femoral) bypass in moribund patients as a means of maintaining the circulation while the patient and the equipment are prepared to get on to full bypass.[7] There has been no randomised trial of embolectomy versus thrombolytic treatment and it is unlikely that one of value will ever be performed because of the relative scarcity of these patients.

The main predictor of operative death is cardiac arrest with the need of resuscitation before the operation. Provided the patients reach the operating room without requiring external cardiac massage the mortality is in the range of 0–33%, but it is between 43–84% in those resuscitated. Postoperative complications include acute respiratory distress syndrome (ARDS), mediastinitis, acute renal failure and, of particular concern, severe neurologic sequelae. Late morbidity of patients successfully operated upon is principally neurological in nature; late mortality is low.[7]

Catheter transvenous embolectomy

An alternative technique in patients with massive pulmonary embolism who still can sustain a blood pressure with vasopressor support is catheter embolectomy employing a large steerable catheter with a suction cup on its end, inserted via cutdown in the femoral or jugular vein. Syringe suction captures the embolus in the cup and holds it there while the catheter and the embolus are withdrawn. However, this procedure is rarely undertaken. The results of the only two studies published show that embolus extraction is achieved in about two thirds of the patients, and the mortality in these studies was about 30%.[7]

An alternative manoeuvre of attempting to fragment the embolus is certainly much easier. If angiography shows massive emboli in the main pulmonary arteries it may be possible to break these up, using a pigtail catheter and a guide wire or an angiographic basket. The rationale is that the cross sectional area of the pulmonary vascular bed increases progressively from proximal to distal. Thus the fragmented clot obstructs a smaller percentage of the whole cross sectional area of the pulmonary vascular bed when displaced distally. The pulmonary vascular resistance will thus decrease and the pulmonary blood flow increase. A further advantage of this mechanical disruption of emboli would be enhanced clot exposure to lytic treatment by creation of multiple channels within the emboli.

A number of rotational devices for percutaneous mechanical thrombolysis has been experimentally evaluated; they work by high speed clot fragmentation and aspiration. Embolectomy can also be accomplished with the use of a catheter that delivers high velocity jets of saline that draw the clot toward the catheter tip and subsequently pulverise it. None of these devices has been extensively used in patients to date.

Oral anticoagulants

Oral anticoagulants act in the liver by inhibiting the synthesis of four vitamin K dependent coagulant proteins (factors II, VII, IX, and X), and at least two vitamin K dependent anticoagulant factors, proteins C and S. They do not act immediately because time is required for coagulation factors already present in the plasma to be cleared. It is therefore essential to overlap oral anticoagulants with heparin for at least five days, even if the prothrombin time reaches the target range sooner (the level of protein C declines quickly after initiation of oral anticoagulants, creating a thrombogenic potential).

The prothrombin time, used to adjust the dose of oral anticoagulation, should be reported according to the INR, not the prothrombin time ratio or the prothrombin time expressed in seconds. The INR is essentially a "corrected" prothrombin time that adjusts for the many different assays used. Effective treatment of venous thromboembolism is reflected by an INR of 2.0–3.0. Every effort should be made to maintain the patient in this range. This is facilitated by always aiming for an INR level that is in the mid-level of the INR range (that is, 2.5). Patients with the antiphospholipid syndrome may require a higher INR (2.5–3.5). In some settings, home monitoring of INR is convenient and cost-effective, and may ultimately improve anticoagulation control.

The duration of oral anticoagulation must be tailored to the individual patient. One should balance the risk of bleeding against the risk of recurrence when treatment is discontinued. The later risk includes not only the likelihood of recurrence but also its potential clinical effect; patients with cardiopulmonary disease might tolerate recurrent pulmonary embolism poorly. For most patients, provided there is no persisting risk factor, six months' treatment is indicated. In patients whose risk factors can be interrupted—for example, transient immobilisation or oestrogen use—treatment may be shorter, but additional clinical trials to test this are needed. Certain groups may require longer or indefinite treatment, including patients with active tumours, thrombophilic disorders, those with proven recurrence of venous thromboembolism, and patients who have chronic thromboembolic pulmonary hypertension. The single best predictor of an increased risk for venous thromboembolism is a prior episode. Patients who have had one episode are at high risk to have another, whether or not they have a defined thrombophilic state.[9]

The risk of haemorrhage is always present and with long term treatment the cumulative risk of serious bleeding is not inconsiderable (6–22 per 1000 patient months). The major determinants of oral anticoagulant induced bleeding are the intensity of the anticoagulant effect, the length of treatment, the patient's underlying clinical disorder (past gastrointestinal bleeding, hypertension, cerebrovascular disease, renal insufficiency), advanced

Oral anticoagulants after pulmonary embolism

- Treatment with oral anticoagulants can be started together with UFH or LMWH

- Patients with reversible or time limited risk factors should be treated for 3–6 months with a INR target range of 2.0–3.0

- Patients with a first episode of idiopathic venous thromboembolism should be treated for at least six months

- Patients with recurrent venous thromboembolism, active cancer, antiphospholipid syndrome, inhibitor deficiency states, or homozygous factor V Leiden should probably be treated indefinitely

- When oral anticoagulation is either contraindicated (pregnancy) or inconvenient, an adjusted dose of LMWH or UFH to prolong the aPTT to a time corresponding to a therapeutic plasma heparin concentration can be used

age, and the concomitant use of drugs that interfere with haemostasis, above all aspirin. The risk of bleeding increases dramatically with an INR > 4.0. Increased variation in anticoagulant effect, as indicated by variation in the INR, is associated with an increased frequency of haemorrhage independent of the mean INR. If the patient has serious bleeding, the INR should be reduced to 1.0 as soon as possible. Reduction or reversal of the anticoagulant effect can be achieved by stopping treatment (effective after about two days), by administering 1–5 mg of vitamin K_1 orally or in slow infusion (effective within 24 hours), or immediately by replacement of vitamin K dependent coagulation factors with fresh frozen plasma or clotting factor concentrates.

Other side effects are rare (for example, skin necrosis) but the wide range of interactions with other drugs should never be forgotten. Although some drugs are more likely to interact with oral anticoagulants than others, clinicians should increase the frequency of INR monitoring when initiating, discontinuing, or altering the dose of any drug in patients receiving oral anticoagulants. The most frequent problems occur with broad spectrum antibiotics, most of which can lead to sudden over-anticoagulation by killing the natural gut flora which are an important source of vitamin K. Subjects receiving oral anticoagulants are sensitive to fluctuating concentrations of dietary vitamin K, which is obtained predominantly from plant material. Oral anticoagulants must not be used in the first trimester of pregnancy and if possible should be avoided throughout pregnancy.[9]

At discharge from hospital, the patient should be aware of side effects of anticoagulants and interactions with other drugs, and should have written information about the treatment, as well as an appointment for anticoagulant supervision.

Venous interruption

Venous interruption procedures are designed to prevent emboli from reaching the lungs. They have no effect on the thrombotic process and do not prevent DVT. In the past the main methods were ligation, plication or the application of clips to the outside of the inferior vena cava. These procedures carried an appreciable mortality and morbidity, of which lower limb swelling after ligation was the worst. Nowadays the method of choice is the pervenous placement of a filter in the inferior vena cava under fluoroscopic guidance.

There is no evidence that the filters have any advantages over anticoagulation for prophylaxis following an acute pulmonary embolism because the incidence of recurrence with anticoagulation alone is so low. Their place is in the rare case in which intensive and prolonged anticoagulation alone fails or adequate anticoagulation cannot be achieved because of strong contraindications (for example, serious multiple injuries, or during and after surgery). Although caval filtration is probably effective in these indications, there is a remarkable lack of controlled studies to support the use of this procedure.[10 11]

Devices placed in the inferior vena cava may perforate the vessel wall or migrate within and outside the venous system. Thrombosis occurs frequently at the venous access site. Pulmonary emboli, either passing through or around the therapeutic obstruction or originating proximally, have been reported with all these measures. Other late sequelae include caval thrombosis, filter fractures, and leg oedema. Because of the lack of controlled data regarding eventual outcome and the true incidence of complications, if a permanent filter is used long term clinical follow up is appropriate.

Treatment of pulmonary embolism in pregnancy

The management of venous thromboembolism during pregnancy remains controversial because of the lack of prospective trials. Heparin does not cross the placenta, and therefore does not have the potential to cause fetal bleeding or teratogenicity, although bleeding at the uteroplacental junction is possible. Oral anticoagulants cross the placenta and may cause fetal developmental abnormalities, fetal bleeding, spontaneous abortions, and stillbirth. Therefore, oral anticoagulants must not be administered in the first trimester of pregnancy (and preferably throughout the entire pregnancy), and all women of childbearing potential taking oral anticoagulants must avoid becoming pregnant.

Pregnant women with pulmonary embolism are best treated initially with continuous intravenous UFH or weight adjusted dose of

244

subcutaneous LMWH, and then taught to self administer LMWH once daily for the remainder of pregnancy until the onset of labour and further on in the puerperium. If possible, measurement of anti-fXa concentrations approximately four hours after injection and adjustment to a concentration of approximately 0.5–1.2 U/ml should be performed. A high index of suspicion for the development of osteopenia and a two weekly assessment of the platelet count is important. Heparin should be discontinued 24 hours before elective induction of labour. If spontaneous labour occurs in women receiving adjusted dose heparin, careful monitoring of the aPTT is required and, if it is prolonged near delivery, protamine may be required to reduce the risk of bleeding.[10] [11]

Another acceptable approach is to give oral anticoagulants between the 13th and 36th week of gestation, and switch to heparin during the last two weeks of pregnancy. If the mother is admitted in premature labour while still on oral anticoagulants she should be given fresh frozen plasma. Treatment with oral anticoagulants can be resumed immediately after delivery, and continued for at least six weeks postpartum. Their effect on the baby persists for 7–14 days after they are stopped and therefore the baby should be given vitamin K at the time of delivery. Breast feeding is not contraindicated.

Current evidence suggests that thrombolysis is appropriate treatment for massive pulmonary embolism during pregnancy, but not within six hours of delivery or in the early postpartum period because of the high risk of bleeding complications.

The future

A widespread use of LMWHs for the treatment of acute pulmonary embolism is certain. Cost savings should prove substantial and will be directly proportional to the number of hospital days avoided. It is likely that heparinoids and specific thrombin inhibitors will replace UFH or LMWH for some indications, provided that their costs are not prohibitive. Decreased bleeding and less thromboembolic recurrence may also result as we gain experience with these new agents. It is also possible that synthetic thrombin inhibitors will be developed for oral use; this would open up the possibility for long term use. Optimal duration of anticoagulant treatment in different subgroups of patients with venous thromboembolism have yet to be determined. The risk:benefit ratio of the treatment of small subsegmental pulmonary embolism without residual DVT in the absence of persisting risk factors should be tested. Inhalation of nitric oxide or prostacyclin might prove to be a useful adjunct in the treatment of acute massive pulmonary embolism.

1. **Hirsh J, Warkentin TE, Raschke R,** et al. Heparin and low-molecular-weight heparin. Mechanisms of action, pharmacokinetics, dosing considerations, monitoring, efficacy, and safety. Chest 1998;**114**:489S–510S.
• Recommendations of the ACCP consensus conference on antithrombotic treatment.

2. **Hyers TM, Agnelli G, Hull RD,** et al. Antithrombotic therapy for venous thromboembolic disease. Chest 1998;**114**:561S–78S.
• Further recommendations of the ACCP consensus conference on antithrombotic treatment.

3. **Théry C, Simonneau G, Meyer G,** et al. Randomized trial of subcutaneous low-molecular-weight heparin CY 216 (fraxiparine) compared with intravenous unfractionated heparin in the curative treatment of submassive pulmonary embolism. A dose-ranging study. Circulation 1992;**85**:1380–9.
• The first study showing that LMWH (nadroparin) is as effective and safe as UFH in the treatment of submassive pulmonary embolism.

4. **The Columbus Investigators.** Low-molecular-weight heparin in the treatment of patients with venous thromboembolism. N Engl J Med 1997;**337**:657–62.
• In this randomised trial on 1021 patients, fixed dose subcutaneous reviparin given twice daily was as effective and safe as dose adjusted intravenous UFH for the initial management of venous thromboembolism, regardless of whether the patient had pulmonary embolism or a history of venous thromboembolism.

5. **Simonneau G, Sors H, Charbonnier B,** et al. A comparison of low-molecular-weight heparin with unfractionated heparin for acute pulmonary embolism. N Engl J Med 1997;**337**:663–9.
• In a randomised study involving 612 patients with acute pulmonary embolism, initial subcutaneous treatment with tinzaparin in a dose of 175 U/kg once daily was as effective and safe as dose adjusted intravenous UFH.

6. **Hull RD, Raskob GE, Brant RF,** et al. Low-molecular-weight heparin vs heparin in the treatment of patients with pulmonary embolism. Arch Intern Med 2000;**160**:229–36.
• In this double blind randomized trial on 200 patients, tinzaparin given in a dose of 175 U/kg once daily subcutaneously was probably more effective than dose adjusted intravenous UFH for preventing recurrent venous thromboembolism in patients with pulmonary embolism associated with proximal DVT.

7. **Riedel M.** Therapy of pulmonary thromboembolism. Part I: acute massive pulmonary embolism. Cor Vasa 1996;**38**:93–102.
• An analysis and review of all reports on pulmonary embolectomy and of all randomised trials of thrombolysis in pulmonary embolism.

8. **Konstantinides S, Geibel A, Olschewski M,** et al. Association between thrombolytic treatment and the prognosis of hemodynamically stable patients with major pulmonary embolism. Results of a multicentre registry. Circulation 1997;**96**:882–8.
• This study demonstrates a survival advantage and reduced risk of recurrence with thrombolytic treatment in patients with pulmonary embolism but without shock. Because of its non-randomised design and selection bias, however, this study has several important limitations.

9. **Hirsh J, Dalen JE, Anderson DR,** et al. Oral anticoagulants. Mechanism of action, clinical effectiveness, and optimal therapeutic range. Chest 1998;**114**:445S–69S.
• Recommendations of the ACCP consensus conference on antithrombotic treatment.

10. **British Thoracic Society, Standards of Care Committee.** Suspected acute pulmonary embolism: a practical approach. Thorax 1997;**52**(suppl 4):S1–24.
• Comprehensive guidelines with practical algorithms on diagnosis and management.

11. **Task Force on Pulmonary Embolism, European Society of Cardiology.** Guidelines on diagnosis and management of acute pulmonary embolism. Eur Heart J 2000;**21**:1301–6.
• A comprehensive and authoritative "consensus" review with extensive literature references.

Abbreviations
APSAC: anisoylated plasminogen streptokinase activator complex (anistreplase)
ATIII: antithrombin III
aPTT: activated partial thromboplastin time
DVT: deep venous thrombosis
fIIa: activated factor II (thrombin)
fXa: activated factor X
INR: international normalised ratio
LMWH: low molecular weight heparin
rt-PA: alteplase
UFH: unfractionated heparin

34 Anatomic basis of cross-sectional echocardiography

Robert H Anderson, Siew Yen Ho, Stephen J Brecker

There can be little doubt that the cross-sectional echocardiographer will be tomorrow's anatomist. The level of discrimination of modern day echocardiographic machines is such that all but the finest details of cardiac structure are revealed in real time. Advances in three dimensional reconstruction now amplify the information obtained, and make it more amenable to clinical interpretations. It remains true, nonetheless, that the information available to the echocardiographer will be more accurately interpreted if the investigator has a good working knowledge of cardiac anatomy. This is not difficult to obtain. The basic rules and principles are exactly as we set them out in 1983.[1] As with any three dimensional structure, so as to determine the interrelationships of the cardiac components, it is necessary to obtain details as seen in the three orthogonal planes. These planes, at right angles to each other, are the equivalent of the floor plan, the frontal elevation, and the side elevation of any building. When considering the heart, however, the information obtained must be interpreted taking account of the fact that the orthogonal planes of the heart itself are very malaligned relative to the orthogonal planes of the body. The steps involved in gaining the basic knowledge, therefore, are to begin by reviewing the orthogonal planes of the body. It is then essential to understand the usual position of the heart within the body, along with the orientation of its own orthogonal planes. Thereafter, it is necessary to understand the usual positions of the cardiac chambers and valves within the cardiac silhouette. The basic anatomic information must then, self-evidently, be understood in sectional format. There are, of course, no standard sections which will always deliver the necessary information, since no two individuals have exactly identical relations of the cardiac components. So, it is not always possible to reveal cardiac structure using "standard" echocardiographic windows. The skilled echocardiographer will use any section, obtained from any echocardiographic window, to delineate the desired findings. It helps, nonetheless, to illustrate certain typical sections. The focus, however, should not be on obtaining the given section, but rather on demonstrating the required anatomy.

Anatomic position

Structures within any part of the body are traditionally described on the basis that the

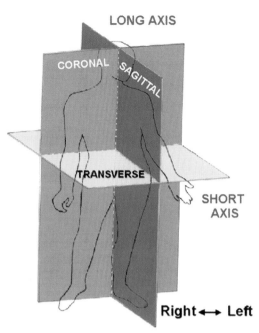

Figure 34.1. The so-called "anatomical position". The subject is upright and facing the observer. Any structure within the body can be described within the references of the three orthogonal planes—two in the long axis and the third in the short axis.

subject is standing upright and facing the observer (fig 34.1). Within the body as thus seen, there are three basic orthogonal planes. Two are in the long axis of the body. One of these cuts the body from right to left, and produces sections in the frontal, or coronal, plane. The second plane along the long axis cuts from the front, or anterior, to the back, or posterior. This is the sagittal plane. These are, of course, any number of frontal and sagittal planes, each at right angles to the other. There are then infinite intermediate planes in the long axis, but no single one is at right angles, and hence also orthogonal. Instead, the third series of orthogonal planes is in the short axis. This series extends from the head, or superiorly, to the feet, or inferiorly. Any number of intermediate planes are similarly to be found between each of the short axis and the long axis planes, but none of these is orthogonal. It is knowledge of the three basic orthogonal planes which is sufficient to build up the three dimensional configuration of the body.[2]

Location of the heart

The heart lies in the middle mediastinal compartment of the thorax, enclosed within its pericardial sack, and sandwiched between the two pleural cavities. When projected to the frontal projection, the cardiac silhouette is trapezoidal, with two thirds of its bulk to the left and one third to the right of the midline (fig 34.2). The right side of the trapezoid is more-or-less straight, and is positioned just to the right of the sternum. The left side is pointed, and extends out to the apex, which is located in the left mid-clavicular line in the normal individual. The short upper, and long lower, borders are both horizontal. The lower border

Long axis of body

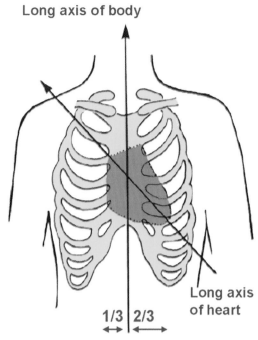

1/3 | **2/3**

Long axis of heart

Figure 34.2. The heart lies in the mediastinum with its own long axis tilted relative to the long axis of the body. Appreciation of this discrepancy is important in the setting of cross-sectional echocardiography.

lies on the diaphragm, while the upper border is at the sternal angle.

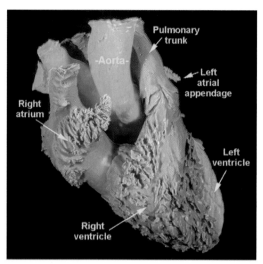

Figure 34.3. The heart has been prepared by making casts of its "right" and "left" sides, shown in blue and red, respectively. When viewed from the front, it can be seen that the so-called "right heart" chambers are really anterior to the "left" sided counterparts.

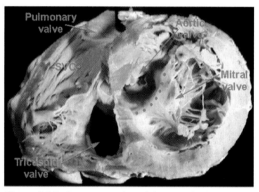

Figure 34.4. A cross-section of the ventricular mass is shown as viewed in left anterior oblique orientation. The right ventricle is anterior to the circular left ventricle, to the left hand as viewed in the section. Note the fibrous continuity of the valvar leaflets in the roof of the left ventricle (dotted line), in contrast to the situation in the right ventricle where the supraventricular crest (SVC) separates the leaflets of the tricuspid and pulmonary valves.

Arrangement of the cardiac chambers and valves

The biggest problem to be overcome in understanding cardiac anatomy is to appreciate that the adjectives "right" and "left" are used inappropriately when describing the cardiac chambers. In reality, the so-called "right" chambers are more-or-less anterior to their purported left sided counterparts, while the atria are essentially to the right of their respective ventricles. Thus, in the frontal silhouette, it is the right atrium and right ventricle which occupy most of the cardiac surface (fig 34.3). Viewing the heart from its apex, corresponding to the left anterior oblique angiographic projection (fig 34.4), then reveals the crucial interrelation of the cardiac valves. The pulmonary trunk is the most superior valve, with the leaflets supported on the free standing muscular infundibulum. The tricuspid valve is the most anterior valve, but is also the most inferior. The aortic valve forms the centrepiece of the heart, and is located directly in front of, and just above, the mitral valve.[3] The leaflets of the aortic and mitral valves are in fibrous continuity, a feature of crucial importance in understanding the complications of endocarditis of the aortic root. Via the substance of the membranous part of the septum, the aortic valvar leaflets are also in continuity with those of the tricuspid valve. When seen in the frontal silhouette, only a thin strip of left ventricle projects to the cardiac margin, and only the appendage of the left atrium is visible. This is important information for the echocardiographer, since it means that, if approached anteriorly, it is necessary to

traverse the cavities of the right atrium or ventricle before it becomes possible to interrogate the left sided structures.

The echocardiographic windows

Access to the heart is limited because the sound beam emitted by the echocardiographic transducer does not readily pass through either bone or the pulmonary parenchyma. There are, therefore, strictly limited windows through which the heart can be interrogated transthoracically. Two of these windows permit the heart to be cut along its own long or short axes. From each window, the heart can be cut in only two of the orthogonal planes, albeit that multiple intermediate planes can be obtained. Once again, nonetheless, it is knowledge of the images obtained in the orthogonal planes which provides the key to understanding. The parasternal windows, usually obtained from the third or fourth interspaces, permit the heart to be cut from front to back, and also in short axis. Traditionally, the slices from front to back are orientated as they would be seen in lateral projection, with the cardiac apex pointing to the left hand of the observer (fig 34.5). The short axis slices are orientated as they would be seen from inferiorly (fig 34.6). The long axis slice from front to back can also be obtained from

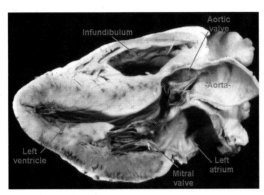

Figure 34.5. The heart has been sectioned to simulate the parasternal long axis plane. This is shown with the cardiac apex to the left hand of the observer. The anterior surface is to the top of the panel.

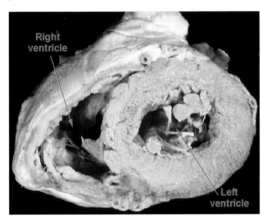

Figure 34.6. This is a short axis cut across the middle of the ventricular mass—compare with the section shown in fig 4.

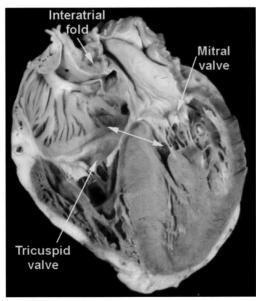

Figure 34.7. This section, taken to replicate the so-called "four chamber cut", is orientated in attitudinally correct position. It makes little sense to show this slice in upside down orientation. Note the off-setting of the septal hinges of the tricuspid and mitral valves (yellow double headed arrow). Note also the superior interatrial fold (shown again in fig 9).

the cardiac apex, but the apical window provides the crucial slice in which the heart is cut from side to side, giving the so-called four chamber section (fig 34.7). In fact, because of the deeply wedged location of the aortic root, most sections obtained from the cardiac apex which slice the heart from right to left also cut through the aorta, giving the so-called "five chamber" cut (fig 34.8). These cuts show well the arrangement of the septal components, particularly the membranous septum, which forms an integral part of the aortic root. For traditional reasons, it is customary for echocardiographers dealing with adult subjects to display these "four chamber" sections as though the patients are standing on their head. There seems no logical reason to continue this practice, other than familiarity, since echocardiographic machines permit the operator to produce the images in whatever orientation is desired. Correlations with other imaging modalities, and with anatomy itself, are surely facilitated if the images are shown in attitudinally appropriate fashion.

The other echocardiographic windows permit the heart to be cut in the orthogonal planes of the body. Thus, from subcostal position the heart can be sliced in paracoronal and parasagittal fashion. Similar slices, and intermediate planes, can be obtained from the suprasternal notch. Information obtained from these windows supplements that obtained using the parasternal and apical windows, and is particularly valuable for the echocardiographer examining neonates and infants with congenitally malformed hearts. The basic knowledge concerning the overall cardiac structure, nonetheless, is usually obtained from the classical windows. Using these limited points, it is usually possible to obtain information concerning not only the dimensions and structure of the chambers and

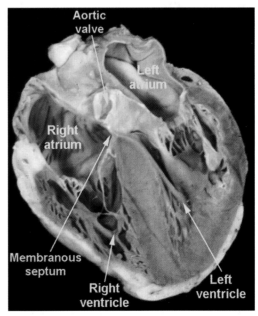

Figure 34.8. This four chamber section comes from the same heart as the one shown in fig 7, but is cut more anteriorly. It shows how the subaortic outflow tract is interposed between the leaflets of the mitral valve and the septum, with the so-called membranous septum forming an integral part of the aortic root, separating the outflow tract from the right-sided chambers.

248

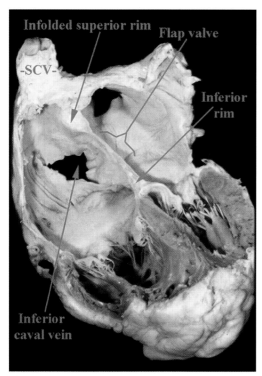

Figure 34.9. When studied with prior knowledge, the echocardiographer should be in a position to demonstrate all the features shown in this angled four chamber section. Thus, it should be possible to confirm that the so-called "septum secundum" is no more than a deep infolding between the venous attachments to the right and left atria. The true atrial septum is the flap valve, anchored on the muscular inferior rim.

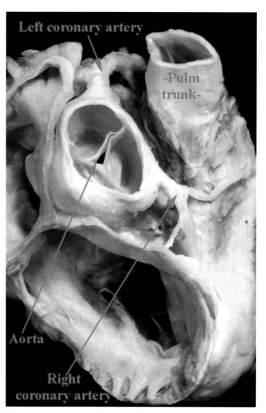

Figure 34.10. With modern day equipment, particularly when combined with Doppler interrogation, it should be possible to show all the details of coronary arterial origin from the aortic root, illustrated here in the right posterior oblique projection.

valves, along with the outflow tracts and the arterial trunks, but also the origins and patency of the proximal coronary arteries. By combining cross-sectional examination with Doppler interrogation, it is also possible to reveal the patterns of the flow of blood throughout the heart. With the advent of harmonic and contrast imaging, the patterns of contraction of the ventricles can be determined, permitting recognition of subtle abnormalities of wall motion.

The clinical echocardiographer must be versatile and opportunist. Not all views will be optimal, or even obtainable, in all patients. In most patients, nonetheless, all the necessary information can be obtained. The parasternal long axis views are particularly useful for displaying the left atrium, the mitral valve, the inflow and outflow tracts of the left ventricle, and the aortic valve. The apex of the left ventricle is often amputated in the parasternal long axis cut, but is well shown by an apical "two chamber" view. This latter view should always be interrogated in patients with poor parasternal windows. The parasternal short axis views show to best effect any abnormalities of ventricular wall motion, and are invaluable in determining overall ventricular function. The central location, and precise anatomy, of the aortic valve is best appreciated from this approach. The apical four chamber view is the "cardiologist's friend". It is the view most readily interpreted without much knowledge of cardiac anatomy! The information would be the more amenable if the images were orientated in attitudinal fashion. This view is essential for the Doppler assessment of flow across

the aortic and mitral valves. When combined with harmonic and contrast imaging, it is used for identification of abnormalities of wall motion during stress echo.

Echocardiography, without doubt, is an immensely and increasingly powerful tool. To take full advantage, it helps if the investigator is fully conversant with the detailed structure of the heart, particularly such features as the precise arrangement of the atrial septum (fig 34.9), the origin and proximal course of the coronary arteries (fig 34.10), and the structure of the aortic root.[3] Detailed descriptions of these features are beyond the scope of this brief review, but the structure of the atrial septum will be addressed in a subsequent article in this series of anatomic reviews. The simple rules as set out here, nonetheless, should provide the information needed to display the echocardiographic manifestations of clinically significant cardiac structure.

Professor Anderson is supported by the Joseph Levy Foundation and he and Dr Ho are supported by the British Heart Foundation.

1. **Silverman NH, Hunter S, Anderson RH,** *et al.* Anatomical basis of cross-sectional echocardiography. *Br Heart J* 1983;**50**:421–31.
• *This review, now nearly 20 years old, sets out the philosophy summarised in the current article. Nothing has changed in the meantime, except that the echocardiographic machines are now much more powerful, and demonstrate the anatomy in even greater detail.*

2. **Cosio FC, Anderson RH, Kuck K,** *et al.* Living anatomy of the atrioventricular junctions. A guide to electrophysiological mapping. A consensus statement from the Cardiac Nomenclature Study Group, Working Group of Arrhythmias, European Society of Cardiology, and the Task Force on Cardiac Nomenclature from NASPE. *Circulation* 1999;**100**:e31–7; *Eur Heart J* 1999;**20**:1068–75; *J Cardiovasc Electrophysiol* 1999;**10**;1162–70.

- *This article sets out the obvious, but highlights a problem that we had ignored even though, for many years, we had professed to illustrate the heart as seen by the clinician. We had failed to observe that the terms used to describe the heart reflects its position as standing on its apex, rather than its true position within the thorax. This means that there is, in general, a deficiency of almost a right angle in current descriptions. Those structures presently said to be "anterior" are, in reality, superior, and so on. The article emphasises the deficiencies of the current* approach for the electrophysiologist, but they are equally applicable to description of the coronary arteries.

3. **Anderson RH.** Clinical anatomy of the aortic root. *Heart* 2000;**84**:670–3.
- *This review was the forerunner to this article in our contributions to "Education in Heart". We discussed the structure of the aortic root, emphasising clinical features, and pointing to problems in defining the enigmatic "annulus".*

SECTION IX: HYPERTENSION

35 Matching the right drug to the right patient in essential hypertension

Morris J Brown

In most hospitals, it is cardiologists to whom patients with difficult hypertension are referred. Although these patients may appear a distraction from the sicker patients in cardiac clinics, cardiologists will recognise hypertension as the most common cause of strokes, the most common reversible cause of cardiac failure, and more important than hypercholesterolaemia as a preventable cause of ischaemic heart disease in diabetes.[1] The purpose of this review is to let cardiologists reap some of the fruits of the last two years in the hypertension world, where we now have more answers than questions about the objectives of treatment and how to achieve these, and (with a little didactic licence) we can relate treatment choices to a logical understanding of hypertension itself.

Absolute versus relative risks of hypertension: indications for treatment

Paradoxically, one gulf in our knowledge that remains is that separating our extensive knowledge that hypertension is a major risk factor for stroke and ischaemic heart disease, from an understanding of why hypertension causes these conditions. So unimpressive was the evidence for prevention of ischaemic heart disease in early outcome trials of drugs in hypertension that the question became not *why* but *if* hypertension causes ischaemic heart disease. If treating X fails to prevent Y, maybe X is not a cause of Y after all. This argument has now proven flawed, the fallacy being a confusion between the absolute and relative risks of hypertension. This subtle but vital point is illustrated in fig 35.1. More patients with hypertension succumb to a myocardial infarction than stroke. But this is simply because myocardial infarction is almost twice as common as stroke in the population at large, and it is only the increased risk from hypertension—the slope of the curves in the graph—which is amenable to antihypertensive treatment.[2 3] The distinction between absolute and relative risk, illustrated in fig 35.1, has also become central to recent guidelines for the treatment of hypertension.[4] Patients' absolute risk—the y axis in fig 35.1—depends not only on blood pressure but also on their other risk factors (age, sex, lipids, diabetes), and its calculation is used to postpone the need for treatment in the majority of patients with borderline hypertension (< 160/100 mm Hg). The full British Hypertension Society (BHS) criteria are shown in fig 35.2.[4] As well as the

emphasis on absolute risk in treatment decisions, there should be increasing emphasis in older patients on systolic pressure: more doctors would be inclined to treat patients with a blood pressure of 150/95 mm Hg than 150/85 mm Hg, although the latter carries a higher risk.[5]

However, the emphasis on absolute rather than relative risk has a down side. If one compares a 35 year old and 75 year old man with a blood pressure 150/95 mm Hg, there is an age paradox.[6] The 75 year old has protection factors to have made it beyond his 70 years, but is at high absolute risk of an event in the next decade. The 35 year old is at low risk of an event within the same period, but at high risk compared to his normotensive peer of failing to reach his 70th birthday. For similar reasons, terms like mild, moderate or severe hypertension are misleading in isolation.[1] The 35 year old has severe hypertension for his age, meaning that he will become the resistant hypertensive of tomorrow, and for this reason should be treated now.

Long term benefits of treatment

The contribution of risk factors other than hypertension itself to absolute risk has long raised the possibility that antihypertensive drugs might vary in their long term efficacy, depending on ancillary actions (for example, desirable or undesired metabolic effects). However, recent outcome trials in hypertensive patients have now shown clearly that there is no difference in the primary composite outcome of stroke and major coronary events between any two classes.[7–11] A rigorous meta-analysis of these, undertaken by the World Health Organization and International Society of Hypertension, confirms this. It also shows that possible differences between classes in cause specific outcomes, of approximately 10%, are minor compared to the difference in outcome between regimens achieving different degrees of blood pressure control.[12] Overall, the conclusion must be that the blood pressure achieved

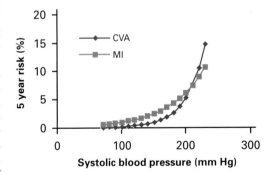

Figure 35.1. Absolute versus relative risk of myocardial infarction and stroke. Data from MacMahon et al[2] and Collins et al[3] are used to illustrate how myocardial infarction (MI) appears a more common complication of hypertension than stroke (cerebrovascular accident, CVA), because its incidence starts higher in the normal part of the blood pressure distribution. However, stroke has a higher relative risk (plotted as 40% v 25% for each 10 mm Hg increase in systolic blood pressure), and overtakes myocardial infarction as an absolute risk in severe hypertension.

Table 35.1   Compelling and possible indications and contraindications for the major classes of antihypertensive drugs. Reproduced from Ramsay et al[4] with permission of the BMJ Publishing Group

Class of drug	Indication		Contraindications	
	Compelling	Possible	Possible	Compelling
α Blockers	Prostatism	Dyslipidaemia	Postural hypotension	Urinary incontinence
ACE inhibitors	Heart failure, left ventricular dysfunction, type 1 diabetic nephropathy	Chronic renal disease*, type 2 diabetic nephropathy	Renal impairment*, peripheral vascular disease†	Pregnancy, renovascular disease
Angiotensin II receptor antagonists	Cough induced by ACE inhibitor‡	Heart failure, intolerance of other antihypertensive drugs	Peripheral vascular disease†	Pregnancy, renovascular disease
β Blockers	Myocardial infarction, angina	Heart failure§	Heart failure§, dyslipidaemia, peripheral vascular disease	Asthma or chronic obstructive pulmonary disease, heart block
Calcium antagonists (dihydropyridine)	Isolated systolic hypertension in elderly patients	Angina, elderly patients	–	–
Calcium antagonists (rate limiting)	Angina	Myocardial infarction	Combination with β blockade	Heart block, heart failure
Thiazides	Elderly patients	–	Dyslipidaemia	Gout

*Angiotensin converting enzyme (ACE) inhibitors may be beneficial in chronic renal failure but should be used with caution. Close supervision and specialist advice are needed when there is established and significant renal impairment.
†Caution with ACE inhibitors and angiotensin II receptor antagonists in peripheral vascular disease because of association with renovascular disease.
‡If ACE inhibitor indicated.
§β Blockers may worsen heart failure, but in specialist hands by be used to treat heart failure.

on treatment is more important than the choice of initial therapy. An exception might be the benefit from the angiotensin converting enzyme (ACE) inhibitor ramipril in the HOPE (heart outcomes prevention evaluation) study.[13] However the mean starting pressure in HOPE, 138/78 mm Hg, was the same as the best blood pressure achieved on treatment in any of the trials in hypertensive patients, and the mechanism of benefit of ACE inhibitors in normotensive patients—including post-myocardial infarction, heart failure or diabetes—may not be relevant to their use in hypertension. This review will therefore concentrate on the optimisation of blood pressure control and how this can be improved by an understanding of hypertension pathogenesis.

Antihypertensive drugs and short term measurement of response

Compared with the three types of drug used in the treatment of angina or heart failure, the range of drugs for hypertension can seem bewildering, and the range of indications and contraindications in the BHS guidelines proves unhelpful in most individual patients (table 35.1). Although, however, there are eight classes of drugs available—ACE inhibitors, β blockers, calcium channel blockers, diuretics, angiotensin receptor blockers, α blockers, centrally acting drugs, and direct vasodilators—the first four of these are sufficient to account for most current prescribing in hypertension in almost equal measure (if only treatment initiations are counted). There are two coincidences. One is that the first four are also the ones used in angina or heart failure, whereas some of the others would be contraindicated (changing a

hypertensive patient from β blockade to α blockade, for example, is quite an effective provocation test for angina). The second is that the names of these four classes start with the first four letters of the alphabet. The felicity of this coincidence is accentuated by the antithesis between the AB and CD pairs, as will become apparent, giving rise to a mnemonic "AB/CD" rule introduced later that forms the

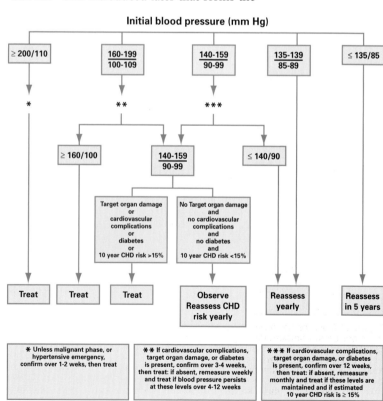

Figure 35.2. Blood pressure indications for treatment (British Hypertension Society guidelines). Reproduced from Ramsay et al,[4] with permission of BMJ Publishing Group.

basis of our approach to the treatment of hypertension.[14]

If the long term objectives in hypertension treatment are prevention of the cardiovascular complications, the short term objectives measurable in every patient are simply reduction in blood pressure and avoidance of adverse effects. The only room for controversy here concerns the blood pressure target and whether treatment that avoids adverse effects actually improves quality of life in apparently asymptomatic patients. Two large studies—TOMHS (treatment of mild hypertension study) and HOT (hypertension optimal treatment)—do indeed support the latter notion.[15 16] Coupled to the evidence, from one outcome trial, that blood pressure treatment prevents dementia,[17] we have the beginnings of a story that patients compliant with treatment will have improved mental and physical well-being. This story is weaker than the main argument for treatment, but perhaps it can become a useful adjunct for patients for whom prevention of a stroke in future decades seems insufficient incentive to take daily treatment for an asymptomatic condition.

The question of blood pressure targets is probably more important, but one which engenders more heat among protagonists than enlightened interest in the minds of readers. The observational data strongly suggest that the lower the blood pressure the better.[2 3] When one turns to the evidence from individual outcome trials, only analyses in diabetics have successfully shown the value of more rather than less blood pressure reduction, and even these do not come close to justifying the targets recommended by diabetes associations.[10 18–20] The methodological problem is that of dissociating lower blood pressure on treatment from a lower blood pressure before treatment (about whose predictive value there is no argument). The situation is compounded by confusion between systolic and diastolic targets, and the recognition that in older patients there is an *inverse* relation between diastolic pressure and risk.[5] The recommended target is 140/85 mm Hg, with a "minimum audit standard" of 150/90 mm Hg.[4] This duality may sound like first and second class post, but it is a sensible recognition that first class post cannot be delivered in all patients. Although the guidelines recommend that both the systolic and diastolic targets are achieved, in practice doctors will accept success with one of them—most likely the diastolic target. It has therefore been suggested that target setting be unified by dropping the diastolic altogether.[21] Certainly it is important to involve the patients in the process of target setting: they must be told both what their blood pressure is and what it should be, and chances of their remembering are doubled by adhering to a single figure.

A unitary scheme for pathogenesis of hypertension, and implications for rational choice of treatment

In turning from the objectives to mechanics of antihypertensive treatment, we are now in the fortunate position of having both evidence and a logical basis for what we recommend. In the 1970s and early '80s it was fashionable to propose unitary hypotheses for hypertension. One of those was centred on the renin system, which seemed to be more important in young, white patients and gave way to other systems of blood pressure control in older patients.[22 23] As molecular genetics came of age, it became clear that hypertension is one of the "common complex disorders", and the involvement of multiple genetic variants—probably most in yet unknown genes—has now been confirmed on a genome wide scan.[24] We therefore sought evidence that different patients have a different "best" drug, depending on the genetic basis for their hypertension. The possibility of this had been suggested by previous crossover comparisons.[25–28] Surprisingly, however, when we rotated patients through all four of the main classes, there was a clear pattern that most patients responded well to one or other of the AB and CD pairs mentioned earlier[11]; we have recently repeated this study double blind, incorporating also α blockade and a placebo control.[29] I believe now that, while there is great heterogeneity at the molecular level, this should not blind us to the central part of one or two systems, in which these molecules play a part.

The key lies in one of the fundamental laws of cardiovascular physiology—that blood pressure is the product of cardiac output and peripheral resistance—and this gave rise many years ago to the concept that there are separate volume and vasoconstriction phases or types of hypertension.[30] Figure 35.3 seeks to satisfy both the lumpers and splitters' approach to a complex disorder like hypertension. Noradrenaline (NA) and salt (Na$^+$) are better contenders

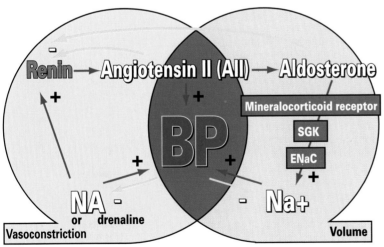

Figure 35.3. NA or Na in hypertension? The principal initiating factors in hypertension are noradrenaline (NA) released from sympathetic nerves, which causes vasoconstriction, or sodium (Na$^+$) which increases blood volume. Since blood pressure = peripheral resistance × cardiac output, hypertension cannot occur until vasoconstriction by noradrenaline and its stimulation of renin secretion fails to be offset by pressure natriuresis. Apart from the key players of NA, Na$^+$, renin and angiotensin, there are a very large number of molecules involved in the synthesis, secretion or response to these, which provide candidate genes to explain inherited susceptibility to hypertension. The figure illustrates just three of these, relevant to the cell signalling of aldosterone. ENaC, epithelial sodium channel; SGK, serum glucocorticoid kinase.

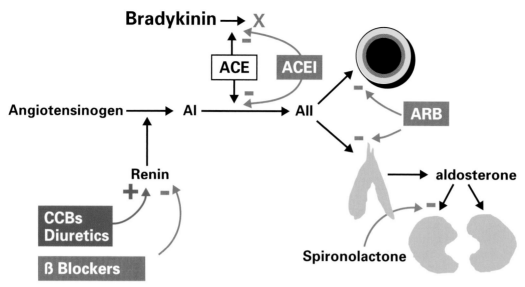

Figure 35.4. Drugs acting on the renin-angiotensin-aldosterone system. Drugs which suppress the system are shown in red, those which activate the system are in green. ACEI, angiotensin converting enzyme inhibitor; ARB, angiotensin receptor blocker; CCBs, calcium channel blockers.

than renin itself for initiating the processes leading to hypertension, but it is the renin system which should be arraigned when explaining either the raised peripheral resistance in established hypertension or how this responds to the different drug treatments (fig 35.4). A large number of molecular candidates up and downstream of renin will probably be found to harbour genetic variants which illuminate understanding of hypertension in individual patients; but measurement of plasma renin is likely to remain the best single guide to the type of hypertension and choice of treatment.[22]

Some attempt is required to overcome the paradox that we *can* control blood pressure when following a rational protocol,[10 20] but in everyday practice fail to achieve this in 90% of patients.[31] Diabetologists have successfully separated diabetes in doctors' minds into types 1 and 2, with clear therapeutic implications, without having a clear idea about the cause of either other than the relative lack or excess, respectively, of insulin. It would be wrong to press the analogy with hypertension too far. Nevertheless, a similar notional division of hypertension into types 1 and 2 may help promote more rational and effective drug treatment. Type 1 would be the vasoconstrictor, high renin type of hypertension seen in younger white patients; type 2 would be the volume dependent, low renin hypertension seen in African Caribbean and older white patients. Taking figs 35.3 and 35.4 together, it is apparent that type 1 (high renin) hypertension should be treated with a renin suppressing drug, A or B (ACE inhibitor or β blocker), whereas type 2 (low renin) hypertension should be treated with C or D (calcium channel blocker or diuretic).

It also follows that salt is not, in whites, a major influence early in hypertension, and dietary advice should focus on reducing fat, and increasing fruit and fibre intake.[32] In the early stages of hypertension development—recognisable clinically as a phase of labile hypertension, where the negative feedback loops in fig 3 are still operative—sole treatment

with a β blocker is the most effective. It is likely that at this stage increased cardiac output contributes to the raised blood pressure, and β blockade blocks the action of noradrenaline both upon the heart and upon renin release.[33] Once hypertension is sustained, the role of renin becomes predominant and ACE inhibitors can be the most effective treatment. It is interesting to speculate whether this transition from what might be considered a high flow to high pressure system has any useful analogy with that recognised on the right side of the circulation in patients with congenital cardiac left to right shunts. At the least, such patients demonstrate the long period of time over which structural changes can develop in the vasculature, and support the view that even young patients with established hypertension already have an end stage disease. Two years after using the AB/CD strategy to lower blood pressure in 37 patients (mean age 41 years) to 125/75 mm Hg, we stopped treatment. Blood pressure promptly returned to pretreatment values, and estimation of arterial stiffness showed this had remained high despite the "prolonged" period of normotension.[34]

Volume dependent (low renin) hypertension may be primary, typically in African Caribbean patients, in Conn's syndrome,[35] and in a rare group of monogenic syndromes caused by activating mutations in a Na^+ transporter[36] or the aldosterone pathway.[37-39] Indeed the latter patients illustrate well the principle of fitting the treatment to the cause of hypertension, with spironolactone or amiloride, respectively, being particularly effective in patients with increased stimulation of the mineralocorticoid receptor or epithelial sodium channel (ENaC, fig 35.3), respectively. However, most white patients do not have primarily volume dependent hypertension, and the transition to this may be secondary to renal or renovascular consequences of the hypertension. These patients may need a combination of a calcium channel blocker or diuretic (C or D), which is the preferred initial treatment in low renin hypertensives, with a renin suppressing drug—ACE

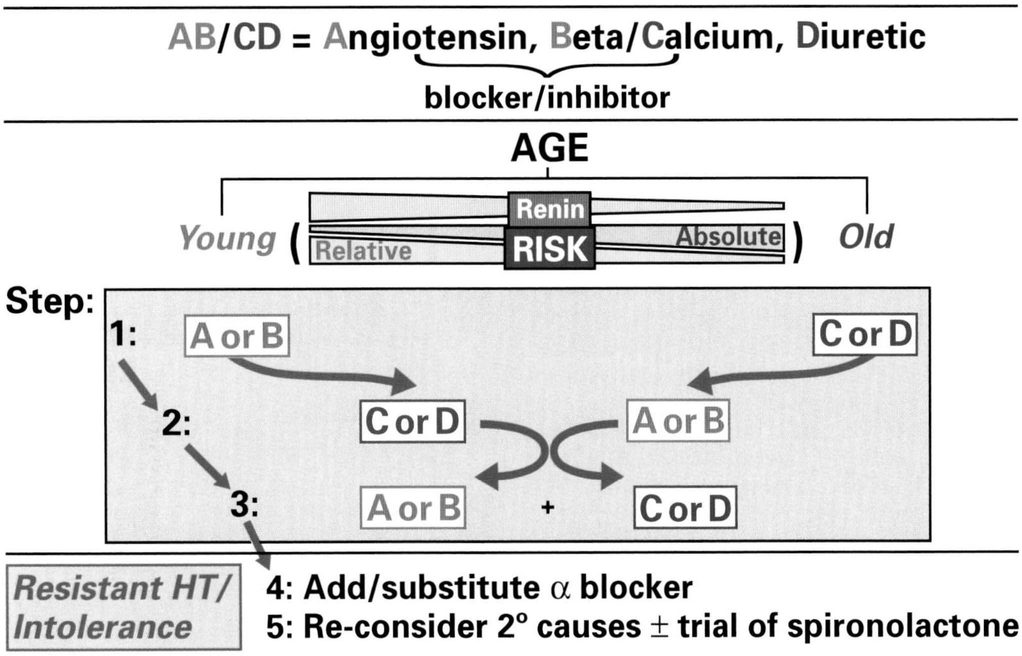

AB/CD = Angiotensin, **B**eta/**C**alcium, **D**iuretic

blocker/inhibitor

AGE

Young (Relative | Renin **RISK** | Absolute) *Old*

Step:

1: A or B   C or D

2: C or D — A or B

3: A or B + C or D

Resistant HT/ Intolerance | **4: Add/substitute α blocker**
5: Re-consider 2° causes ± trial of spironolactone

Figure 35.5. AB/CD schema for optimisation of antihypertensive treatment. In choosing initial treatment—step 1—age in a white population is used as a surrogate for plasma renin, which falls with age. The typical younger patient (aged < 55 years) responds better to ACE inhibition or β blockade, whereas in the older patient (aged > 55 years) calcium channel blockade or diuretic is the preferred starting treatment; angiotensin receptor blockade can substitute for ACE inhibition in intolerant patients. Because the response of patients to the two drugs within each pair is well correlated, there is usually no point in switching an unresponsive patient to the other of the pair (for example, A to B); therefore step 2 in such a patient is to switch to one of the other pair. If the blood pressure is still above target, step 3 is to combine one drug from each pair.

inhibitor or β blocker (A or B). In effect, C or D not only lowers the blood pressure but converts a previously low renin patient into a higher renin patient who can respond to the addition of A or B. Given that the older patients, in whom C or D are the initial drugs of choice, are also those at higher absolute risk of complications, combination therapy should increasingly be the norm. Diabetics in particular require more drugs than other patients, and may not achieve the stiff targets set for them.[18 40] It is time therefore to cease the arguments over whether ACE inhibitors or calcium channel blockers are preferable among the newer classes, and instead ensure that any patient with microalbuminuria is receiving both. Among all patients, it is also time to encourage greater use of combination formulations, in recognition of patients' desire to minimise their tablet intake.

the initial dose is mainly placebo response or will increase with dose. The advice of a pharmacologist, whenever there is doubt about efficacy or tolerability, is to try doubling the dose—true drug effects follow a dose-response curve.

The schema also skirts the issue of whom to treat. Current British guidelines recommend treatment in patients with a blood pressure > 160/100 mm Hg, or > 140/90 mm Hg if there is >2% annual risk of stroke or coronary heart disease (fig 35.2). As discussed already, systolic pressure alone may be preferable; more doctors would be inclined to treat a patient with a blood pressure of 150/95 mm Hg than 150/85 mm Hg, although the latter carries a higher risk.[5] As the schema also suggests, the younger hypertensive patient is likely to have high renin hypertension and the renin may itself be a risk factor for coronary heart disease.

The AB/CD rule

At this point the recommendations and arguments can be summarised in the form of an AB/CD rule (fig 35.5). This arises not only from the small rotation studies, but also from previous observations on the influence of age upon drug response in parallel groups studies.[23 41–43] The somewhat arbitrary age definitions are based on the two studies which initially suggested the rule: a rotation through all four drug classes in patients aged < 50 years,[14] and a randomised comparison of C and D, with addition of A or B, in patients aged > 55 years.[10] The schema shown in fig 35.5 does not advise on dose; clinical judgement is still required to assess whether a small response to

Investigation and treatment of resistant hypertension: importance of aldosterone

One term which the AB/CD rule helps to define is resistant hypertension; this is a blood pressure above target despite a combination of [A or B] + [C or D]. This is helpful to recognise as a discrete entity because resistance to a conventional therapeutic attack on the volume and vasoconstriction elements of hypertension implies an extra, or unusual, stimulus to one of these. Alcohol is the most common curable cause of resistant hypertension. Reflex sympathetic activation requiring α blockade is another, and may be suggested if slightly raised noradrenaline excretion is found during the tests to exclude phaeochromocytoma as a secondary causes of hypertension.[44] In the presence of impaired renal function, bilateral renal artery stenosis should be sought by magnetic resonance imaging. Of most interest now is hyperaldosteronism. There is no doubt that primary hyperaldosteronism, or Conn's syndrome, is underdiagnosed.[45 46] In a survey of 800 unselected patients in primary care, we have found almost 10% of patients to have raised aldosterone to renin ratios and blood pressure more responsive to spironolactone than other drugs. This prevalence is comparable with findings from hospital based studies, and the outstanding finding is that in many cases the plasma potassium (K^+) concentration is normal, even > 4.0 mmol/l. Only a handful of these patients have adrenal adenomas.

In such a cross-sectional study, it is not possible to know whether hyperaldosteronism in the absence of an adenoma is the primary cause of the hypertension, or a tertiary development after long standing hyper-reninaemia. From a therapeutic standpoint, this is academic. Although a single outpatient sample is sufficient for measurement of renin and aldosterone, the infrequency of adenomas suggests that the response to spironolactone can be undertaken first as a therapeutic test. At a dose of 1 mg/kg daily (to the nearest 25 mg), gynaecomastia is rare, and should be avoided altogether with the advent of more specific aldosterone antagonists.

What about the really resistant patient, the one uncontrolled on four or five drugs? Assuming that none of the above strategies has worked, the ultimate "weapon" is minoxidil. This is the most powerful vasodilator, almost guaranteed to normalise blood pressure provided patients can tolerate β blockade and high doses of a loop diuretic. However, side effects such as hirsutism and coarsening of facial features render this the treatment of last resort, though patients who have endured the adverse effects of other drugs can be surprisingly resilient. One promising alternative is the combination of second generation angiotensin and aldosterone receptor blockade; this appears the most effective way of targeting the whole of the renin system, blocking both the vasoconstrictor and volume drivers of hypertension.

Emergency reduction of blood pressure

This article has concentrated on the hypertensive outpatient, but there are rare occasions when emergency treatment for high blood pressure is indicated. It is important to differentiate these indications from the similarly rare occurrence of accelerated phase hypertension; the latter is almost a contraindication to emergency reduction of blood pressure because of the loss of cerebral autoregulation and consequent risk of cerebral infarction. The three indications for emergency reduction are hypertensive encephalopathy (of which eclampsia is the most common cause),

---

Key points

- Community surveys show that less than 10% of patients have a blood pressure at target

- Recent outcome trials show that achieved blood pressure is much more important than choice of initial drug in preventing stroke and myocardial infarction. Therefore strategies for optimising blood pressure control in the individual patient are paramount

- In more than 90% of patients, the cause of hypertension remains unknown

- Primary hyperaldosteronism (Conn's syndrome) accounts for at least 5% of hypertension, and usually presents with normal plasma electrolytes

- Numerous molecular variants are being found which contribute a small amount to the development of hypertension. Patient response to different drugs may depend in part on which of these is inherited

- The main determinant of response pattern is the patient's age. This probably reflects the dominant role of the renin system in blood pressure regulation

- Younger patients have relatively high renin concentrations and respond well to drugs which suppress the renin system—ACE inhibitors, angiotensin receptor blockers (A), and β blockers (B)

- Older patients have low renin concentration, and respond well to drugs which do not suppress renin—calcium channel blockers (C), and diuretics (D). These drugs actually cause reflex activation of the renin system, and therefore make patients more sensitive to A or B

- Target blood pressure is 140/85 mm Hg, or 135/80 mm Hg in diabetics. Less than 50% of patients are likely to reach these targets on one drug

- The best combinations have complementary actions on the renin system—that is, one of [A or B] + one of [C or D]

- Resistant hypertension is a blood pressure > 140/85 mm Hg despite treatment on such a combination. Such patients should be screened for secondary causes. Treatment options include addition of an α blocker, or a trial of spironolactone ± an angiotensin blocker.

- Rarely, patients require treatment with minoxidil, the most powerful vasodilator available

left ventricular failure, and dissecting aneurysm. Parenteral treatment with nitroprusside for a maximum of 2–3 days is advisable for the first two conditions, whereas more prolonged treatment with parenteral nitrate and labetalol are preferable for the latter; this combination is also useful for any other patients requiring excellent blood pressure control and parenteral treatment. Accelerated phase hypertension is best treated with low dose oral β blockade. In none of these circumstances is short acting nifedipine advisable, but long acting calcium channel blockade may be started as cover for parenteral treatment that can be down titrated as the oral treatment starts to be effective.

Conclusion

Hypertension describes the upper end of the blood pressure distribution, in which there is a high relative risk of cardiovascular disease. It is a complex disorder in that a variety of genetic and environmental factors, many as yet unknown, determine an individual's point in the blood pressure distribution. However, the main physiological and biochemical systems controlling blood pressure are well understood, as are their responses to the drugs used for treating hypertension. Hypertension occurs when excessive vasoconstriction and/or volume are not compensated, respectively, by adequate pressure natriuresis or suppression of the renin-angiotensin-aldosterone system. The AB/CD rule for treatment minimises the steps required in individual patients to achieve these compensatory adjustments. Possible differences between drug classes in prevention of stroke or coronary heart disease are minor compared to the importance of blood pressure control. This is ideally assessed by 24 hour ambulatory monitoring of blood pressure and its impact on left ventricular mass.

1. **Joint National Committee.** The sixth report of the Joint National Committee on prevention, detection, evaluation, and treatment of high blood pressure. *Arch Intern Med* 1997;**157**:2413–46.

2. **MacMahon S, Peto R, Cutler J,** *et al.* Blood pressure, stroke, and coronary heart disease. Part 1. Prolonged differences in blood pressure: prospective observational studies corrected for the regression dilution bias. *Lancet* 1990;**335**:765–74.
   - *Definitive overview of long term risks from hypertension. Authors dispute whether there is any safe level of blood pressure, showing a straight line relation between blood pressure and incidence of stroke or myocardial infarction, when risk is log transformed.*

3. **Collins R, Peto R, MacMahon S,** *et al.* Blood pressure, stroke, and coronary heart disease. Part 2. Short-term reductions in blood pressure: overview of randomised drug trials in their epidemiological context. *Lancet* 1990;**335**:827–38.
   - *The sister article of the one above, this was the first paper to establish that antihypertensive treatment does significantly reduce risk of myocardial infarction, but less effectively than it reduces risk of stroke.*

4. **Ramsay LE, Williams B, Johnston GD,** *et al.* British Hypertension Society guidelines for hypertension management 1999: summary. *BMJ* 1999;**319**:630–5.
   - *Current recommendations for antihypertensive treatment. Introduces concept of using absolute risk for deciding who needs treatment.*

5. **Franklin SS, Khan SA, Wong ND,** *et al.* Is pulse pressure useful in predicting risk for coronary heart disease? The Framingham heart study. *Circulation* 1999;**100**:354–60.

6. **Dickerson JE, Brown MJ.** Influence of age on general practitioners' definition and treatment of hypertension. *BMJ* 1995;**310**:574–81.

7. **Hansson L, Hedner T, Lund-Johansen P,** *et al.* Randomised trial of effects of calcium antagonists compared with diuretics and beta-blockers on cardiovascular morbidity and mortality in hypertension: the Nordic diltiazem (NORDIL) study. *Lancet* 2000;**356**:359–65.

8. **Hansson L, Lindholm LH, Niskanen L,** *et al.* Effect of angiotensin-converting-enzyme inhibition compared with conventional therapy on cardiovascular morbidity and mortality in hypertension: the captopril prevention project (CAPPP) randomised trial. *Lancet* 1999;**353**:611–16.

9. **Hansson L, Lindholm LH, Ekbom T,** *et al.* Randomised trial of old and new antihypertensive drugs in elderly patients: cardiovascular mortality and morbidity. The Swedish trial in old patients with hypertension-2 study. *Lancet* 1999;**354**:1751–6.
   - *First outcome comparison of old and new drugs in hypertension, showing no difference between ACE inhibitor, calcium channel blocker and "conventional treatment" (diuretic or β blockade).*

10. **Brown MJ, Palmer CR, Castaigne A,** *et al.* Morbidity and mortality in patients randomised to double-blind treatment with once-daily calcium channel blockade or diuretic in the International nifedipine GITS study: intervention as a goal in hypertension treatment (INSIGHT). *Lancet* 2000;**356**:366–42.
    - *First double blind outcome comparison of two antihypertensive drugs. Emphasises the importance of blood pressure control rather than choice of initial drug in determining outcome.*

11. **ALLHAT Collaborative Research Group.** Major cardiovascular events in hypertensive patients randomized to doxazosin vs chlorthalidone: the antihypertensive and lipid-lowering treatment to prevent heart attack trial (ALLHAT). *JAMA* 2000;**283**:1967–75.

12. **Blood Pressure Lowering Treatment Trialists' Collaboration.** Effects of angiotensin converting enzyme inhibitors, calcium antagonists and other blood pressure lowering drugs on mortality and major cardiovascular morbidity. *Lancet* 2000;**356**:1955–64.
    - *Overview of all outcome trials of newer antihypertensive drug classes. No difference in overall outcome between any two classes. Possible small differences in incidence of stroke (less on calcium blockers) and coronary heart disease (less on ACE inhibition and older drugs).*

13. **Yusuf S, Sleight P, Pogue J,** *et al.* Effects of an angiotensin-converting-enzyme inhibitor, ramipril, on cardiovascular events in high-risk patients. The heart outcomes prevention evaluation study investigators. *N Engl J Med* 2000;**342**:145–53.

14. **Dickerson JEC, Hingorani AD, Ashby MJ,** *et al.* Optimisation of anti-hypertensive treatment by crossover rotation of four major classes. *Lancet* 1999;**353**:2008–13.
    - *Crossover comparison of the main drug groups. Demonstrates inter-individual variation in response, and led to formulation of the AB/CD rule.*

15. **Grimm RH, Jr, Grandits GA, Cutler JA,** *et al.* Relationships of quality-of-life measures to long-term lifestyle and drug treatment in the treatment of mild hypertension study. *Arch Intern Med* 1997;**157**:638–48.

16. **Hansson L.** The hypertension optimal treatment study and the importance of lowering blood pressure. *J Hypertens* 1999;**17**(suppl):S9–13.

17. **Forette F, Seux ML, Staessen JA,** *et al.* Prevention of dementia in randomised double-blind placebo-controlled systolic hypertension in Europe (Syst-Eur) trial. *Lancet* 1998;**352**:1347–51.

18. **American Diabetes Association.** Clinical practice recommendations 2000. *Diabetes Care* 2000;**23**(suppl 1):S1–116.

19. **UK Prospective Diabetes Study Group.** Tight blood pressure control and risk of macrovascular and microvascular complications in type 2 diabetes: UKPDS 38. *BMJ* 1998;**317**:703–13.

20. **Hansson L, Zanchetti A.** Effects of intensive blood-pressure lowering and low-dose aspirin in patients with hypertension: principal results of the hypertension optimal treatment (HOT) randomised trial. *Lancet* 1998;**351**:1755–62.
    - *Removed doubts about dangers of aiming at a normal blood pressure—end of the U shaped curve.*

21. **Sever P.** Abandoning diastole. *BMJ* 1999;**318**:1773.

22. **Laragh JH, Letcher RL, Pickering TG.** Renin profiling for diagnosis and treatment of hypertension. *JAMA* 1979;**241**:151–6.
    - *Introduced concept of high and low renin hypertension.*

23. **Buhler FR, Burkart F, Lutold BE,** *et al.* Antihypertensive beta blocking action as related to renin and age: a pharmacologic tool to identify pathogenetic mechanisms in essential hypertension. *Am J Cardiol* 1975;**36**:653–69.

24. **Sharma P, Fatibene J, Ferraro F,** *et al.* A genome-wide search for susceptibility loci to human essential hypertension. *Hypertension* 2000;**35**:1291–5.

25. **Attwood S, Bird R, Burch K,** *et al.* Within-patient correlation between the antihypertensive effects of atenolol, lisinopril and nifedipine. *J Hypertens* 1994;**12**:1053–60.

260

26. **Laragh JH, Lamport B, Sealey J,** *et al.* Diagnosis ex juvantibus. Individual response patterns to drugs reveal hypertension mechanisms and simplify treatment. *Hypertension* 1988;**12**:223–6.

27. **Menard J, Serrurier D, Bautier P,** *et al.* Crossover design to test antihypertensive drugs with self-recorded blood pressure. *Hypertension* 1988;**11**:153–9.

28. **Bidiville J, Nussberger J, Waeber G,** *et al.* Individual responses to converting enzyme inhibitors and calcium antagonists. *Hypertension* 1988;**11**:166–73.

29. **Deary AJ, Schumann A, Murfet H,** *et al.* Double-blind, placebo-controlled crossover rotation of the five principal classes of antihypertensive drugs. *Am J Hypertens* (in press)

30. **Laragh J, Sealey J.** Renin system understanding for analysis and treatment of hypertensive patients: a means to qualify the vasoconstrictor elements, diagnose curable renal and adrenal causes, access risk of cardiovascular morbidity, and find the best-fit drug regimen. *Hypertension: pathophysiology, diagnosis, and management*, 2nd ed. New York: Raven Press, 1995:1813–36.

31. **Colhoun HM, Dong W, Poulter NR.** Blood pressure screening, management and control in England: results from the health survey for England 1994. *J Hypertens* 1998;**16**:747–52.

32. **Appel LJ, Moore TJ, Obarzanek E,** *et al.* A clinical trial of the effects of dietary patterns on blood pressure. *N Engl J Med* 1997;**336**:1117–24.

33. **Lund-Johansen P.** Twenty-year follow-up of hemodynamics in essential hypertension during rest and exercise. *Hypertension* 1991;**18**:III54–61.

34. **Dickerson JEC, Brown MJ.** Withdrawal of antihypertensive treatment after two years of blood pressure normalisation in young patients. *J Hum Hypertens* 1999;**13**:885.

35. **Stewart PM.** Mineralocorticoid hypertension. *Lancet* 1999;**353**:1341–7.

36. **Shimkets RA, Warnock DG, Bositis CM,** *et al.* Liddle's syndrome: heritable human hypertension caused by mutations in the β-subunit of the epithelial sodium channel. *Cell* 1994;**79**:407–14.

37. **Geller DS, Farhi A, Pinkerton N,** *et al.* Activating mineralocorticoid receptor mutation in hypertension exacerbated by pregnancy. *Science* 2000;**289**:119–23.

38. **Lifton RP, Dluhy RG, Powers M.** A chimaeric 11 beta-hydroxylase/aldosterone synthase gene causes glucocorticoid remediable aldosteronism and human hypertension. *Nature* 1992;**355**:262–5.

39. **Stewart PM, Krozowski ZS, Gupta A,** *et al.* Hypertension in the syndrome of apparent mineralocorticoid excess due to mutation of the 11β-hydroxysteroid dehydrogenase type 2 gene. *Lancet* 1996;**347**:88–91.
 • *Finding of the molecular basis for a previously recognised rare inherited type of hypertension, which also explains the hypertension in patients consuming excess liquorice.*

40. **Brown MJ, Castaigne A, De Leeuw PW,** *et al.* Influence of diabetes and type of hypertension on the response to antihypertensive treatment. *Hypertension* 2000;**35**:1038–42.

41. **Philipp T, Anlauf M, Distler A,** *et al.* Randomised, double blind, multicentre comparison of hydrochlorothiazide, atenolol, nitrendipine, and enalapril in antihypertensive treatment: results of the HANE study. *BMJ* 1997;**315**:154–9.

42. **Materson BJ, Cushman WC, Reda D,** *et al.* Single-drug therapy for hypertension in men—a comparison of six antihypertensive agents with placebo. *N Engl J Med* 1993;**328**:914–21.

43. **Brown MJ, Dickerson JEC.** Synergism between α_1 blockade and angiotensin converting enzyme inhibition in essential hypertension. *J Hypertens* 1991;**9**:S362–3.

44. **Brown MJ.** Phaeochromocytoma. In: Weatherall D, Ledingham J, Warrell D, eds. *Oxford textbook of medicine.* Oxford University Press, 1995:2553–7.

45. **Gordon RD, Stowasser M, Tunny TJ,** *et al.* High incidence of primary aldosteronism in 199 patients referred with hypertension. *Clin Exp Pharmacol Physiol* 1994;**21**:315–18.

46. **Lim PO, Rogers P, Cardale K,** *et al.* Potentially high prevalence of primary aldosteronism in a primary-care population. *Lancet* 1999;**353**:40.

36 Essential hypertension: the heart and hypertension

K E Berkin, S G Ball

Hypertension:

- Is a common risk factor for ischaemic heart disease and heart failure

- Is suboptimally detected and treated

- In the elderly is often systolic only, and treatment reduces risk of coronary heart disease

The heart and hypertension are intimately linked. Hypertension predisposes to coronary heart disease, myocardial hypertrophy, and cardiac dysfunction. Other organs and systems are also important in hypertension but this article concentrates on the effect of hypertension on the heart. The impact of hypertension on the heart is much more important than its effect in causing stroke and renal failure in terms of numbers of patients affected. There is still undue emphasis on diastolic pressure, with little attention paid to isolated systolic hypertension, and treatment remains inadequate for many patients. Cardiologists have a responsibility in this regard. The perspective taken in this article is that of the physician in the outpatient clinic.

Background

General practitioners deal with most hypertension. Patients are usually sent to the hospital clinic because the blood pressure has not been controlled despite multiple drug treatment, for loss of previously good control, where it is felt that a cause for hypertension should be sought, or because of an overt cardiovascular event. The extent and tempo of investigation of the elevated pressure are determined by the clinical situation. Hypertension also presents as an incidental finding in other clinical situations and as a result is often suboptimally managed or even ignored. Attention to blood pressure is surprisingly cavalier in cardiac clinics given its importance as a risk factor. Undoubtedly, it is more difficult to deal with than the measurement of cholesterol and the reflex—albeit appropriate—prescribing of a statin in the patient with known ischaemic heart disease. In light of the cost of coronary angioplasty and bypass graft surgery, especially to the patient, it seems inappropriate not to pursue rigorously the best management of hypertension. Blood pressure recordings after myocardial infarction, revascularisation, and rest in hospital are unlikely to be representative of subsequent levels. Follow up is essential.

Even when undertaken, the measurement of blood pressure is sometimes casual and imprecise. Nonetheless, attaching a number to the reading is important. Inspection of the hospital notes for previous recordings can be useful in determining past levels and the need for treatment. The British Society of Hypertension (BSH) guidelines have been incorporated into the joint British guidelines on the prevention of coronary heart disease,[1] and recommend formal assessment of 10 year coronary heart disease risk as a guide to the treatment of high blood pressure.[2] Cardiac hypertrophy can alter that risk and is not accounted for in the standard risk tables currently in use for primary prevention. Other articles in this series deal with risk assessment and drug treatment.

The level of the pressure and time of exposure appear to be key factors in determining the effect on the heart. However the response of the individual seems varied and the length of exposure is rarely known accurately. This leads to an imprecise relation between the level of pressure recorded in the office and the state of the heart. The underlying *cause* of the hypertension seems unimportant in the development of cardiac problems, except in the rare case of phaeochromocytoma. Here a cardiomyopathy may ensue of such severity that the patient may no longer have raised blood pressure. All patients with cardiomyopathy, irrespective of blood pressure, should therefore have a 24 hour urine collection for measurement of noradrenaline and adrenaline (norepinephrine and epinephrine). Renal artery stenosis should be sought in hypertensive patients with vascular disease, particularly if presenting with recurrent pulmonary oedema and relatively preserved left ventricular systolic function.

Isolated systolic hypertension

Elevation of systolic pressure not accompanied by the expected diastolic rise carries cardiovascular risk, which can be reduced with treatment. In large population surveys systolic pressure continues to rise whereas diastolic pressure peaks in the sixth decade (50–59 years). Systolic pressure is the major determinant of the workload of the heart and cardiac hypertrophy. The wider pulse pressure associated with isolated systolic hypertension (ISH) is associated with an increase in risks from cardiovascular disease and mortality[3] (fig 1). Systolic pressures continue to be ignored by some practitioners and patients, but in numerical terms ISH is probably responsible for more morbidity than the less frequent diastolic hypertension.

262

Pathophysiology

Coronary artery disease is one of the most frequent accompaniments of raised arterial pressure. Atheroma is not seen in the pulmonary arteries unless there is pulmonary hypertension, indicating a central role for pressure itself in the genesis of atherosclerotic lesions. Even so, the importance of large vessel coronary heart disease complicating hypertension has probably been underestimated. Modest pressure elevation is common in the population. In this substantial group coronary heart disease, not stroke, is the major clinical issue. In severe pressure elevation the problems of stroke and cardiac failure dominate. Framingham data showed that hypertension was the most common cause of heart failure, but this reflects the poor detection and treatment of hypertension 30–50 years ago. Hypertension is now second to ischaemic heart disease as a cause of heart failure.[4] However, the two conditions frequently co-exist. High pressure initially induces useful compensatory hypertrophy but later decompensation results in heart failure. Myocardial infarction may also play an important part in this decompensation.

Structural changes

Increase in left ventricular mass is a consistent feature of hypertension. Cardiac myocyte cell number does not increase but there is cell hypertrophy. In addition there is considerable interstitial change and fibroblast proliferation. The myocytes account for 70% of the normal cardiac mass but represent only 25% of the cell content.

The changes in small vessel structure are akin to those seen in other tissues in response to pressure elevation, with increase of wall thickness and relative reduction of lumen. However, the haemodynamics of the coronary vessels and the smaller arterioles are different from other organs. Flow is greatest in diastole but the pressure curve in the epicardial coronary arteries follows that of the proximal aorta with which they are contiguous. The smaller intracardiac vessels are subject to extrinsic pressure from contracting cardiac muscle, their feeding pressure and pressure within the ventricular cavity.

An increasing mass of myocardium, made up of larger cells with increased deposition of surrounding collagen, requires more blood supply and relative ischaemia ensues. Exercise tests may indicate ischaemia when the epicardial vessels show no narrowing. Compensatory hypertrophy turns to myocardial failure, with increasing subendocardial ischaemia and subsequent fibrosis.

Additional ischaemia occurs from narrowing of the large epicardial arteries. A stenosis of less than 70% is usually compensated for by dilatation of the smaller arterioles distal to the lesion. However, when the small distal vessels are hypertrophied and subject to increased extrinsic pressure from hypertrophied myocardium, along with raised ventricular pressure, the flow reserve diminishes. Ischaemia occurs at lower workloads. Occlusion of a major vessel may further damage heart muscle and precipitate overt failure in an already compromised vulnerable hypertrophied heart.

Numerous hormonal and neurogenic factors have been postulated to contribute to these changes. The benefit in morbidity and mortality from treatment with both β antagonists and angiotensin converting enzyme (ACE) inhibitors in patients with impaired systolic function, clinical heart failure after myocardial infarction or at high cardiovascular risk suggest at least two important adverse processes amenable to partial correction with treatment. Nevertheless, the reduction of blood pressure itself, irrespective of the mechanism of drug action, appears to both prevent myocardial infarction and reduce the incidence of heart failure.[5]

Hypertrophy is initially concentric. Wall thickness and muscle mass increase, systolic wall stress remains unchanged. At this stage coronary reserve is already compromised. Asymmetric hypertrophy is reported in some 10–15%, affecting the anterior wall, apex, base, and septum. Confusion can then occur with hypertrophic cardiomyopathy, although other distinctive features should be evident on echocardiography. In time the concentrically hypertrophied ventricle dilates and so-called (confusingly) eccentric hypertrophy is observed.

Haemodynamic changes

In young adults with established hypertension, increased heart rate and stroke volume with normal peripheral resistance are reported. Increased peripheral resistance (from the smaller resistance vessels) and loss of compliance (increased stiffness) of large arteries is seen with a consequent increase of mean pressure and pulse pressure, largely through systolic elevation (fig 36.1). Endothelial dysfunction plays a part in flow modulation via impaired nitric oxide synthesis by the coronary endothelium. Coronary reserve decreases. Myocardial compliance (ventricular distensibility),

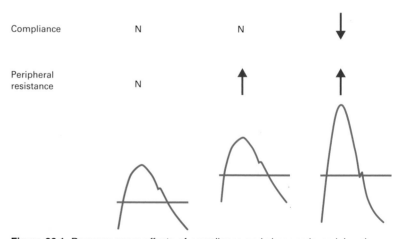

Figure 36.1. Pressure wave effects of compliance and changes in peripheral resistance. Increase in peripheral resistance is the major cause of the increase in mean blood pressure (horizontal bar) with age. In addition the loss of "distensibility" of the large vessels—that is, the decrease in compliance with age—leads to the change in shape of the blood pressure curve as shown, with relative enhancement of the systolic pressure (right hand curve). When loss of compliance is severe diastolic pressure may even fall as seen in patients in their last decade of life. N = normal; ↑ = increase; ↓ = decrease.

Raised pressure leads to:
• Myocyte hypertrophy, interstitial changes, and fibrosis
• Reduction in flow in intracardiac vessels and endothelial dysfunction—"small vessel disease"
• Epicardial (large vessel) coronary disease
• Increased peripheral resistance and loss of compliance in arteries

Clinical assessment should:
• Establish presence of sustained hypertension if necessary by 24 hour measurement
• Elicit symptoms and signs of coexistent heart disease
• Include assessment of standard risk factors
• Include an ECG
• Consider need for cardiac ultrasound, stress testing, and coronary angiography

measured by the pressure–volume relation, can remain normal even with severe hypertrophy. Decompensation of the ventricle is associated with loss of compliance. The product of the systolic wall stress and the stroke volume is increased but the forward pump function is lessened. The heart function can be supported by reducing afterload, reducing preload (thereby reducing volume so increasing the mass:volume ratio), and inotropes.

Causes of cardiac and vascular changes

Undoubtedly increased blood pressure itself enhances the vessel and cardiac changes alluded to above. The proof is the reversibility of many of these by the lowering of pressure by a variety of means.[6] What initiates and augments the elevation remains largely unknown though extensively investigated.

> **Clinical approach to the heart in the patient with hypertension**

The patient with high blood pressure should be assessed clinically and with selected investigations. Much of this assessment is rightly directed to the heart and is expanded upon below.

Clinical information

Hypertension should be assessed in the context of all the other standard risk factors. Cardiac symptoms and age are clearly relevant as regards any likely underlying heart disease. Obesity, especially if increasing in recent years, is a common cause of worsening breathlessness and blood pressure control (1 mm Hg systolic for each 1 kg increase in weight). The heart may be enlarged on clinical examination with associated third and fourth heart sounds. The presence of a systolic ejection murmur in the elderly without significant gradient increases the risk of cardiovascular death and myocardial infarction by 50%.[7] An accentuated second heart sound, referred to in standard texts, helps little, but any auscultatory abnormality pointing to cardiac involvement in hypertension should stress the need for good blood pressure control. Hypertension is a common cause of atrial fibrillation, which carries its own risks and requires specific treatment. Concomitant cerebrovascular and peripheral vascular disease

and other evidence of "end organ damage" increase the likelihood of the presence of cardiac involvement.

The ECG

The ECG is inexpensive, informative, and available routinely. However, lead placement is too often approximate, even on the limbs. This can alter interpretation, particularly for voltage measurement but also for ischaemia (poor R wave progression in the chest leads may be caused by incorrect placement of V2–4). Computer algorithms for interpretation can help to alert the clinician to left ventricular hypertrophy (LVH), which is sometimes overlooked. Silent myocardial infarction is surprisingly common in males in the 40–59 year age group and may be more common in the hypertensive population.[8]

Interpretation, particularly for LVH, must take account of the patient's age and build. In particular the chest lead voltages are increased in young, slim, and athletic individuals and reduced in obesity. Racial differences alter the usefulness of the standard ECG criteria of hypertrophy. Specificity is decreased in blacks.[9] See table 36.1 for commonly used voltage criteria and fig 36.2 for ECG examples.

The overall reliability of the ECG in the detection of hypertrophy ranges from less than 10% up to 50% when compared to measurement by cardiac ultrasound, depending on the population screened and ECG criteria chosen. This is well illustrated when electrocardiographic criteria were compared with ultrasound derived evidence of cardiac hypertrophy in 4684 subjects of the Framingham heart study.[10] Voltage criteria combined with borderline and definite repolarisation changes had a sensitivity of only 6.9% but a specificity of 98.8%. Nevertheless, the presence of voltage criteria of LVH *and repolarisation changes* (fig 36.2) on ECG criteria adds a risk similar to that for a patient with a previously documented myocardial infarction.[11] Indeed, investigation of asymptomatic hypertensive patients with ECG LVH strain shows a high prevalence of epicardial coronary disease. Sudden death is claimed to be six times more common for any given level of blood pressure and is thought more likely to relate to ischaemia rather than a primary arrhythmia, although long QT intervals are seen. LVH based on voltage criteria

ECG

- Inexpensive, informative, and available routinely

- Misplacement of leads may mislead

- Normal ECG does not exclude significant coronary heart disease or hypertrophy

- May detect "silent myocardial infarction"

- Voltage criteria for left ventricular hypertrophy (LVH) are reasonably specific (table 1)

- Voltage criteria for LVH with a strain pattern (table 1) carry risk equivalent to a previous myocardial infarction

without ST/T wave change carries less risk and seems to reflect largely the risk associated with the duration and severity of the hypertension. Non-specific ST/T changes alone carry no more risk than the presence of voltage criteria alone and are less clearly related to pressure levels. The finding of left bundle branch block (LBBB) or left axis deviation in hypertension is not uncommon but the significance is uncertain unless caused by ischaemia. Finally, a normal ECG cannot exclude significant ischaemic heart disease or heart failure in the patient with high blood pressure.

The calculation of independent risk associated with ECG change depends on the use of multiple logistic regression analysis to take account of other factors—for example, age—which themselves exert notable effects. The approach has well described limitations and serves to emphasise the importance of the controlled clinical trial to determine best clinical practice. Observational studies support the notion that antihypertensive treatment reduces the prevalence of high blood pressure and ECG voltage evidence of LVH with mild/moderate repolarisation changes.[12]

Chest *x* ray

An enlarged heart shadow may represent LVH but equally may be caused by chamber dilatation, pericardial fat or technical factors such as poor inspiration and projection. Conversely, an apparently normal sized heart may be hypertrophied or have impairment of function, especially if induced through ischaemia. However, chest radiography can still be important in the assessment of the hypertensive patient and may show left atrial enlargement, pulmonary venous hypertension as a consequence of increased left atrial pressure, abnormalities of the aorta and rarely rib notching.

Cardiac ultrasound

Cardiac ultrasound is not generally recommended in the assessment of all hypertensive patients, but it can be informative in certain situations. The assessment of the LVH is an important but difficult task. Modern ultra-

Table 36.1 Commonly used criteria for ECG left ventricular hypertrophy (LV)

25–50% sensitive★
95% specific★

Chest lead
R wave in V_5 or V_6 exceeds 25 mm
S wave in V_1 or V_2 exceeds 25 mm
Tallest R wave in V_5 or V_6 + deepest S wave in V_1 or V_2 exceeds 35 mm
Ventricular activation time (onset of QRS to peak R) exceeds 0.04 s

Limb lead
R in aVL exceeds 11 mm
R in I exceeds 12 mm
R in aVF exceeds 20 mm
R in I + S in III exceeds 25 mm
R in aVL + S in V_3 exceeds 13 mm

Repolarisation changes (see note)
Mildly abnormal:
  ST-T segment flattening, isolated ST depression or T wave inversion
Severely abnormal:
  ST depression with inverted or biphasic T waves
  - V_4 to V_6 (that is, leads facing left ventricle)
  - 1 and aVL (facing left ventricle when heart horizontal) or
  - 11 and aVF (facing left ventricle when heart vertical)

Additional points
LVH results in only slight shift to the left of the frontal plane QRS axis
  Horizontal heart: axis = +30° to −30°
  Vertical axis: axis = +60° to +90°
There is often counterclockwise rotation—that is, qR complexes appear in the chest leads before the usual V_4 to V_6
Prominent u waves may be seen in the mid and right precordial leads in LVH
Remember digoxin can produce ST/T wave changes and u waves

★Vary with criteria used and population screened—see text.
Note: "strain" refers to the *additional* presence of ST/T wave changes, usually definite ST depression (1 mm) and T wave inversion or biphasic T wave, which are of particular prognostic importance in *the presence of* voltage changes—see text.

A

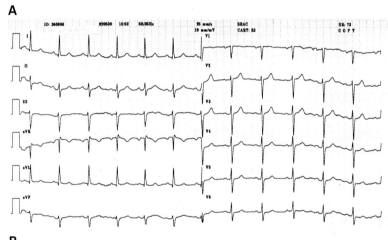

B

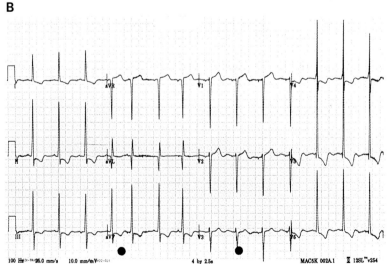

Figure 36.2. (A) Twelve lead ECG showing left ventricular hypertrophy (LVH) in the limb leads only. The patient was obese, which reduces the sensitivity of the chest leads for LVH. (B) Twelve lead ECG showing LVH and widespread strain pattern. The strain pattern denotes a worse prognosis. Ischaemia (large and/or small vessel) is likely to be present.

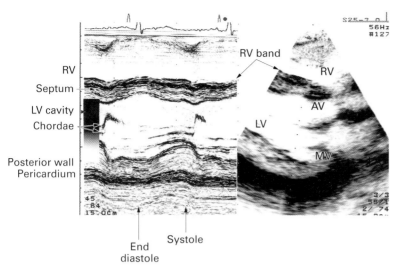

Figure 36.3. M mode (left panel) and two dimensional (right panel) echocardiography (parasternal long axis view) demonstrating concentric LVH in a female patient (septum 13 mm; left ventricular (LV) cavity 48 mm; posterior wall 13 mm). The measurements (leading edge to leading edge) are taken just beyond the tips of the mitral valve (MV) leaflets at end diastole. Care must be taken not to include the right ventricular band in the septal measurement. RV, right ventricle; AV, aortic valve.

sound machines have better capability for endocardial border detection but accurate measurements of wall thickness can still be difficult and involve a degree of subjectivity. The use of harmonic imaging (present on many of the machines currently on the market) improves image quality but can alter the subjective appearance of wall thickness and must be allowed for by the echocardiographer. Measurements of septal and posterior wall thickness at end diastole (fig 36.3) or subjective assessment by an experienced echocardiographer usually suffice, but eccentric hypertrophy (chamber enlargement but left ventricular wall thickness remains within normal units despite increased left ventricular mass) may be missed. Greater accuracy is introduced by estimating left ventricular mass using septal, posterior wall, and left ventricular M mode dimensions in diastole, calculating volumes, and correcting for height or body surface area (table 36.2[13]). Few UK echocardiography laboratories do this routinely because of time constraints and uncertain impact on clinical decisions.

Systolic ejection murmurs are common in the hypertensive. High pressure and loss of vascular compliance can mask the slow rising pulse of aortic stenosis, and echo assessment of the valve and gradient is important. Missed significant aortic incompetence as a cause of systolic hypertension would embarrass most clinicians, but it occurs. Echocardiography is

useful in the assessment of associated atrial fibrillation. Detection of regional wall motion abnormalities is useful confirmatory evidence for associated ischaemic damage and may be found in the absence of a history of coronary ischaemia.[14] Increased left atrial size and pulmonary artery pressure may indicate hypertensive damage but are not specific. Non-invasive estimates of left atrial or end diastolic ventricular pressures are not sufficiently robust for clinical use. Calcified aortic cusps—"aortic sclerosis"—are found more frequently in the hypertensive and may be a marker of increased risk through coronary disease.[7]

The ultrasound examination may also give useful information on cardiac function and consequently prognosis. Should the presence of myocardial dysfunction influence the choice of treatment or management? Impaired systolic ventricular function was a major reason to justify treatment with an ACE inhibitor and perhaps to avoid treatment with a β blocker. The recent HOPE (heart outcomes prevention evaluation) study has emphasised that high cardiovascular risk alone is sufficient to warrant use of an ACE inhibitor.[15] The recent β blocker studies[16] now mandate the use of β blockade in patients with heart failure, assuming clinical stability and careful titration of dose. Thus knowledge of left ventricular systolic function does not necessarily influence treatment decisions.

Cardiac ultrasound can sometimes help sort out the breathless hypertensive patient, particularly if there is clear cut evidence of systolic dysfunction or significant valve disease. Patients may, however, be more breathless than expected for a given level of systolic dysfunction, raising the possibility of associated diastolic dysfunction, particularly if LVH is present. Patients with hypertension are often old, and age and hypertension are particularly associated with "stiff ventricles" and consequent breathlessness. The assessment of diastolic dysfunction is controversial and has been the subject of many reviews.[17] Its reported frequency ranges from 10–40%, depending on selection criteria and measurement techniques. Diastolic dysfunction is difficult to establish using current echocardiography techniques, many of which are unduly influenced by fluid loading conditions in the patient. The finding of an apparently normal heart or one with obvious hypertrophy, dilatation or impaired systolic function on echocardiography is helpful in assessing the breathless hypertensive patient. Indeterminate findings are more difficult to interpret clinically.

Magnetic resonance imaging

Assessment of left ventricular wall thickness and overall left ventricular mass using magnetic resonance imaging (MRI) is probably the most accurate non-invasive method for the assessment of LVH. Assessment of left ventricular systolic function and tissue blood flow at rest and with pharmacological stress can also be undertaken. However, there are no substantial studies linking measurements by this approach to outcome. Limited availability and patient acceptance restrict its use at present, but future

Table 36.2   Echo criteria for LVH and formula for left ventricular mass calculation

Septal and posterior wall thickness are measured just beyond the tips of the mitral valve leaflets
Abnormal S > 13 mm men; > 12 mm women
Abnormal PW > 12 mm men; >11 mm women

Left ventricular mass formula (using American Society of Cardiology guidelines, measuring
  leading edge to leading edge)
Left ventricular mass (g) = 0.83 [(S + PW + LVDD)^3 − LVDD^3] + 0.6

*Left ventricular mass > 134 g/m^2 (men)
*Left ventricular mass > 110 g/m^2 (women)

*Corrected for body surface area. Correction by height in metres is preferred in Framingham outcome studies.
S, septal thickness; PW, posterior wall thickness; LVDD, left ventricular diastolic diameter.

protocols may allow for a single complete investigation of the hypertensive patient, giving information not only on the presence of LVH, but also coronary disease, myocardial structure and function, valve disease, and other important pathology including evidence of renal artery narrowing or adrenal pathology (fig 36.4).

Ambulatory blood pressure measurement

It seems logical that multiple measurements of blood pressure give a better estimate of "hypertensive load" than a single measurement.[18] This is borne out in the consistency of such 24 hour readings, which have allowed definitions of day and night time normality, and exhibit a closer relation to ventricular mass estimates and coronary events.[19] The daytime average is most usefully compared with the clinic reading. Guidelines suggest adding 10/5 mm Hg to accord with clinic/office readings. The early readings after initial cuff application, if unduly elevated, indicate the presence of the "alerting reaction"; it may be seen again in the hour preceding return of the pressure measuring device. This measurement seems most useful when clinic readings show unusual variability, when blood pressure is resistant to treatment, when there are symptoms suggestive of *hypotension* in the absence of an obvious postural fall, or when "white coat hypertension" is suspected.

Stress testing and the hypertensive

Exercise ECG can be helpful in the diagnosis of associated ischaemia. Generally, the stress test should not be undertaken if the blood pressure is very high (> 220 mm Hg systolic or 115 mm Hg diastolic, or both) and should be stopped if the pressure increases greatly during exercise. It may not be possible to stop antihypertensive drug treatment before exercise testing, thus reducing the sensitivity of the test. The prognostic value of the increase in blood pressure with exercise does not seem greater than for resting blood pressure, even though it is claimed to relate more closely to cardiac hypertrophy. A fall in the level of the patient's usual pressure (in contrast to the "settling" of pressure elevated by anxiety) with increased workload can indicate serious cardiac impair-

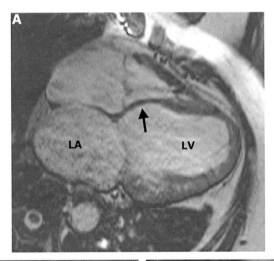

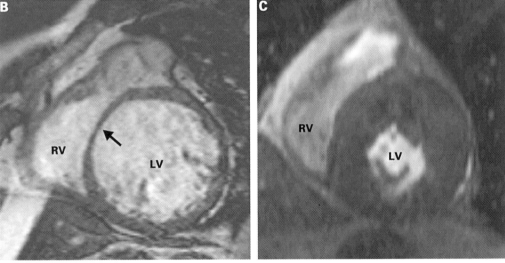

Figure 36.4. Magnetic resonance images. (A) Long axis view showing pronounced left ventricular dilatation and thinning of the interventricular septum (arrow) (True-FISP acquisition). (B) Mid-ventricular short axis view of the same patient as in (A), showing the dilated left ventricle with thinning (arrow) of the septum (True-FISP acquisition). (C) Another patient but a similar view to (B) acquired from a single phase gradient echo cine and in contrast showing pronounced hypertrophy of the left ventricle. The thin walled right ventricle can be seen wrapping around the left ventricle, lying superiorly and to the left on the cross sectional views. The views are similar to a cross sectional two echo view. Note the clarity of the endocardial border, allowing accurate estimation of left ventricular volume and mass. LA, left atrium; LV, left ventricle, RV, right ventricle. (Images provided by Dr U M Savananthan.)

ment. The test can be repeated after improved blood pressure control or an alternative stress test method used. The ECG may be difficult to interpret if repolarisation abnormalities or LBBB are present, but the exercise time, symptoms, and blood pressure response can still provide useful information. Alternative stress tests using either pharmacological agents or exercise with echocardiography or nuclear imaging can improve the sensitivity and specificity of ischaemia detection, but are more costly and generally less available. ST segment depression, abnormal response of ejection fraction, and perfusion defects occur without evidence of obstructive epicardial vessel disease in the presence of hypertrophy.[20] Stress echo techniques may be more specific than nuclear techniques for epicardial vessel as opposed to small vessel narrowing.

Coronary and left ventricular angiography

This can be undertaken when significant coronary and/or valve disease is suspected. Blood pressure control should be optimised before arterial puncture. LVH and dysfunction may be evident from the left ventricular angiogram, but in general the non-invasive tests provide this information. Increases in left atrial and left ventricular end diastolic pressures may indicate cardiac involvement in hypertension. Small vessel disease is inferred when stress tests are abnormal but no narrowing of major vessels is seen on angiography.

Left ventricular hypertrophy

How important is the presence of LVH? The relation of LVH with the level of pressure is complex. In part this may relate to never knowing how long blood pressure elevation has been present at any particular level in an individual. The prevalence of hypertrophy increases considerably with age. Many other factors are involved in its development. Black patients were thought to be more at risk for developing LVH for a given level of pressure, but Lee[9] has shown reduced specificity for ECG criteria for LVH in black patients. In general, hypertensive black patients have a lower incidence of cardiac events than whites.[19] In 3220 subjects in the Framingham heart study, apparently free of cardiovascular disease and over the age of 40 years at enrolment, the relative risk of an increment in cardiac mass of 50 g per metre height (substantial), adjusted for age, diastolic blood pressure, pulse pressure, antihypertensive treatment, cholesterol, cigarette smoking, diabetes, body mass index, and ECG evidence of LVH with repolarisation change, was associated with a 49% risk increase in cardiovascular disease in men but at the same time a 49% risk increase in mortality from all causes. For women the cardiovascular and all cause mortality rates were doubled.[21] Given that the accepted clinical approach is to produce optimal pressure reduction in all patients, especially encouraged by the findings of the recent HOT (hypertension optimal

treatment) trial,[5] how useful is the knowledge about the presence of LVH in the individual patient? There are no drugs currently to treat cardiac hypertrophy itself, even if echo diagnosed hypertrophy is accepted as carrying risk additional to the pressure measurement. Its findings may encourage the physician and patient to try harder and with more drugs, and sway a treatment decision for "borderline" pressure recordings, but the guide will remain the level of pressure achieved. At the moment there is no convincing trial evidence that reduction of hypertrophy carries any more benefit than that from reduction of the blood pressure per se. It is difficult to see how this hypothesis can be tested without the use of agents that reduce ventricular hypertrophy independent of their effect on blood pressure.

Reduction of blood pressure leads to regression of hypertrophy, measured by a variety of techniques. Extrapolation from animal studies suggests that the reversal is only partial both in the quantity of mass reduced and the quality of the remaining myocardial tissue compared with a normal heart. The dominating factor is the extent of blood pressure reduction. Claims for the superiority of one agent compared with another in reducing hypertrophy, particularly the effectiveness of ACE inhibitors as a group compared with other agents, continue to be debated.[11]

Choice of drug in the hypertensive with concomitant heart disease

---

Modern treatment of hypertension is centred on the concept of treating according to risk, not simply the pressure level. Traditional trials in hypertension are characterised by the low cardiac event rates, and the evidence for reduction in myocardial infarction or death has been disappointing compared to prevention of stroke. However, the consensus now from many studies is that reduction of blood pressure reduces not only the occurrence of heart failure but also myocardial infarction rates. Fears associated with the J shaped curve and reduction of blood pressure have been largely allayed by the HOT study.[5] Nevertheless patients with a critical stenosis of a coronary vessel, especially if flow reserve is compromised by LVH and its accompanying pathological changes, can develop worsening ischaemia if pressure is greatly lowered.

The HOPE population carried a risk of death, stroke or myocardial infarction of about 4% per year.[15] Those included with hypertension were treated with conventional drugs excluding an ACE inhibitor. Overall blood pressure control was better in the ACE inhibitor treated patients, but those randomised to the ACE inhibitor showed a significant reduction in cardiac event rates well beyond that predicted from the small added blood pressure fall. Previous trials to find superiority of one drug over another have not found differences; the reduction of pressure rather than the agent seems paramount. However, this does not sit

268

easily with the studies after myocardial infarction and in heart failure patients where clear benefit has been seen from ACE inhibitors and β blockers in reducing cardiovascular mortality and myocardial infarction rates. The recent CAPP (captopril prevention project) study specifically compared treatment including or excluding the ACE inhibitor captopril and found no difference in events.[22] However, the study has been heavily criticised. The Swedish STOP-2 (Swedish trial in old patients with hypertension 2) study superficially also appeared to find no difference between agents on event rates.[6] Nevertheless, subgroup analysis does suggest that a regimen including an ACE inhibitor might be beneficial in reducing rates of myocardial infarction.[6] Furthermore the doxazosin arm of the ALLHAT (antihypertensive and lipid lowering treatment to prevent heart attack) study has been stopped, on the basis that fewer patients in the diuretic arm developed heart failure than those on doxazosin. Whether this is because of "pretreatment" of heart failure by the diuretic or a genuine lack of effect of doxazosin is speculative.[23] The overall mortality and cardiovascular risk is not reduced by treatment to the level of the normotensive.[24] Clearly attention to other risk factors (diabetes, smoking, increased cholesterol) is also important and absolute risk varies widely between populations.[25]

Most patients require at least two agents to control blood pressure adequately, and some three or more. A regimen that includes a β blocker and an ACE inhibitor might be expected to offer some cardiac protection when risk is present. The β blocker will also help control the symptoms of angina. Addition of a vasodilating calcium antagonist may improve symptoms and further reduce pressure. Diuretics remain unequalled for symptom control in the patient breathless from heart failure, offer blood pressure control equal to other agents used alone, combine well with other drugs, and—although they have side effects—are remarkably well tolerated by the majority of patients. Spironolactone no longer has a licence in the UK for the treatment of hypertension, but the recent findings of benefit from this drug in those with severe stable chronic heart failure would justify its use in the hypertensive with heart failure.[26] Lifestyle measures are also important in the reduction of blood pressure levels and thereby LVH.

Aspirin and heart disease

Aspirin is usually prescribed in those with known ischaemic heart disease. Clopidogrel is an alternative in patients genuinely intolerant of aspirin. Aspirin as primary prevention is controversial. The HOT study suggests a relative risk reduction of about 15% for major cardiovascular events, but at the cost of an excess of major bleeding events.[5] When the individual's overall absolute cardiovascular risk is high then the 15% relative risk reduction becomes worthwhile when set against the risk of a serious bleed. The BHS guidelines[2] advocate statin prescription to those with angina or previous myocardial infarction at a total

---

Treatment of hypertension:

- By any agent, if effective, will reduce risk of ischaemic heart disease (IHD)

- Should include β blocker or ACE inhibitor, or both, if heart disease present

- Usually requires two or more agents

- Should include attention to lifestyle and modifiable risk factors

- Should include aspirin for those with IHD, or at high risk of developing IHD

---

cholesterol concentration of 5 mmol/l or higher under the age of 75 years.

Summary

The effect of hypertension on the heart and therefore prognosis is highly variable and depends not only on the pressure level but also on other factors including age, sex, cholesterol, and smoking. High blood pressure can severely damage the heart, reducing the quality of life as well as longevity. Significant protection is offered to the heart by good control of blood pressure and other risk factors. The higher the risk the greater the absolute benefit the patient can expect. Doctors should not exaggerate the risks of pressure elevation to the individual patient and thereby over claim the benefit likely to accrue from treatment; however good the treatment, it cannot be expected to more than compensate for the associated risk. Understanding of these concepts by both patients and physicians should lead to improved care and protection of the heart through the early detection and rigorous control of high blood pressure.

1. **British Cardiac Society, British Hyperlipidemia Association, British Hypertension Society.** Joint British recommendations on prevention of coronary heart disease in clinical practice. *Heart* 1998;**80** (suppl 2):S1–29.

2. **Ramsay LE, Williams B, Johnston DG,** *et al.* Guidelines for management of hypertension: report of the third working party of the British Hypertension Society, 1999. *J Hum Hypertens* 1999;**13**:569–92.
- *The latest guidelines emphasise that the 10 year risk of coronary heart disease (> 15%), diabetes, and target organ damage should be taken into account rather than isolated blood pressure levels. The target level of 140/85 mm Hg should be achieved by standard treatment and lifestyle measures, and control of other risk factors is important.*

3. **Blacker J, Staessen JA, Girerd X,** *et al.* Pulse pressure not mean pressure determines cardiovascular risk in older hypertensive patients. *Arch Intern Med* 2000;**160**:1085–9.
- *A meta-analysis of three large trials in systolic hypertension showed that after controlling for mean pressure, a 10 mm wider pulse pressure increased the risk of cardiovascular mortality by 20%. The probability of a cardiovascular end point increased with lower diastolic pressures for any given systolic pressure suggesting that the wider pulse pressure is driving the risk of major complications.*

4. **McMurray JJ, Stewart S.** Epidemiology, aetiology, and prognosis of heart failure. *Heart* 2000;**83**:596–602.

5. **Hansson L, Zanchetti A, Carruthers SG,** *et al* **for the HOT Study Group.** Effects of intensive blood-pressure lowering and low-dose aspirin in patients with hypertension: principal results of the hypertension optimal treatment (HOT) randomised trial. *Lancet* 1998;**351**:1755–62.

6. **Hansson L, Lindholm LH, Ekbom T,** *et al.* Randomised trial of old and new antihypertensive drugs in elderly patients: cardiovascular mortality and morbidity. The Swedish trial in old patients with hypertension-2 study. *Lancet* 1999;**354**:1751–6.
• *A prospective randomised trial in 6614 patients comparing traditional (β blocker, diuretics) with newer (ACE inhibitor and calcium antagonists) drugs on cardiovascular events and mortality found a significant and similar decrease in both groups.*

7. **Otto CM, Lind BK, Kitzman DW,** *et al.* Association of aortic-valve sclerosis with cardiovascular mortality and morbidity in the elderly. *N Engl J Med* 1999;**341**:142–7.

8. **Kannel WB, Dannenburg AL, Abbott RD.** Unrecognized myocardial infarction and hypertension: the Framingham study. *Am Heart J* 1985;**109**:581–5.

9. **Lee DK, Marantz PR, Devereux RB,** *et al.* Left ventricular hypertrophy in black and white hypertensives. *JAMA* 1992;**267**:3294–9.

10. **Levy D, Labib SB, Anderson KM,** *et al.* Determinants of sensitivity and specificity of electrocardiographic criteria for left ventricular hypertrophy. *Circulation* 1990;**81**:815–20.
• *The sensitivity and specificity of ECG LVH in 4684 subjects in the Framingham heart study was examined, using echo estimates of left ventricular mass. The sensitivity of the ECG was low, and further reduced in females, obese individuals, and smokers, but increased with age.*

11. **Dunn FG, Pfeffer MA.** Left ventricular hypertrophy in hypertension. *N Engl J Med* 1999;**340**:1279–80.
• *A recent editorial reviewing the risks associated with ECG LVH and the likelihood of regression of LVH with blood pressure control.*

12. **Mosterd A, D'Agostino RB, Silbershatz H,** *et al.* Trends in the prevalence of hypertension, antihypertensive therapy, and left ventricular hypertrophy from 1950 to 1989. *N Engl J Med* 1999;**340**:1221–7.
• *Almost 40 years of follow up on over 10 000 subjects in the Framingham heart study! Over the observation period the use of antihypertensive medication increased, and the prevalence of hypertension (blood pressure > 160/100 mm Hg) reduced as did the prevalence of ECG LVH/strain. It is suggested that the improved detection and treatment of hypertension has contributed to the decline in mortality from cardiovascular disease observed in the USA.*

13. **Devereux RB, Alonso DR, Lutas EM,** *et al.* Echocardiographic assessment of left ventricular hypertrophy: comparison with necropsy findings. *Cardiol* 1986;**57**:450–8.

14. **Gardin JM, Siscovick D, Anton-Culver H** *et al.* Sex, age, and disease affect echocardiographic left ventricular mass and systolic function in the free-living elderly. The cardiovascular health study. *Circulation* 1995;**91**:1739–48.

15. **Heart Outcomes Prevention Evaluation Investigation.** Effects of an angiotensin converting enzyme inhibitor, ramipril, on cardiovascular events in high risk patients. *N Engl J Med* 2000;**342**:145–53.

16. **MERIT-HF Study Group.** Effect of metoprolol CR/XL in chronic heart failure: metoprolol CR/XL randomised intervention trial in congestive heart failure (MERIT-HF). *Lancet* 1999;**353**:2001–7.

17. **Brutsaert DL.** Diagnosing primary diastolic heart failure. *Eur Heart J* 2000;**21**:94–6.
• *This editorial reviews the "minefield" of diastolic dysfunction and failure, emphasising that ventricular relaxation times used for assessment are very variable and dependent on systolic contraction times. Hence abnormal relaxation times are probably caused by early systolic dysfunction, and "pure" diastolic dysfunction is rare (and difficult to measure with current echo techniques).*

18. **O'Brien E, Coates A, Owens P,** *et al.* Use and interpretation of ambulatory blood pressure monitoring: recommendations of the British Hypertension Society. *BMJ* 2000;**320**:1128–34.
• *This recent position paper gives clear guidelines on the application and interpretation of ambulatory pressure, reviews devices available, and includes references to the advantages of ambulatory blood pressure monitoring.*

19. **Khattar RS, Swales JD, Senior R,** *et al.* Racial variation in cardiovascular morbidity and mortality in essential hypertension. *Heart* 2000;**83**:267–71

20. **Frohlich ED.** State of the art lecture. Risk mechanisms in hypertensive heart disease. *Hypertension* 1999;**34**:782–9.
• *An up-to-date review of the contributory factors and pathophysiology of hypertensive heart disease from a world authority.*

21. **Levy D, Garrison RJ, Savage DD,** *et al.* Prognostic implications of echocardiographically determined left ventricular mass in the Framingham heart study. *N Engl J Med* 1990;**322**:1561–6.
• *A total of 3220 subjects in the Framingham heart study with no apparent clinical heart disease had left ventricular mass determined by echo. Over a four year follow up a strong correlation was found with left ventricular mass and adverse outcome, despite correcting for age, blood pressure, treatment, smoking, diabetes, obesity, cholesterol, and ECG LVH. There was a 50% increase in risk for each 50 g per metre in left ventricular mass (corrected for height). Echo is a more sensitive method for the detection of LVH than ECG, and left ventricular mass > 140 g/m indicates a higher risk of adverse events.*

22. **Hansson L, Lindholm LH, Niskanen L,** *et al.* Effect of angiotensin-converting enzyme inhibition compared with conventional therapy on cardiovascular morbidity and mortality in hypertension: the captopril prevention project (CAPP). *Lancet* 1999;**353**:611–5.

23. **Ball SG.** Discontinuation of doxazosin arm of ALLHAT. *Lancet* 2000;**355**:1558.

24. **Andersson OK, Almgren T, Persson B,** *et al.* Survival in treated hypertension: follow up study after two decades. *BMJ* 1998;**317**:167–71.
• *Over 20 years follow up on 686 treated hypertensive men, compared with 6810 non-hypertensives. Despite treatment the hypertensives had increased cardiovascular and total mortality. Regression analysis suggested that the incidence of coronary heart disease was related only to cholesterol concentrations.*

25. **MacMahon S.** Blood pressure and the risk of cardiovascular disease. *N Engl J Med* 2000;**342**:50–2.

26. **Pitt B, Zannad F, Remme WJ,** *et al.* The effect of spironolactone on morbidity and mortality in patients with severe heart failure. *N Engl J Med* 1999;**341**:709–17.

Index

Page numbers in **bold** type refer to figures; those in *italic* refer to tables or boxed material

Index

Index

Thank you for purchasing *Education in Heart* Volume II

This purchase entitles you to online access to ALL *Education in Heart* material on the *Heart* website—www.heartjnl.com—for one year (US$50 value).

Education in Heart was launched in January 2000 and publishes three articles per issue (36 articles per year), which have associated multiple choice questions—these are also available online through BMJ Publishing Group Online Learning (www.bmjonlinelearning.com).

The *Heart* website has full text (HTML) and pdf full text versions. There is additional material available only through the website.

To access these articles online you need to complete and return the order form below—THERE IS NO ADDITIONAL CHARGE FOR THIS SERVICE.

Once you receive your customer number you should activate your subscription online and choose a user name and password (www.bmjjournals.com/sub/activate/basic).

Please provide my customer number for FREE ACCESS to *Education in Heart* Online

Name: _____

Address: _____

_____

County: _____   Zip/Postcode: _____

Email address: _____   Telephone: _____

Place of work (optional) _____   Level, eg, Consultant (optional): _____

Return this form by mail to:
Subscriptions Department
BMJ Publishing Group
PO BOX 299
London WC1H 9TD, UK

For enquiries please telephone: +44 (0) 20 7383 6270 or email: subscriptions@bmjgroup.com

The *Education in Heart* articles published during 2000 are also available as a compilation
Further details available from www.bmjbookshop.com